MRCP
PACES
MANUAL

Pastes⁺

MRCP PACES MANUAL

Louise Pealing MA Hons (Cantab) MBBS MSc MRCP MRCGP
General Practitioner and Clinical Research Fellow, Nuffield Department of Primary
Care Health Sciences, University of Oxford

Benjamin Mullish MB BChir MA (Cantab) MRCP AFHEA
Specialty Registrar/Academic Clinical Fellow, Gastroenterology and Hepatology,
St Mary's Hospital, London

Philip J Smith BMedSci (Hons) BMBS (Hons) MRCP MSc (Nutrition)
Gastroenterology Specialist Registrar and MRC Clinical Research Training Fellow
Gastroenterology Department, University College London Hospital, London

Edited by
Douglas C Macdonald BM (Hons) BSc (Hons) MRCP PhD
Consultant Hepatologist, Royal Free London NHS Foundation Trust
Royal Free Hospital, London

Pastes⁺

© 2015 PASTEST LTD
Egerton Court
Parkgate Estate
Knutsford
Cheshire
WA16 8DX

Telephone: 01565 752000

A percentage of material was previously published in *Success in PACES, 2nd edition.*

First Published 2015

ISBN: 978 1905 635 757

A catalogue record for this book is available from the British Library.

The information contained within this book was obtained by the authors from reliable sources. However, while every effort has been made to ensure its accuracy, no responsibility for loss, damage or injury occasioned to any person acting or refraining from action as a result of information contained herein can be accepted by the publishers or author.

PasTest Revision Books and Intensive Courses

PasTest has been established in the field of postgraduate medical education since 1972, providing revision books and intensive study courses for doctors preparing for their professional examinations.

Books, courses and online revision available for:

Medical undergraduates, MRCP Parts 1 and 2, MRCS, MRCPCH Parts 1 and 2, MRCOG, DCH, FRCA, MRCGP, Dentistry.

For further details contact:

Tel: 01565 752000 Fax: 01565 650264

www.pastest.co.uk enquiries@pastest.co.uk

Text prepared by Keytec Typesetting Ltd, Bridport, Dorset
Printed and bound in the UK by Page Bros (Norwich) Ltd.

Contents

Preface

PACES textbooks face a difficult challenge. Reading a book will not make you the deft examiner, sharp-eyed observer, keen listener and eloquent presenter you need to be to pass, no matter how well you understand or retain the information therein. PACES is not a knowledge-based assessment, yet the solitary and sedentary rituals acquired from years of revising for written exams can be difficult to unlearn.

To pass PACES you need to move. You need to examine patients, take histories and tackle difficult communication scenarios *under the scrutiny of a third party*. This need not be a senior colleague with MRCP exam expertise. In fact, a revision partner who shares your sense of urgency and enthusiasm is often far superior and more reliable. Fortunately, you and your revision partner can be rendered expert by referring to this text.

This manual describes structured approaches and strategies for any clinical scenario you might encounter in PACES. Five years in the making, it draws upon decades of PACES teaching experience shared by its authors. They have set out to correct the common deficiencies of existing texts:

- irrelevant knowledge that satisfies 'revision thirst' but does little to enhance the prospect of passing
- a lack of strategic guidance tailored to each station
- scant materials to facilitate hands-on practice
- an Integrated Clinical Assessment section (Station 5) bearing uncanny resemblance to the obsolete 'Skin, eyes, locomotor, endocrine' format of the old exam.

This latter issue is a recurring bug-bear of candidates. Station 5 is a difficult, time-pressured part of the exam in which candidates are assessed on all aspects of the marking scheme. It deserves a thoughtful, comprehensive and tailored approach and that is what the authors have delivered here and throughout this book.

The PACES Manual is an unashamedly exam-focussed text. As such, you will find each section organised around the marking scheme structure. The PACES examination has benefitted from revision and refinement by Royal College examiners over many decades and its current iteration is a relevant, robust and discriminating assessment of a physician's ability. Candidates invariably report a step-change improvement in their clinical ability and confidence after getting through MRCP PACES. The pursuit of an outstanding performance in the PACES exam and excellent clinical practice are thus one and the same.

Professor Thomas Powles
Clinical Professor of Oncology
Barts Cancer Institute

Introduction

Your PACES examiners will be looking for a doctor suitable for specialist training to whom they would entrust the care of a relative. They want to know you will not miss an important clinical sign or alarm symptom, that you will order the most appropriate investigations, institute a sensible management plan and that you are able to talk a patient through a difficult decision without causing distress or antagonism. These requirements are directly reflected in the marking scheme and the structure of each topic in this book.

However, there is a performance element to PACES with which some candidates struggle, especially if they are nervous. Some find it harder than others to come across as friendly rather than over-familiar, confident but not patrician or arrogant. These are not fixed personality traits but rather skills that can be learnt just as easily as others, *but only if you seek feedback on your performance from an observer.*

Such feedback can sometimes be difficult to hear. We all have elements of our clinical repertoire of which we are particularly proud. This perception may result from genuine talent but equally from a lack of insight into our shortcomings. Time and time again, examiners report candidates declaring phantom signs with utter conviction, or taking a clumsy and incomplete history and presenting it with bemused bafflement at the simplicity of the case.

The remedy for our poor insight into our own abilities is a revision partner (or several). This is essential for PACES. Practising your examination, history taking, presentation and communication skills under the scrutiny of a peer should be the bedrock of your preparation. The occasional performance in front of a group of peers or a senior with experience in the relevant system is of course also very valuable. The more feedback you can get on your performance, the better.

In the introduction to each section of this book you will find specific strategies and approaches tailored to that station. In this overall introduction, we highlight some common pitfalls – common to both PACES and clinical practice – for which you should be on the lookout. This can be used to give structured feedback to your revision partner; it can be as difficult to offer criticism as it is to receive it.

Faulty perception, failed heuristics and biases

Errors of diagnosis, clinical judgement and communication are increasingly studied areas of medicine. The dual-process theory has emerged as the dominant model for the interpretation of information and formulation of diagnoses and management plans. If a pattern of signs is immediately recognised, so-called 'Type 1' automatic processes ensue leading to a likely diagnosis and investigation plan. If not, then more 'Type 2' processes are employed which require an effortful systematic approach. Both processes may be used in assessing a patient. In general, Type 1 processes allow us to make quick decisions with minimal cost and anxiety but are more susceptible to errors of perception, failed mental shortcuts (heuristics) and biases. With the help of a revision partner, you can start to gain insight into the types of errors you make most frequently both in PACES and in your wider clinical practice.

Importantly, with greater use of 'Type 2' processes one can systematically avoid and overcome many of these errors.

Physical examination and identifying physical signs

An important strategy in successfully identifying physical signs is minimising simple systemic errors. Having a well-practised routine for the physical examination of each system is crucial. This may seem obvious – a systematic examination is less likely to miss signs – but in fact the *degree* to which you have practised beyond simply 'knowing the routine' is essential. Educational psychologists commonly talk of the following sequential phases in learning a new skill; 1. unconscious incompetence (a lack of competence or knowledge of what competence entails); 2. conscious incompetence (understanding what competence entails but skills falling short); 3. conscious competence (having to focus on one's actions in order to sustain a competent performance) and 4. unconscious competence (the ability to perform competently without conscious attention to what one is doing). You can perform a fluent physical examination without having to think about each step (or how you are going to modify your examination around a chest drain/ascitic drain/temporary pacing wire/urinary catheter) if you have done it a hundred times before and are unconsciously competent. This frees up your mind to think about the signs you are looking at and formulate a coherent narrative about the diagnosis, severity and aetiology before you turn to the examiner to present your findings.

Being a fluent and thorough examiner does not guarantee successful identification of signs, however. There is a growing literature surrounding the causes of 'looking without seeing' in specialities which demand well-developed visual recognition skills, for example radiology and histopathology. A number of biases may affect this process. One common source of error is **anchoring bias** which describes relying on an initial impression and failing to adjust this in light of subsequent information. An example of this in PACES would be identifying changes associated with rheumatoid arthritis in a patient's hands, deciding that this is a case of rheumatoid arthritis, then ignoring or diminishing the significance of psoriatic plaques at the elbows. **Framing bias** describes the influence upon the observer of the way in which a problem is worded or framed. This is particularly salient in the brief clinical consultations (Station 5) where some details are given about a patient before you have the opportunity to examine them. This information is often a helpful starting point, but if not read carefully can lead to mistaken emphasis on trivial physical signs. Another common error in examining a patient is **search satisficing** – the tendency to stop looking for abnormalities once a likely diagnosis has been made. An example of this would be identifying a transplant kidney, but then failing to look for signs of its dysfunction (e.g. oedema, raised JVP, crepitations in the lung bases). A similar and very powerful bias is **confirmation bias** – the tendency to actively look for evidence to confirm a hypothesis rather than evidence to refute it. It typically originates from a personal favouritism of one hypothesis over another. A scientist, for example, might only pursue experiments which confirm or extend a narrative for which they are renowned. In PACES, one might search for signs that confirm a diagnosis about which one is confident and knowledgeable. For example, having found an ejection systolic murmur at the left sternal edge a candidate might detect radiation into the carotid region simply because they are more confident talking about investigations and management of aortic stenosis than a VSD.

Differential diagnosis

Sutton's law takes its name from the Brooklyn bank robber, Willie Sutton, whose famous response to the judge's question "Why do you rob banks?" was: "Because that's where the money is." Going for the obvious ('common things are common') is an efficient means of reaching a diagnosis in medicine, but a series of quick diagnoses that are rewarded by a good patient outcome can lead to a habitual failure to look for other possibilities. Working in departments that do not follow patients through to their final outcome tends to cultivate this approach. The application of Sutton's law is often associated with **shoe-horning** – the tendency to ignore signs or symptoms that do not fit with a commonly occurring diagnosis. Sutton's law is sometimes confused with **Occam's razor**, but the latter is validated by Bayesian probability and is more likely to lead to diagnosis of a rarer condition if it accounts for all the signs and symptoms that would otherwise require several common conditions occurring together. **Playing the odds** is a similar heuristic failure to Sutton's law in which a physician gives greater value to their perception of the likelihood of a diagnosis than the objective evidence to hand. Like Sutton's Law, it is a strategy frequently rewarded if the odds calculation is accurate, but it will not detect unusual but serious conditions with non-specific presentations. People with migraines also suffer subarachnoid haemorrhages. 'Sutton's slip' in PACES can be countered with a **ROWS approach** – Rule Out the Worst-case Scenario. For example, you might tell the examiners "*I did notice some splinter haemorrhages. Although this is most likely degenerative or old rheumatic valve disease I would consider investigations to rule out infective endocarditis in the first instance.*" Try to be exhaustive with your differential diagnosis list but emphasise the most likely or important diagnoses and how you might prioritise investigations accordingly.

Clinical judgement and maintaining patient welfare

The process of instigating investigations to shorten a differential diagnosis list is vulnerable to several biases. The **Zebra retreat** occurs when a physician shies away from investigating a potential rare diagnosis on the differential list for fear of inertia in the system (eg the investigation has to be 'sent away') or, more commonly, self-consciousness about seriously considering a remote diagnosis and being branded 'esoteric' by colleagues. **Overconfidence bias** describes the tendency to finalise a diagnosis before sufficient investigations have been performed. It is often an effort to maintain a positive self-image through disproportionately valuing one's 'instinct' and personal contribution to a patient's outcome. Overconfidence is often associated with **hindsight bias** – the 'I-knew-it-all-along' phenomenon. When events are viewed in hindsight, they are frequently attributed a coherence, causality and inevitability that in fact may have been absent. Overconfidence is a dangerous characteristic in medicine and one which your examiners in PACES will be on the lookout for. Prioritise your investigations and use them to demonstrate you are open to multiple possibilities.

Instigating a management plan is similarly vulnerable to errors and biases. **Commission bias** describes the favouring of action over inaction. It appears to fulfil the moral obligation of 'beneficence' by intervening to reverse or prevent harm. Its opposite is **omission bias**, wherein inaction is preferred over action, sometimes through fear of being held personally responsible for the outcome. Omission bias is an attempt to fulfil the obligation of non-maleficence and indicates a preference for a negative outcome being the consequence of a 'natural' event rather than a doctor's intervention. It is often reinforced by the 'regression to the mean' phenomenon, wherein patients often seek help for a condition at the nadir of their symptoms, a point at which homeostatic recovery from an acute insult is likely to have already begun. Candidates in PACES tend to forget that doing nothing is sometimes an option in a management plan. Conversely, it is always sensible to qualify any management plan with the statement that you would seek senior specialist input and advice before proceeding.

Clinical communication skills and managing patients' concerns

Patients' priorities and anxieties rarely align with those of their doctor and each is subject to significant biases. **Value bias**, for example, refers to attributing a stronger likelihood to a desired outcome rather than an undesired one. **Extreme aversion bias**, on the other hand, describes an avoidance of actions which may lead to an outcome that is perceived as catastrophic, even if the chances of this are very small and the alternative course of action incurs a higher risk of a more moderate adverse event. These biases are particularly relevant in communication skills scenarios when you are talking patients through a difficult decision regarding their management.

A patient's processing of risk may seem irrational but in fact may be a logical extension of their belief system and priorities. It is not necessarily the responsibility of the doctor to persuade them of a more 'rational' course of action. Indeed, the assessment of 'rationality' will be strongly influenced by the doctor's own value and aversion biases. A patrician approach, in which the information given to a patient is skewed or selected to increase the chance of a patient making a choice you believe is best will not win over your examiners (and can lead to disaster in clinical practice). Your responsibility is to make sure patients have absorbed adequate information to make an informed decision or understand their condition and prognosis, including the uncertainties. You may choose to challenge their assumptions or biases, particularly if it puts them at risk of harm, but do so in a non-confrontational manner otherwise you are likely to induce **reactance**: the urge to do the opposite of what someone wants you to do to resist a perceived attempt to limit your freedom!

Examination format and marking scheme

You will be assessed in a combination of the skills described above at each station, but only in the brief clinical consultation (Station 5) are you assessed in all of them. For each you will receive a mark (satisfactory = 2, borderline = 1 or unsatisfactory = 0). To pass you will be required to attain a minimum standard in each of the seven skills assessed *and* a minimum total score across the whole exam. Note that the latter is determined each year by the examination board and is *not* the summation of the minimal scores across each skill. A recent example of pass marks was as follows:

Physical examination	14
Identifying physical signs	14
Clinical communication	10
Differential diagnosis	16
Clinical judgement	18
Managing patient concerns	10
Maintaining patient welfare	28
Minimum total score	**130**

Tables 1 and 2 (adapted from the MRCP UK website) describes the skills and the stations in which they are assessed.

Table 1: (adapted from www.mrcpuk.org)

	Clinical skill	Skill descriptor
A	Physical examination	Demonstrate correct, thorough, systematic (or focused in Station 5 encounters), appropriate, fluent, and professional technique of physical examination.
B	Identifying physical signs	Identify physical signs correctly, and not find physical signs that are not present.
C	Clinical communication	Elicit a clinical history relevant to the patient's complaints, in a systematic, thorough (or focused in Station 5 encounters), fluent and professional manner. Explain relevant clinical information in an accurate, clear, structured, comprehensive, fluent and professional manner.
D	Differential diagnosis	Create a sensible differential diagnosis for a patient that the candidate has personally clinically assessed.
E	Clinical judgement	Select or negotiate a sensible and appropriate management plan for a patient, relative or clinical situation. Select appropriate investigations or treatments for a patient that the candidate has personally clinically assessed. Apply clinical knowledge, including knowledge of law and ethics, to the case.
F	Managing patients' concerns	Seek, detect, acknowledge and address patients' or relatives' concerns. Listen to a patient or relative, confirm their understanding of the matter under discussion and demonstrate empathy.
G	Maintaining patient welfare	Treat a patient or relative respectfully and sensitively and in a manner that ensures their comfort, safety and dignity.

Table 2: (adapted from www.mrcpuk.org)

Station	Encounter	Skills assessed
1	Respiratory	A:B:D:E:G
1	Abdomen	A:B:D:E:G
2	History	C:D:E:F:G
3	Cardiovascular	A:B:D:E:G
3	Nervous system	A:B:D:E:G
4	Communication	C:E:F:G
5	New Station 5 (1)	All seven
5	New Station 5 (2)	All seven

The PACES 'carousel' comprises five clinical stations, each assessed by two independent examiners. Candidates start at any one of the five stations and then move round the carousel until they have completed the cycle (Figure 1). There is a 5-minute period between each station.

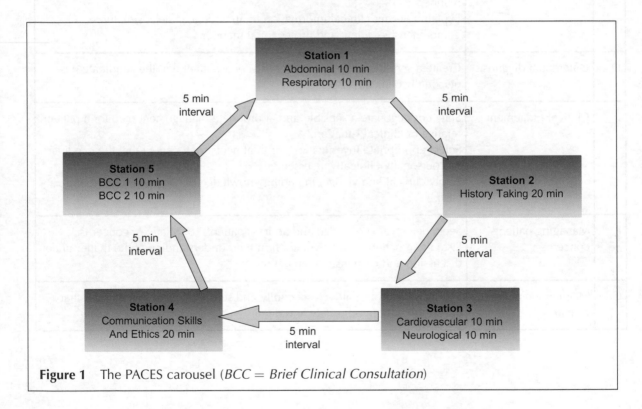

Figure 1   The PACES carousel (*BCC = Brief Clinical Consultation*)

A final thought

There is often a great temptation to dwell on possible mistakes made in the last station while waiting to move on to the next. You will have been given no instant feedback on your performance and this can be unnerving. It is very easy to carry this unease and anxiety into the next station, make further mistakes and risk a spiralling collapse in confidence.

Remember that marks lost with a poor performance in one station can be readily made up in another – you are being marked cumulatively on the skills described above and cannot fail on the basis of a poor performance on one station alone.

Like training for a triathlon, the transitions deserve special attention. It is worth lining up some patients on the ward in a mock exam format with your revision partner, with no feedback on your performance until the very end. Rehearse clearing your head of the mistakes of the last encounter before starting the next. If you have prepared well you will be at the peak of your ability when you go into the exam, but you will not be perfect. Nobody is, including your examiners!

STATION 1

The Abdominal and Respiratory Examinations

THE ABDOMINAL EXAMINATION

Abdominal cases in PACES fall into three main categories:

1. Liver disease, including cirrhosis, portal hypertension, hepatic encephalopathy, right ventricular failure/tricuspid regurgitation, metastatic disease, chronic viral hepatitis, infiltration or inflammation
2. Splenomegaly/hepatosplenomegaly, including myeloproliferative, lymphoproliferative or autoimmune diseases
3. Renal disease, particularly renal replacement therapy and renal transplantation.

The examiner's instructions and general inspection will often indicate into which of the three categories a case is likely to fall from the start. Although patterns of organomegaly are almost always present, most candidates will successfully identify these. The key to a clear pass is spotting peripheral stigmata in order to *identify the cause* of disease and *stage its severity*. Unlike the cardiovascular examination – where most of the important information is gleaned from examination of the precordium – the crucial clues to the abdominal cases are mostly in the periphery.

Examination sequence

Although the examination should follow a well-practised and smooth routine, allow the peripheral stigmata and examiner's instructions to focus your attention on particular elements of your examination, eg the finding of an old fistula in the forearm should prompt a careful search for a multitude of signs: gum hypertrophy (ciclosporin immunosuppression), parathyroidectomy scar (tertiary hyperparathyroidism), insulin injection sites (diabetic nephropathy), hearing aid (Alport's disease, granulomatosis with polyangiitis (Wegener's granulomatosis)), small neck scars (from previous haemodialysis catheters), small abdominal scars (previous Tenckhoff catheters for peritoneal dialysis) and a raised JVP (fluid overload indicating under-dialysis or renal graft failure). All such signs would be easily missed in a 'routine' abdominal examination.

Introduce and expose
- Introduce yourself
- Ask: 'Do you have pain anywhere?'
- Position the patient so that he or she lies supine, with the head resting on one pillow and the arms by the sides
- Expose men from the pubic tubercle upwards. Women should be exposed from the pubic tubercle to the xiphisternum
- Say: 'I'm going to look you over then feel your tummy if that's all right?'

Inspection
General
Many candidates rush this stage (keen to get to the hard signs) and miss important and obvious clues. Stand at the end of the bed and take time to look at the patient.

Ask the patient to take a deep breath in. Look for descending masses, eg liver, spleen or kidneys. Note any obvious scars and assess their likely significance. Look for muscle wasting, loss of subcutaneous fat and oedema – it is important to demonstrate the ability to recognise poor nutritional status whether or not you successfully identify the underlying diagnosis.

Hands
Ask the patient to stretch the arms out in front and cock the wrists back as though pressing against a wall. This is not only a way of looking for a liver flap (asterixis), but also a good way of positioning the hands for examination. Although the hands are a rich source of potential signs, don't waste time examining them exhaustively. Examiners will become quickly irritated if you examine each finger in turn for nailbed fluctuance or Dupuytren's contractures.

Skin
Make a close survey of the skin over the legs and thorax on your way to the face.

Face

Ask the patient to look upwards and look at the conjunctivae (only one side is necessary) for anaemia. Examine the iris for the inflammation of uveitis. Palpate the parotid glands. Ask the patient to open the mouth and warn him or her that you are going to use a tongue depressor. Use a pen torch to examine the oral cavity thoroughly.

Neck and chest

Sit the patient forward at this point and from behind press your fingers firmly into the left supraclavicular fossa, palpating for lymphadenopathy (Virchow's node/Troisier's sign). Examine the neck for scars of previous haemodialysis catheters or parathyroidectomy.

It is not usually necessary to examine the JVP in the abdominal examination. However, you will not be punished for returning to it at the end if you suspect that fluid balance is relevant to the case (ie end-stage kidney disease (ESKD), dialysis or renal transplant cases) or you have detected hepatomegaly in the absence of stigmata of chronic liver disease (suggesting possible right ventricular failure or tricuspid regurgitation).

While the patient is sitting forward, glance down the back looking for far lateral/posterior nephrectomy scars. These are easy to miss on anterior inspection alone.

Examine the breast tissue in men for gynaecomastia and look in the axillae for loss of hair.

Abdomen

Make a closer inspection of the abdomen kneeling at the patient's side.

Palpation

If the patient has pain, begin at the segment furthest from its location.

Look at the patient at all times and not at your hand to ensure that you are not causing discomfort.

Palpate with the wrist in a neutral position and the hand flat on the abdomen, flexing at the metacarpophalangeal joints in a 'dipping' action. You should begin with quick, light palpation to determine if there is any tenderness or obvious masses or organomegaly, then use deeper palpation in each region in turn.

Liver

Start in the right iliac fossa with the hand parallel to the subcostal margin, using the radial border of the index finger to detect any liver edge. Ask the patient to take deep breaths pressing the fingers firmly inwards as he or she does so. Rather than pushing the hand up against the liver edge, you are anticipating the sensation of the edge sliding under the radial border of the hand and gently pushing the hand upwards with inspiration. Avoid the temptation to press more deeply and 'follow' the liver upwards as you feel less resistance with expiration. Advance your hand towards the costal margin 2 cm at a time.

If you feel a liver edge, ask yourself the following

- Is it smooth or nodular?
- Is it soft, firm or hard?
- Is it pulsatile?
- Is it tender?
- Is there a Riedel's lobe (ie a tongue-like projection from the right lobe that can extend as far as the right iliac fossa, a normal anatomical variant)?

Spleen

Start in the right iliac fossa and move diagonally to the left subcostal region. Place your left hand behind the left lower ribs and apply sustained anterior pressure. Ask the patient to take deep breaths and palpate as you would for a liver edge. Finding the spleen is a difficult and often unrewarding experience. If you suspect mild-to-moderate splenomegaly try the following to confirm it

- 'Tipping' the spleen: roll the patient towards you on the right side. Place your left hand under the patient's left ribs while palpating under the costal margin with your right hand. A mildly enlarged spleen may drop below the costal margin and be more readily palpable with this manoeuvre.

- Percuss for dullness between the lower border of the ninth rib and the costal margin in the midaxillary line.
- Percuss the space of Traube: this is over the stomach medial to the left costal margin. It is usually resonant due to a gas bubble in the stomach, but dullness might indicate that the stomach is displaced medially by an enlarged spleen.

All your examiners will have been taunted by many a phantom spleen – a foray into percussion before completion of the palpation sequence is forgivable if you suspect splenomegaly.

Kidneys
Place your left hand under the patient's flank below the twelfth rib lateral to the long strap muscles of the spine and place your right hand anteriorly. Push the bottom hand firmly upwards – an enlarged kidney should be palpable.

If not palpable the kidney may be ballottable. Ask the patient to breathe in deeply and, at maximal inspiration, flex the fingers posteriorly and attempt to 'flick' the kidney upwards against the right hand anteriorly.

Distinguishing between a liver/spleen and a kidney

- Cannot get above the spleen.
- The spleen has a notch.
- The spleen moves inferomedially on inspiration, whereas the kidney moves inferiorly.
- The spleen is not ballottable.
- The spleen is dull to percussion and the kidney is often resonant due to overlying bowel.
- A friction rub may be heard over a spleen but not a kidney.

Other masses
Palpate the aorta bimanually with the tips of the fingers on the midline above the umbilicus. The normal diameter is up to 3 cm.

The bladder and bowel may be felt in normal individuals. Pressure on the bladder, which rises out of the pelvis, may induce a desire to micturate. Pressure on a faecally loaded bowel may leave an indentation.

Percussion
Liver and spleen
A number of studies have investigated the accuracy of percussion in determining liver and spleen size compared with radiological techniques. A recurrent finding is that light percussion is more discriminatory than generating the loudest possible sound. Firm percussion seems to consistently underestimate liver size, for example. Also, percussion of the liver and spleen is best performed in inspiration.

Percussion should follow a similar pattern to palpation. Define the upper border of the liver (around the sixth rib). This determines whether the liver is truly enlarged or displaced inferiorly by a hyperexpanded chest. The normal lower border of the spleen is the ninth rib in the midaxillary line and dullness below this indicates mild splenomegaly. Enlargement of the spleen by 40% or less may be detectable only by this means.

Ascites
Compared with ultrasonography, the sensitivity and specificity of the clinical examination for ascites are very wide ranging and highly dependent on the examiner's experience (50–94% and 29–82%, respectively, in one survey).

Percuss horizontally across the umbilicus through it. If an area of dullness is found in the left flank, ask the patient to roll towards you, keeping the finger in the same position. Wait 20 seconds then percuss again – if it is resonant this is indicative of shifting dullness. Only perform this test if there is definite dullness in the flanks or obvious abdominal distension, otherwise it is a waste of precious time. The absence of dullness in the flanks excludes ascites with 90% accuracy.

If there is tense ascites a fluid thrill may be demonstrable. Ask the patient to place the side of their hand in the midline of the abdomen and press down firmly. With the left hand pressed against the left side of the abdomen flick the near side. This creates a percussion wave that can be felt by the left hand.

Auscultation

Listen with the diaphragm over the abdomen for 30 seconds. A succussion splash may be demonstrated in gastric outlet obstruction by vigorously shaking the abdomen back and forth between both hands.

Bruits may be detectable over an enlarged liver or spleen, over the renal arteries (posteriorly, at the sides of the long strap muscles below the twelfth rib) or over an abdominal aortic aneurysm (in the epigastrium).

Lastly . . .

Palpate the hernial orifices.

Tell the examiner that you would wish to examine the external genitalia, perform a digital rectal examination, test the urine with a dipstick and look at the observations chart.

Thank the patient and re-cover him or her.

Abdominal Scenarios

1. Transplanted kidney

2. Polycystic kidney disease

3. Chronic liver disease

4. Primary biliary cirrhosis

5. Hereditary haemochromatosis

6. Alcohol-related liver disease

7. Chronic viral hepatitis

8. Autoimmune hepatitis

9. Isolated hepatomegaly without stigmata of chronic liver disease

10. Ascites without stigmata of chronic liver disease

11. Hepatosplenomegaly/ splenomegaly without stigmata of chronic liver disease

12. Polycythaemia rubra vera

13. Hereditary spherocytosis

SCENARIO 1. TRANSPLANTED KIDNEY

Identifying clinical signs

Hands

- Forearm fistula
- Nailbed vasculitis
- Half-and-half nails (proximal part white, distal part red or brown with sharp delineation between)
- Finger pulp imprints from blood glucose monitoring.

Face

- Cushingoid
- Anaemia
- Gum hypertrophy
- Hearing aid (Alport's disease, granulomatosis with polyangiitis (Wegener's granulomatosis)).

Fluid status

- Raised JVP
- Sacral or ankle oedema
- Hypertension.

Neck and chest

- Parathyroidectomy scar
- Haemodialysis catheter scars
- Dilated superficial veins (stenosis of central veins secondary to multiple previous lines).

Abdomen

- Peritoneal dialysis scar (midline)
- Mass in iliac fossa
- Hepatomegaly (ADPKD)
- Bilateral renal masses (ADPKD)
- Nephrectomy scar.

Differential diagnosis

Diabetes: insulin injection sites, visual impairment, diabetic foot, BM sticks/glucometer at bedside.

Glomerulonephritis: features of multisystem disease (eg butterfly rash of systemic lupus erythematosus (SLE), purpura of vasculitides or cryoglobulinaemia, scleroderma, rheumatoid arthritis and vasculitis, alopecia, vitiligo, cushingoid in the absence of a renal graft), hearing impairment (Alport's disease, granulomatosis with polyangiitis (Wegener's granulomatosis)), stigmata of infective endocarditis (although rare in PACES).

Renovascular disease: signs of extrarenal embolisation or advanced atherosclerosis (eg focal neurological deficits, previous amputation, ischaemic foot ulcer), stigmata of dyslipidaemia.

Pyelonephritis: nephrectomy scar.

Hypertension: usually no specific stigmata.

Autosomal dominant polycystic kidney disease (ADPKD): hepatomegaly (50–70% will have liver cysts but hepatomegaly is much more common in women and usually present only in the context of severe renal cystic disease), focal neurological deficit (associated intracranial aneurysms in 8%) or nephrectomy scars (20% undergo nephrectomy pre-, post- or during transplantation for recurrent infection, haematuria or chronic pain due to renal bulk).

If you cannot find any stigmata that might indicate the aetiology of ESKD (or there are none), keep in mind the frequency chart (Figure 1.1). These figures were derived from the 2005 Renal Registry Report and indicate the underlying cause of ESKD in 4767 patients started on dialysis that year in the UK. ESKD of unknown cause and renovascular disease are much more common in patients aged >65 years.

Clinical judgement and maintaining patient welfare

Investigations
These should establish cause, severity and chronicity of renal/graft impairment.

1. Establish severity

- urea and creatinine
- potassium
- arterial blood gas (pH)
- bicarbonate
- chest radiograph (fluid overload)

Indications for urgent renal replacement therapy: symptomatic uraemia, refractory hyperkalaemia, refractory acidosis, fluid overload refractory to medical therapies (as well as overdose of certain medications)

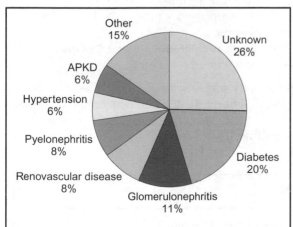

Figure 1.1   Underlying causes of end-stage renal failure

In chronic kidney disease approaching dialysis, the most accurate measure of glomerular filtration rate (GFR) is a ^{51}Cr-labelled EDTA clearance study. A 24-hour creatinine collection and clearance calculation are unreliable and often less accurate than estimates derived by the Cockroft–Gault formula or MDRD (Modification of Diet in Renal Diseases) study equation.

2. Establish cause (see below).

Graft failure
Hyperacute: this is immediate and antibody mediated. The graft must be removed to prevent a severe systemic inflammatory response (hyperacute rejection is unresponsive to immuno-suppressive therapy). The recipient has usually been pre-sensitised to HLA in the donor graft by blood transfusion, pregnancy or previous transplants. Complement-mediated small vessel thrombosis and graft ischaemia characterise the final common pathway of hyperacute rejection.

Acute: T-cell-mediated destruction of the graft is mostly IL-2 mediated and usually responds to increasing immunosuppressive therapy. A patient may have several episodes of acute rejection.

Chronic: antibody-mediated graft destruction can continue insidiously despite apparently adequate immunosuppression. The arterial endothelium is involved, resulting in ischaemia and fibrosis.

Consider **disease recurrence** (5% of graft loss)

Nearly all diseases causing ESKD can recur in the graft with the exception of

- Alport's disease
- Polycystic kidney disease
- Hypertension
- Chronic pyelonephritis
- Chronic interstitial nephritis.

Renal failure of any aetiology should warrant the following investigations.

Urine tests

- **24 hour urine collection**: microalbuminuria: 30–300 mg/day; macroalbuminuria: 300–3000 mg protein/day; nephrotic: >3 g/day proteinuria; nephritic: haematuria and proteinuria
- **Urinary protein:creatinine ratio (uPCR)**: >45 mg/mmol
- **Urinalysis** (red casts: glomerular disease; myoglobinuria: rhabdomyolysis)
- **Blood tests: ANA** (anti-nuclear antibody) and **ENA** (extractable nuclear antigen), and dsDNA: SLE; pANCA: microscopic polyangiitis; cANCA: granulomatosis with polyangiitis (Wegener's granulomatosis)
- **Complement**: decreased C3 and C4: SLE, vasculitis, membranous glomerulonephritis, IgA nephropathy; decreased C4 and normal C3: cryoglobulinaemia (and angio-oedema in C1 esterase inhibitor deficiency)
- **Creatine kinase**: rhabdomyolysis
- **Infectious screen**: anti-streptolysin O titre (ASOT): post-infectious glomerulonephritis; thick/thin film: malaria; blood cultures: infective endocarditis
- **Anti-glomerular basement membrane antibody (anti-GBM)**: Goodpasture's syndrome
- **Cryoglobulinaemia**: note this must be transported at body temperature to lab
- **Chest radiograph**: pulmonary–renal syndromes (granulomatosis with polyangiitis (Wegener's granulomatosis)), Goodpasture's syndrome, microscopic polyangiitis, malignancy, sarcoidosis; more rarely: polyarteritis nodosa, SLE, haemolytic–uraemic syndrome (HUS))

- **Renal tract ultrasonography**: Doppler studies to detect renal artery stenosis or thromboembolism. Large kidneys in diabetes, hydronephrosis, amyloidosis, renal vein thrombosis; small kidneys in chronic kidney disease
- **Renal biopsy**: light and electron microscopy with immunofluorescence.

Always consider **diabetes**, which may cause renal failure through microvascular and macrovascular disease and recurrent infection.

If there is blood in the urine in the context of renal failure, consider papillary necrosis (caused by **p**yelonephritis, **o**bstruction, **s**ickle-cell disease, **t**uberculosis, **c**irrhosis, **a**nalgesic nephropathy (phenacetin and aspirin), **r**enal vein thrombosis and **d**iabetes – POSTCARD).

3. **Establish chronicity**
   - **Renal tract ultrasonography**: small in chronic kidney disease
   - **Calcium and phosphate**: unreliable but hyperphosphataemia and hypocalcaemia usually associated with chronic kidney disease
   - **Parathyroid hormone**: elevated in chronic kidney disease
   - **Haemoglobin**: normochromic/normocytic anaemia secondary to failure of erythropoietin synthesis in chronic kidney disease
   - **Chest radiograph**: annular calcification of mitral or aortic valves.

In the early stages of renal failure due to prerenal causes (Table 1.1), tubular concentrating power

Table 1.1 Values for early stages of renal failure, resulting from prerenal cause or acute tubular necrosis (ATN)

Prerenal cause	ATN
Urine sodium <10 mmol/L Urinary osmolality >500 mosmol/L Urine:plasma osmolality >1.1	Urine sodium >10 mmol/L Urinary osmolality <400 mosmol/L Urine:plasma osmolality <1.1

is retained, whereas in acute tubular necrosis (ATN) it is lost. Prerenal insults will eventually result in ATN, making this distinction impossible.

PTLD: in patients with long-term transplants and evidence of weight loss, anaemia or lymphade-nopathy, consider post-transplantation lympho-proliferative disease (PTLD). The term PTLD includes many tumours, ranging from B-cell hyperplasia to immunoblastic lymphoma. The overwhelming majority are B-cell proliferations associated with Epstein–Barr virus (EBV) infec-tion. All cases carry a high mortality. Around 50% of cases occur in the first year after trans-plantation and have a poorer prognosis. Symp-toms and signs are often non-specific and include fever (about 60%), lymphadenopathy (about 40%), gastrointestinal symptoms (about 30%), glandular fever syndrome (about 20%) and weight loss (about 10%). Nearly all organs and systems can be affected. A high index of suspi-cion is therefore necessary to make the diagnosis.

Management

1. **Make an assessment of the current graft function and include this in the summary of your findings**
    Clues pointing towards a failing transplant include
    *   signs of fluid overload
    *   hypertension
    *   tenderness over the graft (suggesting chronic rejection)
    *   evidence of actively used means of vascular access, eg tunnelled line for haemodialysis, fistula with evidence of recent needling
    *   signs of uraemia ('uraemic frost', excoriation in response to pruritus, fetor, distal sensorimotor neuropathy, signs of uraemic pericarditis)
    *   cushingoid features (evidence of recent high-dose steroid therapy to manage a period of rejection).
2. **Consider how evidence of current immunosuppressive therapy affects management options (Table 1.2).**

All immunosuppressants increase the risk of infection

*   Herpes simplex virus (HSV): dermatomal vesicular rash of shingles
*   Cytomegalovirus (CMV): lymphadenopathy, pyrexia of unknown origin, splenomegaly pneumonitis, retinitis (but often clinically silent)
*   *Pneumocystis jiroveci* infection (formerly termed *Pneumocystis carinii* pneumonia (PCP)) – signs of pneumonia, desaturation <90% on exercise.

Malignancies that occur with increased fre-quency after transplantation

*   Skin and lip squamous carcinomas
*   Lymphoma
*   PTLD.

Dialysis patients (and transplant recipients) bear a storybook of scars from previous dialysis access and its complications. The good candidate will elicit this history from the examination.

Arteriovenous (AV) fistulae: these are typically placed, in order of preference, in the wrist of the non-dominant arm > cubital fossa of the non-dominant arm > wrist of the dominant arm > cubital fossa of the dominant arm. A thrill can be felt over a functioning fistula and a bruit should be easily heard. These are the preferred routes of vascular access for haemodialysis.

Permanent cuffed tunnelled catheters: the right internal jugular is the preferred site for haemodia-lysis catheters. Left-sided catheters follow a more tortuous route to the superior vena cava and this can affect flow rates. Look for multiple scars at both exit sites (over the upper chest) and inci-sions at the base of the neck.

Subcutaneous 'buttonhole' ports: these dialysis catheters have terminals lying just beneath the skin. The skin re-grows over the port between sessions, reducing the likelihood of infection.

Table 1.2 Signs that may be evident in PACES

Immunosuppressant	Signs	Mechanism	Adverse effects
Ciclosporin	Gum hypertrophy Sebaceous gland hypertrophy and acne (especially in males) Alopecia Tremor Hirsutism	Ciclosporin is a polypeptide of 11 amino acids of fungal origin. It acts through calcineurin inhibition thus preventing production of IL-2 and T-helper cell recruitment and activation	Nephrotoxicity (dose related) Hyperlipidaemia Glucose intolerance
Tacrolimus	Few signs (unless levels toxic)	Tacrolimus is a macrolide antibiotic that also works through calcineurin inhibition	Nephrotoxicity Neurotoxicity (encephalopathy syndrome, seizures, tremor, blurred vision) Glucose intolerance (worse than ciclosporin) QT prolongation (patients must avoid grapefruit juice)
Corticosteroids	Cushingoid appearance Proximal myopathy Recent fracture	Corticosteroids inhibit all stages of T-cell maturation and activation. They also prevent IL-1 and IL-6 production by macrophages	Cushing's disease Osteoporosis Avascular necrosis Glucose intolerance Hyperlipidaemia
Azathioprine	Few/none	Azathioprine is an anti-metabolite derivative of 6-mercaptopurine. It reduces DNA and RNA synthesis, thus limiting immune cell turnover	Cholestatic jaundice Pancreatitis Hepatitis and/or cholestasis Myelosuppression – leukopenia, thrombocytopenia, etc Increased risk of skin cancers, lymphoma
Basiliximab and daclizumab	Few/none	Humanised monoclonal antibodies that target the IL-2 receptor	Hypersensitivity reactions have been reported with both

Dacron/PTFE grafts: these have a more uniform shape and a less distensible texture on palpation compared with AV fistulae. They are often sited in the groin if arm sites have been exhausted by multiple previous fistulae.

Tenckhoff catheters: these are usually sited just above the umbilicus in the midline. Look for the scars of previous lines in all patients with evidence of renal disease. Continuous ambulatory peritoneal dialysis (CAPD) is used in the UK to a much greater degree than in the USA.

Complications from previous dialysis will influence future management options

- **Horner's syndrome**: patients who have had multiple lines inserted are at risk of Horner's syndrome due to damage to the cervical sympathetic chain.
- **Dilated superficial veins**: multiple central venous stenoses or thromboses are not uncommon in long-term haemodialysis patients reliant on central venous tunnelled catheters. This can result in distinctive superficial varicosities over the chest wall.
- **Digital ischaemia**: radio-brachiocephalic steal syndromes may occur after an AV fistula fashioned in the arm. Patients with diabetes are particularly vulnerable to impaired blood supply to the fingers if this occurs.
- **Abdominal hernias**: about 15% of patients on long-term CAPD develop abdominal wall hernias. Umbilical hernias occur more commonly than inguinal ones. High-volume exchanges and polycystic kidney disease are key risk factors for herniation.
- **β_2-Microglobulin amyloidosis**: the earliest manifestation is often carpal tunnel syndrome – look for the scars of a previous carpal tunnel release or wasting of the thenar eminence. It may then progress to amyloid arthropathy, which manifests initially in the shoulders, followed by the knees, wrist and small joints of the hands. Chronic joint swelling or evidence of joint destruction may be seen.
- **Malnutrition**: protein loss through peritoneal dialysis is a significant problem. Make a subjective global assessment of nutritional status (estimate BMI, subcutaneous fat and extent of muscle wasting).
- **Bacterial peritonitis**: peritonitis is the most common cause of CAPD failure. Each patient has about a 50% chance of developing peritonitis each year. The earliest warning is often the patient reporting clouding of the drained peritoneal fluid. A white cell count and culture of peritoneal dialysate fluid confirms the diagnosis. Recurrent episodes of peritonitis reduce the efficiency of the peritoneum as a dialysis exchange membrane and the efficacy of dialysis. Recurrent or chronic peritonitis can result in sclerosing encapsulating peritoneal disease and secondary obstruction.
- **Abdominal hernias** (see above).
- **Protein loss and malnutrition** (see above).
- **Diabetes**: CAPD (Table 1.3) conventionally relied upon the osmotic pressure exerted by

Table 1.3 Advantages and disadvantages of continuous ambulatory peritoneal dialysis (CAPD)

Advantages of CAPD	Disadvantages of CAPD
Simple to learn Ambulatory Haemodynamic tolerance Few dietary restrictions	Time-consuming exchanges Peritonitis Protein loss Excessive glucose load Sterile technique needed Peritoneum vulnerable to injury

glucose in the dialysate to remove water across the peritoneal membrane. A significant proportion of this glucose is absorbed, which poses a particular problem for patients with diabetes. New non-glucose peritoneal dialysis solutions have reduced this problem.

- **Mechanical failure**: kinking of the catheter, leakage at the exit site and pain due to contact with the abdominal viscera can all result in unsuccessful CAPD.

SCENARIO 2. POLYCYSTIC KIDNEY DISEASE

Identifying clinical signs

The signs here are similar to 'Scenario 1. Transplanted kidney' plus the following

- Bilaterally (or unilaterally) palpable kidneys OR evidence of renal replacement therapy/transplantation and bilateral or unilateral nephrectomy scar
- Irregular hepatomegaly (50% have associated liver cysts, but these are large volume only in women with severe renal disease)
- Neurological deficit (5–10% prevalence of intracranial aneurysms versus 1% in general population)
- Hypertension – ask to measure the blood pressure.

Differential diagnosis

Make a point of explaining why the mass is not a liver or a spleen

- Can get above it
- Ballotable
- Not notched
- Irregular surface
- Minimal movement inferiorly with inspiration
- Resonant to percussion due to overlying bowel (ie retroperitoneal).

Other cause of a mass in the same region

- **Renal cell carcinoma**: these patients present with haematuria, flank pain and/or a flank mass. The most common form of presentation is as an incidental finding on ultrasonography or CT. Look for associated lymphadenopathy and cachexia, the latter being a common paraneoplastic finding even in non-metastatic disease.
- **Hydronephrosis**: smooth enlargement is clinically detectable only in severe cases. An associated palpable bladder suggests bladder outlet obstruction.
- **Adrenal mass**: phaeochromocytoma and adrenal carcinoma.
- Retroperitoneal soft-tissue tumours.

Causes of renal cysts

Tuberous sclerosis: 20% of patients will develop single or multiple renal cysts but less than 5% develop severe disease with hypertension and ESKD. Renal angiomyolipomas and renal cell carcinomas are also more common in this condition.

Von Hippel–Lindau disease: inherited mutation of the *VHL* tumour-suppressor gene gives rise to cyst formation in the kidney, pancreas, liver and epididymis. Seventy per cent of patients develop renal cell carcinoma. The oncogenesis of renal cell carcinoma in genotypically normal patients involves somatic mutation of the *VHL* gene in 50% of patients.

ADPKD: defects in *PKD1* and *PKD2* genes give rise to faulty polycystin proteins, but a 'second hit' acquired mutation is required in the normal allele to give rise to cyst formation (hence the onset in adulthood).

Autosomal recessive polycystic disease: the gene for fibrocystin (*PKHD1*) is defective, resulting in faulty embryogenesis of the collecting tubule (and biliary defects invariably resulting in liver disease). Neonatal presentation is with pulmonary hypoplasia secondary to oligohydramnios. Childhood presentation is similar to adult polycystic disease, with hypertension and renal insufficiency.

Acquired forms of cystic disease include simple cysts (benign) and medullary cystic disease (which leads to progressive renal failure).

Clinical judgement and maintaining patient welfare

Investigations

1. In all renal cases in PACES, **comment on the presence or absence of renal impairment and its severity or chronicity**, and which investigations you would choose to establish this (see Scenario 1. Transplanted kidney).

2. **Exclude associated disorders**
   - **Liver cysts** occur in up to 70% of cases but significant involvement and hepatomegaly are almost entirely restricted to female patients with severe renal disease.
   - **Intracerebral aneurysms** have up to 15% prevalence, but the relative incidence of subarachnoid haemorrhage is around four times greater than in the general population. However, no studies to date have identified any clear benefit in screening. Invasive tests (eg cerebral angiography) and interventional radiological therapies are not without significant risk of causing more harm than benefit. Patients with a positive family history of subarachnoid haemorrhage should undergo screening.
   - **Hypertension** is almost universal once the kidneys are palpable. It is detectable in 70% of adults before the cysts are detectable on ultrasonography. Cysts overproduce both renin and angiotensin and are often removed for this reason during transplantation to prevent hypertensive damage to the graft.
   - **Mitral valve prolapse** is present in around 25% of patients; significant mitral regurgitation is present in 13%. *If you suspect polycystic kidney disease, tell the examiner during your summing up that you would like to examine the precordium.*

3. **Screen family members**
   Genetic testing is available for family members, but the *PKD1* and *PKD2* genes are large and mutations at multiple different sites can give rise to cystic disease. Mutations in *PKD1* account for the vast majority (85%) of cases. The genetic test is around 70% sensitive.
   The bedrock of screening family members remains ultrasonography after age 18 years. After age 20 this is 99% sensitive for *PKD1* disease, but lower for the rarer *PKD2*.

Management

This is guided by the stage of disease. Approximately 60% of patients develop ESKD by the age of 70 years, with a mean age of onset at 57 years. Of the remaining 40% of patients, at least half will have hypertension.

Look for

- Evidence of renal replacement therapy
- Evidence of either a previous or current kidney transplantation
- Evidence of ESKD (see above)
- Evidence of other organ involvement
- Evidence of longstanding hypertension (eg left ventricular hypertrophy).

The non-hypertensive patient should have regular monitoring of blood pressure, renal function and regular renal tract ultrasonography to anticipate local complications.

Recurrent infections may require antibiotic prophylaxis and infected cysts may require drainage.

Hypertension should be managed aggressively (dual risk of subarachnoid haemorrhage) with ACE inhibitors or angiotensin II antagonists.

Liver disease, if severe, can be managed with ultrasound-guided drainage or surgical de-roofing of cysts. In rare cases, liver transplantation may be required.

Intracranial aneurysms require treatment if there is a history of subarachnoid haemorrhage.

Identifying physical signs

Hands
- Clubbing
- Leukonychia
- Kolionychia
- Palmar erythema
- Liver flap
- *Dupuytren's contracture (alcohol-related liver disease).*

Face
- Yellow sclerae
- Pale conjunctivae
- *Kaiser–Fleischer rings (Wilson's disease)*
- *Xanthelasmas (PBC)*
- *Parotid swelling/squaring of face (alcohol-related liver disease).*

Neck and chest
- Spider naevi
- Scratch marks
- Absence of body hair
- Gynaecomastia
- *Tattoos (viral hepatitis)*
- *Barrel-shaped chest (α_1-antitrypsin deficiency).*

Abdomen
- Hepatomegaly
- Splenomegaly
- Caput medusa
- Venous hum
- Testicular atrophy
- Ascites.

Diagnostic signs italicised.

Differential diagnosis

This is frequently discernible from careful attention to the stigmata (see italicised signs in lists above). Remember that dual pathology is common and alcohol accelerates any cirrhotic process. Say that you would like to take a full history of alcohol consumption whatever the suspected underlying cause.

Clinical judgement and maintaining patient welfare

1. **Establish cause**
   - Viral hepatitis serology
     - hepatitis B surface antigen (HBsAg)
     - hepatitis C antibody (HCV IgG).
   - Metabolic disorder screen
     - haemochromatosis (serum ferritin >500 µg/L, transferrin saturation >50%, total iron-binding capacity (TIBC), free serum iron, followed by *HFE* genotyping
     - Wilson's disease – serum copper/24-hour urinary copper, ceruloplasmin
     - α_1-antitrypsin deficiency – α_1-antitrypsin level followed by genotyping if low.
   - Autoimmune liver disease
     - primary biliary cirrhosis: anti-mitochondrial antibodies (AMAs), anti-nuclear antibody (ANA)
     - autoimmune hepatitis: ANA, anti-smooth muscle antibody (ASMA), anti-liver-kidney microsomal antibody (ALKMA), anti-soluble liver antigen antibody (ASLA), rheumatoid factor.
   - Liver biopsy – if cause remains unclear and clotting permits. Transjugular liver biopsy may be necessary if prothrombin time is prolonged.

2. **Establish severity**
   - Liver function tests: bilirubin, liver enzymes, albumin
   - Full blood count (FBC)
     - haemoglobin: microcytic anaemia in GI blood loss, MCV raised if ongoing drinking or hypersplenism
     - platelets: low in portal hypertension

- white blood cell count: susceptibility to sepsis.
- Clotting profile: prothrombin time measures liver synthetic function.
- Renal function
  - urea: often low even in renal failure.
  - creatinine: hepatorenal failure carries a very poor prognosis.
- Electroencephalogram (EEG) for subclinical encephalopathy – ask the patient to draw a five-pointed star, reverse counting, etc.
- Ultrasonography of the liver and biliary tree – establish abnormal echotexture (signal compared with right renal cortex – if it is more echogenic, this suggests cirrhosis). Exclude focal lesions (in conjunction with α-fetoprotein). Establish if portal hypertension is present (ie splenomegaly).
- OGD – surveillance for varices.
  Any patient with the following is likely to have decompensated liver function
- Jaundice
- Ascites
- Encephalopathy.
  Many candidates wrongly interpret evidence of portal hypertension (splenomegaly, caput medusa) as a sign of decompensation. Liver size is an unreliable indicator of the severity of underlying cirrhosis or liver function – remember, almost any combination of normal or enlarged liver and spleen can occur in cirrhosis.

The Child–Pugh classification, initially developed to assess perioperative mortality in patients with liver disease, is one important way of determining prognosis and determining fitness for treatment in chronic liver disease – particularly with regard to antiviral therapies (Table 1.4).
The individual scores are summed and then grouped as

- <7 = A – associated 10% perioperative mortality rate
- 7–9 = B – associated 30% perioperative mortality rate
- >9 = C – associated 82% perioperative mortality rate.

Class A patients have a >90% 6-month survival rate, whereas class C patients with a score >12 have a 40% 6-month survival rate. Although several of the scores are biochemical, the good candidate can make conclusions as to the minimum Child–Pugh score according to clinical features, eg a jaundiced patient with ascites and a liver flap must have at least Child–Pugh class B disease.

3. **Look for causes of recent decompensation**
   Upper gastrointestinal bleed (varices), spontaneous bacterial peritonitis (SBP), recent additional liver injury (drugs, alcohol, flare in hepatitis) and intercurrent infections (eg bacterial pneumonia).

Table 1.4 The Child–Pugh score

Score	1	2	3
Bilirubin (μmol/L)	<34	34–50	>50
Albumin (g/L)	>35	28–35	<28
PT – control PT (ie seconds prolonged)	<4	4–6	>6
Encephalopathy	Subclinical/none	Grade 1	Grade 2–3
Ascites	None	Moderate	Severe/diuretic resistant

Management

Ascites

An initial therapeutic paracentesis (with salt-poor human albumin replacement) should be performed in patients with tense ascites followed by

- Salt restriction (refer to dietician) of <2 g/day.
- Spironolactone to induce sodium excretion of >78 mmol/day (a spot urine sample can be taken and if the sodium level is greater than the potassium level this corresponds to adequate natriuresis). If this is achieved and ascites persists, furosemide should be added.
- Fluid restriction unnecessary unless serum sodium <125 mmol/L.
- Patients should be considered for liver transplantation if appropriate.

Diuretic-resistant ascites occurs when renal impairment prohibits increasing diuretics or ascites simply does not resolve despite maximal therapy. Serial paracentesis and TIPSS (transjugular intrahepatic portosystemic shunt) are potential therapeutic options while liver transplantation is expedited. Surgically fitted pumps can divert ascitic fluid into the bladder at a programmable rate and may provide significant symptom relief in patients ineligible for transplantation.

Variceal haemorrhage

- Terlipressin, intravenous antibiotics, large-bore intravenous access and resuscitation
- Urgent endoscopy with banding
- Serial variceal banding until obliterated, with regular surveillance thereafter
- If endoscopy fails to control bleeding, consider TIPSS
- Regular β blocker (typically propranolol), aiming for a heart rate of 55–60 beats/min
- Consider transplantation if appropriate.

Hepatic encephalopathy

- Altering gut transit and reducing nitrogenous byproduct-generating microbiota with lactulose is the mainstay of management.
- Non-absorbed antibiotics such as rifaximin have shown promise in clinical trials and are currently being assessed by NICE.
- Refractory or high-grade encephalopathy should trigger consideration for transplantation.

Spontaneous bacterial peritonitis

- All patients with ascites should have a diagnostic tap on admission to exclude SBP (which is often subclinical). Measure neutrophil count (>250/mm^3 defines SBP) and protein level, and inoculate blood culture bottles. If the protein level is <15 g/L, consider antibiotic prophylaxis even in the absence of SBP.
- Treat with empirical intravenous antibiotics while awaiting culture and sensitivity results.
- All patients who have had SBP should be started on antibiotic prophylaxis, eg with norfloxacin.

Hepatorenal syndrome

- For a patient to have hepatorenal syndrome (HRS) he or she must have a creatinine >133 µmol/L, cirrhosis with ascites, and no evidence of hypovolaemia or shock, intrinsic renal disease or recent nephrotoxic drugs.
- Type I HRS is rapidly progressive, and characterised by acute kidney injury (creatinine >233 µmol/L) in the setting of deteriorating liver function or other organ failure. Type II HRS occurs in the context of refractory ascites in association with avid sodium retention.
- Terlipressin and albumin are the mainstay of therapy for patients with HRS, who should also automatically be considered for liver transplantation.

SCENARIO 4. PRIMARY BILIARY CIRRHOSIS

Identifying physical signs

As for chronic liver disease, but the following are usually present

- Middle-aged woman
- Xanthelasma
- Jaundice
- Excoriations
- Sicca syndrome (xerophthalmia, xerostomia).

- systemic sclerosis
- Sjögren's syndrome
- coeliac disease.
All these share 'lethargy' as part of their symptom complex with PBC.
- When estimating liver function, note that, in the Child–Pugh score in patients with PBC, the relative contribution of jaundice is reduced by an upward shift in the ranges that attracts, 1, 2 or 3 points.

Differential diagnosis

Autoimmune hepatitis is the main differential diagnosis, because it is also associated with other autoimmune disease such as sicca syndrome. Cirrhosis from non-alcoholic fatty liver disease may also present with xanthelasma from associated dyslipidaemia.

Clinical judgement and maintaining patient welfare

Investigations
As with all chronic liver disease cases, investigations should establish stage of disease and exclude decompensation as well as establish the cause (see Scenario 3: Chronic liver disease)

- State that you would request AMAs to confirm the diagnosis of PBC and AMA subtype analysis to determine prognosis. Liver biopsy is not necessary if these are positive, because their specificity and sensitivity are >95%.
- Anti-gastric parietal cell antibodies are positive in 60% of cases, ANAs in 20% and ASMAs in 50%.
- It is also worth mentioning that you would have a low threshold for testing for other associated autoimmune conditions, including
  - Hashimoto's thyroiditis

Management
Cholestasis is treated with ursodeoxycholic acid which delays the progression to cirrhosis, improves biochemical markers of cholestasis (bilirubin, ALP, GGT), and can improve symptoms of lethargy and pruritus.

Pruritus is treated initially with cholestyramine (bile acid sequestrant) and antihistamines, but for many patients this is inadequate. Oral naltrexone (an opiate antagonist) is effective second-line therapy. Rifampicin may be of benefit but may cause deterioration in liver function. Plasmapheresis and MARS (molecular adsorbent recycling system) have been used with varying efficacy on severe cases. Finally, severe uncontrollable pruritus in PBC is an indication for liver transplantation.

Hypercholesterolaemia can be safely treated with statins (while monitoring for deterioration in LFTs). Xanthelasmas may regress if cholesterol is successfully lowered.

Osteoporosis occurs in PBC independently of vitamin D malabsorption. The mechanism seems to involve reduced bone deposition rather than more rapid bone resorption. Calcium supplements and bisphosphonates are the mainstays of treatment.

Fat-soluble vitamin deficiency due to poor bile salt excretion (or depletion due to cholestyramine) is present in 20% and treated with oral vitamin supplements. Coeliac disease should be excluded in the presence of steatorrhoea or fat-soluble vitamin deficiency.

A poorer prognosis can be expected in

- Patients with a high bilirubin level
- Females compared with males
- High anti-M2 and anti-M4 AMA subtype concentrations.

Note that PBC in patients with only anti-M9 AMA subtype tends to run a benign, non-progressive course.

SCENARIO 5. HEREDITARY HAEMOCHROMATOSIS

Identifying physical signs

As for chronic liver disease above, but the following may also be present in hereditary haemochromatosis (HH)

- Middle-aged (or older) men – twice as common in men as women
- Slate-grey skin pigmentation
- Evidence of arthritis
- Evidence of diabetes – look for insulin injection sites
- Evidence of cardiomyopathy – displaced apex, signs of congestive cardiac failure
- Venesection marks in the cubital fossae.

Differential diagnosis

- Autosomal dominant: ferroportin deficiency
- Autosomal recessive
  - hereditary haemochromatosis due to *HFE* mutations (most common)
  - hereditary haemochromatosis due to transferrin receptor 2 mutations
  - juvenile haemochromatosis due to hepcidin mutations
  - juvenile haemochromatosis due to haemojuvelin mutations
  - iron overload secondary to transferrinaemia
  - iron overload secondary to ceruloplasminaemia
- Acquired
  - thalassaemia
  - myelodysplasias
  - dyserythropoietic anaemias
  - sickle cell disease
  - red cell enzyme deficiencies
  - multiple blood transfusions.

Clinical judgement and maintaining patient welfare

As with all chronic liver disease cases, investigations should establish stage of disease and exclude decompensation as well as establish cause (see Scenario 3. Chronic liver disease).

1. **Confirming the diagnosis**
   State that you would initially request indirect serological markers of iron stores
   - Fasting serum free iron
   - TIBC
   - Ferritin level.
   The fasting free iron and TIBC determine the transferrin saturation; a value >50% has a sensitivity of 92% and specificity of 93% for HH. If the cut-off is lowered to 45%, the sensitivity increases to 100%, but this also detects liver disease associated with secondary iron overload such as alcohol-related liver disease, hepatitis C and non-alcoholic steatohepatitis (NASH).
   A raised (>50%) transferrin saturation and/or raised ferritin (>1000 ng/mL) warrant *HFE* gene status testing. Of all patients with iron overload
   - 90% will be homozygous for the *C282Y* mutation
   - 5–6% will be compound heterozygotes for the *C282Y* and *H63D* mutations
   - the remainder will have 'non-HFE'-associated iron overload.
   Note that half of cirrhotic patients with HH will have normal LFTs. Liver biopsy was therefore previously indicated in patients aged >40 years (fibrosis is rarely present before this age) or those with raised transaminases in order to rule out other causes of liver disease and assess the degree of hepatic iron concentration and fibrosis (both useful prognostic indicators). However, the role of biopsy is increasingly being

supplanted with MRI, which can assess both fibrosis and iron content.

In patients with the *HFE* gene mutations, a fasting glucose, LH, FSH, testosterone level, AP radiography of both hands and echocardiography are crucial screening tests for extrahepatic manifestation of the disease (see below).

2. **Look for extrahepatic disease (Table 1.5)**

   HH arthropathy typically begins at the first metacarpophalangeal joint (MCPJ), causing a characteristic squaring of the joint. Chondrocalcinosis (calcium pyrophosphate deposition) is seen in the menisci and articular cartilage on radiographs and distinguishes HH arthropathy from osteoarthritis. Unlike osteoarthritis, the arthropathy is usually difficult to control with NSAID therapy. Joint deformity is rare.

Management

- **Regular phlebotomy** (once or twice a week) is the mainstay of treatment, removing one unit of blood on each occasion (approximately 250 mg iron) and aiming for a target ferritin level of 50 ng/mL. This may take many years. Maintenance phlebotomy (approximately one unit a month) then continues lifelong, monitoring carefully for iron deficiency.
- Hypogonadism and arthropathy tend not to improve with phlebotomy, whereas insulin requirements may fall and cardiac function improve.

Table 1.5 Extrahepatic manifestations in hereditary haemochromatosis

Manifestation	Percentage
Skin hyperpigmentation	70
Hypogonadism	50
Amenorrhoea	15
Diabetes mellitus	50
Arthropathy	70
Cardiomyopathy	15–30
ECG abnormalities/arrhythmias	35

- Fibrosis does not reverse after phlebotomy and the risk of hepatocellular carcinoma (HCC) remains. HCC accounts for 30% of all deaths in haemochromatosis, so regular surveillance (ultrasonography and α-fetoprotein levels) is necessary.
- Decompensated liver disease and early HCC are indications for liver transplantation. The survival rates are lower than transplantation for other forms of liver disease due to coexistent cardiomyopathy and susceptibility to infection.
- Cardiac dysrhythmias are a common cause of death in HH and preventive measures should be taken when there is evidence of cardiomyopathy (eg antiarrhythmics and/or implantable cardioverter defibrillator (ICD)).

SCENARIO 6. ALCOHOL-RELATED LIVER DISEASE

Identifying physical signs

As for chronic liver disease but look for

- Parotid swelling and squaring of the jaw
- Dupuytren's contractures
- Peripheral neuropathy (tell the examiner that you would like to exclude this)
- Facial flushing.

It is three to four times more likely to be a man than a woman.

Differential diagnosis

State that you would like to take a full alcohol history and send off a liver screen (see above) to exclude dual pathology. This is crucial not only because viral hepatitis is more prevalent among people with alcohol dependence, but also because alcohol will dramatically accelerate other cirrhotic processes.

Clinical judgement and maintaining patient welfare

Investigations

1. *As with all chronic liver disease cases, investigations should establish the stage of disease and exclude decompensation as well as establish cause (see Scenario 3. Chronic liver disease).*
2. Make an assessment of nutritional status. The evidence that malnutrition is a major factor in the morbidity and mortality of those who use alcohol excessively is vast. Indeed, 30 years ago it was thought to be the principal mechanism of liver cirrhosis.
   Look for muscle wasting, subcutaneous fat loss and oedema. If any of these is present, state that you suspect malnutrition and would like to

- Take a full dietary history (or refer to dietician) and determine if there is a history of weight loss and its time-scale
- Calculate the BMI.

Patients with alcohol-related liver disease may be at risk of re-feeding syndrome.

3. Alcohol dependence has multisystem consequences for which there should be a low index of suspicion. Consider investigations assessing the following

- **Cardiac**
  - **Dilated cardiomyopathy (DC)**: an impaired ejection fraction can be demonstrated in a third of patients drinking ⩾70 g alcohol each day for >20 years. A third of all cases of DC are alcohol related.
  - **Hypertension**: drinking 4 units of alcohol a day doubles the risk of hypertension compared with teetotallers. There is a dose-related increase in blood pressure above this level of consumption. Those with advanced chronic liver disease are protected to some degree by associated hypotension, which may have multiple causes (eg bacterial translocation across the gut, failure to metabolise vasodilatory substances in the liver).
- **Gastrointestinal**
  - **Acute/chronic pancreatitis**: alcohol increases the viscosity of luminal secretions, resulting in ductal obstruction with upstream inflammation, fibrosis and atrophy. Of people using alcohol excessively 5–10% develop chronic pancreatitis, accounting for some 60% of all cases.
  - **Peptic ulcer disease**: alcohol has been shown to increase the risk of developing ulcers and delay ulcer healing.
  - **Oral, oesophageal and gastric cancers** are all more common in those who drink alcohol to excess.

- **Nervous system**
  - **Cerebellar atrophy**: increased sway is found in up to 70% of people with chronic alcohol problems and ataxia in around a third. There seems to be little correlation with peripheral neuropathy, suggesting a different pathogenesis in the loss of cerebellar Purkinje cells compared with peripheral neurons.
  - **Polyneuropathy**: using DSM-IV criteria to define chronic alcohol excess, one study found that 58% of patients had some form of polyneuropathy. Typical features include
    - reduced sensation to pinprick stimulation in a stocking-and-glove distribution
    - reduced tendon reflexes, especially the ankle
    - reduced distal power, eg plantar flexion
    - gait ataxia.
  - **Marchiafava–Bignami disease**: the pathological hallmark of this disease is necrosis of the corpus callosum. The key sign is apraxia of the non-dominant hand, indicating interhemispherical disconnection.
  - **Wernicke's encephalopathy**: alcohol reduces thiamine absorption by up to 50%, which combined with malnutrition can lead to negligible thiamine levels and myelin degeneration in the brain stem. The incidence can be as high as 12% in patients with alcohol dependence. Only the minority of patients (10%) present with the classic triad of global confusion, ophthalmoplegia and ataxia.
  - **Korsakoff's syndrome**: permanent anterograde and retrograde memory loss may remain after the initial confusion characterising Wernicke's encephalopathy has resolved. Patchy retrograde memory loss results in confabulation whereas anterograde formation of memories is often severely impaired.

Management

1. Nutritional support is key, especially during a hospital admission for decompensated liver disease or alcoholic hepatitis. Rapid intravenous replacement of B vitamins is standard management for prevention of Wernicke's encephalopathy.
2. Treatment for alcohol dependence is a two-stage process involving detoxification followed by rehabilitation. Traditionally the former was pharmacologically managed (chlordiazepoxide), and the latter was the domain of support workers and psychotherapists. However, naltrexone and acamprosate have been shown in several trials and meta-analyses to be useful adjuncts to traditional rehabilitative methods.

Naltrexone is an opioid receptor antagonist and is thought to reduce the reward effect of alcohol. Its major drawback is dose-related hepatotoxicity, making it contraindicated in those with active hepatitis or decompensated liver disease.

Acamprosate normalises the altered N-methyl-D-aspartate (NMDA)-mediated glutamatergic excitation that occurs in alcohol withdrawal and early periods of abstinence.

The COMBINE trial completed in 2006 suggested no benefit in combining the two. Its principal finding was that behavioural therapy and naltrexone coordinated by a specialised alcohol dependence team had the best chance of achieving lasting remission.

Identifying physical signs

As for chronic liver disease but look for the following

- Signs of current injecting drug use
- Tattoos/piercings
- Age and nationality (see below).

Differential diagnosis

Some knowledge of the international epidemiology of hepatitis B and C can inform the likelihood of a given patient with liver disease having either aetiology.

Three distinct epidemiological trends in hepatitis C are evident worldwide. In developed western countries, the peak prevalence is among patients aged 30–49 years, consistent with the greatest risk of exposure among injecting drug users 15–20 years ago. In developed countries in the Far East (eg Japan), the hepatitis C-positive population is far older, consistent with exposure in the post-war years – probably due to reuse of medical equipment without sterilisation. Ongoing hepatitis C infection is observed in all age groups in developing countries, due primarily to healthcare-related procedures rather than injecting drug use or high-risk sex.

In hepatitis B, country of birth is a particular risk factor, with high prevalence in south-east Asia and China, sub-Saharan Africa, the Amazon basin region of South America, and areas of Canada and Greenland (people of Inuit origin). A significant (and rapidly rising) proportion of hepatitis B and C in this country is therefore due to immigration rather than the stereotypical groups with high-risk factors. Be wary, therefore, of the traditional tattoo/piercing/injection mark doctrine of hepatitis risk.

Extrahepatic manifestations
Hepatitis B (HBV)
- Polyarteritis nodosa
- Glomerulonephritis and nephrotic syndrome
- 'Arthritis–dermatitis' syndrome
- Palpable purpura.

Hepatitis C (HCV)
- Essential mixed cryoglobulinaemia
- Lymphoma
- Glomerulonephritis
- Porphyria cutanea tarda
- Diabetes mellitus
- Autoimmune phenomena
- Peripheral neuropathy.

Clinical judgement and maintaining patient welfare

As with all chronic liver disease cases, investigations should establish the stage of disease and exclude decompensation as well as establish cause (see Scenario 3. Chronic liver disease).

Investigations: hepatitis C (Figure 1.2)
Once the diagnosis of chronic infection has been established, disease must be staged to assess whether treatment is indicated. The decision of who, when and how to treat is complex and changes rapidly with the emergence of directly acting antiviral agents (DAAs). Current licensed treatment is unpleasant and associated with serious side effects, and more than half of patients with chronic HCV will not progress to cirrhosis. The key factors in the initial assessment are

- HCV genotype: informs likelihood of response to therapy
- Presence of relative/absolute contraindications: informs likelihood of response to or tolerance of therapy

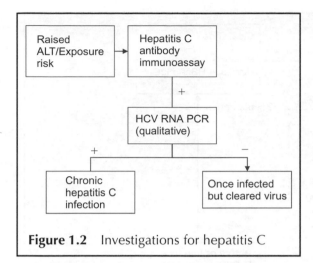

Figure 1.2   Investigations for hepatitis C

- Liver histology: informs likelihood of progression without therapy and response to therapy
- Increasingly full HCV sequencing will indicate presence of viruses resistant to new DAAs in treatment failures.

Contraindications to combination therapy with pegylated interferon and ribavarin

- Depressive illness or psychosis: a past history of these is not an absolute contraindication but requires careful surveillance during therapy
- Untreated autoimmune thyroid disease
- Neutropenia and/or thrombocytopenia
- Organ transplantation other than liver
- Symptomatic heart disease
- Decompensated cirrhosis
- Uncontrolled seizures
- Evidence of ongoing alcohol or injecting drug abuse.

The last of these is controversial, eg some clinicians believe that all ongoing injecting drug users with HCV should be treated because the risk of reinfection is actually low and, without treatment, the risk of infecting others is high.

Management – hepatitis C
This is changing rapidly. The mainstay of therapy for many years has been pegylated interferon-α

(P-IFN) and ribavarin. The former upregulates many hundreds of genes that produce proteins with antiviral functions. The pegylation of interferon results in sustained therapeutic levels and a more convenient once-a-week injection. The addition of ribavarin markedly increased the rates of sustained viral response (SVR) (a cure and the goal of therapy) compared with P-IFN monotherapy. SVR is defined as a negative HCV PCR test 6 months after cessation of treatment.

In 2012 NICE approved the use of either **boceprevir or telaprevir** for first-line therapy of genotype 1 disease or in those who have previously failed P-IFN and ribavarin therapy. These drugs are NS3/4 protease inhibitors. Both are given at the start of P-IFN and ribavarin therapy. They are expensive, up to £30 000 for a course, but have increased response rates in genotype 1 disease to around 80% from 50%.

In 2014 the DAAs sofosbuvir and simeprevir were licensed for use in HCV, which in combination with P-IFN and ribavirin improve SVR rates even further to >90%. More than 20 DAAs are in development (polymerase inhibitors, NS5A inhibitors) and protease inhibitors), with licensing expected in 2015. Used in combination for 6–12 weeks, these can achieve SVR rates >95% across all genotypes without combination with P-IFN and with minimal side effects.

Investigations – hepatitis B
Following acute hepatitis B infection (which may rarely lead to fulminant liver failure), >95% of adult patients will become HBsAg negative and HBsAb positive by 6 months (ie permanently clear the virus and have immunity from further infection). The remainder will go on to have chronic hepatitis B, which follows the phases described in Figure 1.3.

Treatment for hepatitis B
The aim of treatment is to suppress HBV DNA replication, because viral load (not ALT) correlates most closely with progression to cirrhosis and risk of HCC.

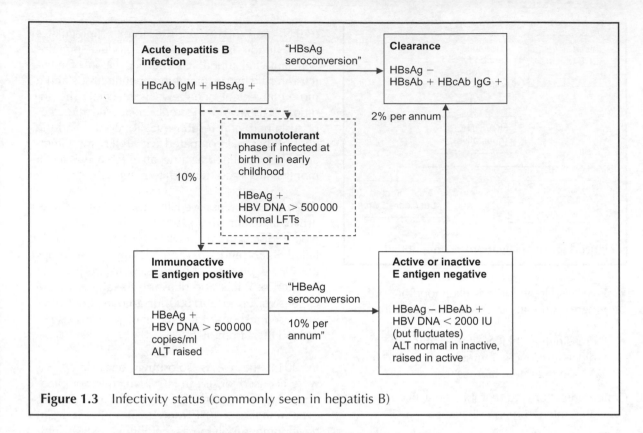

Figure 1.3   Infectivity status (commonly seen in hepatitis B)

There are two ways of achieving this: IFN-α monotherapy and oral antivirals. With the recent introduction of highly effective nucleoside analogue antivirals (such as entecavir or tenofovir), which have a high genetic barrier to resistance (and so can be used as monotherapies) and low side-effect profiles, IFN-α therapy for HBV is being used much less frequently. Treatment with oral antivirals is expensive, however, and of an indefinite duration due to the risk of viral escape if suppression is not maintained.

SCENARIO 8. AUTOIMMUNE HEPATITIS

Identifying physical signs

As for chronic liver disease but look for the following

- Usually a middle-aged woman
- Signs of thyroid disease
- Signs of rheumatoid arthritis
- Signs of scleroderma.

Differential diagnosis

Autoimmune hepatitis may present as

- Acute hepatitis: tender hepatomegaly, fever and jaundice
- Chronic hepatitis: serendipitous finding of abnormal liver enzymes
- Cirrhosis: presenting with decompensation (ascites, jaundice, variceal bleed, encephalopathy).

The latter presentation is the most likely to be encountered in PACES. Such patients are likely to be or have been on corticosteroid therapy so look for

- Cushingoid features
- Evidence of previous fractures
- Steroidal skin purpura.

Clinical judgement and maintaining patient welfare

Investigations

1. As with all chronic liver disease cases, investigations should establish the stage of disease and exclude decompensation as well as establish cause (Scenario 3. Chronic liver disease).
2. **Confirm the diagnosis**

- **Liver biopsy** is the most important test when autoimmune hepatitis (AIH) is suspected. There is a high degree of overlap with other conditions (PBC, PSC, autoimmune cholangitis), which can be differentiated only histologically. It also assesses severity and is used after treatment to determine whether remission has been achieved.
- **Autoantibodies** help differentiate between three main types of AIH.

Type 1	ANA
	Anti-smooth muscle antibody (ASMA)
Type 2	Anti-liver kidney microsomal (ALKM)
Type 3	Anti-soluble liver antigen (ASLA)

Type 2 is rare in adults. Types 1 and 3 have similar responsiveness to steroids, female predominance (80%), rates of other autoimmune disease (40%) and raised polyclonal γ-globulin. Type 3 is, however, more likely to progress to cirrhosis.
- **Serum electrophoresis and immunoglobulins** will detect a polyclonal expansion of IgG.
- **Transaminases** are crucial to the monitoring of response to therapy, although it must be noted that up to 50% of patients with normal LFTs have ongoing inflammation on histology. Histological resolution tends to lag behind biochemical remission by 3–6 months.

3. **Exclude other autoimmune conditions**
   AIH should be regarded as a multisystem disorder associated with a plethora of autoimmune diseases. These can be divided into intrahepatic ('overlap') and extrahepatic.
- **Intrahepatic 'overlap' conditions**
  - PBC about 7%
  - primary sclerosing cholangitis (PSC) about 6%
  - autoimmune cholangitis
  - antibody-negative AIH.

- **Extrahepatic associations**

Rheumatological	Endocrine	Gastrointestinal
Rheumatoid arthritis Sjögren's syndrome Systemic sclerosis	Graves' disease Autoimmune thyroiditis Juvenile diabetes mellitus	Coeliac disease Inflammatory bowel disease
Haematological	**Cardiological**	**Renal**
Haemolytic anaemia Pernicious anaemia	Pericarditis Myocarditis	Glomerulonephritis

Management
Indications for treatment

- AST more than tenfold upper limit of normal or more than fivefold with an IgG level more than twofold normal
- Bridging or multi-acinar necrosis on liver biopsy
- Raised AST below criteria but symptomatic (fatigue, arthralgia, jaundice).

Corticosteroids and azathioprine are the principal agents used. A reducing dose of corticosteroids is used to initiate therapy, followed by maintenance on low-dose steroids with azathioprine or mono-therapy depending on tolerance and side effects. Approximately 65% of patients respond to initial therapy and enter histological remission; however, 80% of these patients relapse after drug withdrawal within 3 years. Some clinicians thus advocate long-term maintenance therapy on azathioprine.

Remission is rarely achieved in the first year of treatment; 80% of patients achieve remission within 3 years. However, with immunosuppressant therapy the prognosis is good, with 10-year survival rates of around 90% irrespective of the presence of cirrhosis at presentation.

SCENARIO 9. ISOLATED HEPATOMEGALY WITHOUT STIGMATA OF CHRONIC LIVER DISEASE

Identifying physical signs

Face
- Flushing: carcinoid
- Pale conjunctivae: anaemia of chronic disease (amyloid, sarcoid) or malignancy.

Hands
- Clubbing.

Neck
- JVP raised/giant V waves
- Lymphadenopathy, Virchow's node.

Precordium
- S3 or murmur of tricuspid regurgitation.

Abdomen
- Hepatomegaly
- Pulsatile?: tricuspid regurgitation
- Smooth?: sarcoidosis, amyloidosis
- Irregular?: malignant infiltration, polycystic, hydatid cysts
- Tender?: acute hepatitis, Budd–Chiari syndrome
- Lymphadenopathy: malignancy
- Ascites: malignant, cardiac failure, Budd–Chiari syndrome
- Sister Mary Joseph nodule.

Other
- Cachexia: malignancy
- Fever: amoebiasis
- Ankle oedema: congestive cardiac failure.

Differential diagnosis

Hepatomegaly without stigmata of chronic liver disease (ie cirrhosis) has a narrow differential diagnosis. The most common causes (in the UK and in PACES) are

- Congestive cardiac failure (± tricuspid regurgitation)
- Metastatic malignancy.

Note that primary liver tumours are rare in the absence of cirrhosis.

Rarer causes of isolated hepatomegaly include

- Budd–Chiari syndrome
- Hydatid cyst
- Riedel's lobe
- Polycystic liver disease (usually with accompanying renal enlargement)
- Sarcoidoisis
- Amyloidosis
- Carcinoid.

Clinical judgement and maintaining patient welfare

Investigations
These usually begin with imaging and liver enzymes.

Irregular hepatomegaly
In the absence of cardiac signs, liver ultrasonography is the best initial investigation. Further imaging may well be needed to distinguish benign from sinister lesions. Biopsy risks upstaging and seeding a malignant lesion in the biopsy tract, and should be undertaken only if

- Tumour markers are negative and imaging has failed to distinguish the nature of the lesion
- The tumour is inoperable anyway.

CT, MRI and laparoscopy with intraoperative ultrasonography are all useful modalities in further characterising hepatic lesions.

Riedel's lobe is a normal anatomical variant. It is not a true accessory lobe but a tongue-like projection of the right lobe of the liver which may extend downwards as far as the right iliac fossa. In one CT-based study that defined Riedel's lobe as a protuberance of the right lobe below the costal margin, the prevalence was 33%, rising to 65% in patients aged >50 years.

Benign lesions of the liver may be confused with malignancy on ultrasonography or CT

- Haemangiomas
- Focal nodular hyperplasia
- Complex liver cysts
- Focal fatty infiltration/focal fatty sparing
- Hepatic adenomas
- Biliary hamartomas.

MRI with gadolinium contrast enhancement is often the best means of distinguishing these lesions from primary or secondary liver malignancies.

Hydatid cyst disease is a parasitic infestation by a tapeworm of the genus *Echinococcus*. In the UK, the most common intermediate host is a sheep, hence a higher incidence of the disease in farming areas. Cysts grow most commonly in the liver (and lung) over many years. **Sequelae** include painful hepatomegaly, obstructive jaundice or rarely acute rupture with an associated anaphylactic response. Secondary infection can also occur. **Diagnosis** is by abdominal CT, which has the highest sensitivity and specificity. Serological tests have a sensitivity of 90% for hepatic echinococcosis and are a useful initial screening test. **Treatment** is with a 6-month course of albendazole and mebendazole.

Liver abscesses are rarely encountered in PACES because the patient is typically systemically unwell with fever and right upper quadrant pain.

Carcinoid syndrome is suggested by irregular hepatomegaly in combination with skin flushing and telangiectasiae. Liver metastases must occur before symptoms develop. A dietary history may reveal specific foods that induce flushing. Investigations include

- Elevated urinary 5HIAA
- Elevated plasma chromogranin A
- Octreotide scanning (scintigraphy with labelled octreotide) is the gold standard diagnostic test. It is highly sensitive and specific, and also predicts the degree to which a patient will respond to octreotide treatment.

Smooth hepatomegaly
Cardiac disease: if there are signs of cardiac failure, initial tests should include

- Echocardiography
- Chest radiograph
- Liver ultrasonography (to exclude other pathologies).

Liver biopsy (not usually warranted) rarely reveals signs of cirrhosis. Only 10% of patients become jaundiced, and encephalopathy is extremely rare. Signs and symptoms of cardiac failure dominate the clinical picture, varying according to whether the underlying cause of hepatic congestion is biventricular failure, cor pulmonale, pericardial disease or tricuspid incompetence.

Budd–Chiari syndrome often presents with ascites and jaundice. Ultrasonography with Doppler flow examination of the hepatic veins reveals thrombus with a high sensitivity and specificity (90%). MRI with pulsed sequencing may clarify the venous anatomy.

Sarcoidosis rarely presents with hepatomegaly alone, yet liver granulomas are present in up to 70% of patients with sarcoidosis *post mortem*. CT may reveal the coalescing granulomas apparent as multiple hypointense or hypoattenuating nodules. In the context of other clinical features of sarcoid (eg pulmonary involvement), no further investigation is necessary to confirm hepatic sarcoid. However, multiple nodules in hepatic sarcoidosis are easily mistaken for metastases or lymphoma and screening for malignancy may be required.

Secondary amyloidosis (AA) due to excessive serum amyloid A secretion in chronic inflammatory conditions is the most common form affecting the liver. By the time there is hepatomegaly there are usually signs of renal impairment (anaemia, hypertension and oedema). The presence of macroglossia, congestive heart failure, peripheral neuropathy or carpal tunnel syndrome suggests AL amyloid. Rectal biopsy with Congo red staining (displaying apple-green birefringence on polarised light examination if amyloid is present) has 80% sensitivity. Liver biopsy is rarely undertaken due to the high risk of bleeding or rupture.

SCENARIO 10: ASCITES WITHOUT STIGMATA OF CHRONIC LIVER DISEASE

Identifying physical signs

Non-cirrhotic ascites, similar to isolated hepato-megaly, is usually due to either congestive **cardiac failure** or **intra-abdominal malignancy**. The signs that one should look for are thus very similar to those in Scenario 4. In younger patients, consider **nephrotic syndrome** (look for ankle oedema, hypertension, evidence of dyslipi-daemia, evidence of deep vein thrombosis).

Differential diagnosis

Rarer causes include

- Budd–Chiari syndrome – look for jaundice and hepatomegaly
- Tuberculous peritonitis – look for lung signs
- Chylous ascites due to lymphatic obstruction.

The most common primary tumours leading to malignant ascites are

- Ovarian (most common)
- Endometrial
- Breast
- Colon
- Gastric
- Pancreatic.

Clinical judgement and maintaining patient welfare

Investigations
A diagnostic tap is the key investigation, request-ing the following

- **The serum–ascites albumin gradient (SAAG)**: this is calculated by subtracting the ascitic fluid albumin level from the plasma value. Values >1.1 g/dL indicate portal hypertensive ascites. Values <1.1 g/dL indicate non-portal hypertensive causes (most often infection or

malignancy). This has almost 100% accuracy in discriminating between these two aetiological categories.
- **Cell count**: lymphocytic infiltrate is suggestive of tuberculous or carcinomatous peritoneal disease, whereas neutrophils suggest bacterial peritonitis.
- **Culture/Gram stain** and stain for acid-fast bacilli (AFBs).
- **Cytology**: if an adequate sample is taken for centrifugation (approximately 500 mL), cytology has up to 75% sensitivity in detecting malignant cells.

Other useful investigations include

- Echocardiography: if congestive cardiac failure is suspected
- Abdominopelvic CT: if malignancy is suspected
- Tumour markers
- Breast exam ± mammography
- Diagnostic laparoscopy.

Ultrasonography is useful for tapping small-volume or loculated ascites.

Management
The management of ascites in congestive cardiac failure is similar to that of chronic liver disease (see above) with salt restriction and diuretics (eg spironolactone).

Malignant ascites is often painful and difficult to treat due to its resistance to chemotherapy and rapid reaccumulation after drainage. The usual life expectancy is <4 months although this varies according to the underlying causes. Serial para-centesis is an appropriate means of controlling symptoms but care must be taken to ensure adequate dietary protein replacement. Permanent exteriorised catheters and peritoneovenous shunts are other therapeutic options in patients with a longer life expectancy. These often be-come infected or blocked within 6 months.

Identifying physical signs

Hands
- Rheumatoid arthritis (Felty's syndrome).

Head and neck
- Lymphadenopathy
- Alopecia (recent chemotherapy)
- Pale conjunctivae (anaemia due to bone marrow failure)
- Tunnelled catheter (for chemotherapy)
- Jaundice (haemolysis)
- Butterfly rash (SLE).

Abdomen
- Smooth enlargement of liver and spleen
- Lymphadenopathy.

Other
- Petechial rash
- Shingles
- Bruises
- Evidence of bone marrow biopsy over iliac crest.

Differential diagnosis

The differential diagnosis is vast and examiners are principally concerned that the candidate has a good grasp of the diagnostic possibilities and their likelihood. It is therefore imperative to have a clear diagnostic algorithm in your mind. A suggested scheme is outlined in Figure 1.4.

The principal causes of hepatosplenomegaly or isolated splenomegaly without cirrhosis are usually

- Haematological
- Infectious
- Storage disorders
- Inflammatory.

Haematological (look for anaemia)

Myeloproliferative
- Chronic myeloid leukaemia
  - massive spleen ± hepatomegaly
  - pallor
- Acute myeloid leukaemia
  - mild-to-moderate splenomegaly ± hepatomegaly
  - pallor
  - petechiae
  - tunnelled line for chemotherapy ± alopecia
- Myelofibrosis
  - massive spleen ± hepatomegaly
  - pallor
  - evidence of gout.

Essential thrombocytosis (often no physical signs)
- Mild splenomegaly
- Bleeding diatheses
- Deep vein thrombosis
- Digital gangrene/ischaemia.

Polycythaemia rubra vera (PRV)
See below.

Lymphoproliferative
- Chronic lymphocytic leukaemia
  - lymphadenopathy
  - mild-to-moderate splenomegaly ± hepatomegaly
  - pallor
  - petechiae
- Acute lymphoblastic leukaemia
  - lymphadenopathy
  - mild-to-moderate splenomegaly ± hepatomegaly
  - pallor
  - purpura, petechiae
  - skin rash
  - fever

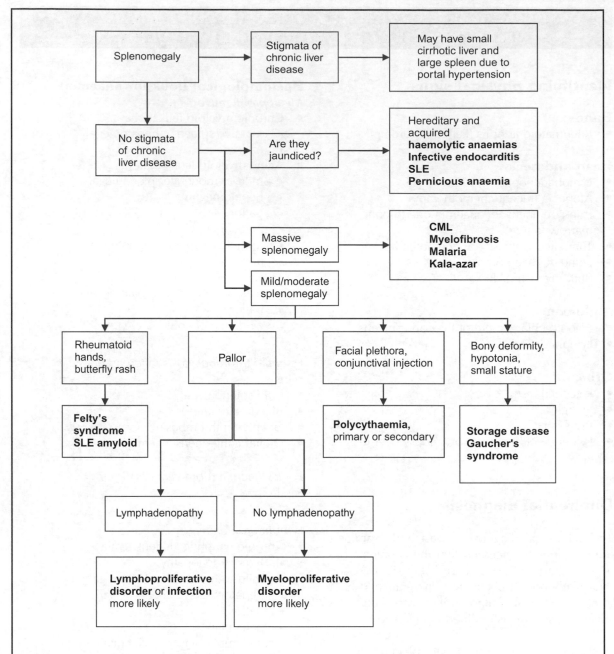

Figure 1.4 Suggested flowchart for determining cause of splenomegaly by clinical type. All entries in bold are diagnoses

- tunnelled line for chemotherapy ± alopecia.

Lymphoma
- Lymphadenopathy
- Mild-to-moderate splenomegaly ± hepatomegaly
- Skin rashes (mycosis fungoides/Sézary's syndrome)
- Abdominal mass (Burkitt's lymphoma).

Acute leukaemias are understandably rare in PACES. Note that, in the presence of marked lymphadenopathy, an underlying lymphoproliferative disorder is more likely than a myeloproliferative one.

The presence of splenomegaly, anaemia and jaundice in the absence of stigmata of chronic liver disease suggests a haemolytic disorder such as **hereditary spherocytosis** (see below).

Infectious
The most common causes of hepatosplenomegaly worldwide are vanishingly rare in PACES

- Malaria
- Kala-azar (abdominal leishmaniasis)

- Schistosomiasis
- Tuberculosis.

In the UK more common infectious causes of hepatosplenomegaly are

- Brucellosis (agriculture worker, neurological signs, skin rash)
- Leptospirosis with Weil's syndrome (jaundice, fever, muscle tenderness, positive Murphy's sign)
- Toxoplasmosis (cervical lymphadenopathy)
- Infectious mononucleosis (lymphadenopathy).

Storage disorders
- Gaucher's disease (bony deformity, previous fractures)
- Glycogen storage disease (small build, hypotonia, muscle atrophy).

Inflammatory
- Felty's syndrome (look for rheumatoid features)
- Amyloid (look for evidence of chronic inflammatory disease).

Extent of splenomegaly can help differentiate the underlying cause (Table 1.6).

Table 1.6 Extent of splenomegaly

Mild (spleen just palpable)	Moderate (up to four finger-breadths)	Massive
Infectious mononucleosis Infective endocarditis	Myeloproliferative disorders Lymphoproliferative disorders Cirrhosis and portal hypertension	CML Myelofibrosis Malaria Kala-azar

Clinical judgement and maintaining patient welfare

Investigations
See Table 1.7.

Table 1.7 Investigations for Scenario 11

Haematological	Myeloproliferative disorders	Chronic myeloid leukaemia	Bone marrow sampling (BMS) cytogenetics: Philadelphia chromosome
		Myelofibrosis	Peripheral blood smear – leukoerythroblastosis with teardrop poikilocytosis BMS – reticular fibrosis
		Acute myeloid leukaemia	BMS >20% blasts
		Essential thrombocytosis	Raised platelets BMS – hypercellular with giant megakaryocytes
		PRV	Increased red cell mass, *JAK2* mutations
	Lymphoproliferative disorders	Chronic lymphocytic leukaemia	Sustained WCC >50 cells/mm^3 with lymphocytosis Lymph node/BMS required if transformation to lymphoma suspected
		Lymphoma	Lymph node biopsy, CT and BMS staging
		Acute lymphoblastic leukaemia	BMS >30% lymphoblasts Cytogenetics for typing
Storage disorders		Glycogen storage disease	Liver/muscle biopsy
		Gaucher's disease	Reduced acid β-glucosidase activity in peripheral blood leukocytes Plain radiography to detect flask deformity of the distal femur
Inflammatory		Amyloid	Rectal biopsy with Congo red stain
		Felty's syndrome	Presence of rheumatoid arthritis, positive rheumatoid factor

(*continued*)

Table 1.7 (*continued*)

Infectious	Schistosomiasis	Urine/stool egg count, serology cannot distinguish past from active infection
	Brucellosis	Serum tube agglutination test (developed in 1887!), blood cultures, PCR
	Toxoplasmosis	Detection of *Toxoplasma gondii* antigen in blood by ELISA
	Kala-azar	Detection of antibodies to recombinant K39 antigen (ELISA) or PCR test for leishmaniasis DNA
	Malaria	Thick and thin blood films
	Infectious mononucleosis	Monospot test followed by EBV serology if negative
	Weil's syndrome	Blood cultures, microscopic agglutination test

Management
See Table 1.8.

Table 1.8 Management of Scenario 11

Haematological	Myeloproliferative disorders	Chronic myeloid leukaemia	Imatinib[a] (Gleevec) is the main treatment for CML. Dasatinib, nilotinib or interferon-based therapy is an alternative should CML prove resistant to imatinib. Bone-marrow transplantation or stem-cell transplantation (SCT) can be curative
		Myelofibrosis	Chemotherapy with thalidomide, hydroxycarbamide and/or melphalan. SCT can be curative. Splenectomy is often performed
		Acute myeloid leukaemia	This depends on subtype but combination chemotherapy and SCT are the main therapeutic modalities
		Essential thrombocytosis	Hydroxycarbamide with low-dose aspirin to reduce thrombosis risk
		PRV	See below
	Lymphoproliferative disorders	Chronic lymphocytic leukaemia	Combination chemotherapy (if treatment is necessary) sometimes combined with rituximab
		Lymphoma	Treatment varies by subtype. Radiotherapy and combination chemotherapy ± SCT remain the mainstay of treatment.
		Acute lymphoblastic leukaemia (ALL)	Depends on subtype and immunotype but combination chemotherapy ± SCT is a primary therapy. Imatinib may be useful in Philadelphia chromosome-positive ALL[b]

(*continued*)

Table 1.8 (*continued*)

Storage disorders	Glycogen storage disease	Treatment is aimed at managing hypoglycaemia, hypertriglyceridaemia, hyperuricaemia and lactic acidosis
	Gaucher's disease	Enzyme (β-glucosidase) replacement therapy
Inflammatory	Amyloid	Depends on underlying aetiology
	Felty's syndrome	Treat underlying rheumatoid disease
Infectious	Schistosomiasis	Praziquantel – a single dose is usually effective
	Brucellosis	Streptomycin and doxycycline
	Toxoplasmosis	Pyrimethamine and sulfadiazine, or azithromycin monotherapy. Most cases are mild and do not require therapy unless the patient is immunosuppressed
	Kala-azar	Liposomal amphotericin is the current treatment of choice for visceral leishmaniasis
	Malaria	Artemisinin in combination with amodiaquine, mefloquine, lumefantrine or sulfadoxine/pyrimethamine. In severe cases, intravenous quinine or artersunate
	Infectious mononucleosis	Steroids for dangerous tonsil enlargement; otherwise treatment is supportive
	Weil's syndrome	Effective antibiotics include doxycycline, penicillin and cefotaxime

[a]Imatinib (Gleevec) is a tyrosine kinase inhibitor that has revolutionised the treatment of CML (and gastrointestinal stromal tumours or GISTs). It works by inducing apoptosis in cells with the *bcr/abl* fusion gene. It induces complete cytogenetic response in almost all patients in the chronic phase with 3-year survival rates around 95%. The results in the accelerated phase of CML are less impressive (30% complete response) but still a vast improvement over combination chemotherapy. Imatinib is also far better tolerated than older treatments.

[b]Chromosomal translocation of the *c-abl* oncogene, which encodes for a tyrosine protein kinase from chromosome 9 to the *bcr* locus of chromosome 22, resulting in markedly increased tyrosine kinase activity. This is the basis for malignant clonal expansion. The fusion gene mRNA can be detected extremely sensitively by PCR, which is useful for monitoring residual disease after therapy.

SCENARIO 12. POLYCYTHAEMIA RUBRA VERA

Identifying physical signs

- Middle-aged/elderly patient
- Splenomegaly/hepatosplenomegaly
- Facial plethora
- Scratch mark
- Hypertension
- Enlarged conjunctival vessels
- (Dilated retinal veins on fundoscopy)
- Evidence of venesection
- Gout.

Differential diagnosis

See Scenario 11. Hepatosplenomegaly/splenome-galy without stigmata of chronic liver disease.

Clinical judgement and maintaining patient welfare

Common pitfalls in understanding and diagnosis of PRV

- Although it takes its name from its associated erythrocytosis, it is an expansion of **three** cell lineages including platelets and leukocytes. These result from the clonal expansion of a multi-potent haematopoietic progenitor cell. The cause of this is unknown.
- The WHO proposed diagnostic criteria for PRV that require two major and one minor or the first major and two minor criteria
  - Major criteria
    - Hb >18.5 g/dL (men), >16.5 g/dL (women) or >25% normal predicted red cell mass
    - Janus kinase 2 (*JAK2*) mutation
  - Minor criteria
    - bone marrow biopsy showing hypercellularity with prominent erythroid, granulocytic and megakaryocytic proliferation

- serum erythropoietin level below normal range
- endogenous erythroid colony formation in vitro.
- Measuring red cell mass (with ^{51}Cr) and the plasma volume (with ^{125}I-labelled albumin) confirms true erythrocytosis and remains a tenet of the Polycythaemia Vera Study Group diagnostic criteria. This will exclude relative erythrocytosis (caused by states of reduced plasma volume, eg diarrhoea) but does not exclude other secondary causes of erythrocytosis.
- Bone marrow examination is not diagnostic.

Evidence of complications or progression

- The principal complication of increased red cell mass and hyperviscosity is thrombosis. As a rule of thumb
  - 40% present with a thrombotic episode
  - 40% of those who present by other means will eventually experience thrombosis
  - 40% die from a thrombotic complication.
- Arterial thrombosis is more common than venous and the central nervous system is most commonly affected (ie stroke).
- PRV is the leading cause of hepatic vein thrombosis (Budd–Chiari syndrome) in the UK.

Look for evidence of previous stroke (asymmetrical weakness, facial droop, inattention, etc).

Other complications include

- Painful organomegaly
- Hyperuricaemia and gout (due to increased cell turnover)
- Haemorrhage (counterintuitively, this probably occurs due to sequestration of von Willebrand's factor by an expanded platelet population).

Conditions that PRV can progress to

- **Myelofibrosis**: occurs in approximately 5% of patients treated with phlebotomy alone and 8.4% of those treated with chemotherapy or radiotherapy. Cases of spontaneous resolution of myelofibrosis have been documented.
- **Acute leukaemias**: may be a consequence of therapy rather than a natural progression of the disease, although this is controversial. Patients treated with radioactive phosphorous and chlorambucil are at greatest risk. Long-term hydroxycarbamide may also increase the incidence of acute leukaemia.

Management

Phlebotomy is the mainstay of therapy, aiming to reduce red cell mass and viscosity. A haematocrit of <45% is the usual goal of therapy (this may require twice-weekly phlebotomy initially).

Hydroxycarbamide (hydroxyurea) in addition to phlebotomy has been shown to reduce the risk of thrombosis compared with phlebotomy alone and is recommended in patients aged >40 years.

The grim prognosis of a 50% survival rate at 18 months if untreated is largely drawn from poorly designed studies in the 1960s. Although referral for treatment should be immediate, PRV generally follows an indolent course. Some groups have presented data for life expectancy, with adequate treatment and follow-up, not dissimilar to normal.

SCENARIO 13: HEREDITARY SPHEROCYTOSIS

Identifying physical signs

Look for the triad of

- Splenomegaly
- Jaundice
- Pallor (anaemia).

The patient is usually of north European origin.

Other typical features

- Cholecystectomy scar
- Splenectomy scar
- Leg ulcers.

HS has mild, moderate and severe phenotypes, which can be differentiated clinically

- **Mild** HS occurs in 20% of cases, but is rare in PACES because patients are asymptomatic and rarely have signs. These patients may present or through family screening with an aplastic crisis precipitated by infection.
- **Moderate** HS accounts for 75% of all HS cases. These patients display the classic triad of splenomegaly, jaundice and anaemia. The inheritance is autosomal dominant.
- **Severe** HS occurs in only 5% of all patients. Patients have commonly undergone splenectomy but the response is usually incomplete, hence they may present in PACES with jaundice and anaemia. This is recessively inherited.

Other causes of anaemia, splenomegaly and jaundice

These are unusual but include

- Infective endocarditis
- SLE
- Pernicious anaemia
- Infectious mononucleosis.

Normally one would expect associated stigmata of these systemic conditions to be apparent.

Clinical judgement and maintaining patient welfare

A number of red cell membrane proteins may be deficient or inadequately integrated. The most common defect in autosomal dominant HS is β-spectrin deficiency. This results in a characteristic spherical structure of erythrocytes, which are rapidly cleared in the spleen leading to (extravascular) haemolysis and splenic hypertrophy.

Initial investigations for HS should include

- Reticulocyte count and haptoglobins
- Lactate dehydrogenase
- Split bilirubin
- Peripheral blood smear: may show megalocytosis and Howell–Jolly bodies (if the spleen has been removed).

The diagnosis is confirmed with an **osmotic fragility test**, which involves incubating blood in saline for 24 hours at 37°C.

If there is evidence of an aplastic crisis

- Vitamin B_{12} and folate stores should be assessed to ensure that recovery is possible.
- HSV, EBV and human papillomavirus type 19 should be tested for as potential aetiological agents.

Complications

- Anaemia is the principal concern in HS and may require serial transfusions.
- Gallstones are found in 50% of patients with HS. Biliary colic and obstruction are frequent complications.
- Aplastic crises occur when bone-marrow suppression (caused most commonly by infection or drugs) means that the high rate of destruction of erythrocytes can no longer be compensated for by increased production.

Although **splenectomy** is clearly indicated in severe cases, the treatment of asymptomatic moderate HS is less straightforward. Splenectomy is curative in such cases but must be balanced against the associated 200-fold increase in mortality risk from sepsis. Partial splenectomy may offer a compromise between sustained immuno-protection and minimal ongoing haemolysis.

Postsplenectomy prophylaxis should include

- Immunisation for pneumococci
- Immunisation for *Haemophilus influenzae* type b
- Immunisation for meningococcus C
- Influenza vaccine annually
- Lifelong oral penicillin prophylaxis.

THE RESPIRATORY EXAMINATION

Data from previous candidates show that the following three presentations account for over 65% of the respiratory examination cases

1. Interstitial lung disease (twice as common as bronchiectasis)
2. Bronchiectasis
3. Pneumonectomy (any cause).

It is therefore essential to know these cases well. Patients with residual signs recovering from pneumothorax, pleural effusion and asthma may feature in this station and the integrated clinical assessment (ICA).

Examination routine

Approach to the patient
Introduce yourself to the patient, wash your hands and ask for permission to examine him or her, which will require exposing the chest. Check that the patient has no pain before you start. Position the patient correctly (sitting up at 45°).

Observation
Look around the bed for

- Oxygen cylinders
- Inhalers
- Nebulisers
- Peak flow meters
- Steroid cards/bracelets/necklaces
- Sputum pots.

Ask the patient to stretch out his or her hands in front and take a deep breath in and out. Look for the following

- Asymmetry of expansion (a useful guide to the side where pathology may be found)
- Dyspnoea at rest (with tracheal tug, intercostal recession, use of accessory muscles or pursed-lip breathing)
- Cyanosis
- Surgical scars (pneumonectomy, previous chest drains)

- Signs of steroid use (bruises, cushingoid appearance, etc)
- Cachexia (malignancy)
- Cough (bronchiectasis or COPD)
- Rashes (autoimmune disease and sarcoidosis)
- Arthropathy (rheumatoid arthritis)
- Bony abnormalities (kyphoscoliosis/pectus excavatum and carinatum)
- Signs of radiotherapy markings or burns.

Record the respiratory rate and estimate the length of the expiratory versus inspiratory phases. Inspiration is usually longer than expiration; this is reversed in obstructive disease.

Hands
With the patient's arms outstretched, examine the hands for the following

- Tar stains (COPD and malignancy),
- Clubbing (idiopathic, fibrosis, malignancy, bronchiectasis, tuberculosis and lung abscess)
- Swelling of the wrists (consider hypertrophic pulmonary osteoarthropathy (HPOA) – a rare paraneoplastic manifestation of lung cancer, with specific radiographic changes)
- Wasting of the small muscles of the hands (suggestive of T1 impingement by an apical tumour)
- Warm vasodilated peripheries (CO_2 retention)
- Cyanosis
- Tremor (β-agonist therapy),
- Asterixis/flap with dorsiflexed wrists and fingers spread out (CO_2 retention)
- Signs of systemic diseases such as rheumatoid arthritis or systemic sclerosis
- Bounding pulse (CO_2 retention)
- Tachycardia (infection and β-agonist therapy).

Face
- Conjunctival pallor
- Cushingoid facies
- Miosis and ptosis – Horner's syndrome
- Plethora
- Lips/beneath tongue – central cyanosis.

Neck
Look for signs of cor pulmonale leading to an **elevated JVP** with a prominent 'a' or 'v' wave. If this is suspected, examine for a left parasternal heave (representing right ventricular hypertrophy (RVH)) and tricuspid regurgitation (a high-pitched pansystolic murmur at the lower left sternal border, accentuated by inspiration and associated with an S3 gallop).

You may examine for **lymphadenopathy** at this point, which requires sitting the patient forward. It may be more efficient to wait until the transition between anterior and posterior chest examination, so that findings in the anterior chest can determine the amount of time that you ration for searching for reactive or malignant lymphadenopathy.

Examine for **deviation of the trachea** by placing index and ring fingers on the sternal notch and the middle finger on the apex of the curve of the trachea. It should rest equidistant from the index and ring fingers if the trachea is central. The trachea may be slightly deviated to the right in a normal examination.

Inspection of the chest
Look closely for any **scars** on the chest, not neglecting the posterior aspect of the patient. Ask the patient to lift the arms up to look at the axillae. Look for lobectomy, thoracotomy, VATS, chest drain and lung biopsy scars. Assess the **shape** of the chest

- Barrel shaped: an increase in the anteroposterior diameter (COPD)
- Pigeon chest (pectus carinatum): outward bowing of the sternum (chronic childhood respiratory illness or rickets)
- Funnel chest (pectus excavatum): developmental defect with depression of the sternum
- Kyphoscoliosis: idiopathic, secondary to polio, neurodegenerative diseases or ankylosing spondylitis.

Palpation
Examine the cardiac apex, which may be difficult to feel in patients with a hyperexpanded chest, or pulled towards the side of collapse/pneumonectomy. Gently palpate any lump or deformity.

Expansion
Assess the upper and lower chest separately

- Upper chest: place hands lightly on the upper chest just below the clavicles. The hands should be felt to rise symmetrically.
- Lower chest: ask the patient to breathe in and out, then place the hands on the lateral side of the lower ribs, with the thumbs pointing towards the midline. The thumbs may touch lightly in the midline. Ask the patient to breathe in again and the thumbs should move symmetrically apart during inspiration. Normal expansion is 4–5 cm.

Percussion
Percuss the clavicles (not directly onto the bone) and then the lung fields. Compare left with right at each point, moving down the chest. Do not forget to specifically percuss the supraclavicular fossae and in each axilla; the latter is the only place where resonance throughout all lobes in the right or left lungs can be assessed.

Tactile vocal fremitus
Assess fremitus by asking the patient to say '99' while placing the lateral border of the hands on the chest wall. Compare the left and right lungs simultaneously, using both hands; move down the chest wall from top to bottom.

Auscultation
Once again, move down in a zig-zag manner from top to bottom, asking the patient to breathe quietly through the mouth. Use the diaphragm of the stethoscope on the chest wall, but the bell for the supraclavicular area because it is smaller.

Characterise the breath sounds

- Vesicular, ie normal

- Bronchial (noise transmitted to the chest wall from a large airway, eg consolidation or along the top of an effusion)
- Decreased, eg emphysema
- Wheeze: always expiratory, mono-/polyphonic
- Stridor: always inspiratory and indicates extrathoracic obstruction
- Crackles: fine/coarse; inspiratory/expiratory; early/late (Table 1.9)
- Pleural rub: pleurisy secondary to a pulmonary embolism or pneumonia.

Vocal resonance
This is analogous to tactile vocal fremitus (TVF) and can be performed as an alternative. One hears bronchophony over consolidation or fibrosis, or at the top of an effusion, because the noise from large airways is transmitted directly to the chest wall. It sounds as if the words are spoken directly into your ear.

Posterior chest
Some candidates choose to feel for cervical lymphadenopathy now as the patient is leaning forward. Repeat observation, percussion, TVF, auscultation (and vocal resonance (VR)) for the back of the chest.

To finish
Examine the ankles for pitting oedema (seen in cor pulmonale or sometimes in COPD without cor pulmonale). Ask to measure the peak expiratory flow rate and look at observation charts. Examine any sputum in a pot, noting quantity and colour.

Thank the patient, help him or her to dress and WASH YOUR HANDS.

Table 1.9 Signs in common cases

Signs	ILD/fibrosis	Bronchiectasis	Pneumonectomy/ lobectomy	COPD	Pleural effusion (see Station 5: Integrated clinical assessment)
General	Breathless Central cyanosis Cushingoid Signs of diseases such as SS or RA Kyphosis with ankylosing spondylitis Rashes with sarcoidosis, SLE, dermatomyositis	Breathless Frequent cough Audible inspiratory clicks	Deformity or flattening of chest wall Scars Cachexia if malignancy	Breathless Pursed lips Central/peripheral cyanosis Using accessory muscles Cushingoid	May be breathless May be cachexia if associated with malignancy
Hands/pulse	Joint/skin changes in SLE, RA or dermatomyositis	Clubbing Yellow nails Tar staining if associated with COPD	Clubbing if malignancy, TB, bronchiectasis or abscess	CO_2 flap Bounding pulse Tar-stained fingers β_2-Agonist tremor	Clubbing if malignancy
Neck/trachea	JVP raised with prominent 'a' and 'v' waves if cor pulmonale Lymphadenopathy if cause is sarcoidosis	JVP raised with prominent 'a' and 'v' waves if cor pulmonale	Trachea deviated towards side of resection	JVP raised with prominent 'a' and 'v' waves if cor pulmonale Tracheal tug and reduced cricosternal distance	Trachea deviated away from side of large effusion

SS: systemic sclerosis; RA: rheumatoid arthritis; SLE: systemic lupus erythematosus; COPD: chronic obstructive pulmonary disease; TB: tuberculosis; EAA: extrinsic allergic alveolitis

(continued)

Table 1.9 (*continued*)

Signs	ILD/fibrosis	Bronchiectasis	Pneumonectomy/lobectomy	COPD	Pleural effusion (see Integrative clinical assessment)
Chest appearance	No change	No change	Deformity or flattening of chest wall. Scars	Hyperexpanded	No change or scars from surgical treatment of malignancy
Expansion	May be bilaterally reduced	No change	Reduced on side of resection	Reduced	May be reduced on side of effusion
Percussion	No change	No change	Dull on side of resection	Hyperresonant with loss of cardiac and hepatic dullness	Stony dull over effusion
TVF/VR	No change	May be increased if areas of consolidation	Reduced on side of resection	Reduced	Absent over effusion, may be increased at top of effusion
Auscultation	Fine end-inspiratory crackles No change with coughing Basal: IPF, connective tissue disease, asbestosis, aspiration, drugs Apical: TB, radiation, sarcoidosis, EAA, ankylosing spondylitis, psoriasis, other pneumoconioses	Early to mid-inspiratory and expiratory crackles, clicks and squeaks. Change with coughing Can be wheeze of local obstructive disease or if associated with COPD	Reduced breath sounds on side of resection May be bronchial breathing over deviated bronchus	Reduced breath sounds and occasional expiratory wheeze	No breath sounds over effusion

Respiratory scenarios

1. Interstitial lung disease

2. Bronchiectasis

3. Lobectomy/pneumonectomy

4. Chronic obstructive
   pulmonary disease

5. Pleural effusion – lung
   cancer

SCENARIO 1. INTERSTITIAL LUNG DISEASE

Identifying physical signs

Functional status
The patient may be dyspnoeic, cyanosed and using oxygen. There may be facial plethora, a cushingoid appearance with striae, and bruising or a steroid card/necklace.

Hands
There may be clubbing and peripheral cyanosis, or signs of systemic disease associated with interstitial lung disease (ILD) such as rheumatoid arthritis, systemic sclerosis or dermatomyositis. An important negative finding may be the absence of tar stains. The patient may be wearing a steroid bracelet.

Neck/chest/periphery
Look for scars from lung biopsy or thoracotomy for single or double lung transplantation. There may be lymphadenopathy in sarcoidosis. The trachea is usually central. Assess for cor pulmonale from pulmonary hypertension, looking for 'a' and 'v' waves in the JVP, a displaced apex and left parasternal heave from RVH, and swelling of the ankles. There is symmetrically reduced chest expansion, bases are dull to percussion and there is reduced VR/TVF over the areas of fibrosis.

Auscultation
There are fine end-inspiratory crackles that are basal or apical depending on the underlying cause of the ILD. There may be associated squeaks. There is no change with coughing. There could be occasional wheeze if there is an obstructive element to disease, such as may be found in sarcoidosis. Listen for a split second heart sound and loud P2 indicating advanced disease with pulmonary hypertension.

Basal crackles: idiopathic pulmonary fibrosis (IPF), connective tissue disease (CTD), asbestosis, aspiration, drugs.

Apical crackles: tuberculosis (TB), radiation, sarcoidosis (mid-apical), extrinsic allergic alveolitis/hypersensitivity pneumonitis, ankylosing spondylitis and psoriasis (other rheumatological diseases cause basal disease), and pneumoconioses (except asbestosis).

Differential diagnosis

ILD may be idiopathic (idiopathic interstitial pneumonia (IIP)) or associated with another underlying disease process.

Known associations

- Rheumatological/connective tissue disease: rheumatoid arthritis, systemic sclerosis, SLE, ankylosing spondylitis, dermatomyositis
- Vasculitides such as polyarteritis nodosa (PAN), Churg–Strauss syndrome and granulomatosis with polyangiitis (Wegener's granulomatosis)
- Sarcoidosis
- Occupational pneumoconioses: coal-workers' lung, asbestosis, metal dusts including berylliosis, silicosis (associated with sand-blasting and quarrying, and a strong risk factor for TB) (coal-workers' lung can be simple or complicated/massive pulmonary fibrosis. Simple coal-workers' lung does not cause fibrosis. Caplan's syndrome is fibrosis associated with coal dust exposure and rheumatoid factor positivity)
- Hypersensitivity pneumonitis (extrinsic allergic alveolitis): bird-fanciers' lung, malt workers' lung, farmers' lung, bagassosis (work with molasses), wood-workers' lung and humidifier lung
- Medication/drugs: sulfasalazine, methotrexate, gold, amiodarone, ACE inhibitors, bleomycin, cyclophosphamide
- Radiation/radiotherapy
- Smoking

- Tuberculosis (this tends to cause asymmetrical fibrosis)
- Genetic: familial forms and HPS (Hermansky–Pudlak syndrome).

Idiopathic interstitial pneumonias

- IPF: this is the most common form of IIP (60%), occurs in the sixth to seventh decades, and is associated with radiological and histological changes known as usual interstitial pneumonia (UIP) (peripheral, subpleural, basal, reticular–nodular honeycomb changes more than the ground-glass changes seen with other IIPs). Although by definition it is idiopathic, it is associated with smoking, metal and wood dusts, hairdressing and gastro-oesophageal reflux disease (GORD). There is no medical therapy of proven benefit
- NSIP (non-specific interstitial pneumonia)
- COP (cryptogenic organising pneumonia or BOOP – bronchiolitis obliterans organising pneumonia)
- LIP (lymphocytic interstitial pneumonia)
- RB-ILD (respiratory bronchiolitis–interstitial lung disease)
- DIP (desquamative interstitial pneumonia)
- AIP (acute interstitial pneumonia, formerly known as Hamman–Rich syndrome).

Specific pathologies that are not IIP

- LAM (lymphangioleiomyomatosis – a rare disorder of smooth muscle proliferation around small airways)
- PAP (pulmonary alveolar proteinosis).

Clinical judgement

Causes

A thorough history should be taken for occupation, hobbies, other exposures, past and current medications, systemic disease or symptoms associated with undiagnosed systemic diseases and past or current smoking.

Investigations

In the first instance

- Blood tests: FBC, rheumatoid factor, anti-CCP (cyclic citrullinated peptide), ANA, ANCA, anti-GBM, CK, serum ACE (for sarcoidosis – but this is not sensitive or specific), precipitins
- Chest radiograph: reduced lung volumes, reticular nodular pattern of fibrosis, either midapical or basal depending on underlying cause. There might be bilateral hilar lymphadenopathy with sarcoidosis, joint changes with RA or a dilated oesophagus with systemic sclerosis
- Arterial blood gases (ABG): type 1 respiratory failure.

Key diagnostic/prognostic tests

- Pulmonary function tests: there is a restrictive pattern with forced expiratory volume in 1 second (FEV_1)/forced vital capacity (FVC) >0.8, reduced TLC and reduced gas transfer (K_{CO}). Sarcoidosis may show an obstructive pattern.
- Functional status can be measured with 6MWT (six-minute walking test looking at desaturation timings).
- High-resolution CT (HRCT): is essential for diagnosis and follow-up for pattern and extent of fibrosis.
- Bronchoalveolar lavage (BAL): lymphocyte-predominant washings are associated with better prognosis because these are steroid responsive. Also look for eosinophils and malignant cells.
- Lung biopsy: this can be transbronchial, VATS (video-assisted thoracic surgery) or open, and may be needed for diagnosis of specific IIP subtype.
- Echocardiography and right heart catheterisation may be requested if cor pulmonale is suspected.

Management

Treatment of any underlying disease

Patient education and modification of lifestyle risk factors, eg smoking cessation, avoidance of precipitants and certain medications. Patients should seek prompt medical attention if they have symptoms of respiratory infection or worsening breathlessness. Pulmonary rehabilitation exercises can increase cardiovascular fitness and help the patient manage symptoms of breathlessness.

Immunisation against pneumococcal disease and annual seasonal flu immunisation.

Corticosteroids (up to 6 weeks in first instance), possibly combined with steroid-sparing agents such as azathioprine, may be of benefit but this depends on underlying cause, stage of disease and subsequent response. There is no evidence that any specific treatment helps with symptoms or mortality in IPF.

Long-term oxygen therapy (LTOT) is started if the patient has low oxygen saturation at rest.

Clinical trial enrolment may be offered if appropriate.

Single/double lung transplantation may be of benefit if aged <65 years and in the context of severe disease.

Prognosis

This is very variable depending on the cause. Patients with sarcoidosis tend to make a full recovery and those with connective tissue disorders or more inflammatory lung changes can respond very well to steroids. IPF has a poorer prognosis with a median survival time of 2–3 years after diagnosis. There is an increased risk of bronchogenic carcinoma.

Maintaining patient welfare

Try to move the patient as little as possible because many will be dyspnoeic. Keep to a minimum the number of breaths performed on auscultation; you do NOT need to listen between each intercostal space to confirm your findings, and this could make the patient more breathless and make you appear unsure and unpractised. Patients may have joint pain from associated arthritis so remember to ask before palpation or movement.

Always cover the patient and wash your hands before turning to the examiner.

SCENARIO 2. BRONCHIECTASIS

Identifying physical signs

Functional status
The patient may be dyspnoeic, cyanosed, coughing (look for a sputum pot) and cachectic.

Hands
Look for clubbing, and yellow, thickened, curved nails (yellow-nail syndrome is very rare; if seen look for lymphoedema). Look for tar staining which may signify concomitant COPD.

Neck/chest/periphery
It may be possible to hear inspiratory 'clicks' from the end of the bed. Look for signs of cor pulmonale including shortness of breath (SOB) in advanced widespread disease. There may be lymphadenopathy if bronchiectasis is secondary to local obstruction from lung cancer, sarcoidosis or TB.

Auscultation
There are mixed coarse mid-end inspiratory and expiratory crackles. These can change with coughing. Occasionally there are clicks and there may be wheeze if there is an obstructive element. Up to a third of those with COPD will also have bronchiectactic changes. Assess location and extent of the disease. Is a single lobe affected or is it more widespread?

Signs of treatment
There may be a β-agonist-induced tremor or signs of surgical resection for severe localised disease.

Differential diagnosis

Venturing a plausible underlying cause of bronchiectasis distinguishes a candidate from the majority who will pick up the characteristic signs. Bronchiectasis describes dilatation of the airways resulting from proximal obstruction caused by one of the following.

Mechanical: obstruction secondary to congenital defects of large airways (including yellow-nail syndrome), bronchial malignancy, foreign body, traction fibrosis, or lymphadenopathy associated with cancer, sarcoidosis or TB.

Chemical: chronic gastric aspiration or inhalation of toxic chemicals and resultant hypersecretion with obstruction.

Recurrent childhood infection: TB, whooping cough, measles.

Chronic adult infection: TB, opportunistic mycobacteria, severe pneumonia. These may occur in the context of immunosuppression (HIV and hypogammaglobulinaemias).

Ciliary dyskinesias: Kartagener's syndrome (autosomal recessive condition with immotile cilia, upper respiratory infections, dextrocardia, situs inversus and azoospermia).

Cystic fibrosis (CF): an autosomal recessive condition producing thick secretions affecting upper and lower airways, endocrine and exocrine glands, and gastrointestinal system.

Autoimmune associations: rheumatoid arthritis, Sjögren's syndrome, IBD.

Hypersensitivity: allergic bronchopulmonary aspergillosis (ABPA) – this is caused by hypersensitivity to inhaled aspergillus antigen in a group of patients with asthma or cystic fibrosis, leading to an eosinophilic pneumonia. CT shows bronchiectasis of larger central airways and blood tests are positive for *Aspergillus*-specific IgE and IgG and eosinophils are raised.

Clinical judgement

Causes

Tell the examiners that you would seek a corroborative history of persistent productive cough or frequent lower respiratory tract infections, either recently or in adulthood. You would then ask targeted questions seeking associated features of the underlying diseases above. Questions would then focus on clarifying the patient's functional status.

Investigations

In the first instance

* Blood tests: ESR, CRP, serum ACE (sarcoidosis), HIV serology
* Immunology: aspergillus precipitins, skin tests, RAST, immunoglobulins, ANA and rheumatoid factor
* Sputum: MC&S including culture for mycobacterial disease
* Chest radiograph: ring shadows and tramlines.

Key diagnostic/prognostic tests

* HRCT: diagnosis is made by HRCT. Signet-ring sign – thickening and dilatation of bronchi and bronchioles, appearing thicker than their adjacent pulmonary artery. Localisation of disease can also be assessed and investigation for any obstructing lesion carried out.
* PFTs: there may be an obstructive or restrictive pattern. Reversibility suggests COPD.
* Ciliary function tests: if there is a history of symptoms since childhood and persistent URTIs including otitis media.
* Bronchoscopy and biopsy: this may be required for localised disease to exclude proximal disease and malignancy, or if HRCT suggests atypical mycobacterial infection.

* CF investigations: if aged <40 years, history of infertility, features of malabsorption (sweat chloride test and *CFTR* genotyping).

Management

Treatment of any underlying disease

Patient education and modification of lifestyle risk factors: smoking cessation, avoid exposure to precipitins in ABPA. Patients should seek prompt medical attention if they have symptoms of respiratory infection or worsening breathlessness. Pulmonary rehabilitation exercises can increase cardiovascular fitness and help the patient manage symptoms of breathlessness.

Immunisation against pneumococcal disease and annual seasonal influenza immunisation.

Physiotherapy will help with airway clearance techniques including postural drainage and active cycle breathing. There is some evidence supporting the use of nebulised physiological (0.9%) or hypertonic saline or β_2 agonists before airway clearance techniques. There is currently no evidence to support use of mucolytics such as recombinant human DNase.

Bronchodilators and anticholinergics for those with associated reversible airflow obstruction who have symptomatic improvement.

There is currently no evidence to support use of inhaled corticosteroids unless there is concomitant asthma.

Antibiotics for acute or chronic infective exacerbations: common infections are with *Streptococcus pneumoniae*, *Haemophilus influenzae*, *Staphylococcus aureus* (more common if ABPA or CF), *Pseudomonas aeruginosa* and *Burkholderia cepacia*. It is crucial to send sputum samples before starting antibiotic therapy. First-line empirical therapy is amoxicillin unless previous bacteriological results are available or there is allergy. Ciprofloxacin can be used in patients colonised with *Pseudomonas aeruginosa*. Long-term oral or nebulised antibiotics can be considered for patients with more than three exacerbations per year or in those with CF.

Burkholderia cepacia is resistant to many antiseptic cleaning agents and is usually treated with co-trimoxazole.

Surgical resection may be considered for those with localised disease not controlled by medical management. Bronchial artery embolisation may be required for massive haemoptysis.

LTOT is started if the patient has low oxygen saturations at rest.

Prognosis

Prognosis is very variable depending on the underlying cause and extent of lung disease. Average life expectancy has now increased to the sixth decade. Massive haemoptysis is a serious complication with high associated mortality.

Maintaining patient welfare

Always cover the patient or help him or her to dress and wash your hands before turning to the examiner.

SCENARIO 3. LOBECTOMY/PNEUMONECTOMY

Identifying physical signs

Functional status

These patients are usually not dyspnoeic or cyanosed unless there is underlying bronchiectasis.

Hands

There may be clubbing (malignancy, bronchiectasis, lung abscess or TB). Consider malignancy if there is evidence of smoking, eg tar stains. See above for signs of underlying diseases associated with bronchiectasis.

Neck/ chest/ periphery

There may be scars and associated flattening of the chest wall. Scars may be evident only when moving around to the back of the chest, so remember to ask the patient to lift the arms away from the chest when observing the anterior chest wall and ask him or her to lean forward to look at the back. The trachea and apex beat may be deviated towards the side with the thoracotomy, signifying mediastinal shift. If there has been a lower/middle lobectomy this deviation may be less obvious or not present. Look for reduced expansion on the side of the thoracotomy scar and try to assess if there has been an upper or lower lobectomy, or full pneumonectomy. Beware the case of a single lung transplant where there is a thoracotomy scar, but a normal respiratory examination on that side and possible lung disease changes still present on the contralateral side. There will be reduced percussion and TVF/VR on the side of the thoracotomy; again, try to assess if this is localised representing lobectomy, or if the entire hemithorax is involved with a pneumonectomy.

Auscultation

There will be reduced or missing breath sounds over the removed lobe or hemithorax in the case of a pneumonectomy. Occasionally you can hear bronchial breathing if you listen over a deviated bronchus. There may be abnormal breath sounds over any remaining lung that could give clues to the underlying disease and an indication for surgery.

Signs of treatment

There may be radiotherapy markings in patients who have undergone lobectomy for malignancy. Rib removal (thoracoplasty), previously performed for TB, results in deformity and flattening of the upper chest. This can mimic thoracotomy because the lobe underneath collapses and in the past polystyrene balls were inserted into the cavity to encourage this (plombage). Look for lymphadenopathy and clubbing. A supraclavicular scar from a phrenic nerve crush is easy to miss. This will cause a rise in the ipsilateral hemidiaphragm, resulting in reduced expansion, a dull percussion note and no breath sounds at the base.

Differential diagnosis

In most cases thoracotomy will have been performed for malignancy (non-small cell lung cancer), bronchiectasis, lung abscess or TB.

Malignancy

This is supported by the following findings

- Clubbing and nicotine staining
- Pancoast's syndrome with Horner's sign and wasting of the small muscles of the hand
- Superior vena caval obstruction (SVCO) or lymphadenopathy
- Signs of metastatic disease (jaundice, hepatomegaly, cachexia, etc).

Bronchiectasis

Thoracotomy is indicated for severe local disease or large or recurrent haemoptysis. Clubbing and coarse inspiratory crepitations on the contralateral side or signs of associated diseases (eg malabsorption in cystic fibrosis) may be found.

Lung abscess

These patients often have no other signs (assuming that the underlying infection has resolved), although clubbing may persist.

TB

It used to be common to perform upper lobe thoracotomy for apical disease. This is making a comeback with the emergence of extended drug-resistant (XDR) TB strains. Thoracoplasty and phrenic nerve crush also suggest previous TB.

Clinical judgement

Investigations and management will focus on determining whether the underlying disease indicating thoracotomy is now quiescent or recurrent.

A patient's exercise tolerance is decreased after pneumonectomy or lobectomy, but to a much lesser degree than the decline in lung function tests. The compensatory factors that allow relative preservation of exercise tolerance are unclear.

In the rare post-pneumonectomy syndrome, there is a dramatic mediastinal shift, which results in shortness of breath and dysphagia. This is usually corrected with insertion of silicon implants to correct the mediastinal position.

Maintaining patient welfare

- Always cover the patient and wash your hands before turning to the examiner.
- Patients with malignancy may be dyspnoeic, easily fatiguable or have bone pain, so move them gently and ask if they have pain before any palpation.

SCENARIO 4. CHRONIC OBSTRUCTIVE PULMONARY DISEASE

Identifying physical signs

Functional status
The patient may be dyspnoeic, using accessory respiratory muscles, have a prolonged expiratory phase, pursed lips, cyanosis and/or cachexia. Look around the bed for inhalers, oxygen cylinders and sputum pots.

Hands
Look for tar staining, a carbon dioxide retention flap, a bounding pulse and a β-agonist tremor. COPD alone will not give finger clubbing; if this is present consider lung cancer or bronchiectasis (30% of COPD sufferers have evidence of bronchiectasis on HRCT).

Neck/chest/periphery
A key sign is a hyperinflated chest with reduced chest expansion. There may be a tracheal tug and reduced cricosternal distance. There will be an increased respiratory rate, indrawing of the lower ribs, hyperresonant percussion with loss of cardiac and hepatic dullness, with an impalpable or weak apex beat. If there is pulmonary hypertension there may be a raised JVP, parasternal heave, loud P2 and ankle swelling.

Auscultation
There is usually wheeze and reduced breath sounds throughout. This may be more marked in the bases in α_1-antitrypsin deficiency.

Signs of treatment
Look for signs of steroid use with purpura, striae, cushingoid appearance, proximal myopathy and a steroid bracelet/necklace. There may be a thoracotomy scar if there has been lung volume reduction surgery (LVRS) or the small scars of chest drain insertion for pneumothorax.

Differential diagnosis

The main differential diagnoses for COPD are asthma, bronchiectasis, congestive cardiac failure and α_1-antitrypsin deficiency. As COPD and lung cancer share smoking as a strong common risk factor, it is prudent to state whether there is evidence of malignancy.

Asthma
In clinical practice, episodic obstruction is described in the history and is impossible to diagnose by examination alone. Asthma sufferers tend to be younger with a non-smoking history. It is uncommon to have a productive cough; breathlessness is highly variable and there is a diurnal pattern of symptoms with dry cough/wheeze/SOB worse at night and in the mornings. Peak-flow measurements show diurnal variation >20% and reversible airflow obstruction with >400 mL response to bronchodilators. Signs of atopy (eg eczema) may support the diagnosis of asthma.

Bronchiectasis
There is a productive cough with large volumes of sputum, clubbing, mid-end-inspiratory crackles and clicks with a varied distribution, and usually no chest hyperexpansion. Wheeze is less commonly present.

Lung cancer
There is cachexia, clubbing, cervical and supraclavicular lymphadenopathy, SVC and wheeze only where there is local obstructive disease from endobronchial lesions.

α_1-Antitrypsin deficiency
Prominent signs are seen at the bases with stigmata of liver cirrhosis. It classically presents in a younger person with rapidly progressive disease and a non-smoking history.

Clinical judgement

Candidates often forget to make an assessment of the severity of disease. This can be estimated without taking a full history. Approximate the patient's breathlessness during the examination to the Medical Research Council (MRC) dyspnoea scale

1. Not troubled by breathlessness except on strenuous exercise.
2. Short of breath when hurrying or walking up a slight hill.
3. Walks slower than contemporaries on level ground because of breathlessness, or has to stop for breath when walking at own pace.
4. Stops for breath after walking about 100 metres or after a few minutes on level ground.
5. Too breathless to leave the house, or breathless when dressing or undressing.

Investigations

There is no single diagnostic test; instead the diagnosis is based on a combination of history, physical examination and spirometry.

Consider the diagnosis if the patient is aged >35 years, with a risk factor. Patients are usually (ex-)smokers presenting with chronic cough, SOB on exertion, regular sputum production, and/or winter bronchitis episodes or wheeze.

Pulmonary function tests

A post-bronchodilator obstructive pattern with FEV_1/FVC <0.7 and FEV_1 <80% predicted for age, height and sex. If FEV_1 >80%, a diagnosis of mild COPD can still be made in the presence of typical symptoms. GOLD (Global Initiative for Chronic Obstructive Lung Disease) stages are a measure of airflow obstruction, but measures of disease severity take many other factors into account including disability and frequency of exacerbations

- GOLD 1: FEV_1 ⩾80%
- GOLD 2: FEV_1 50–79%
- GOLD 3: FEV_1 30–49%
- GOLD 4: FEV_1 <30%

Gas transfer tests typically reveal a reduced TL_{CO}.

Blood tests

High WCC/CRP/ESR in infective exacerbations (although neutrophilia may be due to steroids), polycythaemia in hypoxia, liver enzymes and α_1-antitrypsin levels if deficiency suspected.

ABGs

These are used for assessment of acute exacerbations and in stable disease for assessing the need for LTOT (see below).

Chest radiograph

The lung fields are hyperinflated with a flattened diaphragm, increased lucency in upper lobes (reversed in α_1-antitrypsin deficiency) and more than six anterior ribs visible above the diaphragm, and there is a lack of vascular markings towards the lung periphery. There may be signs of acute exacerbation with consolidation or pneumothorax.

ECG

This could show signs of cor pulmonale and right heart strain with right axis deviation, p pulmonale and right bundle-branch block (RBBB).

Echocardiography

In early disease this might show RVH and later dilatation with functional tricuspid regurgitation. Echocardiography can help differentiate if any left-sided heart failure is contributing to the clinical presentation.

HRCT

This is helpful in the diagnosis of suspected bullous disease or malignancy.

Sputum

MC&S is prudent before starting antibiotics in acute exacerbations in order to inform antimicrobial therapy.

Body mass index

Body mass index (BMI) can be a marker of severity of the disease and has prognostic value.

Management

Stable disease

Smoking cessation is the single most important intervention. At every opportunity, at every stage of disease, offer follow-up and nicotine replacement therapy.

Immunisation against pneumococcal disease and annual seasonal influenza immunisation.

Optimise inhaled therapy along NICE guidance 2010, www.nice.org.uk guidance/CG101.

NICE guidelines for optimised inhaled therapy

Step 1: (if breathlessness or exercise limitation)
SABA or SAMA
Step 2: (persistent breathlessness or exacerbations)
Continue SABA as needed and
FEV_1 >50%: LABA or LAMA
FEV_1 <50%: LABA + ICS (use combined preparation) or LAMA
Step 3: (still persistent breathlessness or exacerbations)
Continue SABA as needed and
'Triple therapy': LABA + ICS (combined prep) + LAMA
ICS, inhaled corticosteroid; LABA, long-acting β_2 agonist; LAMA, long-acting muscarinic antagonist; SABA, short-acting β_2 agonist; SAMA, short-acting muscarinic antagonist.

Mucolytic therapy can be initiated for a chronic productive cough but there is little evidence that it reduces frequency of exacerbations.

Candidates to be considered for **LTOT**

- FEV_1 <30% predicted
- Cyanosed

- Polycythaemia
- Peripheral oedema
- Raised JVP
- Oxygen saturations <92% in air when stable.

LTOT is indicated when two ABG measurements 2 weeks apart show

- PaO_2 <7.3 kPa OR
- PaO_2 <8 kPa with one of: secondary polycythaemia, nocturnal hypoxaemia (O_2 sats <90% for >30% time), peripheral oedema and/or pulmonary hypertension.

Those who fulfil these criteria will have improved survival with >20 h/day of LTOT given by nasal cannulae.

Surgery: can be considered for isolated large bullous disease, for lung volume reduction or transplantation in selected cases.

A **multidisciplinary approach** is essential. Refer to pulmonary rehabilitation, a combination of educational talks and exercises (for those who consider themselves functionally disabled and are usually MRC dyspnoea grade ⩾3). 'Breathe Easy' patient support programmes are available through the British Lung Foundation. Depression and anxiety are highly prevalent among patients with COPD so ask about associated symptoms.

Acute exacerbations

Provide controlled oxygen therapy at 24% with regular ABGs, monitoring for type 2 respiratory failure (PaO_2 <8 kPa and $PaCO_2$ >6 kPa).

Start empirical antibiotics if an infective exacerbation is suspected (mucopurulent sputum and/or febrile) according to local protocols.

Consider pneumothorax, left ventricular failure, pulmonary embolism, upper airway obstruction and pleural effusion as causes of exacerbation.

Provide nebulised therapy, including short-acting β_2 agonist and short-acting muscarinic antagonist.

Give 100 mg intravenous hydrocortisone and start 7–14 days of 30 mg oral prednisolone.

Consider intravenous theophylline if not improving with nebulised therapy (beware interaction with macrolide antibiotics).

Consider non-invasive ventilation (NIV) in the form of bilevel positive airway pressure (BiPAP) within the first 60 min of hospital arrival, when there is ongoing decompensated acute respiratory acidosis (pH <7.35 and $PaCO_2$ >6 kPa) despite maximal medical therapy.

Before NIV treatment starts there should be a clearly documented plan for what is to occur if NIV fails: what will be the ceiling of treatment and whether intubation and mechanical ventilation with admission to the ICU is planned.

Decisions for NIV are informed by the patient's pre-morbid state, severity of physiological disturbance, reversibility and prognosis of the acute episode, the presence of relative contraindications (eg impaired consciousness or facial trauma) and the patient's wishes where possible.

NIV can also be used outside the acute setting in chronic hypercapnic respiratory failure in selected patients.

Prognosis

COPD is the fifth leading cause of death in the UK and globally COPD is set to become the third leading cause of death by 2020, only behind ischaemic heart disease and stroke. In those requiring LTOT or nebulised therapy, the 5-year mortality rate is approximately 30%.

Maintaining patient welfare

- Try to move the patient as little as possible because many will be dyspnoeic, so examine the front and then the back of the chest only once.
- Try to keep to a minimum the number of breaths performed on auscultation.

Always cover the patient and wash your hands before turning to the examiner.

SCENARIO 5. PLEURAL EFFUSION – LUNG CANCER

See Station 5 (Integrated Clinical Assessment).

Identifying physical signs

Functional status
The patient may be dyspnoeic, coughing (look for a sputum pot) and cachectic.

Hands
Look for tar staining and clubbing. There may be swollen, tender wrists if there is hypertrophic pulmonary osteoarthropathy (HPOA). There may be wasting of the small muscles of the hand in Pancoast's tumour with axillary invasion.

Neck/chest/periphery
On closer inspection of the patient, starting with the face there may be signs of Horner's syndrome with apical Pancoast's tumour, giving rise to a ptosis, miosis and anhidrosis, and ipsilateral wasting of the small muscles of the hand. If this is suspected, go on to test sensation in the C8–T1 dermatomes. There could be signs of SVC obstruction with locally invasive disease, giving rise to facial oedema and plethora, and fixed engorged neck veins. Inspection of the chest might reveal scars of previous lobectomy or pneumonectomy, lung or pleural biopsy, or pleuradhesis. There may be tattoos and burns from previous radiotherapy. Examine for cervical and supraclavicular lymphadenopathy. The trachea could be displaced either away from a contralateral pleural effusion or towards an ipsilateral collapsed lung. Chest expansion may be reduced on the side of collapse or pleural effusion or previous lobectomy/pneumonectomy. The percussion note will be reduced over consolidation, pleural effusion, collapse or lobectomy. VF/TVR will be increased over any areas of consolidation.

Auscultation
There will be reduced breath sounds over areas of collapse, pleural effusion or lobectomy. There may be bronchial breathing above a pleural effusion.

Signs of treatment
Again look for scars or radiotherapy markings. Look for signs of steroid treatment with cushingoid facies, striae, bruising and MedicAlert bracelets/necklaces.

Signs of disseminated disease
If there is time, then show the examiner that you are looking for signs of disseminated disease with a cranial nerve examination, dermatomal examination in the arms, examining for hepatomegaly, feeling for bony tenderness along the spine and testing for cord compression signs in the legs.

Signs of paraneoplastic phenomena
Look for a dermatomyositis rash on the hands and face and acanthosis nigricans in the axillae, cerebellar signs, peripheral neuropathy and signs of Lambert–Eaton myasthenic syndrome in the cranial nerve and limb examinations, and examine male patients for gynaecomastia.

Finishing points
State that you would enquire about voice hoarseness (recurrent laryngeal nerve palsy from left-sided mediastinal masses) and dysphagia/odynophagia (from oesophageal compression).

Differential diagnosis

COPD
This could present with chronic cough and chest signs including pleural effusion complicating a pneumonia, but there would not be clubbing or cervical/supraclavicular lymphadenopathy and chest signs would tend to be symmetrical.

Remember that there could be both COPD and malignancy signs because they share the common risk factor of cigarette smoking.

Sarcoidosis

This may present with cough and weight loss and cervical/supraclavicular lymphadenopathy, but chest signs tend to be absent or symmetrical and there is no clubbing.

Bronchiectasis

This could present with clubbing and prolonged cough, with bilateral or localised chest signs, but would not usually present with lymphadenopathy and chest signs would tend to be more disseminated and with inspiratory/expiratory squeaks and clicks.

Pulmonary TB

This could present with prolonged cough, weight loss, clubbing and localised chest signs or pleural effusion and/or collapse. It may be difficult to differentiate on examination alone but there may be differentiating risk factors and more prominent fever symptoms in the history.

Clinical judgement

Types of lung cancer

- Lung cancer is broadly divided into two main groups: small-cell lung cancer (SCLC) and non-small-cell lung cancer (NSCLC). NSCLC accounts for approximately 85% of cases and SCLC for the remaining 15%.
- SCLC is an aggressive disease and typically two-thirds of cases have disseminated disease (to nodes, brain, bone, liver or adrenals) at time of diagnosis, so surgical resection is seldom appropriate. It is most commonly seen in older adults who are (ex-)smokers. It is sensitive to chemotherapy and radiotherapy. SCLC can produce several peptide hormones that give rise to various paraneoplastic syndromes.

NSCLC can be further divided into

- Adenocarcinoma: this accounts for 40% of all lung cancers and is the most common subtype in non-smokers, usually presenting with a peripheral lesion.
- Bronchoalveolar carcinoma: this is actually a subtype of adenocarcinoma. It can present with copious amounts of frothy sputum in advanced disease.
- Squamous cell carcinoma (SCC): this accounts for 30% of all lung cancers and in contrast to adenocarcinomas presents more centrally with cavitating lesions; it is the subtype most commonly associated with hypercalcaemia.
- Large cell carcinoma: this accounts for 5–10% of all lung cancers and typically presents as a large peripheral lesion.
- Risk factors for lung cancer include: smoking (most commonly associated with SCLC and squamous subtype of NSCLC), asbestos exposure (most commonly associated with malignant pleural mesothelioma), ionising radiation, radon gas exposure, vinyl chloride and chromium exposure.

Paraneoplastic syndromes

Lung cancer, particularly SCLC, is the most common malignancy causing paraneoplastic syndromes.

Neurological
- Peripheral neuropathy (see neurological examination)
- Subacute cerebellar degeneration (see neurological examination)
- Lambert–Eaton myasthenic syndrome (see neurological examination).

Endocrine
- SIADH (ectopic production of antidiuretic hormone causing hyponatraemia)
- ACTH (ectopic production of adrenocorticotrophic hormone causing Cushing syndrome)

- Hypercalcaemia (ectopic production of parathyroid hormone-related peptide (PTHrP), most commonly seen with SCC)
- Gynaecomastia (ectopic production of hCG).

Rheumatological
- Dermatomyositis/polymyositis (see Station 5 Integrated Clinical Assessment)
- Clubbing
- HPOA (with swelling of the distal ulnar and radius and classic radiographic changes).

Investigations
These are aimed at making the diagnosis and staging the disease so that treatment can be appropriately tailored.

- Blood tests: FBC (anaemia or low platelets), U&Es (hyponatraemia of SIADH), LFTs (liver metastases), bone profile (bone metastases or hypercalcaemia from PTHrP secretion), clotting if considering biopsy.
- Chest radiograph: this may show a central mass or coin lesion, hilar lymphadenopathy, pleural effusion or collapse.
- HRCT: with contrast and including chest, liver and adrenals. This can determine the location, size and spread of the primary tumour, and with SCLC will show whether there is extensive disease, which includes spread to the contralateral hemithorax.
- Sputum cytology: specificity is high (>90%) but sensitivity can be low. Most likely to yield a sample in centrally placed (eg SCLC) and shedding lesions (eg SCC).
- Pleural aspirate: a low-pH, low-glucose exudate, which can give cytological diagnosis in some cases.
- Brain CT/MRI: in certain groups it is appropriate to stage disease with brain imaging.
- Bronchoscopy: endobronchial lesions can be directly biopsied and bronchial washings, brushing and BAL obtained.

- Mediastinoscopy and VATS: these can be used to assess mediastinal and other intrathoracic lymph node status, respectively.
- Positron emission tomography (PET): complementary to CT, PET can further assess mediastinal disease and distant spread.
- Bone scan: not necessary if PET is available because the latter is more accurate, but should be requested where ALP is raised or if there is new bony pain.
- PFTs: these are necessary when considering surgical treatment to ensure adequate lung function where FEV_1 >1.2 L for lobectomy or FEV_1 >1.5 L for pneumonectomy.

Management
This is dependent on stage of disease at diagnosis. NSCLC uses the traditional TNM staging model, whereas SCLC is broadly divided into limited and extensive disease

- Surgical resection: this is first-line treatment for early stage NSCLC but is usually not suitable for SCLC that has usually disseminated by the time of diagnosis.
- Chemotherapy: cisplatin-based agents are the first-line treatment for limited SCLC. Chemotherapy can also be used as an adjunct pre- or post-surgery in NSCLC.
- Radiotherapy: this can be used as adjunctive or alternative treatment for both SCLC and NSCLC, and can be administered as external beam, including stereotactic delivery using CT-guided beams or internally with brachytherapy. Side effects include oesophagitis and pulmonary fibrosis.

Palliative and ongoing treatments
- Endobronchial treatments: these include photodynamic therapy, brachytherapy and laser ablation
- Palliative radiotherapy: used in symptom control for bone pain, haemoptysis, dysphagia and bronchial obstruction, and SVCO
- Analgesia: for local disease or bony pain

- Corticosteroids: to help increase appetite
- Mental health support: this can include the use of antidepressants or anxiolytics and psychological therapies
- Thoracocentesis with pleurodesis: for recurrent symptomatic malignant pleural effusions using graded talc or bleomycin.

Prognosis

- Prognosis is dependent on stage at diagnosis and ability to undergo standard treatments.
- For NSCLC 5-year survival rates range from 65% with stage IA to 25% with stage IIIA.
- For SCLC 5-year survival rates are approximately 20% for limited stage and 1–5% for extensive stage.

Maintaining patient welfare

- Try to move the patient as little as possible because many will be dyspnoeic, so examine the front then the back of the chest smoothly.
- Be gentle when moving the patient because there may be painful bony disease and weakness.
- Try to keep to a necessary minimum the number of breaths performed on auscultation.
- When first giving your differential diagnosis, use the term 'neoplastic disease'.
- Always cover the patient and wash your hands before turning to the examiner.

STATION 2

The History Station

1. Abnormal liver function tests

2. Alcohol dependence and abdominal pain

3. Abdominal pain

4. Chronic cough

5. Chest pain

6. Breathlessness

7. Falls

8. Diarrhoea

9. Hypertension

10. Back pain

11. Acute-onset headache

12. New headache of recent onset

13. Chronic/intermittent headache

14. Weak legs

15. Painful joints of the wrist and hand

16. The patient with HIV

HISTORY TAKING FOR PACES

Strategy for history taking in PACES

Before launching into the history make sure that you

- introduce yourself
- read out the details provided to the patient and confirm that these are correct.

Within PACES, limited time and the specific demands of the marking sheet mean that the strategy for history taking that should be adopted is very different from what you might find in a standard textbook on medical examination. The candidate who simply progresses through the usual stations of the history eliciting facts under each heading will often fail, irrespective of whether the recited history is accurate or the proffered differential diagnosis reasonable.

The key point is to build a final **problem list** and plan of action as you go along. There is an important intermediary 'processing' stage in doing this and arranging the information elicited under the following subheadings can be useful.

Volunteered problems (and important symptoms that the patient ignores) help you build a picture of the patient's own perception of the condition. At least once during the history-taking process you should directly explore the patient's viewpoint, eg 'What are your own thoughts about this?' or 'Is there something worrying you in particular?'. Patients will focus on the most troublesome symptoms, not the most diagnostically useful ones. However, failing to address these symptoms in your problem list – whether or not they are central to the condition – is invariably disastrous for the subsequent therapeutic relationship and is marked negatively.

Alarm symptoms are often elicited in the review of systems. The presence or absence of these has a major impact on the urgency of investigation and treatment. Some alarm symptoms are common to all conditions (eg weight loss), but it is imperative that once you have a differential diagnosis in mind (which can usually be quickly divined from the provided vignette) you should prepare a mental list of the 'emergencies' associated with those disease categories. For example

- The patient with cancer: symptoms of cord compression, hypercalcaemia, superior vena caval (SVC) obstruction, neutropenia
- The patient with heart disease: chest pain at rest, syncope, family history of sudden death
- The patient with liver disease: ascites, melaena, confusion, jaundice
- The patient with abdominal pain: weight loss, jaundice, family history of intra-abdominal malignancy
- The patient with back pain: loss of bladder or bowel control, leg weakness.

Disease interaction
Multiple pathology is common in the PACES history case. Examiners will be specifically assessing your ability to recognise interactions between new conditions and established ones, eg the patient with ascending weakness after a bout of diarrhoea may well require admission to a ward and daily forced vital capacity (FVC) monitoring, but a patient with the same symptoms and established chronic obstructive pulmonary disease (COPD) may require urgent admission to the intensive care unit (ICU) and plasma exchange to avert rapid respiratory failure.

Therapeutic successes and failures
Keep in mind the following questions once you have made a list of medications. Time does not necessarily allow questions about each medication. Focus on the important medications relevant to the presenting problems

- How effective is the medication/drug at alleviating the problem for which it was prescribed?
- How often does the patient actually take it (general compliance rates are often estimated to be less than 50%)?

- What are the side effects?
- What symptoms does the patient rightly or wrongly attribute to the drug?
- Which drugs are being taken unnecessarily for conditions that have resolved?

Similar questions can be applied to any previous therapeutic procedures.

Risks to others

You have a responsibility for the health of others besides the patient in front of you, eg if you suspect a condition that is known to be hereditary, it is crucial to identify which members of the family may be affected and should undergo screening.

Daily life and disease

The social and occupational history is often the crux of the story and a nod to the 'psychosocial' with one quick question about 'daily activities' is a short cut to failure at this station. It is poorly addressed problems in this territory (and not clinical misdiagnoses) that lead to most delayed discharges and readmissions, so they are rightly given high importance in the exam. The following list of key areas (six Ps) is a useful aide-memoir but it is not usually necessary to explore every area in detail – the history so far should give you an idea which areas to focus on

- **People**: marital status, other family members and their proximity, other dependants
- **Place**: accommodation type, numbers of stairs, ownership
- **Profession**: details of occupation, potential exposures/hazards, risk to themselves or others if their professional skills are impaired (eg drivers of large vehicles)
- **Pocket**: financial status and if it is threatened by the current illness
- **Public**: social services, disability allowance, unemployment benefits, home help, meals on wheels, district nurse, twilight nursing
- **Pleasure**: smoking (how many pack-years, previous attempts to stop), alcohol (see below), risk factors for sexual transmitted

infection (STI) (where appropriate), contacts who may need tracing, illicit drug use.

Concluding

Try to have a moment to summarise the history to the patient, thereby checking the details and jogging his or her memory for anything that may have been missed. Ask yourself why the examiners have chosen this case – there is likely to be at least one of the following

- Complex interaction of medical and social issues
- Alarm symptoms that have not been addressed
- Complex symptomatology that requires prioritised investigation
- Additional iatrogenic disease burden
- Implications beyond the patient (contact tracing, notifiable diseases, genetic testing for family members, etc).

If there are none of these it is likely that you have missed something. Identifying the likely diagnosis from a string of subtle cues is rarely the task at hand. If the history was not completed during the consultation do not panic; all one can do is take a structured history in a polite and competent manner and endeavour to use the time effectively.

Using this chapter

The history station is frequently neglected when candidates revise for PACES. One of the reasons for this is that many misguidedly feel their history-taking skills are already sufficient (as supposedly evidenced by the successful clerking of several thousand patients to date). The other frequently cited reason is that finding patients with appropriately challenging problems is much more time-consuming than finding patients with interesting physical signs.

However, it is just as useful (if not more useful) to practise in pairs with a revision partner. The following sections are specifically designed for this. Using the 'Differential diagnosis' and 'Clinical judgement and maintaining patient welfare' that follow, one revision partner can concoct an appropriately challenging scenario while the other has 14 minutes to take the history. Designing the history and acting as the patient gives you a useful insight into the viewpoint of the patient (often an actor in the real exam) and the examiner. Most importantly, generic history-taking skills (eg responding to subtle cues, summarising information gathered so far, using open and closed questions) are best improved and polished by watching other people do them both well and badly.

There are five components to the marking scheme in the history-taking section

1. Clinical communication skills.

2. Managing patients' concerns: these are covered in the flowchart before each section which suggests key areas of focus according to the presenting complaint, gives examples within key 'intermediate' categories of information that should be sought (eg alarm symptoms) and suggests a problem list and plan of action.

3. Differential diagnosis: this is covered in the left column of the table that follows each flowchart. Here, key features of a typical history that have high diagnostic utility are described.

4. Clinical judgement.

5. Maintaining patient welfare: this is covered in the right column of the tables after each flowchart. Here the key investigations and management plan salient to each differential diagnosis are described.

1. Verify the information provided
Check the provided information with the patient and then say: 'Tell me in your own words what the problem is.'

2. History of the presenting complaint (HPC)
Progress from open to closed questions, keeping in mind the **differential diagnosis** There is usually more than one problem. For each, pursue specific symptom characteristics that limit the diagnostic possibilities

3. Previous investigations and treatments for the same problem

4. Systems review (SR)

5. Past medical history (PMH)
What are the current follow-up arrangements?

6. Drug history (DH) and allergies

7. Family history (FH)

8. Social and occupational history (SH)
Cover any points that have been missed so far (see the six 'Ps' above)

9. Summarise
'Is there anything else we haven't discussed that you feel is important?'

10. Thank the patient

Overview: the history station

Volunteered problems
What does the patient's response to open questions reveal about the fears, expectations and beliefs surrounding the condition and how are these best addressed?

Alarm symptoms

Disease interaction:
How do new problems interact with established conditions?

Therapeutic successes and failures

Risks to others

Daily life and disease
What is the impact of disease on daily life? How will treatment and investigation impact further? What is the impact of lifestyle/occupation on the disease?

Final problem list and plan of action

1. Address patients' fears, expectations and understanding of their condition. What are the key symptoms causing most misery and how can they be dealt with?

2. Triage the urgency of further investigation and treatment (eg does the patient require admission?) and determine which sources of expertise need to be called upon

3. Devise a feasible plan for therapy and investigations that is consistent with the limitations of established co-morbidities

4. Anticipate potential problems for compliance with the treatment or investigation regimen

5. Consider the need to treat people other than the patient who might be at risk of disease

6. Outline the impact of the disease on the patient's life (and vice versa) and devise a strategy for improving the key areas

STATION 2

HISTORY-TAKING SCENARIOS

1. **Abnormal liver function tests**
- Gallstones
- Hepatitis A
- Hepatitis B
- Hepatitis C
- Epstein–Barr virus
- Primary biliary cirrhosis
- Drug-induced liver injury
- Autoimmune hepatitis
- Haemochromatosis
- Non-alcoholic steatohepatitis

2. **Alcohol dependence and abdominal pain**
- Pancreatitis
- Peptic ulcer disease
- Spontaneous bacterial peritonitis
- Hepatocellular carcinoma
- Alcohol-induced hepatitis

3. **Abdominal pain**
- Gastro-oesophageal reflux disease
- Peptic ulcer disease
- Gastric cancer
- Chronic pancreatitis
- Functional dyspepsia

4. **Chronic cough**
- Asthma
- Postnasal drip
- Sarcoid
- Drug side effect
- Gastro-oesophageal reflux disease (GORD)
- Lung cancer
- TB
- Bronchiectasis

5. **Chest pain**
- Unstable angina
- Stable angina
- Pulmonary embolism
- Pericarditis
- Pleurisy
- Oesophageal spasm

- GORD
- Costochondritis
- Anxiety

6. **Breathlessness**
- Congestive cardiac failure
- COPD
- Lung cancer
- Cryptogenic fibrosing alveolitis
- Recurrent pulmonary emboli

7. **Falls**
- Syncope
- Postural hypotension
- Epilepsy
- Vertebrobasilar ischaemia
- Parkinson's disease
- Myopathies

8. **Diarrhoea**
- Irritable bowel syndrome
- Inflammatory bowel disease
- Infective diarrhoea/small bowel overgrowth
- Lactose intolerance
- Bile salt malabsorption
- Coeliac disease
- Diverticulitis
- Chronic pancreatitis
- Carcinoid
- Colorectal cancer

9. **Hypertension**
- Essential hypertension
- Conn syndrome
- Cushing syndrome
- Phaeochromocytoma
- Renovascular hypertension
- Coarctation of the aorta

10. **Back pain**
- Bony metastases (without cord compression)
- Cord compression
- Osteoporotic vertebral fracture
- Mechanical lower back pain

11. Acute-onset headache
- Subarachnoid haemorrhage
- Haemorrhagic stroke
- Viral meningitis/encephalitis
- Bacterial meningitis
- Cryptococcal meningitis

12. New headache of recent onset
- Subdural haematoma
- Brain neoplasm (primary or secondary)
- Brain abscess
- TB meningitis
- Temporal arteritis

13. Chronic/intermittent headache
- Migraine
- Cluster headaches
- Trigeminal neuralgia
- Analgesia overuse headache
- Sinusitis

14. Weak legs
- Guillain–Barré syndrome
- Myopathy
- Multiple sclerosis/transverse myelitis

- Lambert–Eaton myasthenic syndrome
- Cord compression
- Familial hypokalaemic periodic paralysis
- Motor neuron disease

15. Painful joints of the wrist and hand
- Rheumatoid arthritis
- Systemic lupus erythemastosus (SLE)
- Osteoarthritis
- Crystal arthropathy

16. The patient with HIV
- Diarrhoea
- Weight loss
- Abdominal pain
- Headache
- Confusion
- Weak legs
- Jaundice/abnormal LFTs
- Breathlessness
- Skin rash/lesion
- Chest pain
- Arthralgia/myalgia
- Visual disturbance

SCENARIO 1. ABNORMAL LIVER FUNCTION TESTS

'A 40-year-old business woman, who drinks alcohol only occasionally, has been referred by the A&E officer for having abnormal LFTs. The woman was alert and oriented but did have some right upper quadrant (RUQ) tenderness. Her past medical history is unremarkable apart from an underactive thyroid. Please take a history.'

'This 50-year-old man has a strong family history of heart disease. He is obese and has a high LDL-cholesterol level. He also has hypertension. Since he was first seen by his new GP 3 months ago, his liver function tests (LFTs) have deteriorated. Please take a history.'

'I would be grateful for your further input regarding this 44-year-old man. He gives a 4-month history of worsening shortness of breath (SOB) and palpitations. He also complains of profound lethargy but attributes this to stress after his recent divorce. I had previously treated him for sexual dysfunction before the separation. On routine tests I found that he had a mildly raised ALT and slightly prolonged INR. Please advise.'

'A 50-year-old woman has been referred by her GP for pruritus. This seems to be resistant to standard treatment. The bilirubin, ALP and γ-GT are slightly raised but the other LFTs are normal. Please take a history.'

'Please would you see this 24-year-old woman who developed RUQ pain suddenly 4 days ago. The pain has now reduced significantly but on routine testing I note a raised ALP and γ-GT level. She thinks that she may have had a similar episode 6 months ago.'

'I would be grateful for your opinion on this 18-year-old young woman. She complains of extreme tiredness and low mood, and is worried about her performance in an imminent exam. On routine testing I noticed that her ALT and γ-GT were slightly raised.'

'This 40-year-old dentist has become jaundiced. She complains of general malaise only. She is concerned that this might be related to an extra-marital affair she had some 6 weeks ago. Please take a history.'

'I was about to start this 55-year-old obese man, who has a past history of ischaemic heart disease, on a statin. However, I note that his AST and γ-GT are slightly raised. I would be grateful for your advice.'

CLINICAL COMMUNICATION SKILLS AND MANAGING PATIENT'S CONCERNS

1. Verify the information provided: 'Tell me in your own words what the problem is.'

2. HPC
Open → closed questions bearing in mind the following **differential diagnoses**
Gallstones
Acute viral hepatitis
EBV
PBC
Autoimmune hepatitis
Drug induced
Non-alcoholic steatohepatitis (NASH)
Haemochromatosis

3. Previous investigations
Liver ultrasound? Upper GI endoscopy?

4. SR
Liver failure screen – jaundice, encephalopathy (eg daytime somnolence and night-time insomnia), bruising, melaena/haematemesis

5. PMH
Autoimmune disease (PBC, PSC, AIH)
DVT/PE (Budd–Chiari syndrome/portal vein thrombosis)
Blood transfusions (viral hepatitis)
Obesity, high cholesterol, hypertension, diabetes (NASH)

6. DH
Paracetamol (unintentional overdose?), herbal remedies, other common culprits (see below)

7. FH
Autoimmune disease? Gallstones?

8. SH
Travel history (HAV), sexual history (HAV, HBV, HCV), background alcohol consumption (may compound other pathologies)

9. 'Is there anything else we haven't discussed that you feel is important?'

Abnormal liver function tests

Volunteered problems

Alarm symptoms
Weight loss, any decompensation symptoms, previous malignancy

Disease interaction
Any ongoing illnesses that may interact unfavourably, eg HIV, established liver disease

Therapeutic successes and failures
If drug induced can the offending drug be safely stopped? Potential contraindications to antiviral therapy with IFN (eg depression, renal failure)

Risks to others
Are there any contact-tracing issues (explore these **sensitively**)?

Daily life and disease
eg restrictions on health professionals with HBV or HCV

Final problem list and plan of action

1. Address patient's anxiety about cirrhosis or cancer (many patients interpret jaundice as a harbinger of doom)

2. Triage urgency of investigation or treatment depending on the likely underlying condition and clinical correlates of liver function

3. Monitor for complications of cirrhosis in patients with established chronic liver disease (eg hepatoma and varices surveillance)

4. Arrange regular surveillance after or during treatment to assess response and pick up complications of therapy

5. Identify transplant candidates in end-stage or fulminant disease and refer early to a transplant centre for assessment

6. Contact tracing issues/screening of family members for viral hepatitis or genetic disorders

Differential diagnosis	Clinical judgement and maintaining patient welfare
Gallstones	
HPC Often asymptomatic Postprandial (30 min to 2 h) RUQ pain, rising to a crescendo then fading Transient dark stools and pale urine if stone passed through duct Ongoing epigastric or RUQ pain suggestive of pancreatitis or cholecystitis (Charcot's triad: RUQ pain, fever and jaundice) **PMH**: Saint's triad – peptic ulcer disease, diverticulitis and gallstones commonly occur together (this may just be a statistical phenomenon arising from three common conditions) **Risks**: obesity, hypercholesterolaemia, sickle cell disease (pigment stones), oral contraceptive pill, multiple pregnancies, rapid weight loss (eg after bariatric surgery) **FH**: one in four has a first-degree relative with gallstones	Management is determined by the presence or absence of stones in the duct and whether the LFTs are improving If there is no clear duct dilatation on transabdominal ultrasonography, leaping in with ERCP is increasingly unpopular even in the presence of obvious stones in the gallbladder (due to the approximately 4% risk of pancreatitis). Endoscopic ultrasonography and MRCP are the best means of visualising stones if transabdominal ultrasonography is normal while the LFTs remain obstructive If a stone in the duct is confirmed then ERCP is usually indicated. Rarely, a cholecystectomy and on-table duct clearance are performed Arrangements need to be made for routine cholecystectomy (usually within 3 months) after a successful stone removal at ERCP and sphincterotomy Warn the patient of the risk of recurrent pancreatitis/cholecystitis and to return if pain persists or if he or she develops a fever
Hepatitis A	
RUQ discomfort/generalised abdominal pain (40%) Elderly or very young patient Flu-like prodrome and/or diarrhoea is common Jaundice (80% – often noticed by partner rather than patient) Dark urine and pale stools Nausea, anorexia, vomiting, fever Rash affecting lower extremities Recent travel (2–6 weeks' incubation period) to an endemic area without immunisation **SH**: elderly patients in institutional care at greater risk, men who have sex with men (MSM), foreign travel, IVDU	Confirm diagnosis with appropriate investigations (eg hepatitis A IgM) Requires notification to the CDSC (Communicable Disease Surveillance Centre) Can usually be managed as outpatient Other causes of an acute hepatitis must be excluded (eg HBV, HEV, autoimmune hepatitis) Very elderly people often require considerable supportive medical care Fulminant hepatitis A is very rare but INR should be monitored in the unwell patient until the LFTs have repeatedly improved Symptoms and infection can relapse in very elderly people – close follow-up is necessary to pick this up

(*continued*)

Differential diagnosis	Clinical judgement and maintaining patient welfare
Hepatitis B	
The patient may present during acute or chronic infection Acute infection • Jaundice, fatigue, anorexia, nausea and vomiting • An arthritis/dermatitis prodrome is seen in a third of cases of acute infection Fulminant acute infection is characterised by encephalopathy (night-time insomnia progressing to confusion and coma) Chronic active hepatitis (± cirrhosis): similar symptoms to the acute phase but less marked Screen for symptoms of decompensated liver disease or portal hypertension: encephalopathy, melaena, ascites Risk factors for hepatitis B: IVDU, MSM, ethnic origin, occupational hazards Extrahepatic manifestations: eg symptoms of nephrotic syndrome, polyarteritis nodosa, cryoglobulinaemia. These conditions often manifest as oedema, palpable purpura, weakness and arthralgias **DH**: may have had previous IFN-α therapy that failed to induce seroconversion Older drugs (adefovir, lamivudine) should be switched to newer drugs with a lower likelihood of resistance (tenofovir, entecavir) **SH**: ongoing risks of infecting others. Occupational history (eg doctor, dentist, nurse)	Need to confirm stage of disease (acute versus chronic). Of acutely infected patients (positive anti-HBc IgM) 90% will develop surface antibodies within a year and require no further treatment or surveillance Follow up to check for HBsAg-negative HBsAb-positive status required For chronic active hepatitis: refer to a hepatologist for treatment. The aim is to suppress viral replication and reduce the risk of cirrhosis or hepatocellular carcinoma (HCC) Fulminant hepatitis needs to be managed in a specialist liver unit A high level of suspicion is required to pick up extrahepatic syndromes There may be contact tracing issues – family members (vertical transmission) and sexual contacts Routine screening for HIV advisable

(*continued*)

Differential diagnosis	Clinical judgement and maintaining patient welfare
Hepatitis C	
Acute infection is usually asymptomatic May present with symptoms of chronic decompensated liver disease (see above) Risk factors are key (IVDU, high-risk sexual practice, first-degree relatives, tattoos, blood products pre-1985 or abroad) Previous episodes of jaundice **PMH**: HIV co-infection? Previous psychiatric history (can complicate IFN-α therapy) **DH**: previous IFN-α and ribavarin therapy for known HCV **SH**: sexual contacts and family members tested? Careful occupational history. Ongoing IVDU? Ongoing alcohol abuse/dependence?	Need to genotype virus (hepatitis C), and refer to hepatology to determine optimal timing for treatment New drugs are available (telaprevir, boceprevir) which achieve high response rates in patients who have previously failed IFN-α/ribavarin therapy, so re-refer previous non-responders Manage decompensated liver disease/HCC if present. This precludes IFN-α/therapy, as does ongoing alcohol abuse/dependence Contact tracing sexual contacts/screening of first-degree relatives Assess likely compliance with further investigation and treatment. Refer to hepatology for consideration of new IFN-α-free therapies Exclude contraindications to IFN-α antiviral therapy Patients with HIV co-infection progress to cirrhosis more rapidly and often need input from tertiary HIV/hepatology centres Routine screening for HIV is recommended There are high rates of mood disorders and depression among HCV patients. These need to be treated and followed up
Epstein–Barr virus (EBV)	
Prolonged lethargy and malaise Sore throat Raised lymph nodes Low-grade fever, anorexia **SH**: may recall close contact with person with pharyngitis	IgM monospot to confirm acute infection Monitor LFTs – these are disrupted in most cases to some degree and may take many months to resolve (especially γ-GT) May need long period of time off work due to profound lethargy Beware rare complications: splenic rupture, meningoencephalitis, chronic fatigue syndrome Supportive management as an outpatient is usually sufficient

(*continued*)

Differential diagnosis	Clinical judgement and maintaining patient welfare
Primary biliary cirrhosis	
Long indolent history of lethargy (65%), pruritus (55%), RUQ pain (20%) Jaundice (often disproportionate to other indicators of chronic liver disease) **PMH**: hypercholesterolaemia, other autoimmune disease	Confirm diagnosis with an anti-mitochondrial antibody test. If positive, liver biopsy is usually unnecessary and liver disease can be staged clinically Exclude other autoimmune causes of symptoms (eg hypothyroidism) Asses the implications of profound lethargy for patient's career, family and social life Treatment is with ursodeoxycholic acid Pruritus is often extreme and difficult to control. It also leads to insomnia and depression. There are documented cases of suicide attributed to this symptom alone Treat hypercholesterolaemia if present Regular follow-up and surveillance for HCC if cirrhosis is established
Drug-induced liver injury	
See Table 2.1 Has the patient used alternative/herbal remedies and does he or she still have them? Illicit drug use	Stop offending agent and monitor LFTs. A rising INR requires immediate discussion with a liver transplant unit Exclude background liver disease of alternative aetiology Determine alternative treatments for original problem, eg anti-tuberculous therapy, immunosuppression for transplantation There are frequently medicolegal issues surrounding iatrogenic injury
Autoimmune hepatitis	
AIH can present as an acute hepatitis (RUQ pain, anorexia, lethargy) or chronic decompensated liver disease (see above) **PMH**: other autoimmune disease; especially Sjögren's syndrome, SLE, autoimmune thyroid disease	Confirm the diagnosis/exclude other causes Liver biopsy nearly always indicated when the ANA is positive and no other cause is obvious Refer to hepatology for treatment (steroids and a steroid-sparing agent) AIH may interact unfavourably with other autoimmune disease (eg hypothyroidism) Consider bone protection for extended steroid therapy

(*continued*)

Differential diagnosis	Clinical judgement and maintaining patient welfare
Haemochromatosis	
Patients may present with manifestations of arthritis, cardiomyopathy, diabetes and/or chronic liver disease The most common symptoms are • Profound lethargy • Arthralgia • Impotence/reduced sex drive/amenorrhoea Arthritis: painful second and third MCP joints are characteristic Cardiomyopathy: younger patients, palpitations, increasing SOB on exertion, ankle oedema, syncope Diabetes (50%): poluyria, polydipsia, weight loss, chance finding of glycosuria Chronic liver disease (see above). Rates of HCC are high in haemochromatosis	Diagnosis requires confirmation of *HFE* mutations after assessment of transferrin saturation (>55%). Ferritin is usually >1000 ng/mL A multidisciplinary approach is crucial (endocrinology, hepatology, rheumatology, cardiology) Regular surveillance (ultrasonography and AFP every 6–12 months) is needed for HCC in patients with established cirrhosis Compliance with twice-weekly venesection is often problematic (especially in needle-phobic patients) All first-degree relatives must be screened Alcohol cessation advice and support may be necessary
Non-alcoholic steatohepatitis (NASH)	
Abnormal LFTs are often a chance finding on routine blood tests **PMH**: obesity, diabetes, hypertension, dyslipidaemia **SH**: concomitant alcohol excess is common	Need to exclude other causes of liver disease (may rarely require biopsy) The general strategy is aggressive treatment of causative co-morbidity while monitoring the LFT response Often associated with hypertension, hypercholesterolaemia and insulin insensitivity/diabetes, all of which usually pose a greater threat to morbidity and mortality than the associated liver dysfunction Dietician referral is often useful There is 10% progression to cirrhosis – those who do not improve with modification of risk factors or develop signs of chronic liver disease may require a staging biopsy

Table 2.1 Drug-induced hepatitis: common culprits

Acute necrosis	Chronic injury and fibrosis	Acute cholestasis	Chronic cholestasis	Veno-occlusive disease	Autoimmune hepatitis
Isoniazid		Contraceptives			Sulfonamides
Rifampicin					
Amiodarone		Co-amoxiclav			Nitrofurantoin
Methotrexate		Macrolides	Co-trimoxazole		Methyldopa
Valproate		Cimetidine	Carbamazepine		
Halothane		Hydralazine			
Paracetamol		Allopurinol			
Ketoconazole		Quinolones			

SCENARIO 2. ALCOHOL DEPENDENCE AND ABDOMINAL PAIN

'This 35-year-old man drinks half a bottle of whisky a day. He presented to my clinic with a 24-hour history of severe central abdominal pain. This is similar to an episode he experienced a year ago. Since then he has lost at least 5 kg in weight. His pain is barely controlled with co-codamol and I am concerned that he may have an ulcer. I would be grateful if you would admit him for an endoscopy.'

'This 55-year-old woman with established alcoholic liver disease has been complaining of increased abdominal girth despite the diuretics I prescribed recently. Over the last 24 hours she has had fevers and feels generally unwell. I would be grateful if you could see her and advise about further management.

'This 40-year-old man was previously a heavy drinker but has been dry for 6 months. Despite that he now presents with increasing abdominal distension and right upper quadrant discomfort. He looks emaciated and says he is off his food. Please take a history.'

'This 38-year-old lorry driver had an endoscopy last year which revealed a severe gastritis. His pain improved on a proton-pump inhibitor (PPI) but has now returned. He also tells me that he passed black stools 1 week ago. I would be grateful for your advice about his further investigation.'

This 35-year-old woman, recently divorced, visited my clinic 3 weeks ago feeling generally unwell. She complains of profound lethargy during the day and being unable to sleep at night. She also describes vague RUQ discomfort and today she appears jaundiced. Please take a history.'

CLINICAL COMMUNICATION SKILLS AND MANAGING PATIENT'S CONCERNS

1. Verify the information provided
'Tell me in your own words what the problem is.'

2. HPC
Open to closed questions keeping in mind the following **differential diagnosis**
Pancreatitis
Peptic ulcer disease
Spontaneous bacterial peritonitis
Hepatocellular carcinoma
Acute hepatitis

3. Previous investigations
Varices surveillance (OGD), HCC surveillance (ultrasonography), CT of the abdomen (pancreatitis)

4. SR
Decompensation screen: ascites, encephalopathy (eg altered sleep–wake cycle), bruising, melaena/haematemesis, fever

5. PMH
Withdrawal seizures/syndrome
Neurological sequelae (stroke, Wernicke's syndrome, etc)
Cardiomyopathy
Pancreatitis, peptic ulcer disease
Coping strategy for other chronic illness, eg depression

6. DH
Multivitamins
Acamprosate?
Propranolol for varices prophylaxis?

7. FH:
Children with fetal alcohol syndrome?

8. SH
Impartial exploration of quantity of alcohol consumption. CAGE questionnaire for alcohol dependence. Impact of alcoholism on work/relationships/financial status

9. Summarise
'Is there anything else we haven't discussed that you feel is important?'

10. Thank the patient

Alcohol dependence and abdominal pain

Volunteered problems

Alarm symptoms
Weight loss, any symptoms of decompensation, previous malignancy

Disease interaction
Impact of acute illness on other alcohol-related pathologies and further detriment to social circumstances and chances of cessation

Therapeutic successes and failures
Interactions with alcohol, eg warfarin, antiepileptics, benzodiazepines.
Compliance with prescribed therapy

Risks to others
Is the patient violent or continuing to drive?

Daily life and disease
Is the patient drinking and driving? What are his or her occupational prospects? Sympathetic employer? Homeless? Vulnerable to abuse or risk to other dependants?

Final problem list and plan of action

1. Need to assess severity of disease and triage level of care (eg most complications of alcoholic liver disease are potentially life threatening).

2. Is the patient likely to comply with further investigation and treatment?

3. Need to screen for alcohol-related damage to other organs

4. Alcohol abuse has massive socioeconomic impact – are others at risk (eg does the DVLA need to be informed?)

5. Encourage referral to alcohol cessation services (Alcoholics Anonymous, community drugs and alcohol team) after resolution of acute episode

Differential diagnosis	Clinical judgement and maintaining patient welfare
Pancreatitis	
Severe central abdominal pain Nausea Fever Loose, pale stools Recent alcohol binge **PMH**: alcoholic liver disease/cardiomyopathy/neuropathy **DH**: opiate use for recurrent episodes of pancreatitis **Note this may be non-alcohol related, eg gallstone pancreatitis**	CT is the best diagnostic modality Glasgow criteria staging for acute pancreatitis to triage level of care Risk of opiate addiction in chronic pancreatitis Possible pancreatic insufficiency – diabetes? malabsorption? Fasting glucose and faecal elastase/faecal fat estimation are useful adjunctive tests Chronic pain and alcoholism usually interact unfavourably Prophylactic treatment for alcohol withdrawal (reducing dose of chlordiazepoxide) unless encephalopathic
Peptic ulcer disease	
Postprandial gnawing epigastric pain radiating through to back Duodenal ulcer: hunger pains before eating Nausea and vomiting (stricture and outlet obstruction) Anorexia, weight loss Melaena, haematemesis Recent alcohol binge **PMH**: established cirrhosis **DH**: NSAIDs, steroids (recent alcoholic hepatitis?)	The patient may have other risk factors besides alcohol that need to be addressed, eg NSAIDs/*Helicobacter pylori*? Recent stress or surgery? In patients with alcohol problems who present with a GI bleed for the first time, a variceal source must be suspected until proven otherwise Triage urgency/necessity of upper GI endoscopy. Exclude perforation Lifelong PPI may be necessary, especially if alcohol cessation is unlikely *H. pylori* infection rates higher among those with alcohol problems so test and eradicate if positive
Spontaneous bacterial peritonitis	
A third of cases asymptomatic Abdominal distension, generalised pain, fevers Worsening confusion/drowsiness **PMH**: established chronic liver disease **DH**: diuretics	An urgent ascetic tap is needed in all patients with ascites and chronic liver disease. Antibiotic treatment while awaiting results Exclude and treat encephalopathy/hepatorenal syndrome/varices Nutritional status often poor and requires support Antibiotic prophylaxis on discharge Is the patient a liver transplant candidate?

(*continued*)

Differential diagnosis	Clinical judgement and maintaining patient welfare
Hepatocellular carcinoma (HCC)	
Weight loss, malaise, RUQ pain, newly decompensated liver disease (abdominal distension, symptoms of encephalopathy, etc) Ascites often develops quickly due to portal vein thrombosis on top of cirrhosis **PMH**: higher rates of HCC	Stage liver disease to determine whether liver transplantation or resection is necessary/feasible Multidisciplinary approach (hepatobiliary surgeon, interventional radiologist, oncologist, hepatologist) Tumour markers Avoid biopsy if candidate for transplantation Exclude and treat encephalopathy/hepatorenal syndrome/varices
Alcohol-induced hepatitis	
RUQ pain, recent binge OR recent cessation (withdrawal hepatitis) Evidence of decompensation: jaundice, bruising, encephalopathy (eg nocturnal insomnia)	Exclude other concurrent causes of liver disease Exclude and treat encephalopathy/hepatorenal syndrome/varices Long-term HCC and varices surveillance crucial Surveillance for varices with OGD once recovered Condition carries a high mortality rate (50% at 6 months) – should be managed by hepatology team. Steroids and pentoxyphylline may be appropriate

For all diagnoses: consider financial status, ability to work/drive and likelihood of alcohol/IVDU cessation, and encourage self-referral to AA or community drugs and alcohol team.

The important features of an alcohol consumption history

An impartial approach is crucial (any hint of judgement will provoke a dishonest answer) eg 'Lots of people drink more than the recommended amount without it affecting their day-to-day life. Do you drink more than is recommended?'

How much and what type (spirits, wine, beer)?

If she is drinking much more than the recommended limit ask the following

Where, when and with whom?
How does it affect your

- Domestic life: relationship, friends, home and children
- Work life: recent redundancies, drinking at work

- Financial situation: jobs, mortgages, etc.

Other questions
- Precipitating factors: relationship, work?
- Binge drinking?
- Has he or she sought help before?
- Violence or trouble with the police?

CAGE questionnaire

An affirmative reply to **two or more** of these four questions has a high sensitivity and specificity for alcohol dependence syndrome

1. Have you tried to **c**ut down the amount you drink?
2. Do you get **a**ngry if people tell you that you drink too much?
3. Do you feel **g**uilty about how much you drink?
4. Do you ever drink in the mornings (**e**ye opener)?

C – cut down
A – angry
G – guilty
E – eye opener

SCENARIO 3: ABDOMINAL PAIN

'This 55-year-old male car salesman has recently been made redundant. He has been suffering from epigastric pain for the last few months that has not responded to antacids. Please advise.'

'This 34-year-old woman has persistent heartburn despite using a PPI for many weeks. A recent endoscopy revealed mild oesophagitis. She is keen to explore surgical options for her problem but I thought referral to your clinic to ensure that we had maximised medical therapy would be prudent.'

'This 74-year-old man has just been diagnosed with a microcytic anaemia. He has also lost weight over the past 4 months. Please take a history.'

'This 40-year-old woman is now on Oramorph to control her recurrent abdominal pain. A recent upper GI endoscopy was normal. I would be grateful for your further advice.'

'This 18-year-old young man has had a lot of time off work recently due to recurrent abdominal pain. This is only partially relieved by a PPI. He has noticed his symptoms are much worse when at work. Please take a history.'

CLINICAL COMMUNICATION SKILLS AND MANAGING PATIENT'S CONCERNS

1. Verify the information provided
'Tell me in your own words what the problem is.'

2. HPC
Progress from open to closed questions keeping in mind the **differential diagnosis**
GORD
Peptic ulcer
Gastric cancer
Pancreatitis
Functional dyspepsia

3. Previous investigations
Cardiac investigations?
Previous therapeutic trial of PPI/H_2-receptor antagonist?

4. SR
SOB (anaemia)? Depression/anxiety?

5. PMH
Cardiac disease, liver disease, pancreatitis. Functional (non-ulcer) dyspepsia has higher proportion of psychological co-morbidity

6. DH
NSAIDs, bisphosphonates, aspirin, clopidogrel
Previous PPIs/H_2-receptor antagonists

7. FH
Gastric cancer, peptic ulcer disease

8. SH
Alcohol consumption in units, smoking in pack-years. Recent stress?

9. Summarise
'Is there anything else we haven't discussed that you feel is important?'

10. Thank the patient

Abdominal pain

Volunteered problems
Alarm symptoms

Weight loss, GI bleeding, jaundice, dysphagia,

Disease interaction:
There may be an organic problem (eg gastritis) exacerbating a functional problem (eg postprandial distress syndrome)

Therapeutic successes and failures
Is the pain relieved by a PPI?
Side effects: gynaecomastia, diarrhoea, interactions (CYP450 induction by some PPIs)
Is aspirin really needed or can an alternative anti-platelet be used?

Risks to others

Daily life and disease
What is the impact of disease on daily life? How will treatment and investigation impact further? What is the impact of lifestyle/occupation on the disease?

Final problem list and plan of action

1. Beware interminable over-investigation of patients with functional disorders

2. Malnutrition and undernutrition need to be corrected – a dietician's opinion is often very useful

3. Patient may be very reluctant to undergo invasive endoscopic investigations

4. Referral to a surgeon may be appropriate if there is gastric outlet obstruction/cancer/ treatment-resistant GORD

5. Patients may not be willing to take a medication lifelong, even if effective

6. Diet and lifestyle factors often need to be addressed to prevent recurrent disease

Differential diagnosis	Clinical judgement and maintaining patient welfare
Gastro-oesophageal reflux disease (GORD)	
Retrosternal burning pain Dysphagia Odynophagia Associated epigastric pain Waterbrash Regurgitation of food Acid in the back of throat Often worse at night lying flat Exacerbated by: large meals, tight belt, stooping over, fruit juice, spicy food, chocolate, caffeine, smoking **PMH**: diabetes (gastroparesis), co-morbidity precluding laparoscopic fundoplication **DH**: PPI (effective?), motility agents (eg domperidone)	Need to establish the efficacy of current therapy and whether all basic advice is being followed (tilt bed towards feet slightly, eat evening meal early, avoid tight clothing, avoid alcohol and spicy food, etc) Those with symptoms despite a PPI (or with new unexplained onset aged >55) should have an upper GI endoscopy Use of pH manometry is helpful to confirm reflux after a normal OGD (non-erosive reflux disease) and/or before referral for laparoscopic fundoplication Patients may have well-controlled symptoms with a PPI but do not like the idea of lifelong medication and would prefer to have surgery. They need to be aware of the failure rate (15%) and complications (eg oesophageal stenosis and dysphagia in 5%) of surgery
Peptic ulcer disease	
Postprandial, gnawing, epigastric pain radiating through to back Duodenal ulcer: hunger pains before eating Nausea and vomiting (stricture and outlet obstruction) Anorexia, weight loss Melaena, haematemesis Recent alcohol binge **PMH**: established cirrhosis, previous ulcer disease **DH**: NSAIDS, steroids (recent alcoholic hepatitis?)	Identify and treat causative factors: NSAIDs, *Helicobacter pylori* infection, alcohol, steroids Triage urgency/necessity of upper GI endoscopy. Exclude perforation if unwell Need follow-up endoscopy to confirm healing of *gastric* ulcers only Non-healing ulcers need to be biopsied. Benign non-healing ulcers and pain despite a PPI raise the possibility of Zollinger–Ellison syndrome
Gastric cancer	
Constant abdominal pain Weight loss Nausea and vomiting (there may be gastric outlet obstruction) Anorexia Ethnic origin (very high incidence in Far East) **PMH**: previous gastric surgery (higher incidence of cancer). Known *H. pylori* infection **FH**: people with blood group A have a higher incidence	Urgent endoscopy required if cancer suspected A multidisciplinary approach to staging and treatment. CT of the chest/abdomen/pelvis, endoscopic ultrasonography Post-gastrectomy vitamin B_{12} replacement Consider co-morbidity and fitness for surgery Regular surveillance for recurrence

(*continued*)

Differential diagnosis	Clinical judgement and maintaining patient welfare
Chronic pancreatitis	
Relapsing–remitting severe central abdominal pain Weight loss, fatty stools Fat-soluble vitamin deficiency: vitamins A, D, E and K **PMH**: post-ERCP, known gallstones, recent mumps, EBV, pancreatic cancer, osteoporosis, fractures **DH**: azathioprine, steroids, sulfonamides, methyldopa **SH**: alcohol consumption	Investigate and treat aetiology Nutritional status and support (eg enzyme supplements) Malabsorption and vitamin deficiency screen Alcohol dependence and screening for other alcohol-related disease Opioid dependence is common. In chronic severe pain, input from a chronic pain specialist is useful. Consider coeliac plexus ablation in resistant cases
Functional dyspepsia	
Rome III criteria for functional dyspepsia At least 3 months, with onset at least 6 months previously, of one or more of the following • Bothersome postprandial fullness • Early satiation • Epigastric pain • Epigastric burning • No evidence of structural disease (including at upper endoscopy) that is likely to explain the symptoms Exacerbation of symptoms with stress and anxiety is common **PMH**: depression and anxiety more common	Difficult to distinguish from FAPS (functional abdominal pain syndrome), which is not a primary dysmotility problem but an abnormal neuropsychological response to normal visceral stimuli Patients often require repeated reassurance that their symptoms do not result from serious pathology Spasmolytics, dietary modification, low-dose antidepressants and hypnotherapy are acknowledged treatment modalities

Clinical guideline (NICE 2004)

Which patients with dyspepsia should be referred for endoscopy?

- Symptoms despite cessation of provoking factors (alcohol, NSAIDs, steroids, bisphosphonates, nitrates, calcium antagonists)
- Unintentional weight loss*
- GI bleeding*
- Iron deficiency anaemia*
- Dysphagia*
- Persistent vomiting*
- Epigastric mass*
- Suspicious barium meal result*
- Patients aged >55 with persistent symptoms with no obvious cause*

*Warrants urgent endoscopy

If endoscopy is not indicated, patients should be screened for *H. pylori* (a 2-week washout period off PPIs is required before breath tests) and treated if positive.

If *H. pylori* test is negative or treatment does not relieve symptoms, a therapeutic trial of a PPI can be tried, starting at the higher dose for 1 month then stepping down to the lowest dose that controls symptoms. Unsuccessful treatment or weaning off a PPI warrants referral to a gastroenterologist (who will almost always arrange an endoscopy).

SCENARIO 4. CHRONIC COUGH

'This 24-year-old woman is troubled by a persistent cough, worse at night. She says it always seems to be a problem during the summer months. Please take a history.'

'This 30-year-old painter and decorator has been increasingly wheezy. His usual inhalers do not control his symptoms. I would be grateful for your further assessment.'

'This 60-year-old man is normally fit and well. He complains of paroxysmal coughing fits that can come on at anytime. He is an ex-smoker and his past history is unremarkable apart from hypertension.'

'This 50-year-old woman with a 5-year history of asthma now complains of a chronic cough with occasional haemoptysis. Her asthma is becoming increasingly difficult to control. Please take a history.'

'I recently saw this 70-year-old retired builder when he attended my clinic with his wife (who was consulting for anxiety and insomnia). It emerged that he has had a nocturnal cough for the last 4 months which is keeping his wife awake at night. Furthermore, he has lost 4 kg in weight over that period which, although he seems unconcerned, is causing his wife considerable anxiety. I would be grateful for your further assessment of the man's problem.'

'This 35-year-old ex-intravenous drug user works in a shelter for homeless people. Over the last 2 weeks he has been troubled by a persistent productive cough and night sweats. Please take a history.'

'This 40-year-old woman recently returned home after visiting relatives in Jamaica. She feels that she caught a chest infection abroad but a course of antibiotics has not improved her symptoms. She has a persistent cough and complains of general malaise and anorexia. In the last few days she has noticed a painful skin rash over her legs. Please take a history.'

CLINICAL COMMUNICATION SKILLS AND MANAGING PATIENT'S CONCERNS

1. Verify the information provided
'Tell me in your own words what the problem is.'

2. HPC
Open to closed questions keeping in mind the **differential diagnosis**
Asthma
Postnasal drip
Sarcoid
Drugs
GORD
Lung cancer
TB
Bronchiectasis

3. Previous investigations
Chest radiograph? Bronchoscopy? Nasal endoscopy?

4. SR
GORD symptoms

5. PMH
Childhood asthma, atopy, nasal polyps, sinus problems, previous TB, recurrent pneumonias

6. DH
NSAIDs (as precipitant of asthma), ACE inhibitors (chronic cough)
Current inhaler regimen if known to have asthma
Any known allergies?

7. FH
Asthma, atopy, lung cancer, TB exposure

8. SH
Smoking history in pack-years, working conditions (recent dust/paint/solvent exposure), living conditions (damp, decorating work), pets, asbestos exposure, travel to TB endemic areas. Financial status. HIV risks (TB co-infection)

9. Summarise
'Is there anything else we haven't discussed that you feel is important?'

10. Thank the patient

Chronic cough

Volunteered problems

Alarm symptoms
Weight loss, haemoptysis, night sweats, progressive SOB, chest pain

Disease interaction
eg GORD exacerbating asthma, steroid therapy in established osteoporosis

Therapeutic successes and failures
Has condition improved with inhalers/steroids?
Did symptoms coincide with a change in medication?
How is the patient's inhaler technique?

Risks to others
TB exposure risk to close contacts

Daily life and disease
Does the patient require a change in occupation or accommodation?
Are there legal/ compensation issues?

Final problem list and plan of action

1. Patient anxiety about cancer is common irrespective of the most likely underlying diagnosis

2. Triage urgency of further investigation and treatment

3. Exclude and treat non-respiratory conditions that may be exacerbating symptoms

4. Encourage compliance with maintenance therapy when well

5. Check inhaler technique

6. Infection control issues and their enforcement

7. Help with smoking cessation

8. Occupational lung disease and employment/financial/ compensation issues

Differential diagnosis	Clinical judgement and maintaining patient welfare
Asthma	
Wheeze, cough and nasal congestion (polyps) are classic symptoms Identify triggers: animal dander, dust, cold, exercise, pollutants, infection, emotion Duration, severity and frequency of attacks Green sputum? Reduced exercise tolerance? Previous skin testing? **PMH**: previous ICU admission, atopy, nasal polyps **FH**: atopy or asthma **SH**: smoking, occupational exposure to precipitants (eg sawdust, animal dander, solvents), living conditions and recent refurbishment, pets. Time off work/school	Examination to assess severity (eg peak flow) and triage urgency of further investigation and management Current inhaler technique adequate? Current inhaler regimen may be inadequate – need to step up therapy Repeat courses of steroids – has bone density been checked? Working conditions may be exacerbating symptoms and a change of profession may be inevitable. What is the financial situation and what can the doctor do to assist (eg letters to employers for change of role at work)? Compliance with treatment between attacks is a major issue. Specialist nurses have time to reinforce patient education Patients with brittle asthma should be included on an at-risk register to ensure rapid assessment and treatment in primary and secondary care
Postnasal drip	
Unpleasant taste in mouth Nocturnal cough Nasal congestion Headache common (associated sinusitis) **PMH**: atopy, asthma **DH**: symptoms usually improve with topical steroids	Need to exclude chronic sinusitis (CT of the sinuses indicated?) ENT referral may be necessary May need to exclude a more sinister cause of cough
Sarcoid	
Fever, anorexia and arthralgias SOB on exertion Persistent cough **SR** Cardiac: cardiomyopathy, heart block, neurological – lymphocytic meningitis, cranial nerve palsies Skin: erythema nodosum, lupus pernio Eye: uveitis FH: African–Caribbean or Scandinavian origin (Löfgren's syndrome)	Diagnosis: serum ACE, CT of the chest, bronchoscopy and transbronchial biopsy Assess severity: pulmonary function tests, transfer factor (DLCO) A multidisciplinary approach is frequently needed to identify and treat all involved systems Patient may require simple monitoring or aggressive steroid therapy

(*continued*)

Differential diagnosis	Clinical judgement and maintaining patient welfare
Drug side effect	
ACE inhibitors	All antagonists may reduce cough, or choose alternative antihypertensive
GORD	
Retrosternal burning pain Dysphagia Odynophagia Associated epigastric pain Waterbrash Regurgitation of food Acid in the back of throat Cough worse at night or lying flat for extended periods Exacerbated by: large meals, tight belt, stooping over, fruit juice, spicy food, chocolate, caffeine, smoking **PMH**: diabetes (gastoparesis), co-morbidity precluding laparoscopic fundoplication **DH**: cough may improve with PPI	Poorly controlled asthma exacerbated by GORD may warrant laparoscopic fundoplication even if the oesophagitis or heartburn is minimal A normal OGD does not exclude asthma exacerbation by 'microdroplet' aspiration; pH manometry may be more useful Inhaled/oral steroid use for asthma may cause oesophageal candidiasis and symptoms of GORD
Lung cancer	
Local disease: cough, haemoptysis, non-resolving chest infection **Metastatic**: weight loss, anorexia, headache (most common cancer leading to brain metastases), behavioural change, SVC obstruction, recurrent laryngeal nerve palsy **Paraneoplastic** (Lambert–Eaton myasthenic syndrome) weakness, hypercalcaemia, DVT/PE **SH**: smoking history, occupational asbestos exposure	Multidisciplinary approach: oncology (clinical and medical), cardiothoracic surgeons, histopathology, respiratory physician, neurosurgeon Staging disease: staging CT of the brain/chest/abdomen. PET scan. Bronchoscopy or CT-guided biopsy. Endoscopic ultrasound for hilar lymphadenopathy Does the patient qualify for compensation for asbestos exposure? Financial status and time off work for investigations/treatment Patient expectations may differ wildly from the likely prognosis

(*continued*)

Differential diagnosis	Clinical judgement and maintaining patient welfare
TB	
Symptoms often non-specific Fever, anorexia, weight loss, haemoptysis, night sweats **Risks**: potential exposure to TB, recent travel to TB endemic area, ethnic origin **PMH**: HIV/AIDS **DH**: immunosuppressant therapy for another condition?	Need to screen for HIV co-infection Isolation and infection control. Screening/prophylaxis of close contacts – implications for work and family life Stigma affects acceptance of diagnosis and compliance with investigations (often invasive) and long-term therapy. The patient's family may not always be supportive due to perceived risk of infection Screen for other organ involvement, eg abdominal TB, bone marrow infiltration, TB meningitis Monitor for adverse effects of anti-tubercular medications (see section below table) Nutritional status may be poor and require correction Reduced efficacy of the oral contraceptive pill on rifampicin – recommend barrier contraception
Bronchiectasis	
Productive cough, SOB, wheeze, haemoptysis, weight loss Causes (anything that obstructs mucociliary clearance) **Young's syndrome** (mild variant of cystic fibrosis presenting in middle-aged men) **Cystic fibrosis** **Primary ciliary dyskinesia** **Allergic bronchopulmonary aspergillosis** (asthmatic prodrome) **HIV-related lung disease (chronic infection)** **Inhaled foreign objects**	Diagnosis: chest radiograph and CT of the chest Investigate and treat the underlying cause if treatable Most causes are chronic progressive conditions that have major implications for the patient's future HIV and contact tracing, treatment, etc

Common adverse reactions to anti-TB medications

Isoniazid: raised liver enzymes (20%), acute hepatitis approximately 2%, peripheral neuritis, seizures, drug-induced lupus.

Rifampicin: hepatitis, reduced efficacy of CYP450-metabolised drugs, orange discoloration of body fluids.

Ethambutol: optic neuritis, gout, rash, peripheral neuritis.

Pyrazinamide: gout, hepatitis.

Streptomycin: ototoxicity (audiovestibular disturbance), nephrotoxicity.

SCENARIO 5. CHEST PAIN

'Please would you see this 49-year-old man who has recently been complaining of chest pain when walking upstairs? His examination reveals a blood pressure of 140/96. Many thanks.'

'This 24-year-old, 30-week pregnant woman has been experiencing sharp chest pains for the last 48 hours. Please take a history.'

'I would be grateful for your opinion regarding the further investigation of this 28-year-old professional footballer. He has been complaining of severe chest pain after a recent match. He also describes a flu-like illness 2 days previously.'

'This 62-year-old woman responded well to a course of antibiotics for a recent chest infection. However, she now complains of severe right-sided chest pains. Please take a history.'

'This 50-year-old man continues to suffer from angina despite a recent successful coronary by-pass operation. This is usually postprandial and associated with low-grade nausea. Please take a history.'

'I would be grateful for your opinion about this 30-year-old woman who complains of palpitations and chest pains which are worse at night. A recent ECG, 24-hour tape and exercise tolerance test were reported as normal.'

CLINICAL COMMUNICATION SKILLS AND MANAGING PATIENT'S CONCERNS

1. Verify the information provided
'Tell me in your own words what the problem is.'

2. HPC
Open to closed questions keeping in mind the **differential diagnosis**
Unstable/stable angina
Myocardial infarction
Pulmonary embolism
Pericarditis
Pleurisy
Oesophageal spasm
GORD
Costochondritis
Anxiety

3. Previous investigations:
Chest radiograph?
ECG?
Exercise tolerance test (ETT)?
Coronary angiogram?

4. SR
Risk factors for coronary disease
Associated SOB, nausea, palpitations, headache

5. PMH
Known ischaemic heart disease (IHD), CVA, diabetes, dyslipidaemia, hypertension, autoimmune disease, DVT/PE

6. DH
Contraindications to anti-platelet therapy/thrombolysis/β blockers/heparin/ACE inhibitors
Current therapy for IHD, hypercholesterolaemia, hypertension

7. FH
Premature IHD

8. SH
Smoking history in pack-years, limitation of work by pain, recent travel (DVT/PE), Canadian Cardiovascular Society status, stress

9. Summarise
'Is there anything else we haven't discussed that you feel is important?'

10. Thank the patient

Chest pain

Volunteered problems

Alarm symptoms
Chest pain at rest/minimal exertion, crescendo symptoms

Disease interaction
Is there more than one cause or more than one type of chest pain?

Therapeutic successes and failures
Has the condition improved with medications?
Did symptoms coincide with a change in medication?
Side effects (eg β blockers and impotence)

Risks to others
Familial dyslipidaemia?

Daily life and disease
What is the impact of symptoms on daily tasks and vice versa?
Are stress and anxiety exacerbating symptoms or resulting from them?

Final problem list and plan of action

1. Triage urgency of further investigation and treatment

2. Identify the best means of investigation (eg ETT or myocardial perfusion scan for suspected angina, endoscopy or pH manometry for suspected reflux disease)

3. Consider long-term secondary prevention and likely compliance, eg treatment of hypercholesterolaemia, hypertension, smoking cessation, exercise, weight loss

4. Compliance with investigations and treatment (especially primary or secondary prevention)

5. 'Atypical' chest pain syndromes and abnormal disease behaviour may require clinical psychology input

Differential diagnosis	Clinical judgement and maintaining patient welfare
Unstable angina	
Cardiac pain at rest or minimal exertion Typical or atypical (atypical more common in elderly people and women) Associated SOB/nausea Prevalence of other features (GUARANTEE study 1996 [1]) ● Hypertension about 60% ● Previous angina about 60% ● Hypercholesterolaemia about 40% ● Family history of CAD about 40% ● Previous MI about 40% ● Previous angioplasty about 25% ● Previous CABG about 25% ● Diabetes mellitus about 25% ● Current smoker about 25% ● Previous CVA about 9%	Urgent risk stratification, eg ECG and troponin to collate a TIMI score (see below) ETT or myocardial perfusion scan to further risk stratify Contraindications to ETT Anti-platelet, antihypertensives, statins, β blockers and other secondary prevention medications Consider DVLA rules and driving after an MI Debilitating chest pain may impair ability to work and impact on other areas of life
Stable angina	
Exercise tolerance before onset of pain Pain not affected by respiration or position Crescendo angina (falling exercise tolerance, increasing frequency of attacks) Pain abates with rest Risk factors for cardiac disease	Assess current antianginal therapy and potential for escalation Repeat risk stratification if not done previously Impact on working and social life Side effects of medications (depression, impotence, etc) Anti-platelet, antihypertensives, statins, β blockers and other secondary prevention medications
Pulmonary embolism	
PIOPED study ● SOB (about 70%) ● Pleuritic chest pain (66%) ● Cough (about 33%) ● Haemoptysis (about 10%) ● Swollen calf/known DVT ● Risk factors for DVT (previous DVT/PE, hypercoagulable states, immobility, malignancy, smoking, OCP, pregnancy)	Urgent investigation and therapy if needed Ventilation–perfusion scan versus CTPA Investigations and treatment in pregnancy (ventilation–perfusion scan > CTPA) Long-term anticoagulation and potential contraindications (eg falls) and risks

(*continued*)

Differential diagnosis	Clinical judgement and maintaining patient welfare
Pericarditis	
Chest pain • Severe ('devil's grip') • Worse on lying flat, deep inspiration and swallowing Fever/flu-like prodrome SOB is common **PMH**: autoimmune disease, TB, renal failure, known malignancy	Exclusion of acute MI and other causes of pain Investigations to identify cause (see below) and implications for long-term treatment and risk of constrictive pericarditis
Pleurisy	
Chest pain on inspiration Fever SOB **PMH**: TB, recent/recurrent chest infection, known autoimmune disease, eg rheumatoid arthritis	Exclusion of PE Coxsackie virus B infection: are other family members affected? (Intrafamiliar spread of echoviruses and Coxsackie virus is common) NSAIDs unless contraindicated Need to provide adequate analgesia Time off work Postviral fatigue syndrome
Oesophageal spasm	
Chest pain (80%) Dysphagia (50%) Heartburn (20%) Globus and regurgitation are common	Need for pH manometry Diffuse oesophageal spasm (random contractions) vs nutcracker oesophagus (coordinated spasm of excessive amplitude) Treatment (eg Botox injection, PPI, calcium channel antagonists) Exclusion of cardiac pain
GORD	
See above	Exclusion of concomitant cardiac pain if cardiac risk factors are prominent

(*continued*)

Differential diagnosis	Clinical judgement and maintaining patient welfare
Costochondritis	
Insidious onset Movement-related, deep inspiration Recent activity at unaccustomed level of exertion **PMH**: osteoarthritis elsewhere, inflammatory arthropathy, chest deformity (eg pectus excavatum)	Exclusion of PE/angina Address patient anxiety about heart/lung disease
Anxiety	
Palpitations, diaphoresis, sense of impending doom, SOB, dizziness, paraesthesiae History of depression/post-traumatic stress disorder/ other anxiety disorder	Exclusion of underlying organic disorder Identification of precipitant factors Need for psychiatric review and likely compliance

The TIMI score

The thrombolysis in myocardial infarction (TIMI) score predicts adverse outcomes in non-ST-segment elevation MI (NSTEMI) and correlates well with the degree of coronary artery stenosis.

Each of the following scores 1 point (Table 2.2)

- Aged ⩾65 years
- Use of aspirin in the last 7 days
- Known coronary stenosis of ⩾50%
- ST deviation on ECG >0.5 mm
- Severe anginal symptoms (two or more anginal events in the last 24 h)
- At least three risk factors for coronary disease
- Elevated serum cardiac markers (eg troponin I).

Clinical assessment of angina

The Canadian Cardiovascular Society grading scale for classification of angina

- Class I: angina only during strenuous or prolonged physical activity

Table 2.2 TIMI scores and risk of death from ischaemic heart disease (IHD)

Score event	Risk of death from IHD (%)
0–1	4.7
2	8.3
3	13.2
4	19.9
5	26.2
6–7	40.9

- Class II: slight limitation, with angina only during vigorous physical activity
- Class III: symptoms with everyday living activities, ie moderate limitation
- Class IV: inability to perform any activity without angina or angina at rest, ie severe limitation.

'Please see this 60 year old who has been complaining of nocturnal cough and breathlessness for the past 4 months. It is becoming increasingly debilitating these last few days such that he can no longer get about the house. Many thanks.'

'This 75-year-old man with a history of ischaemic heart disease has been increasingly breathless over the last 2 weeks. Please take a history.'

'This 50-year-old woman complains of worsening shortness of breath on exertion. This seems to improve then worsen again. Her past medical history is unremarkable apart from three miscarriages in her 20s. Please take a history.'

'This 45-year-old man has worsening shortness of breath. This is now impeding his ability to work as a postman. I would be grateful for your further advice.'

CLINICAL COMMUNICATION SKILLS AND MANAGING PATIENT'S CONCERNS

1. Verify the information provided
'Tell me in your own words what the problem is.'

2. HPC
Open to closed questions keeping in mind the **differential diagnosis**
Congestive cardiac failure (CCF)
COPD
Lung cancer and effusion
Cryptogenic fibrosing alveolitis
Recurrent pulmonary emboli
Asthma (see above)

3. Previous investigations
Echocardiogram, coronary angiogram, lung function tests, CT of the chest

4. SR
Reactive depression very common in CCF

5. PMH
Known heart or lung disease
Rheumatic fever
DVT/PE
Number of previous admissions to hospital with exacerbations

6. DH
ACE inhibitors, β blockers, diuretics
Drugs causing fibrosis, eg amiodarone, nitrofurantoin
Home oxygen

7. FH
α_1-Antitrypsin deficiency
Looking after a sick relative?

8. SH
Occupational exposure to agents causing fibrotic lung disease, alcohol and dilated cardiomyopathy, smoking in pack-years, NYHA grade and specific limitations on hobbies, family life, ability to travel, etc

9. Summarise
'Is there anything else we haven't discussed that you feel is important?'

10. Thank the patient

Breathlessness

Volunteered problems

Alarm symptoms
Syncope or chest pain
Haemoptysis
Weight loss

Disease interaction
eg COPD and CCF commonly occur together

Therapeutic successes and failures
Symptoms despite maximal medical therapy, treatment limited by side effects, compliance with secondary prevention (eg inhaled steroids)

Risks to others
Oxygen at home and continued smoking

Daily life and disease
What is the impact of symptoms on daily tasks and vice versa? Is stress and anxiety exacerbating symptoms or resulting from them?

Final problem list and plan of action

1. Triage urgency for further investigation and treatment

2. Assess likelihood of compliance with investigations and treatment

3. What is the degree of disability and need for additional help at home?

4. Optimise medical therapy and investigate potential complications (eg steroids and osteoporosis)

5. Ongoing smoker despite need for home oxygen?

6. Offer help with smoking cessation

7. End-of-life decisions in patients with end-stage disease – set an appropriate ceiling of therapy

Differential diagnosis	Clinical judgement and maintaining patient welfare
Congestive cardiac failure	
SOB at rest or on exertion Paroxysmal nocturnal dyspnoea Orthopnoea Peripheral oedema Nocturia Confusion, lethargy Establish NYHA status **PMH**: IHD, hypertension, alcohol, valvular disease **DH**: diuretics, β blockers, ACE inhibitors	Failing independence at home requiring additional support with activities of daily living (ADL) Inadequate/over-medication Medications that may exacerbate heart failure (eg β blockers, rosiglitazone) Possible reversible coronary insufficiency not investigated Reactive depression is common and often overlooked On maximal therapy but deteriorating – are palliative care measures warranted? Heart transplant candidate?
COPD	
SOB on minimal exertion > than 3 consecutive months for >3 years Wheeze Previous lung function tests? Consultation with a respiratory physician? **PMH**: previous hospitalisations and weight loss with anorexia imply a poorer prognosis **DH**: on home oxygen? Nebulisers? **SH**: usually >20 pack-years smoking. Occupational lung disease	Further investigations to stage disease and identify cause Adequacy of current treatment Occupational lung disease and compensation Adequacy of current social support services Contraindications to home oxygen (eg ongoing smoker) Are the nebulisers helping? They may encourage patient to struggle on at home and present to hospital in a much worse state Exclude coexistent CCF or cor pulmonale
Lung cancer	
See Scenario 4	See Scenario 4
Cryptogenic fibrosing alveolitis (CFA)	
Insidious onset of SOB Flu-like symptoms and arthralgia common Wheeze and fever unusual Weight loss common **PMH**: chronic microaspiration from GORD may be implicated in some cases **SH**: smoking and occupational exposure to wood and metal dust slightly more common in CFA	Need to exclude other known causes of interstitial lung disease (eg drugs, occupational exposure) High-resolution CT of the chest and transbronchial biopsy usually necessary Progressive condition – need to assess stage and plan long-term support

(*continued*)

Differential diagnosis	Clinical judgement and maintaining patient welfare
Recurrent pulmonary emboli	
May have no documented previous PEs (all subclinical) Risk factors for DVT (previous DVT/PE, hypercoagulable states, immobility, malignancy, smoking, OCP, pregnancy) **PMH**: known prothrombotic disorder (anti-thrombin III deficiency, protein C/S deficiency, factor V Leiden mutation, anti-phospholipid syndrome)	May require cardiac catheterisation to determine pulmonary artery pressures if pulmonary hypertension suspected Risk of paradoxical embolism (history of stroke?) Anticoagulation and its contraindications Management of pulmonary hypertension (diuretics, prostaglandins, endothelin antagonists, home oxygen therapy)

SCENARIO 7: FALLS

'Please see this 69-year-old woman, who has had three falls. Apart from feeling a little more tired than normal over the last few months she has been well. I could find no injury and her examination is normal except for a pulse of 46 beats/min.'

'You are referred a 28-year-old right-handed woman by the accident and emergency STI. She attended today having had an episode of loss of consciousness 2 days ago. The mother feels that she has not recovered completely as her daughter is not herself. She has a headache that has been present for the preceding 2 weeks.'

'This 78-year-old man is struggling to cope at home. His warden tells me that he is increasingly slow and hesitant on his feet and he has had two falls in the past month. I would be grateful for your further assessment.'

'This 66-year-old woman with rheumatoid arthritis had a blackout at the hairdressers. An ambulance was called but she felt fine when it arrived and was not keen to go to hospital (she is the main carer for her husband).'

'This 60-year-old woman has been finding it increasingly difficult to get around the house. She had a fall when climbing the stairs 2 days ago. Please take a history.'

'This 50-year-old man with longstanding diabetes and hypertension (well controlled on medication) complains of periodic dizziness. Please take a history.'

CLINICAL COMMUNICATION SKILLS AND MANAGING PATIENT'S CONCERNS

1. Verify the information provided
'Tell me in your own words what the problem is.'

2. HPC
Open to closed questions keeping in mind the **differential diagnosis**, eg
Loss of consciousness (LOC)
Syncope
Postural hypotension
Epilepsy
Vertebrobasilar ischaemia
No LOC
Parkinson's disease
Myopathies

3. Previous investigations
24-hour tape? Carotid Doppler scans? CT/MRI of the head? EEG? Echocardiogram?

4. SR
Memory loss, ankle swelling, hypothyroid symptoms, tremor

5. PMH
Hypertension, hyperlipidaemia
Epilepsy
Rheumatic fever as a child
Previous fractures
Known movement disorder

6. DH
Sedatives, antiarrhythmic, β blockers, antihypertensives, ACE inhibitors

7. FH
Cardiac risk factors?

8. SH
Layout of house, support at home, support from outside immediate family, driving, alcohol, isolation, depression social responsibility (caring for others). Smoker? Driver?

9. Summarise
'Is there anything else we haven't discussed that you feel is important?'

10. Thank the patient

Falls (with or without loss of consciousness)

Volunteered problems
Is the patient's insight intact?

Alarm symptoms
LOC rather than loss of postural tone, exertional syncope, family history of sudden death, serious injury following fall, socially isolated, injured, unclear/no collateral history (unable to triage risk)

Disease interaction
eg osteoporosis and aortic valve stenosis – is there adequate secondary prevention of hip fracture?

Therapeutic successes and failures
Iatrogenic hypotension/sedation/arrhythmias/long QT

Risks to others
Continuing to drive after a syncopal event?

Daily life and disease
Loss of confidence and independence very common after injurious falls

---

Final problem list and plan of action

1. Triage urgency of further investigations and treatment

2. Inpatient vs outpatient investigation depending on risk of injury

3. Early involvement of occupational therapist and physiotherapist

4. Preserved insight into dangers of further collapse?

5. Level of risk of injury given social/home/occupational circumstances

6. A spell in a rehabilitation centre may be warranted

7. Need to improve social support – is the patient amenable to this?

8. Dependants may also need additional support while the patient is incapacitated

Differential diagnosis	Clinical judgement and maintaining patient welfare
Loss of consciousness	
Syncope	
Dysrhythmias Palpitations before or after fall Previous pacemaker and recent checks Family history of sudden death **Structural heart disease** (eg aortic stenosis) Exertional syncope Rheumatic fever as child Previous valve disease Cardiomyopathy/CCF	24-hour tape has low sensitivity: is the patient suitable for an implantable Holter loop recorder? Assess need for urgent pacing/pacemaker Are antiarrhythmics optimised? Risk assessment of further injury Get collateral history/witness Address loss of confidence after the fall and rehabilitation with an early physiotherapy regimen Syncope is a harbinger of rapid deterioration and the need for surgery in aortic valve disease On an ACE inhibitor with aortic valve disease?
Postural hypotension	
Fall after standing Altered vision before fall Recent change in medications (eg antihypertensives) Other autonomic disturbance, eg micturition syncope or associated diseases (eg diabetes, Parkinson's or Alzheimer's disease) Cognitive impairment	Need for autonomic testing if a cause cannot be found and symptoms are severe Exclusion of metabolic causes (eg Addison's disease) Triage between inpatient and outpatient investigation and treatment (frequency of falls more important than severity of injury) Associated cognitive impairment and its further investigation and management

(*continued*)

Differential diagnosis	Clinical judgement and maintaining patient welfare
Epilepsy	
Pre-seizure 'aura' Post-ictal confusion or weakness (Todd's paresis) Injury (eg tongue biting) Incontinence Provoking factors Previous abnormal neuroimaging **PMH**: stroke, meningitis/encephalitis, alcohol excess **DH**: benzodiazepine/alcohol withdrawal? Side effects on anticonvulsants	Focus investigations on 1. Is it true epilepsy? 2. What kind of epilepsy? 3. What is the cause? MRI is superior to CT of the head (CT misses half of the lesions detected by MRI) but sometimes an urgent need to rule out serious pathology may make CT preferable EEG most sensitive within 24 h of a seizure; sleep-deprived EEGs are more sensitive (50%) but should not be used to 'exclude' epilepsy because false positives are common Consider DVLA rules and implications for the patient Address anxiety regarding recurrence: 'sword of Damocles' syndrome Assess need for anticonvulsant therapy. Risk of recurrent seizure higher if: night-time seizures, family history of epilepsy, prior seizures, Todd's paresis, known abnormal neuroimaging, abnormal EEG
Vertebrobasilar ischaemia	
Symptoms provoked by head position **Vertigo** is the cardinal symptom Hemifacial numbness or paraesthesiae with contralateral symptoms in the extremities Dysphagia, dysarthria Previous strokes in posterior territory Arm claudication suggests subclavian steal syndrome Risk factors: hypertension, smoking, etc	MRI superior to CT for posterior fossa imaging Surgical options far more limited than in carotid stenosis but angioplasty and stenting may be of benefit (but high risk of stroke) Assessment of swallow reflex crucial Extra caution needed with new or changed antihypertensives – this may precipitate a hypoperfusion injury Anti-platelets (unless contraindicated) should be started

(*continued*)

Differential diagnosis	Clinical judgement and maintaining patient welfare
No loss of consciousness	
Parkinson's disease	
Asymmetrical resting tremor Clumsiness/reduced dexterity Stop–start symptoms Cognitive impairment Sleep disturbance Autonomic dysfunction: sexual dysfunction, constipation, sweating Depression in up to 40% Drug induced: neuroleptics, antiemetics **DH**: side effects of established L-dopa therapy, eg dyskinesias, hallucinations, impulse control disorders	Investigation by a specialist MRI and CT are not diagnostic but can exclude multi-infarct disease, normal pressure hydrocephalus (ataxia, incontinence, dementia) and Wilson's disease Single photon emission computed tomography (SPECT) useful if available Level of disability and implications for long-term care especially if cognitive impairment is present (eg Lewy body dementia). A key challenge is balancing effective control of rigidity versus peak-dose-induced dyskinesias
Myopathy	
Proximal muscle weakness Difficulty getting up stairs or out of the bath Fatigue No sensory symptoms Dark urine (myositis) **Timing** Over hours: toxic/metabolic cause Over days: dermatomyositis, rhabdomyolysis Over months: polymyositis, steroid induced, thyroid disease Drugs and rhabdomyolysis (eg statins)	Establish cause with appropriate investigations (CK, ANA, TFTs, fasting cortisol, anti-Jo-1 antibodies, muscle biopsy, nerve conduction studies) Supportive care while awaiting response to treatment If drug induced (eg steroids) can drug be safely stopped? Muscle biopsy crucial if polymyositis suspected Occupational therapist and physiotherapist referral

Note: with the exception of vertebrobasilar ischaemia, transient ischaemic attacks (TIAs) do NOT cause loss of consciousness, but rather focal neurological impairment resolving within 24 h.

SCENARIO 8. DIARRHOEA

'Dear colleague, This 39-year-old woman with a family history of colon cancer has suffered from intermittent diarrhoea over the last few months. Would you be kind enough to see her and advise on management?'

'Please assess this 25-year-old woman who has severe diarrhoea and some associated abdominal pain. She has noticed that this is worse during her periods. It is becoming increasingly difficult to continue her work as a shop-floor sales person. Many thanks.'

'This 30-year-old man has lost 2 stone (12–13 kg) over the past 3 months. He complains of loose stools with occasional blood mixed in. Please take a history.'

'This 50-year-old man has longstanding alcohol problems. He recently suffered from a fractured humerus after a fall. Today he presents with diar-rhoea that has been troubling him for 6 months and is worsening. I would appreciate your advice regarding further investigation of this problem.'

'This 30-year-old woman presents with diarrhoea. She noticed this worsened significantly on holiday in Italy, where she also developed an itchy rash. Please take a history.'

'This 28-year-old man had a small bowel resection 5 years ago after a gunshot wound. He now presents with weight loss and diarrhoea but a healthy appetite. Please could you assess him further.'

'This 70-year-old woman has had a recent change in bowel habit. She frequently has to rush off to the loo to open her bowels and on occasions has suffered from faecal incontinence. She is understandably very distressed about these symptoms. Please advise.'

CLINICAL COMMUNICATION SKILLS AND MANAGING PATIENT'S CONCERNS

1. Verify the information provided
'Tell me in your own words what the problem is.'

2. HPC
Open to closed questions keeping in mind the **differential diagnosis**, eg
Irritable bowel syndrome (IBS)
Inflammatory bowel disease (IBD)
Infective diarrhoea/small bowel overgrowth
Lactose intolerance
Bile salt malabsorption
Coeliac disease
Chronic pancreatitis/insufficiency
Diverticular disease
Carcinoid
Colorectal cancer

3. Previous investigations
Endoscopies? CT of the abdomen? Stool collection? Blood tests?

4. SR
Skin rash (eg erythema nodosum in IBD, dermatitis herpetiformis in coeliac disease)
Joint pains, eye inflammation
Fistulae: vaginal discharge, pneumaturia
IBS: symptoms worse with period, dyspareunia common
Infective: foreign travel, fever, HIV risks?

5. PMH
Previous acute pancreatitis
Itchy skin rash (dermatitis herpetiformis – DH)
Arthritis
Thyroid disease

6. DH
A multitude of drugs cause diarrhoea.
Laxative abuse?

7. FH
Colon cancer: which relatives and their age at diagnosis? IBD, coeliac disease

8. SH
Does diarrhoea interfere with work (eg taxi driver) or social life? Smoking (exacerbates Crohn's disease), alcohol consumption and pancreatitis, other stressful events precipitating IBS symptoms

9. Summarise
'Is there anything else we haven't discussed that you feel is important?'

10. Thank the patient

Overview: diarrhoea

Volunteered problems
Is the patient worried about cancer?

Alarm symptoms
Weight loss
PR bleeding
Flushing/palpitations (thyroid disease or carcinoid)

Disease interaction
Staggered presentation of multisystem disease? For example, IBD-associated arthropathy

Therapeutic successes and failures
Inappropriate use of anti-diarrhoeals in infective or IBD. Non-compliance with therapy for established condition

Risks to others
Infectious diarrhoea and need for isolation (eg *Clostridium difficile*). Colorectal cancer and screening of relatives

Daily life and disease
Is removing caffeine, alcohol and stress easily achieved given the daily demands on the individual?

Final problem list and plan of action

1. Identify and address any anxieties about cancer

2. Judge impact of symptoms and risk of sinister pathology and triage urgency of investigations accordingly

3. Assess willingness to have a colonoscopy if indicated

4. Determine if any relatives may require colonoscopic screening

5. Impact of diarrhoea on work and social life (eg long-distance lorry driver)

Differential diagnosis	Clinical judgement and maintaining patient welfare
Irritable bowel syndrome	
Abdominal pain Usually relieved by defecation Mucus PR Bowels open several times in morning and not throughout the day Rarely open bowels at night No alarm symptoms Worse during periods Dyspareunia common Symptoms worse with anxiety Episode of infective gastroenteritis within past year (post-infectious IBS) Relapsing and remitting Intermittent constipation	Set an appropriate limit of investigative depth when IBS suspected If the patient is aged <45 with normal examination and blood tests, endoscopic tests are not required Abnormal inflammatory markers or alarm symptoms in patient aged <45: flexible sigmoidoscopy usually adequate The patient may fulfil surveillance criteria for colonoscopy due to family history of colorectal cancer Avoid repeating previously normal invasive investigations Diet with high fat, high caffeine, high alcohol, spicy foods or low fibre requires modification Associated anxiety disorder or depression Poor response to previous medications (eg spasmolytics, loperamide/Imodium)

(*continued*)

Differential diagnosis	Clinical judgement and maintaining patient welfare
Inflammatory bowel disease	
Diarrhoea >300 g/day Bowels open at night PR blood and mucus mixed in with stool Abdominal pain Anaemia and fatigue Weight loss Malaise Triggering factor: stress, infection Factors favouring Crohn's disease over ulcerative colitis: intermittent bloating (partial obstruction), perianal fistulae and fissures (perianal pain worsened by defecation), vesicoureteric fistulae (pneumaturia, recurrent UTIs), anaemia (can also occur in ulcerative colitis but less common), less faecal urgency (rectal sparing), surgical intervention more common, less responsive to 5-ASAs (5-aminosalicylic acid derivatives) **SR**: extra-articular manifestations, eg uveitis, arthropathy, erythema nodosum **PMH**: previous operations, previous TB (contraindication to anti-TNF agents), heart failure (also a contraindication to anti-TNF agents), chronic renal failure (contraindication to ciclosporin) **DH**: 5-ASA maintenance therapy, azathioprine, 6-mercaptopurine, methotrexate (Crohn's disease), previous anti-TNF agents **SH**: symptoms began with smoking (Crohn's disease) or worsened on stopping (ulcerative colitis)	If IBD suspected then colonoscopy superior to flexible sigmoidoscopy What is the extent of disease? May require small bowel imaging, eg MR enteroclysis, small bowel follow-through, capsule endoscopy, white cell scan Need for screening colonoscopy if total colitis for >10 years Assessment for malabsorption if small bowel Crohn's disease suspected Involvement of surgeons if unresponsive to medical therapy: planned surgery preferable to emergency Admission if symptoms severe (and/or undiagnosed) Need for steroid-sparing agents if recurrent flares on weaning steroids (eg azathioprine) Immunomodulators and their side effects Anti-TNF agents for poorly controlled disease and contraindications Assessment of bone density if on long-term malabsorption and/or steroids
Infectious diarrhoea/small bowel overgrowth	
Chronic infection: travel abroad (*Microsporum, Giardia, Cryptosporidium* spp. or amoebiasis endemic areas), weight loss, depression HIV status: cryptosporidia, microspora, CMV colitis, HSV proctitis, lymphogranuloma venereum, colonic TB, drug side effect Small bowel overgrowth: vitamin B_{12}/folate deficiency (anaemia symptoms, neurological symptoms), previous bowel surgery/blind loop/jejunal diverticulum, weight loss	Need to obtain three stool samples – for giardia stool ELISA **or** therapeutic trial of metronidazole Replace vitamin deficiency, correct nutritional deficiencies and exclude other non-infective causes Dietician review – low-carbohydrate diet may be helpful in bacterial overgrowth Recurrent disease due to structural abnormality/jejunal diverticulum may require surgical correction HIV-related diarrhoea often requires colonoscopy and biopsy (with CMV and Ziehl–Neelsen stains) due to wide differential diagnosis

(*continued*)

Differential diagnosis	Clinical judgement and maintaining patient welfare
Lactose intolerance	
Ethnic origin (80–90% of adults of Asian/African origin) Diarrhoea induced by dairy products/relieved by stopping dairy products Bloating, nausea, abdominal pain	Trial of dairy-free diet (lactose hydrogen breath test often positive but poorly predicts response to lactose restriction) Dietician consultation Need for supplemental calcium in patients at risk of osteoporosis (eg Asian women)
Bile salt malabsorption	
Diarrhoea, watery and nocturnal Previous small bowel surgery/known short bowel/ terminal ileal disease eg Crohn's disease Also associated with: small bowel overgrowth, irritable bowel of the diarrhoea type (33% have bile salt malabsorption), coeliac disease	Successful trial of cholestyramine usually sufficient to make the diagnosis SeHCAT test useful for complex cases where diarrhoea may have multiple causes Need to identify any underlying small bowel pathology
Coeliac disease	
Oily light stools Weight loss Fatigue Abdominal pain Itchy papulovesicular rash (dermatitis herpetiformis) Bleeding diatheses (vitamin K deficiency) Treatment for iron deficiency anaemia in the past Bony pain, weakness, paraesthesiae (hypocalcaemia) Improves with cutting out gluten-containing products and worsens when gluten is reintroduced	If transglutaminase antibodies positive (see below) then proceed to duodenal biopsy to confirm the diagnosis Check total IgA levels (selective IgA deficiency may give a false-negative transglutaminase antibody result). Patients should be eating gluten-containing foods when tested May need repeat antibody testing while consuming wheat products if they stopped before previous test (patients often try wheat exclusion before consultation) Correct nutritional deficits Dietician support and problems with compliance (especially young females who may use gluten to effect weight control) Exclude complications if deteriorating despite gluten-free diet

(*continued*)

Differential diagnosis	Clinical judgement and maintaining patient welfare
Diverticulitis	
Episodic diarrhoea associated with LIF pain and PR bleeding Fever Longstanding constipation **Fistulae**: dysuria, pneumaturia, vaginal discharge	Need to involve surgeon if patient having recurrent bouts/fistulating disease/abscess/acute abdomen Usually resolve with conservative management (fluids, antibiotics) Need to exclude other causes of PR bleeding (usually occurs in patients aged >50) High-fibre diet may reduce flares
Chronic pancreatitis	
Abdominal pain (unpredictable, sometimes severe) Steatorrhoea Weight loss Bleeding diatheses (vitamin K deficiency) **PMH**: alcohol excess, previous abdominal trauma hyperlipidaemia, diabetes (endocrine insufficiency), osteoporosis (vitamin D deficiency) **DH**: opiate dependence for chronic pain	Need to exclude other end-organ damage from alcohol dependence if this is the likely cause Correct nutritional deficits Asses osteoporosis with bone densitometry Referral to alcohol cessation clinics Chronic pain team Enzyme replacement therapy may need increasing Diabetes management
Carcinoid	
Diarrhoea (80%) Weight loss Skin flushing (80%) if metastatic Abdominal pain Wheeze Palpitations	Logistics of diagnosis often tricky: 24-hour urine collection and avoidance of foods with high tryptophan beforehand Multidisciplinary approach to staging and treatment: radiology, oncology, surgery, gastroenterology and endocrinology input Adequacy of symptomatic control with octreotide/other medications

(*continued*)

Differential diagnosis	Clinical judgement and maintaining patient welfare
Colorectal cancer	
Abdominal pain (50%) Diarrhoea/constipation (about 33%) Anaemia/bleeding (about 33%) Weight loss Anorexia **PMH**: IBD, colonic polyps, other cancers, acromegaly **FH**: HNPCC, FAP (Table 2.3) Smoking and alcohol powerful risk factors	May fulfil colonoscopic screening guidelines for patients with a positive family history Other diagnostic modalities may be preferable to the patient (eg CT pneumocolon) Multidisciplinary approach to staging Address anxiety and investigate need for screening of other relatives Co-morbidity and fitness for potential surgery Colorectal cancer surveillance Patients who fulfil the following criteria should be offered a colonoscopy at age 35 or at presentation, whichever is later • At least one affected first-degree relative aged <45 years • Two affected first-degree relatives diagnosed at any age Screening by faecal occult blood testing is now offered to all those between ages of 60 and 70 in the UK. One positive sample in three indicates screening colonoscopy

Table 2.3 Lifetime risk of colorectal cancer

	Lifetime risk
Population average	1:50
Any family member	1:17
One affected first-degree relative aged <45	1:10
Two affected first-degree relatives	1:6

'This previously healthy 38-year-old woman felt unwell at work today with a headache and attended my walk-in centre. I have found a blood pressure of 230/110 mmHg and would value your opinion.'

'This 40-year-old man complains of ankle oedema and facial swelling. I also noted that his blood pressure was high (for the second time in the last month) last week. Please advise.'

'This 60-year-old woman was recently diagnosed with hypertension which has been difficult to control. This seems to be associated with profound lethargy and she is struggling to get her day-to-day tasks done around the house. I would be grateful for your further assessment.'

'I would be grateful for your opinion about this 38-year-old man with intermittent headache associated with sweating and palpitations. I took his blood pressure today during an episode and it was 200/106. Please could you advise about his further investigation and management?'

CLINICAL COMMUNICATION SKILLS AND MANAGING PATIENT'S CONCERNS

1. Verify the information provided
'Tell me in your own words what the problem is.'

2. HPC
Open to closed questions keeping in mind the **differential diagnosis**, eg
Essential hypertension
Conn syndrome
Cushing syndrome
Phaeochromocytoma
Renovascular hypertension
Coarctation of the aorta

3. Previous investigations
Previous blood pressure recordings?

4. SR
Visual symptoms (retinopathy), headache, heart failure (strain)
Paroxysmal headache or palpitations, panic attacks
Leg claudication
Lethargy/confusion

5. PMH
Renal disease
Diabetes
Endocrine disease
Stroke/IHD

6. DH
Current antihypertensives, steroids, sympathomimetics, OCP

7. FH
Renal disease (eg cystic), multiple endocrine neoplasia (MEN) type

8. SH
Smoking history (cessation ameliorates hypertension-associated mortality and morbidity more than antihypertensives). Caffeine consumption. Alcohol raises BP in dose-dependent fashion. Regular cocaine use has a similar effect

9. Summarise
'Is there anything else we haven't discussed that you feel is important?'

10. Thank the patient

Overview: hypertension

Volunteered problems

Alarm symptoms
Visual loss
Confusion
Severe headache

Disease interaction
Hypertension perpetuating other diseases (eg renal function, IHD)

Therapeutic successes and failures
Adequacy of current antihypertensives.
Drug interactions?
Side effects?
Compliance?

Risks to others
MEN syndromes will require family screening

Daily life and disease
Is removing caffeine, alcohol, stress and smoking easily achieved given the daily demands on the individual?

Final problem list and plan of action

1. Triage between potential malignant hypertension and chronic non-malignant hypertension (note that a diagnosis of malignant hypertension requires retinopathy)

2. Assess compliance with therapy (compliance for an asymptomatic condition is often poor)

3. Screen for end-organ damage

4. Assess previous ability to adopt lifestyle changes

Differential diagnosis	Clinical judgement and maintaining patient welfare
Essential hypertension	
Usually asymptomatic Symptoms resulting from end-organ damage (stroke, TIA, angina, cardiac failure, etc) Cardiovascular risk factors Alcohol intake Cocaine use Current medications for high BP Headache *less* common in essential hypertension than general population	Need to document high BP on three separate occasions Screen/examine for end-organ damage Hypertension is the most important modifiable risk factor for IHD, stroke, CCF, end-stage renal failure and peripheral vascular disease. Implement treatment with clear follow-up arrangements
Conn syndrome	
Alkalosis and hypokalaemia: weakness, myalgia, polyuria, fatigue, palpitations Symptoms resulting from end-organ damage	Need for high index of suspicion (up to 10% of patients with hypertension may have Conn syndrome) Need to stop ACE inhibitors/diuretics before checking renin levels Need to differentiate bilateral adrenal hyperplasia from a solitary adenoma (CT) Referral to a surgeon if appropriate
Cushing syndrome	
Weight gain (in characteristic distribution) Striae, easy bruising, amenorrhea, depression, new diabetes, easy fractures Hirsutism in women, feminisation in men Symptoms resulting from end-organ damage Visual loss, polyuria, headaches, galactorrhoea (Cushing's disease) Difficult to control hypertension Exogenous Cushing syndrome – long-term steroid use	Differentiating Cushing syndrome from Cushing's disease (see below) Difficulty in diagnosis when other conditions disturb the hypothalamic–pituitary axis (see below) Associated depression/cognitive impairment and life impact Multisystem consequences of steroid excess

(*continued*)

Differential diagnosis	Clinical judgement and maintaining patient welfare
Phaeochromocytoma	
Diagnosis not excluded if asymptomatic Classic triad of episodic headaches, sweating and palpitations Tremor, nausea, weakness, weight loss, flank pain, constipation Symptoms resulting from end-organ damage Resistant to antihypertensives **PMH**: MEN type 2, neurofibromatosis, von Hippel–Lindau disease **FH**: MEN 2	Identification and treatment of hypertensive emergencies – encephalopathy, retinopathy, seizures, worsening renal function, aortic dissection Multidisciplinary approach to staging and treatment Logistics of 24-hour urine collection for creatinine, catecholamines, vanillylmandelic acid Rule out a familial syndrome, eg MEN 2 α Blockade and compensatory volume expansion with fluids and increased salt intake α and β blockade before surgery
Renovascular hypertension	
Age <65 years with abrupt-onset hypertension Resistant to antihypertensives Recurrent sudden-onset SOB (flash pulmonary oedema) **PMH**: stroke, IHD, peripheral vascular disease. **SH**: smoker	Exclude fibromuscular dysplasia rather than atherosclerosis as the cause Established chronic renal failure (note hypertensive insult to unaffected contralateral kidney if unilateral) and risk of contrast-induced failure after renal artery angiography Angioplasty vs surgical revascularisation Smoking cessation crucial Need aggressive BP control
Coarctation of the aorta	
Often asymptomatic Headache, palpitations, leg pain, cold feet, muscle cramps **PMH**: Turner syndrome. Known structural heart disease, eg VSD. Previous subarachnoid haemorrhage	High index of suspicion required Impact of claudication on day-to-day life Risks of surgery and associated co-morbidity Women contemplating pregnancy will need surgical intervention beforehand Unfavourable interaction with aortic valve disease or poor ejection fraction

Differentiation of Cushing syndrome and Cushing's disease

Differentiation of ACTH-dependent and ACTH-independent hypercortisolaemia is usually straightforward; a plasma ACTH level <10 pg/L suggests cortisol secretion by an autonomous site (Cushing syndrome) rather than a pituitary adenoma or ectopic ACTH production (Cushing's disease).

Eighty-five per cent of cases of Cushing's disease are due to pituitary adenomas. Ectopic ACTH secretion compared with a pituitary adenoma is usually associated with higher ACTH levels, an obvious lung lesion, hypokalaemia and a rapid onset of symptoms. Small carcinoids (<1 cm) may secrete ACTH ectopically and prove very difficult to identify. The cortisol-releasing hormone (CRH) test (which looks for a rise in ACTH after CRH administration) is a useful means of differentiating ectopic ACTH production (no change in ACTH) from a pituitary adenoma (further rise in ACTH levels).

SCENARIO 10. BACK PAIN

'A 72-year-old man with known prostate cancer has been referred to A&E with sudden-onset back pain when loading the washing machine. Current oral analgesia is no longer sufficient and the patient is now less mobile. Please take a history.'

'A 50-year-old woman with a previous history of breast cancer has been referred to the clinic with worsening back pain. She is otherwise completely well. Please take a history.'

'I would be grateful if you could see this 64-year-old man urgently. He has had back pain for many months but now complains of weakness in his left leg. He has also been unable to pass urine today.'

'This 36-year-old courier has recently been made redundant. He complains of lower back pain, which began after lifting a heavy package. His pain is no longer controlled with NSAIDs or paracetamol. I have arranged radiographs of his spine and would be grateful for your further assessment.'

CLINICAL COMMUNICATION SKILLS AND MANAGING PATIENT'S CONCERNS

1. Verify the information provided
'Tell me in your own words what the problem is.'

2. HPC
Open to closed questions keeping in mind the **differential diagnosis**: eg
Spinal metastases
Vertebral fracture (osteoporotic/pathological)
Cord compression
Mechanical lower back pain

3. Previous investigations
Previous bone scan? Bone densitometry? Spine radiograph/MRI? Mammogram?

4. SR
Hypercalcaemia (constipation, renal colic, depression, bone pain)?
Bladder and bowel control
Leg weakness
Paraesthesiae/numbness

5. PMH
Previous malignancy and stage when treated
Other conditions limiting mobility
Dates of the menopause

6. DH
Calcium/vitamin D supplements
Hormone replacement therapy
Bisphosphonates

7. FH
Breast/prostate cancer, osteoporosis, coeliac disease

8. SH
Limitation of function in ADL. Degree of improvement when pain controlled. Assistance from social services/family/friends. Smoking history

9. Summarise
'Is there anything else we haven't discussed that you feel is important?'

10. Thank the patient

Back pain

Volunteered problems

Alarm symptoms
Leg weakness, paraesthesiae, numbness, symptoms of hypercalcaemia, faecal/urinary incontinence

Disease interaction
Fall in performance status and reduced fitness for further treatment or chemotherapy
Combined osteoporosis and metastatic disease

Therapeutic successes and failures
Pain score and how it changes with activity/analgesia
Side effects (eg opiates and constipation, bisphosphonates and oesophagitis)

Risks to others

Daily life and disease
May now be unable to care for other dependants. If normally working, will financial status be affected by current problem?

Final problem list and plan of action

1. Potential oncological emergencies (hypercalcaemia, cord compression, SVC/IVC obstruction)

2. Identify patient's reservations about opiate analgesia (eg fear of addiction)

3. Does the patient require your help with arranging time off work (or even a lawsuit against employers) and is this appropriate?

4. Assess loss of independence and explore willingness to accept help from external agency

5. Does the patient require admission for pain control and/or OT/physiotherapy assessment?

Differential diagnosis	Clinical judgement and maintaining patient welfare
Bony metastases (without cord compression)	
Severe pain, worse at night and after prolonged immobility/recumbent Persistent pain after minimal injury/lifting Multiple areas of pain, eg ribs and back Impairment of mobility Associated hypercalcaemia symptoms **PMH**: known breast, prostate, lung or renal cancer. Myeloma **DH**: side effects of analgesia especially NSAIDs (gastritis, peptic ulcer disease) and/or opiates (constipation, nausea)	Consider the need for urgent radiotherapy and/or treatment of hypercalcaemia Implications for prognosis and further treatment Associated depression and anxiety Analgesia and the logistics of drug delivery at home (eg fentanyl patch, syringe driver) and follow-up (eg Macmillan service) Formal assessment of disability and need for help at home
Cord compression	
Gradually worsening back pain (90%) Radicular pain Worse lying flat Leg weakness or paraesthesiae Loss of bladder/bowel control **PMH**: known breast, prostate, lung or renal cancer *Pain often precedes neurological symptoms by many months*	Need for urgent investigation and treatment Availability of urgent MRI is a frequent problem Urgent radiotherapy/decompressive surgery Implications for long-term care if neurological deficit permanent Litigious issues (if symptoms previously dismissed) are common
Osteoporotic vertebral fracture	
History of minimal trauma suggests severe osteoporosis or pathological fracture **Date of menopause** **PMH**: previous fractures to hip, pelvis, proximal humerus and distal forearm Smokers, high alcohol consumption **DH**: previous steroid use, hormone replacement therapy **SH**: prolonged inactivity Residence in TB endemic areas (Pott's disease)	Need to minimise risk of further injury (eg hip protectors) Exclude cord injury/unstable fractures – refer to orthopaedic surgeons Exclude myeloma, malignancy, Pott's disease Vitamin D and calcium supplementation (after assessment for deficiency) Resulting immobility and acquisition of new problems during bed rest (pressure sores, pneumonia, DVT, PE) Physiotherapy and OT assessment for discharge planning

(continued)

Differential diagnosis	Clinical judgement and maintaining patient welfare
Mechanical lower back pain	
Pain after twisting back while lifting a heavy object or after road traffic accident/operating vibrating machinery/a fall Normal spinal imaging Radicular pain, leg weakness, paraesthesiae, numbness – consider a possible associated disc herniation **PMH**: previous back surgery/injury/physiotherapy Psychiatric co-morbidity **SH**: if a work-related injury, has there been time off work/poor job satisfaction/legal action against employer?	Important to exclude sinister pathology but a thorough examination is usually adequate in the absence of alarm symptoms or trauma Protracted symptoms may nevertheless require MRI to exclude herniated disc Access and compliance with physiotherapy Patient dissatisfaction without 'full scan' Opiate dependence Poor prognosis when patient is involved in litigation against injurious party

SCENARIO 11. ACUTE-ONSET HEADACHE

'An HIV-positive male has referred himself to A&E with a headache. His partner thinks that he has been behaving slightly bizarrely recently. Please take a history.'

'A 34-year old-man presents to A&E with a headache that began earlier that day. It is now unbearable. Please take a history.'

'This 74-year-old man had a sudden-onset headache earlier today. He thinks that he may have lost consciousness for a moment and has been bed-bound since. Please take a history.'

'This 18-year-old young woman is suffering from a severe headache that woke her up in the early hours of the morning. Please take a history.'

CLINICAL COMMUNICATION SKILLS AND MANAGING PATIENT'S CONCERNS

1. Verify the information provided
'Tell me in your own words what the problem is.'

2. HPC
Open to closed questions keeping in mind the **differential diagnosis**: eg
Subarachnoid haemorrhage (SAH)
Haemorrhagic stroke
Viral meningitis/encephalitis
Bacterial/crypytococcal meningitis

3. Previous investigations
Previous CT/MRI? HIV test? Renal imaging?

4. SR
HIV risk factors. Symptoms of polycystic kidney/liver disease
Symptoms of AIDS-defining illnesses, meningism, photophobia, neck stiffness, non-blanching rash, fevers, rigors, seizures, cold sores (HSV)

5. PMH
HIV and CD4 count
PCKD
Previous headaches
Previous splenectomy ± prophylaxis (pneumococcal meningitis)
Base-of-skull fracture /trauma (pneumococcal meningitis)

6. DH
Analgesia and efficacy
Anticoagulation and SAH
Immunosuppressants

7. FH: SAH, renal cyst/renal failure

8. SH
Risk factors for HIV (IVDU, high-risk sex), contact with birds (*Cryptococcus* sp.), contact with other case of meningitis.

9. Summarise
'Is there anything else we haven't discussed that you feel is important?'

10. Thank the patient

Acute-onset headache

Volunteered problem

Alarm symptoms
Impaired cognition/loss of consciousness
Neurological impairment
Meningism
HIV/high risk of HIV

Disease interaction
eg recognition of sinister pathology on a background of frequent migraine

Therapeutic successes and failures
Adequacy of current analgesia. Symptom control leading to prolonged delay in diagnosis
Opioids and drowsiness – jeopardises recognition of a fall in GCS
New AIDS-defining disease and implications for possible resistance to HAART

Risks to others
Meningitis and treatment of close contacts
Contact tracing in HIV-related disease

Daily life and disease
May need a long recovery period including rehabilitation. This may exacerbate existing financial/social problems

Final problem list and plan of action

1. Such cases always require urgent investigation and treatment

2. Early involvement of neurosurgeon in appropriate cases

3. Screening for other organ disease/ complications of sepsis/AIDS-defining illnesses

4. Consent for investigation and treatment in the cognitively impaired patient

5. Medicolegal issues surrounding late presentations after missed diagnosis

6. HIV contact tracing

Differential diagnosis	Clinical judgement and maintaining patient welfare
Subarachnoid haemorrhage	
Sudden-onset, 'worse headache ever', similar to being hit over the head Nausea and vomiting Neck stiffness, back pain Sudden loss of consciousness (about 40%) Sentinel bleeds (about 35%) – severe headaches that resolve quickly (usually around 2 weeks before a major bleed) Neurological deficit evolving after headache onset Mass effect symptoms – falling GCS, nerve VI palsy **PMH**: renal cystic disease, hypertension, vasculitis, blood dyscrasias, fibromuscular dysplasia **FH**: intracranial aneurysm/early stroke/polycystic kidney disease **DH**: headache not responding to analgesia	Need for urgent investigation (CT of the head 93–98% sensitive) and treatment Early involvement of neurosurgeons in all cases Timing of lumbar puncture – greatest sensitivity 12 h after headache onset Close monitoring and surveillance for rising intracranial pressure (especially with blood in the fourth ventricle) Prophylaxis for re-bleeding and vasospasm (fluids to keep hypervolaemic, nimodipine) Also need to anticipate other complications • Seizures (25%) • Hydrocephalus (25%) • Neurogenic pulmonary oedema (up to 90%) • Arrhythmias A quarter have residual neurological deficit and most have transient/permanent cognitive deficit – this has major implications for rehabilitation/career/support at home Emotional lability and depression are common after recovery Secondary prevention of another event is crucial
Haemorrhagic stroke	
Sudden-onset headache Nausea and vomiting Seizures Focal neurological deficit. **Alarms**: cerebellar or brain-stem symptoms (double vision, ataxia, slurred speech, vertigo) Loss of consciousness common **PMH**: hypertension, known brain tumour, coagulopathies **DH**: anticoagulant **SH**: cocaine use – in young patients	Complication of another treatment, eg thrombolysis for MI Surgical intervention for cerebellar haematoma (high risk of brain-stem compression) Often decline rapidly – need early decision about resuscitation status support, taking into account co-morbidities Correction of anticoagulation Complex issues surrounding long-term support for survivors with neurological deficit – rehab potential (specialist centre or at home) and need to plan support at home Secondary prevention of another event

(*continued*)

Differential diagnosis	Clinical judgement and maintaining patient welfare
Viral meningitis/encephalitis	
Swift onset of headache within the last 36 h Fever (>90%) Prodromal coryzal symptoms and myalgia 48 h before headache (50%) Nausea and vomiting Photophobia Cognitive impairment Neck stiffness Irritability Rash HIV risk factors (CMV, adenovirus, HIV, HSV encephalitis) Testicular pain – mumps Diarrhoea – enterovirus **PMH**: immunosuppression/HIV Measles/mumps/immunisations Previous viral meningitis (HSV and EBV recur) **DH**: immunosuppressants (CMV, EBV) Analgesia **SH**: HIV risk factors, hamster/mouse/rat as pet – lymphocytic choriomeningitis virus	CT needed before LP (see below)? Need for antibiotics until bacterial meningitis excluded Antiviral therapy (anti-HIV, ganciclovir for CMV, aciclovir for HSV) indicated if evidence of encephalitis (seizures, focal neurology, decreased GCS) Failure to improve after 24 h? Investigate potential HIV, toxoplasmosis or tubercular meningitis which may give similar LP results Long-term prognosis excellent unless concomitant encephalitis Barrier contraception for HSV-2-infected individuals HIV contact tracing if first presentation Beware neonatal death in pregnant women with Coxsackievirus B meningitis

(*continued*)

Differential diagnosis	Clinical judgement and maintaining patient welfare
Bacterial meningitis	
Classic triad of headache, neck stiffness and fever in 80% Onset in last 24 h common (25%) Cough/cold within last week (50%) Vomiting (35%) Seizures (30%) Drowsiness Indolent presentations in elderly and immunocompromised patients **PMH**: base-of-skull fracture (pneumococcal meningitis) Recent mastoiditis, sinusitis, otitis media Splenectomy (pneumococcal meningitis) Ventriculoperitoneal shunt? HIV/AIDS Immunised for group C meningococci or *Haemophilus influenzae* type b? **DH**: may be partially treated by GP with course of antibiotics resulting in more indolent presentation Immunosuppressants/recent chemotherapy	Consider the need for urgent treatment before further investigation CT before LP (see below) Vigorous resuscitation if septic Aggressive control of seizures Prophylaxis for close contacts Close surveillance for immediate complications (50%): venous thrombosis, subdural/brain abscess, raised ICP and hydrocephalus, SAH, infarcts A third of survivors have long-term neurological sequelae – need to plan rehabilitation and additional support Surveillance for obstructive hydrocephalus within first month of episode
Cryptococcal meningitis	
Known HIV-positive patient Similar presentation to bacterial meningitis but often less symptomatic in immunocompromised patients Contact with birds	May have a normal LP initially. India ink stain only 30% sensitive. CSF culture and latex agglutination test important Lifelong oral fluconazole after successful treatment with IV amphotericin

Use of CT brain imaging before lumbar puncture

The possibility of herniation after lumbar puncture in the presence of raised intracranial pressure means a CT of the head before a lumbar puncture is usually sensible. No national guidelines exist but most trusts have their own guidelines for out-of-hours CT imaging in suspected meningitis. These are usually based around the findings of a 2001 *New England Journal of Medicine* paper* which prospectively studied 301 patients with suspected meningitis. The absence of any of the following features was associated with a normal CT of the head in 93 of 96 patients (all 96 safely underwent lumbar puncture)

- Age >60 years
- Immunocompromise
- Previous CNS disease
- Seizure within the past week
- Abnormal GCS
- Inability to answer two consecutive questions or follow two consecutive commands
- Gaze palsy
- Abnormal visual fields
- Arm or leg drift
- Dysphasia/aphasia/dysarthria.

The presence of any of these features, or papilloedema, should prompt CT brain imaging before lumbar puncture.

Table 2.4 CSF profiles (protein, white cell count, glucose and opening pressure) associated with the differing pathogens of meningitis

Pathogen	Opening pressure (cmH$_2$O)	WCC (cells/mm^3)	Glucose	Protein	Further tests
Bacterial	20–30	100–5000; >80% PMNs	Low	High	Culture and Gram stain
Viral	10–20	10–300; lymphocytes	Normal	Slightly increased	PCR
TB	20–30	100–500; lymphocytes	Low	High	AFB stain, culture, PCR
Cryptococcus sp.	20–30	10–300; lymphocytes	Low	Increased	India ink, latex agglutination

AFB, acid-fast bacillus; PCR, polymerase chain reaction; PMNs, polymorphonuclear neutrophils.

SCENARIO 12. NEW HEADACHE OF RECENT ONSET

'Please could you see this 70-year-old man who takes warfarin for atrial fibrillation. He has been increasingly frail and slow over the last year. Today he is confused and complaining of a headache.'

'This 24-year-old HIV-positive man is currently on HAART. His latest viral load was undetectable. Today he presents with a 4-day history of worsening headache. He was having difficulty keeping up with a presentation at work. Please take a history.'

'This 70-year-old Asian woman describes an intermittent worsening headache over the past 4 weeks. She speaks little English but her daughter tells me that she has lost weight and has been feeling generally unwell for some time. Please take a history.'

'Please could you assess this 56-year-old woman who has had a throbbing headache for the last 3 days. Today she was concerned to find herself unable to read the newspaper (she normally has perfect vision).'

'This 40-year-old woman has had a persistent cough for 2 months. She now complains of a constant headache (worse in the mornings), which is unbearable when she coughs. She has become increasingly anxious about the cause of her symptoms.'

CLINICAL COMMUNICATION SKILLS AND MANAGING PATIENT'S CONCERNS

1. Verify the information provided
'Tell me in your own words what the problem is.'

2. HPC
Open to closed questions keeping in mind the **differential diagnosis**, eg
Subdural haematoma
Brain neoplasm, primary or secondary
Brain abscess/toxoplasmosis
TB meningitis
Giant cell arteritis (GCA)

3. Previous investigations
Previous CT/MRI? HIV test?

4. SR
Night sweats (lymphoma/TB), nausea and vomiting (raised ICP), weight loss, cough/haemoptysis (TB/bronchial carcinoma with cerebral metastases)
Myalgia (GCA)

5. PMH
Known malignancy?
HIV/AIDS
Recent head injury/recurrent falls
Polymyalgia rheumatica

6. DH
Analgesia and efficacy
Anticoagulation
Immunosuppressants

7. FH
Primary brain tumours

8. SH
Smoking history. TB exposure and recent travel. HIV exposure

9. Summarise
'Is there anything else we haven't discussed that you feel is important?'

10. Thank the patient

New headache of recent onset

Volunteered problems

Alarm symptoms
Morning nausea and vomiting, weight loss, focal neurological deficit, altered mentation, haemoptysis, seizures

Disease interaction
Implications of new illness for established disease (eg tumour progression, HAART resistance)
Co-morbidity and fitness for surgical intervention (subdural haematoma)

Therapeutic successes and failures
Recent medications prolonging warfarin half-life resulting in over-anticoagulation
Non-compliance/adverse effects with anti-TB medications

Risks to others
TB and HIV exposure

Daily life and disease
May need a long recovery period including rehabilitation. This may exacerbate existing financial/social problems

---

Final problem list and plan of action

1. Urgent investigation and treatment

2. Compliance and consent for investigation and treatment in the confused patient

3. Patient anxiety about disease progression

4. Need to determine resuscitation status in metastatic disease through discussion with patient and family

5. Neurological impairment and rehabilitation – implications for long-term self-care and independence

Differential diagnosis	Clinical judgement and maintaining patient welfare
Subdural haematoma	
Acute (<72 h from injury) Subacute (3–20 days since injury) Chronic (>20 days since injury) Insidious onset of symptoms • Headache (90%) – exacerbated by coughing or straining • Cognitive dysfunction (50%) • Irritability • Asymmetrical motor weakness • Aphasia • Double vision on lateral gaze (nerve VI palsy indicating raised ICP) **PMH**: recurrent falls **DH**: warfarin or aspirin **SH**: possibility of non-accidental injury by carer	Urgent investigation (CT of the head) and treatment (referral to neurosurgeon) May need a collateral history Aggressive control of seizures Chronicity of disease, neurological deficit and prognosis are crucial to determining whether neurosurgical intervention indicated Reversal of anticoagulation may not be straightforward, eg in context of metallic heart valve Exclude C-spine fracture Determine underlying cause of falls Non-accidental injury and possible abuse of elderly person
Brain neoplasm (primary or secondary)	
Morning headache and/or vomiting Frontal tumours: depersonalisation, emotional lability, disinhibited behaviour, olfactory hallucinations/anosmia Parietotemporal tumours: seizures (often jacksonian), apraxia, memory loss, dysphasia, cognitive dysfunction, hemiparesis Pituitary fossa: bitemporal visual field loss, symptoms of panhypopituitarism/prolactinaemia/diabetes insipidus Posterior fossa: ataxia, headache onset earlier in disease Brain stem: dysphagia, facial weakness, double vision Symptoms relating to primary tumour elsewhere: eg cough with haemoptysis (lung cancer most common site of primary in metastatic brain disease) **PMH**: HIV/immunocompromised – primary cerebral lymphoma Known malignancy **SH**: smoker	Multidisciplinary approach crucial (clinical and medical oncologist, radiologist, histopathologist, neurosurgeon, neurologist) Staging and treatment of extracerebral primary Control of seizures paramount to quality of life Patient wishes are key – for metastatic lesions treatment is usually palliative (testicular cancer is a notable exception) and may have profound side effects

(*continued*)

Differential diagnosis	Clinical judgement and maintaining patient welfare
Brain abscess	
Headache (about 70%), altered mental state (about 65%), focal neurological impairment (65%), fever (50%), seizures (33%) Nausea and vomiting (40%) Neck stiffness (25%) Headache may worsen suddenly if the abscess ruptures Localised symptoms depending on location of abscess (see Brain neoplasm above) Symptoms from source of infection: sinusitis, otitis media, other chronic purulent focus **PMH**: immunocompromise (toxoplasmosis) Congenital heart disease, endocarditis, recent dental surgery, penetrating trauma, transplantation **DH**: immunosuppressants **SH**: HIV risks (toxoplasmosis, listeriosis, mycobacteria, *Nocardia* spp., cryptococci), exposure to cats (toxoplasmosis)	Urgent treatment and investigation. Blood cultures before antibiotics LP usually avoided Biopsy of lesion crucial Surgical excision for single lesions, multiple decompressive aspirations for multiple lesions Cover for *Toxoplasma gondii* infection if HIV suspected (treated with pyrimethamine and sulfadiazine) Good prognosis if onset of symptoms within a week. Otherwise residual deficit is likely and rehabilitation/additional support should be anticipated Treat underlying source of infection/immunocompromise
TB meningitis	
Immunocompetent: fever, headache, confusion, neck stiffness for several weeks Immunocompromised: <5% have meningism Sudden-onset neurological impairment, including blindness Fever, weight loss, anorexia, night sweats **PMH**: previous TB, known immunocompromise (HIV/AIDS), no BCG immunisation, positive PPD test **FH**: contact with TB *Infections that can mimic tuberculous meningitis in their clinical presentation* ***Bacterial***: partially treated bacterial meningitis, brain abscess, *Listeria*, *Neisseria* spp. ***Viral***: herpes, mumps, HIV ***Fungal***: cryptococci, histoplasmosis, *Actinomycetes*, *Nocardia*, *Candida* spp. ***Spirochaetes***: *Borrelia burgdorferi* (Lyme disease), syphilis, leptospirosis Brucellosis ***Parasitic***: toxoplasmosis, cysticercosis	Requires urgent differentiation from other causes of meningitis Diagnostic difficulties are frequent, especially when CD4 count is low (acellular CSF) Screening of close contacts for TB Exclusion of other organ involvement HIV staging and treatment, including contact tracing Patient issues with stigma, relatives/partners fear of infection, compliance with long-term treatment Management of long-term neurological sequelae: rehabilitation, additional support

(*continued*)

Differential diagnosis	Clinical judgement and maintaining patient welfare
Temporal arteritis	
Unilateral temporal headache, often worse at night Jaw claudication (50%) Pain on combing hair/wearing hat/glasses Transient (amaurosis fugax in 10%) or complete visual loss Proximal myalgia, low-grade fever, malaise **PMH**: known polymyalgia rheumatica. Recent deterioration in vision **DH**: steroids (breakthrough vasculitis rare) **Diagnostic criteria for giant cell arteritis** Patients should have at least three of the following five criteria for a diagnosis of GCA 1. Age >50 years 2. New localised headache 3. Tenderness or decreased pulse of the temporal artery 4. ESR >50 mm/h 5. Biopsy of artery characteristic of giant cell arteritis	Need to commence steroid therapy urgently to protect against (further) visual loss Non-urgent plan for temporal artery biopsy (but sensitivity decreases the longer steroid therapy continues) Maintenance therapy ± steroid-sparing agents, eg azathioprine. Long-term consequences of steroids and need for bone-protecting agents (patients often elderly and at risk of osteoporosis) Monitoring for bone marrow suppression and hepatitis on azathioprine

SCENARIO 13: CHRONIC/INTERMITTENT HEADACHE

'This 28-year-old woman is known to suffer from migraines. Recently she has developed a tingling sensation in her right arm and difficulty with word finding just before the headache begins. In light of these features I thought I should refer her for your opinion.'

'This 34-year-old woman has had a series of severe headaches over the last 3 weeks. She experienced a similar episode 2 years ago and a CT of the head was organised. I have been told that this was normal. She is currently unable to work because of the severity and frequency of her headaches. I

would be grateful for your urgent investigation and further management of this problem.'

'I would be grateful if you could see this 33-year-old man who rarely attends my clinic except for a few exacerbations of asthma. He has had fevers and a severe frontal headache for the last week. He also describes some flu-like symptoms. Many thanks.'

'This 50-year-old woman has suffered from tension headaches for many years. She thinks that they are getting worse. Please advise.'

CLINICAL COMMUNICATION SKILLS AND MANAGING PATIENT'S CONCERNS

1. Verify the information provided
'Tell me in your own words what the problem is.'

2. HPC
Open to closed questions keeping in mind the **differential diagnosis**, eg
Migraine
Cluster headache
Trigeminal neuralgia
Analgesia overuse headache
Sinusitis

3. Previous investigations
Previous CT/MRI? Previous echocardiography?

4. SR
Visual ticlopsia, lacrimation, nausea and vomiting, postnasal drip, nasal congestion

5. PMH
Previous sinus surgery
Known structural heart disease/patent foramen ovale

6. DH
Analgesia and efficacy
$5HT_1$-receptor agonists

7. FH
Migraine

8. SH
Elicit any recent stress/bereavement. Time off work, financial problems

9. Summarise
'Is there anything else we haven't discussed that you feel is important?'

10. Thank the patient

Chronic/intermittent headache

Volunteered problems

Alarm symptoms
Morning nausea and vomiting, weight loss, persistent focal neurological deficit, seizures

Disease interaction
Co-morbidity: would the patient be fit for invasive interventional cardiac procedures (severe migraine) or trigeminal nerve decompression (trigeminal neuralgia)?

Therapeutic successes and failures
Analgesics may be contributing to headache rather than attenuating it
Interaction between $5HT_1$-receptor agonists and SSRIs

Risks to others

Daily life and disease
Chronic pain and its impact on daily life – is there any secondary gain from symptoms?

Final problem list and plan of action

1. Patient acceptance of diagnosis/anxieties about more sinister pathology

2. Exclusion of sinister pathology, especially if focal neurological impairment

3. Involvement of ENT surgeon where appropriate

4. Referral for specialist management of chronic pain

5. Impact of debilitating pain on day-to-day life and how this can be assuaged

Differential diagnosis	Clinical judgement and maintaining patient welfare
Migraine	

Preceding aura (one in five)
 • Scotoma
 • Zig-zags (fortifications)
 • Scintilla (flashing lights)
 • Headache, usually unilateral
 • Nausea (80%) and vomiting (about 40%)
 • Photophobia (about 80%)
 • Aversion to loud noise (about 70%)
 • *Migraine variants*
   • Hemiplegic migraine
   • Aura without headache
   • Basilar migraine (vertigo and ataxia)
   • Ophthalmoplegic migraine (double vision)
   • Cyclical vomiting syndrome (nausea without headache)
 • Precipitating food or alcohol
 PMH: previous episodes
 FH: migraine (80% have positive family history)
	Rule out sinister pathology
	 CT is indicated in atypical cases or where there is focal neurology
	 Abortive therapy (eg $5HT_1$-receptor agonists, high-flow oxygen) and prophylaxis (eg β blockers)

Cluster headaches	
Short-duration, severe periorbital headaches Episodes of frequent attacks, separated by at least 2 pain-free weeks Triggers: stress, extreme temperatures, sexual activity **SR**: autonomic periphenomena common (eg palpitations)	Psychosocial maladaptation to this lifelong condition is common Abortive therapy similar to migraine therapy Neurosurgical ablation of cavernous sinus plexus in severe/resistant cases
Trigeminal neuralgia	
Hemifacial, lancinating pain Usually episodic with increasing frequency as the condition progresses Usually women aged >40 Often triggered by sensory stimulation of trigeminal nerve territory **PMH**: ophthalmic zoster, trauma to trigeminal nerve	Referral for microvascular decompression (surgical correction of vascular compression of the trigeminal nerve) if medical therapy fails (eg carbamazepine) Management of chronic pain by specialists Other neurological symptoms/signs raises possibility of MS which should be investigated further Address associated depression. This is common – many cases of suicide are known

(*continued*)

Differential diagnosis	Clinical judgement and maintaining patient welfare
Analgesia overuse headache	
Headache present for >15 days each month (by definition) Headache reverts to less severe pattern when analgesics stopped	Persuading patient to reduce analgesia to attenuate pain often difficult
Sinusitis	
Nasal congestion, postnasal drip, anosmia, sore throat, chronic cough **PMH**: nasal polyps, septal deviation, allergic rhinitis, Wegener's granulomatosis **DH**: smoker	CT imaging usually diagnostic and excludes other pathology Referral to ENT surgeon may be required for correction of osteomeatal obstruction

SCENARIO 14: WEAK LEGS

'This 40-year-old choreographer was recently treated by another practice doctor for a chest infection. She now represents with weak legs. She tells me that she has fallen twice at work when they seemed to just give way. I would be grateful for your urgent assessment and opinion.'

'Please could you assess this pleasant 60-year-old man who has a longstanding history of COPD. He is becoming increasingly weak and his daughter (his main carer) is having difficulty looking after him. He can no longer manage the stairs. Many thanks.'

'I would be grateful if you could see this 30-year-old artist. She had a seizure last year, which was thoroughly investigated but no underlying cause could be found. Last week she developed shoot-ing pains down her left arms and today, on getting out of the bath, she found that her legs were very wobbly. Many thanks for your further assessment of these worrying symptoms.'

'This 44-year-old man fell down the stairs last week. He feels increasingly weak in both legs and has also started to drop things. His wife tells me that she is concerned that he is more irritable than usual and recently nearly lost his job after an altercation with a senior colleague. I would be grateful for your opinion.'

'This 24-year-old Asian man describes being ex-tremely weak on two occasions in the last month. On one of these episodes he was unable to get out of bed. The problem only lasted a few hours. Please take a history. '

CLINICAL COMMUNICATION SKILLS AND MANAGING PATIENT'S CONCERNS

1. Verify the information provided
'Tell me in your own words what the problem is.'

2. HPC
Open to closed questions keeping in mind the **differential diagnosis**, eg
Guillain–Barré syndrome
Myopathy
Multiple sclerosis/transverse myelitis
Lambert–Eaton myasthenic syndrome
Cord compression
Motor neuron disease (MND)
Familial hypokalaemic periodic paralysis

3. Previous investigations
Previous CT/MRI? Previous EMG/nerve conduction studies?

4. SR
Visual disturbance, bladder dysfunction, emotional lability, cognitive impairment, myalgia, recent coryzal symptoms

5. PMH
Known malignancy
Previous spinal surgery
Recent upper respiratory tract infection
Established COPD

6. DH
Long-term steroids
Thyroxine

7. FH
Periodic paralysis, thyroid disease

8. SH
Alcohol consumption. Smoking history

9. Summarise
'Is there anything else we haven't discussed that you feel is important?'

10. Thank the patient

Weak legs

Volunteered problems

Alarm symptoms
Ascending weakness, weight loss, haemoptysis, back pain, loss of bowel/bladder control, visual disturbance

Disease interaction
Implications of new episode on projected course of disease (eg primary progressive vs relapsing–remitting MS, progression of MND)
Interaction between new respiratory muscle weakness and established lung disease

Therapeutic successes and failures
Drugs may well be causative/precipitant
Is thyroxine therapy adequate?
Drug therapy available on the NHS (IFN-β1a)
Steroids can cause myopathy and treat it (eg polymositis)

Risks to others
Care of other dependants may be jeopardised

Daily life and disease
There are very few areas of one's life not affected by weak legs!

Final problem list and plan of action

1. Diagnosis of some of these conditions may take many months and patients need to be aware of this

2. Many of these are devastating diseases affecting young individuals with young children. The socioeconomic impact must be anticipated and attenuated wherever possible (eg letters to employer, DSS for disability allowance, council for unpaid rent, etc)

Differential diagnosis	Clinical judgement and maintaining patient welfare
Guillain–Barré syndrome	
Symmetrical lower limb weakness spreading proximally A benign respiratory or gastrointestinal illness some 2–4 weeks previously Double vision (ophthalmoplegia – Miller–Fisher variant) Falls (impaired proprioception) and inability to walk SOB Paraesthesiae (also beginning distally and moving proximally) Shooting pains Palpitation, dizziness on standing, facial flushing (autonomic dysfunction common) **PMH**: recent immunisation **DH**: recent treatment for diarrhoea or chest infection **Note that no sensory loss/rising sensory level is found in Guillain–Barré syndrome**	Investigations: LP may show raised protein and CT often performed to exclude other pathology. Neither is diagnostic Stool culture for *Campylobacter jejuni* may support the diagnosis Alert ICU – one in three requires ventilatory support Cardiac monitoring if autonomic features/heart block/arrhythmias present – the major cause of mortality after respiratory failure Need to monitor FVC at least twice a day (<20 mL/kg is concerning) DVT prophylaxis crucial due to immobility Early referral for plasma exchange or IV immunoglobulin Most take months to recover – major implications for discharge planning and home support/financial status Residual neurological damage in about 25%, often mild – need for careful OT and physiotherapy rehabilitation planning
Myopathy	
Difficulty standing from chairs or bath, difficulty climbing stairs, shaving, combing hair Distal muscle weakness: dropping objects, tripping over small obstacles, problems writing Falls Timing of onset crucial • Over hours: toxic/periodic paralysis • Over a few days: dermatomyositis, rhabdomyolysis • Over weeks: endocrine myopathy (hypo/hyperthyroidism, hyperparathyroidism, Cushing's disease, Addison's disease), steroid myopathy, polymyositis, alcohol, infectious (HIV, cysticercosis) • Malaise, fatigue **PMH**: endocrinopathy, renal failure, autoimmune disease, alcohol dependence **DH**: steroids, statins, colchicine, AZT **SH**: heroin/cocaine use	Investigation and treatment of underlying cause with 'myopathy screen': TFTs, 24-h urinary cortisol, CK, ESR, ANA, serum myoglobin EMG and nerve conduction studies sometimes useful Muscle biopsy may be indicated Exclusion of acute rhabdomyolysis and its complications (renal failure, fulminant hepatic failure) is crucial in weakness of recent onset OT and physiotherapy to plan rehabilitation and support while recovering/on treatment For alcohol dependence will need screen for liver/pancreas/heart disease and encourage self-referral to alcohol cessation groups (Alcoholics Anonymous, community drugs and alcohol team)

(*continued*)

Differential diagnosis	Clinical judgement and maintaining patient welfare
Multiple sclerosis/transverse myelitis	
Acute **partial** loss of motor, sensory, autonomic (bladder and bowel control) and reflex function below a particular vertebral level	Confirmation of MS as a diagnosis often requires prospective monitoring. There is no diagnostic test, although MRI is crucial to reveal demyelinating disease
Accompanying acute onset visual blurring and decreased acuity ('Devic's syndrome' when occurring with a transverse myelitis)	CT is usually performed before LP to rule out mass lesions
Uthoff's phenomenon: symptoms worsen after a hot bath or exercise	Need to monitor over time for prognostic indicators Primary progressive or relapsing–remitting?
Profound fatigue	Neurological recovery is rarely complete between attacks – a step-wise decline (secondary progressive MS) is common and has great implications for rehabilitation and social/medical support
Depression, mild cognitive impairment or low concentration span, sensory loss, psychiatric disturbance, ataxia, seizures (5%)	
Lhermitte's sign: neck movement results in shock-like pain radiating to extremities	Although early assessment and ongoing management by a neurologist are obviously crucial, a multidisciplinary approach is often required (urologist, gastroenterologist, colorectal surgeon, stoma nurse, etc)
Symptoms distributed in space and time are the prerequisite of a diagnosis of MS	
A history of recent spinal injury suggests compressive spinal injury rather than MS	Identify and treat precipitants aggressively (eg early antibiotics for infections)
PMH: other causes of transverse myelitis: autoimmune (sarcoid, SLE, vasculitis), post-infectious (Lyme disease, *Mycoplasma pneumoniae*, syphilis, TB, viral)	High-dose steroids often indicated for non-MS transverse myelitis (eg post-infectious). May require concomitant bone protection and surveillance for side effects
	IFN-β1a, glatiramer acetate, natalizumab therapy for relapsing–remitting MS

(*continued*)

Differential diagnosis	Clinical judgement and maintaining patient welfare
Lambert–Eaton myasthenic syndrome (LEMS)	
Weakness of the proximal leg muscles is the most common complaint – difficulty rising from chairs, getting out of bath, climbing stairs, etc More rarely • Oropharyngeal muscles: difficulty chewing, swallowing, dysarthria • Ocular muscles: diplopia, ptosis A dry mouth and symptoms of autonomic dysfunction (eg impotence) may be prominent Symptoms may have been progressing over many years Patient may describe facilitation: strength improving after repeated action Weight loss, anorexia, haemoptysis, cough Note that **myasthenia gravis** is an important differential diagnosis. This tends to present the other way around, with ocular palsies first followed by leg weakness much later in the disease **PMH**: known or suspected malignancy (usually lung or ovarian)	Urgent investigation and treatment of the underlying malignancy (found in 75%) Anti-acetylcholine (Ach) receptor antibodies, EMG and nerve conduction studies crucial to the diagnosis Exclude ectopic ACTH as a cause of proximal myopathy if there are features of Cushing syndrome Avoid magnesium, calcium channel blockers, aminoglycosides The prognosis is usually determined by the underlying disease, but LEMS has major implications for day-to-day independence and end-of-life palliative support
Cord compression (see Scenario 10)	
Familial hypokalaemic periodic paralysis	
This may present in adulthood (but usually before age 16) Attacks of symmetrical weakness, usually in the morning. Can develop complete paralysis Mild attacks may just affect a small group of muscles, often in the legs Weakness usually lasts a few hours but can last up to 3 days Precipitants: high-carbohydrate meal, vigorous exercise the day before Permanent muscle weakness later on in the disease **DH**: may be precipitated by any drugs that cause hypokalaemia, eg salbutamol, steroids, insulin **FH**: usually hereditary	Exercise EMG and nerve conduction studies crucial in diagnosis. May require hypokalaemic provocation (with a glucose and insulin bolus) to induce the characteristic changes Avoidance of precipitating factors Carbonic anhydrase inhibitors for prophylaxis, oral potassium supplements to manage attacks Screening of family members is controversial: the genetic defect is heterogeneous with incomplete penetrance

(*continued*)

Differential diagnosis	Clinical judgement and maintaining patient welfare
Motor neuron disease	
Insidious-onset weakness, atrophy and fasciculation Symptoms often begin distally and progress proximally Common complaints include reduced manual dexterity, wrist drop, foot drop or cramps of the small muscles of the hand and/or foot Bulbar involvement leads to speech difficulties or difficulty swallowing. Tongue fasciculations are common Cognitive impairment, with frontal lobe symptoms, sometimes reported	Diagnosis is usually arrived at after exclusion of other pathology over several months or years During this time clinicians will have to address patient anxieties about a devastating progressive disease EMG (fibrillation and fasciculations) and nerve conduction studies more useful than imaging in diagnosis It is important to discuss end-of-life decisions with the patient, who may wish to instigate an advanced directive/living will. Advanced directives and the degree to which they should influence clinical decisions are a controversial area

SCENARIO 15. PAINFUL JOINTS OF THE HAND AND WRIST

'Please could you see this 50-year-old painter and decorator who complains of a swollen, painful index finger. This came on abruptly 5 days ago and is barely controlled with NSAIDs. He is overweight and drinks fairly heavily.'

'This 34-year-old architect complains of joint stiffness in her hands that is particularly troubling in the morning. She is concerned that she is not able to keep up with her workload. Radiographs of the hand were reported as normal. I would be grateful for your advice about further investigation.'

'This 30-year-old woman from Nigeria, who has previously attended my clinic for reactive depression after a miscarriage, now complains of painful wrists and knees. She is having trouble looking after her young daughter. She was very distressed and tearful about this when she attended my clinic today. Please advise regarding her further investigation and management.'

'The lawyer of this 50-year-old-secretary recently contacted me requesting a medical report about possible repetitive strain injury. The secretary has attended once before complaining of painful wrists and joints while typing. Radiographs showed some small osteophyte formation, but were otherwise normal. I have informed her solicitor that a rheumatology opinion would be more appropriate.'

CLINICAL COMMUNICATION SKILLS AND MANAGING PATIENT'S CONCERNS

1. Verify the information provided
'Tell me in your own words what the problem is.'

2. HPC
Open to closed questions keeping in mind the **differential diagnosis**, eg
Rheumatoid arthritis (RA)
SLE
Osteoarthritis
Crystal arthropathy

3. Previous investigations
Previous radiographs? Blood tests? Seen by a rheumatologist?

4. SR
Symptoms of serositis (pericarditis, pleuritis, scleritis) or vasculitis (eg neuropathies). Recent gastroenteritis or an STI (reactive arthritis). Loin pain (urate renal stones). Fatigue, weight loss, myalgia, rash

5. PMH
Cardiovascular disease, peptic ulcer disease (NSAIDs), previous TB (planned anti-TNF-α treatment?)
Previous DVT/PE (SLE)

6. DH
NSAIDs and complications, DMARDs and side effects

7. FH
RA, spondylarthropathies

8. SH
Occupational history and assessment of level of disability. Smoking. Sexual history may be important in reactive arthritis

9. Summarise
'Is there anything else we haven't discussed that you feel is important?'

10. Thank the patient

Painful joints of the hands and wrist

Volunteered problems

Alarm symptoms
Leg/arm/hand weakness, sensory loss, anuria, chest pain

Disease interaction
Impact of multisystem inflammatory disease on other organs or established disease (eg rheumatoid arthritis and high mortality from cardiac disease)
High mortality from non-arthritic disease (eg cardiac, pulmonary)

Therapeutic successes and failures
Adverse events and monitoring after introduction of new immunomodulator (eg azathioprine and leukopenia)
Non-compliance with medication when well

Risks to others
eg now unsafe in the workplace due to a new disability

Daily life and disease
How do specific disabilities translate into limitations on daily life and work?

Final problem list and plan of action

1. Any features of RA should prompt urgent referral to a rheumatologist for early DMARD therapy to prevent deformity and disability

2. Exclusion of other organ involvement

3. Management of risk factors for associated disease (especially cardiac disease in RA)

4. Step-down approach to therapy in inflammatory arthropathies increasingly popular

5. Immunosuppresants and their side effects/ risks

6. Steroids and bone protection/ osteporosis risk assessment

7. Secondary prevention for cardiac risk factors (RA)

Differential diagnosis	Clinical judgement and maintaining patient welfare
Rheumatoid arthritis	
Establishing criteria for urgent rheumatology referral • Morning joint stiffness lasting ≥30 min • Swelling of three or more joints • Involvement of the metocarpophalangeal or metatarsophalangeal joints Constitutional symptoms: malaise, fatigue, symptoms of anaemia, weight loss, muscular aches and pains The minority have an abrupt onset of symptoms (about 15%) If the diagnosis is already established, look for symptoms suggestive of disease activity • Worsening joint pain • Increased duration of morning joint stiffness • Increased fatigue • Worsening limitation of function **SR**: other system involvement: pleuritis, pericarditis, neurological deficit (mononeuritis multiplex), ischaemic heart disease, dry mouth/eyes (Sjögren's syndrome) **PMH**: cardiovascular disease and risk factors (cholesterol, BP) **DH**: DMARDs and adverse effects. Steroids – frequency and duration of use **SH**: level of disability, occupational impact, alcohol and DMARDs (eg methotrexate). Smoking (further risk of cardiac disease)	**Need for immediate referral to rheumatologist for DMARD therapy to prevent joint disability** Surgical intervention may be necessary, eg to improve joint function/stabilise joints/tendon repair/carpal tunnel release Exclusion of rheumatoid emergencies (renal failure, vasculitis, atlantoaxial subluxation) Management of long-term immunomodulators and their adverse effects (hepatotoxicity, nephrotoxicity, pneumonitis, infections) Assess for changes in level of ability and adjust social support accordingly Aggressive management of cardiac risk factors Management of other organ involvement (eg pulmonary fibrosis, pericarditis, pleurisy) and associated autoimmune disease (eg Sjögren syndrome, Raynaud's disease) Steroid-sparing therapy, bone protection and monitoring for osteoporosis

(*continued*)

Differential diagnosis	Clinical judgement and maintaining patient welfare
SLE	
Joint pain is the most frequent presenting complaint Small joints of the hands commonly affected Disability is mostly due to pain that often migrates from joint to joint Other features General: malaise, fever, lethargy Skin: malar rash, photosensitivity, discoid lupus, alopecia, Raynaud's disease Renal disease (50%): nephritic/nephritic syndromes Pericarditis/pleuritis Anaemia, thrombocytopenia (bleeding diatheses) **PMH**: recurrent infection, neuropsychiatric disease, more than two recurrent miscarriages, previous DVT/PE (anti-phospholipid syndrome) **DH**: immunosuppressants – dose and duration important Note drug-induced lupus (procainamide, hydralazine, quinidine and 35 other drugs)	A multidisciplinary approach is crucial – several systems are frequently affected Exclusion of SLE-associated emergencies: vasculitis, glomerulonephritis, severe neurovasculitis, diffuse alveolar haemorrhage, profound thrombocytopenia Assessment of disease activity: C3 and C4 complement levels, CRP, ESR and dsDNA are all markers of activity Management of long-term immunomodulators and their adverse effects (hepatotoxicity, nephrotoxicity, pneumonitis, infections) Monitor for renal disease with regular urinalysis Similar to RA, cardiac disease is more common and treatable risk factors should be attenuated aggressively (smoking cessation, cholesterol-lowering medications, BP control, etc) Steroid-sparing therapy, bone protection and monitoring for osteoporosis Anticoagulation for patients with previous DVT/PE and positive anti-phospholipid antibodies
Osteoarthritis	
Pain and stiffness (<1 h) in any joint Distal interphalangeal joint commonly affected Often asymmetrical History of excessive use/load bearing of affected joint **PMH**: previous orthopaedic operations **SH**: occupational history and limitation of work. Any legal action in process against employer (eg for repetitive strain injury) may worsen prognosis	Assessment of level of disability by OT and physiotherapist Referral to orthopaedic surgeon where appropriate Encourage weight loss, exercise, occupational adjustments Pain control with NSAIDs, paracetamol and steroid injection for analgesia-resistant joint disease

(*continued*)

Differential diagnosis	Clinical judgement and maintaining patient welfare
Crystal arthropathy	
Acute onset (often at night) of a hot, swollen, exquisitely tender joint, often the metatarsophalangeal joint of the great toe Pseudogout may have a more insidious onset than gout Fevers, rigors, malaise – common to both crystal arthropathies and septic arthritis **PMH**: renal calculi, haemoproliferative disorders, renal impairment **SH**: alcohol consumption	Always treat for septic arthritis until it is excluded (this may not be necessary in recurrent identical episodes of known gout or podagra) Establish adequate prophylaxis and lifestyle changes to prevent future attacks Low-purine diet

SCENARIO 16. THE PATIENT WITH HIV

A 34-year-old man was diagnosed with HIV 5 years ago and commenced on HAART shortly afterwards. He is troubled by intermittent diarrhoea and occasional faecal leakage which has been very distressing. His weight is stable and he has not noticed any bleeding per rectum.

Please advise on the further investigation of this 44-year-old woman from Ghana. She was diagnosed with HIV when she first came to the UK 14 years ago. She has been taking HAART for 10 years and has steadily lost weight over the past 4 years. Her friends and family have commented on this recently which has upset her. She describes no specific symptoms but does report profound tiredness.

A 56-year-old man describes a taste of blood in his mouth and ulcers that will not heal. He was diagnosed with HIV 4 months ago with a CD4 count of 150 cells/mm^3 at diagnosis. Mouthwashes have not improved his symptoms and he has now developed epigastric pain that will not respond to a proton pump inhibitor. I would be grateful for your further opinion.

I would be grateful for your urgent assessment of this 30-year-old woman who recently tested positive for HIV in her local sexual health clinic. She reports a 2-week history of malaise with a worsening headache. Her family tell me she has been forgetful and behaving strangely over the last three days.

I would be grateful for your opinion on this 67-year-old man with painful legs. He has been on HAART since 2004 and has a normal CD4 count

and a viral load below quantification. Yesterday he fell down the stairs whilst climbing them and he has been having difficulty getting out of the bath.

This 40-year-old HIV positive woman has been complaining of intermittent right upper quadrant pain for 6 weeks. An USS of the liver was normal but liver function tests reveal a raised ALP and GGT. Her adherence to HAART has been poor recently and her last CD4 count was 250 cells/mm^3.

Please see this 42-year-old man with HIV is a lifetime smoker. Over the past 6 months he has developed progressive shortness of breath, worsened by exertion. In addition he describes night-sweats and weight loss.

This 27-year-old man was diagnosed with HIV 2 months ago and commenced on HAART. He has developed some dark skin lesions on his lower limbs. I would be grateful for your further assessment.

A 56-year-old man from Nigeria has been on HAART for 12 years. He has high cholesterol and hypertension. He recently described central chest pain worsened by climbing the stairs. I would be grateful for your further assessment.

This 26-year-old ex-intravenous drug user has recently developed visual difficulties. He describes thread-like dark lines in his field of vision which appear to drift slowly. He first noticed these two weeks ago but they have since increased and now obscure his vision on the left side. Many thanks for your opinion.

CLINICAL COMMUNICATION SKILLS AND MANAGING PATIENT'S CONCERNS

1. Verify the information provided
'Tell me in your own words what the problem is.'

2. HPC
- Establish the current problem
- Establish mode of original presentation and likely mode of infection
- Establish disease history to date focusing on any AIDS-defining illnesses

3. Previous investigations
What is the latest CD4+ count and viral load?

4. SR
Full screen of all systems to pre-empt emerging HIV-related problems (see table below). Depression and anxiety common

5. PMH
HIV-related disease (eg Kaposi's sarcoma) and previous screening for other STIs (eg HCV, HBV, *Chlamydia* sp., gonorrhoea)

6. DH
Antiretrovirals – focus on duration of therapy, recent changes (known viral resistance?), compliance and side effects. Other drugs that interfere with HAART metabolism?

7. FH
Affected relatives/children? Plans for a family?

8. SH
Current occupation and potential risk to others (eg healthcare professional) Sexual history: gender of partners, frequency and nature of sexual contact. Use of barrier contraceptives Previous/ongoing IV drug use.

9. Summarise
'Is there anything else we haven't discussed that you feel is important?'

10. Thank the patient

The patient with HIV

Volunteered problems

Alarm symptoms
Any new symptom should raise suspicion of HIV-related disease and disease progression

Disease interaction
eg HIV and HCV/HBV co-infection (more rapid progression to cirrhosis)

Therapeutic successes and failures
Many patients require at least one modification to their antiretrovirals before the optimum regimen is found
Common side effects: lipoatrophy, dyslipidaemia, dyspepsia/GORD, rash, hypersensitivity reaction Immune reconstitution disease (unmasking of pre-existing infections with immune recovery with HAART)

Risks to others
What is the patient's perception of risk to self and others and is it accurate? Contact tracing issues must be elicited

Daily life and disease
Assess impact of drug regimen, adverse effects and disease burden on life and relationships
How does the current problem further influence the situation?

Final problem list and plan of action

1. Establish stage of disease (CD4 count and viral load)

2. A lower CD4+ baseline (usually at presentation) limits the upper plateau of CD4+ count that can be achieved with therapy. The CD4+ count at presentation thus has prognostic significance

3. Triage urgency of further investigation of new symptoms (should this be done as an outpatient or inpatient?)

4. It is often difficult to disentangle medication side effects from new HIV-related disease – several consultations with changes in medications may be needed

5. New contact tracing issues may arise long after first diagnosis

Differential diagnosis	Clinical judgement and maintaining patient welfare
Diarrhoea	
Consider all the causes of diarrhoea common in the non-HIV population and the following (in approximate order of decreasing prevalence) • HAART side effect: foscarnet – 30% • Interferon-α – 29% • Nelfinavir – 25–30%, didanosine (ddI) 17–28% • Ritonavir – 12–18% • Zalcitabine (ddC) – 10% Cryptosporidia: cholera-like diarrhoea – severity inversely related to CD4 count. Often present with volume depletion *Cyclosporum, Microsporum* spp.: waxing and waning watery diarrhoea, anorexia, fatigue, weight loss. May persist for several months in HIV CMV colitis: abdominal pain, fever, bloody diarrhoea, weight loss *Mycobacterium avium intracellulare* (MAI): CD4 count usually <150, fever, abdominal pain (often RUQ), anorexia, weight loss *Clostridium difficile*: bloody diarrhoea after a course of antibiotics for another infection. More common in HIV population Lymphogranuloma venereum (LGV): *Chlamydia trachomatis*. Can cause bloody diarrhoea in the tertiary phase in MSM, painful inguinal lymphadenopathy is characteristic, fever, chills, malaise HSV proctitis: pain in sacral nerve root distribution, bloody mucus discharge, painful inguinal lymphadenopathy Intestinal TB: fever, weight loss, malaise, diarrhoea, abdominal pain *E. coli, Campylobacter* sp., *Shigella* sp., *Entamoeba* sp. and *Giardia* sp. are all more common in the HIV population IBD is also encountered and easily missed	Colitis: frequent small-volume bloody or mucopurulent stools, lower abdominal pain, tenesmus and faecal urgency Small intestine infection: watery diarrhoea, dehydration, weight loss, abdominal cramps Multiple stool samples for microscopy and culture are key. A high neutrophil count in the stool suggests bacterial infection, eg *Salmonella, Shigella, Listeria, Campylobacter* spp. or *Escherichia coli*. Bloody diarrhoea without a high faecal neutrophil count suggests amoebiasis Specific tests that won't be done unless you ask • Biopsy and staining: *Isospora belli*, CMV, tuberculosis, MAI • Stool culture (non-routine): *E. coli* O157 in McConkey sorbitol medium • Stool antigen test: *Giardia, Cryptosporidium* spp. Empirical therapy should be instituted immediately, eg fluoroquinolone and metronidazole. Both drugs successfully treat the underlying bacterial infections most commonly associated with diarrhoea, ie *Shigella, Salmonella* and *Campylobacter* spp. Treat dehydration, electrolyte imbalance and any nutritional deficit Endoscopic investigation with biopsies is nearly always appropriate, especially if diarrhoea fails to resolve or if the CD4 count <200 (because multiple pathologies may be present) Changing medications may not be advisable even if the side effect of diarrhoea is severe. Loperamide may offer some relief The prevalence of diarrhoea in the HIV-positive population is approximately 40%, higher in developing countries. Rapid and thorough assessment is crucial to minimising the impact on day-to-day life

(continued)

Differential diagnosis	Clinical judgement and maintaining patient welfare
Weight loss	
HIV-associated wasting: involuntary loss of 10% of ideal body weight in the absence of another disease process that could account for it Weakness, lethargy and fever are commonly associated. Can occur despite HAART and a normal CD4 count HAART-related fat redistribution: typically lipoatrophy occurs in the face and extremities with lipotrophy in the trunk and abdomen HAART-related pancreatic insufficiency and malabsorption: bulky, pale, frequent stools. Weight loss despite adequate calorie intake. Nucleoside analogues and protease inhibitors are common culprits	Gaunt appearance can be stigmatising. This can have a major effect on compliance with HAART if the patient feels that this is the cause Degree of weight loss directly proportional to mortality in HIV-wasting syndromes Bioelectrical impedance analysis should be arranged – this is the cheapest and most accurate diagnostic test Patients require careful systematic exclusion of underlying infection or malignancy as a cause of weight loss before diagnosing HIV-associated wasting Full dietician assessment. Lean body mass is often lost before fat – high-protein and high-calorie diets are usually appropriate Thiazolidinediones ('glitazones') may be effective in reversing lipoatrophy Enzyme replacement with meals may counter pancreatic insufficiency
Abdominal pain	
HAART-related GORD and dyspepsia (see above for GORD and dyspepsia symptoms) HAART- or pentamidine-related pancreatitis (see above for pancreatitis symptoms). Combined didanosine and tenofovir therapy carries the highest risk of pancreatitis (about 13%) Cholecystitis (CMV, cryptosporidiosis): RUQ pain, jaundice, fever, pale stools, dark urine GI lymphoma: abdominal pain, weight loss, fever, pruritus, night sweats, alcohol-induced pain, diarrhoea, GI bleed GI Kaposi's sarcoma: abdominal pain, GI bleeding, symptoms of intermittent obstruction (bloating, vomiting and constipation)	Always need to exclude infectious or malignant pathology before attributing symptoms to medications (the most common cause of GI upset in HIV) Often the offending agent cannot be stopped – standard medical management of dyspepsia and GORD is appropriate Pancreatitis, cholecystitis and GI bleeding are emergencies that require immediate investigation and treatment GI lymphoma and Kaposi's sarcoma are difficult to diagnose in the small intestine. Capsule endoscopy and MR enteroclysis are increasingly available and optimise pick-up rates in small bowel malignancy

(*continued*)

Differential diagnosis	Clinical judgement and maintaining patient welfare
Headache	
CNS cryptococcosis: CD4 <100. Indolent onset of headache (75%), fever (70%), neck stiffness (about 30%), altered mental state (20%), photophobia (about 20%) CNS toxoplasmosis: CD4 <200. Constitutional symptoms followed by headache, drowsiness and confusion. Seizures and focal neurological deficits tend to develop later. Can progress to coma within days **CNS lymphoma**: CD4 <100. Similar symptoms to toxoplasmosis but more indolent onset	Early CSF analysis and CT imaging are key in all cases, eg EBV DNA in CSF (detected by PCR) is a useful corollary of CNS lymphoma Exclude extracranial disease Effective prophylaxis against further infection may be appropriate HAART-naïve patients usually benefit from immediate introduction of therapy. This especially improves the prognosis in CNS lymphoma
Confusion	
Progressive multifocal leukoencephalopathy (PML) (demyelination caused by reactivation of endemic JC papovavirus): CD4 <100. Usually presents with focal neurological symptoms, eg behavioural change, speech, cognitive dysfunction, motor weakness and visual impairment. Headaches are rare. It evolves over several weeks but progresses more rapidly than AIDS–dementia complex CMV encephalitis: may have other systemic disturbance due to CMV (eg colitis, hepatitis, pneumonitis) plus three distinct presentations 1. Ventriculoencephalitis characterised by abrupt onset and rapid-onset confusion and lethargy 2. Facial and oculomotor cranial nerve palsies 3. Slowly progressive cognitive impairment similar to the AIDS–dementia complex HIV-1 encephalopathy and AIDS–dementia complex: CD4 <200. Insidious onset of behavioural and/or mood change, apathy and/or loss of interest in social activities. Poor concentration and decreased libido are common. Progresses to global cognitive impairment especially affecting memory and language functions	Other causes of cognitive impairment must be excluded ('dementia screen': eg CT of the head, TFTs, vitamin B_{12}, syphilis serology) Depression and anxiety are commonly associated and need to be addressed Empirical initiation of IV ganciclovir may be appropriate until CMV encephalitis has been excluded Optimised HAART must be achieved to slow progression of AIDS–dementia complex Beware an initial worsening of PML on commencing HAART due to immune reconstitution Often cognitive impairment is permanent, which has major implications for independence and working life. Multidisciplinary input is crucial

(*continued*)

Differential diagnosis	Clinical judgement and maintaining patient welfare
Weak legs	
HIV-1-associated vacuolar myelopathy: CD4 <100. Gradual onset of lower limb leg weakness, numbness and loss of balance are common. Progresses to cognitive decline and sphincter dysfunction HTLV-1-associated myelopathy (tropical spastic paraparesis): this most commonly presents with insidious onset leg weakness. Other symptoms include painful legs, paraesthesiae, back pain and bladder dysfunction. Neurological disability usually stabilises after a few years. An associated sicca syndrome, arthralgias and dermatitis are very common Elicit history of travel to (or originating from) endemic areas: southern Japan, the Caribbean, parts of Central Africa and South America	Early input from occupational therapist and physiotherapist may limit the impact of disability on day-to-day life HTLV-1-associated myelopathy requires long-term surveillance for development of T-cell leukaemias

(*continued*)

Differential diagnosis	Clinical judgement and maintaining patient welfare
Jaundice/abnormal LFTs	
NNRTI-induced hepatitis: concomitant administration of protease inhibitors increases the risk of liver toxicity. There is no clear evidence that prolonged HAART is associated with liver fibrosis HBV and/or HCV co-infection: IV drug use is usually the mode of HIV transmission. Patients may present with features of decompensated liver disease (eg ascites, encephalopathy, jaundice) CMV hepatitis: CD4 usually <100. CMV hepatitis frequently presents with isolated abnormal LFTs. Jaundice is unusual and progression to cirrhosis is rare Biliary tract disease: cryptosporidia, microsporidia, CMV, *Mycobacterium avium intracellulare* can all cause biliary tract infection which may manifest as abnormal LFTs (γ-GT, bilirubin and alkaline phosphatase) rather than acute cholecystitis	Need to stage liver disease (Child–Pugh score, ultrasonography, varices surveillance if cirrhotic, etc) and exclude other causes of liver disease All patients with HIV should be screened for HBV and HCV infection Liver biopsy may be necessary to distinguish NNRTI-induced transaminitis from inflammation due to viral hepatitis in HIV/HBV or HIV/HCV co-infection Patients with viral hepatitis co-infection tend to progress more rapidly to cirrhosis. This has a detrimental affect on HAART tolerance. Early, optimal control of both infections is therefore essential Liver transplantation is an increasingly successful option in HIV-positive individuals with chronic liver disease – survival rates at 1 year are similar to HIV-negative graft recipients. Early assessment for transplantation is crucial (the HIV-positive pre-transplantation population have a higher mortality rate than HIV-negative individuals with a similar severity of liver disease) Treatment regimens for HBV and/or HCV co-infection are sometimes synergistic and sometimes antagonistic. Joint management by a hepatologist and HIV specialist is important

(*continued*)

Differential diagnosis	Clinical judgement and maintaining patient welfare
Breathlessness	
***Pneumocystis jiroveci* pneumonia (PJP; previously *Pneumocystis carinii* pneumonia or PCP)**: CD <250. Progressive exertional dyspnoea, fever and a non-productive cough are almost universal presenting complaints Chest discomfort, weight loss, rigors and (more rarely) haemoptysis are also features Recent chest radiographs may have been normal **PMH**: recent oral thrush (susceptibility to other fungal infection is common) **DH**: not on co-trimoxazole prophylaxis *Mycobacterium avium intracellulare*: CD4 <50. Insidious onset of worsening cough, sputum production, weight loss, fever, lethargy and night sweats. Patients sometimes complain of RUQ pain. Haemoptysis is rare. Breathlessness is unusual unless there is an associated hypersensitivity pneumonitis. May have a history of exposure to MAI from using jacuzzis. Fever of unknown origin is a common presentation **PMH**: pulmonary MAI often associated with established chronic lung disease, eg COPD Lymphocytic interstitial pneumonia: dyspnoea with fever, cough and pleuritic chest pain. May follow an indolent course and present much later as fibrosis and/or bronchiectasis Tuberculosis (see above): CD4 count variable (often normal) CMV pneumonitis: CD4 <150. In addition to breathlessness the patient may have an associated mononucleosis syndrome (fever and lymphadenopathy) *Pseudomonas aeruginosa* infection: CD4 <50. Recent inpatient stay and/or invasive ventilation, productive cough, anorexia, dyspnoea HIV myocarditis/cardiomyopathy: CD4 often <100. Orthopnoea, PND, exertional dyspnoea and ankle swelling HIV-related pulmonary hypertension (no clear relationship with CD4 count): exertional dyspnoea, ankle swelling, lethargy, syncope (about 10%). Kaposi's sarcoma at other sites (human herpesvirus 8 appears to be the pathogenic organism)	Bronchoalveolar lavage (BAL) is often needed for definitive diagnosis of an opportunistic pulmonary infection An elevated LDH is a useful pointer towards PJP in an HIV-positive patient with an acute respiratory illness The severity of PJP needs to be determined by arterial blood gas sampling. This affects management – only severe PJP seems to benefit from adjunctive steroid therapy Diagnostic criteria for MAI lung disease require specific numbers of AFB-staining sputum or BAL and positive mycobacterial culture Anti-mycobacterial therapy may adversely affect organs already impaired by HIV-related disease (eg ethambutol and optic neuritis rifampicin and hepatotoxicity). Close surveillance for complications is necessary Need to exclude extrapulmonary disease (eg disseminated CMV, MAI) Long-term infection with its associated anorexia and a catabolic state often results in undernutrition or malnutrition which should be corrected For all opportunistic infections antimicrobial resistance is a growing problem. Sending repeat specimens for sensitivity testing is important, especially if initial response to therapy is poor Prophylaxis against future infection is key, eg co-trimoxazole for PJP. It may be safe to stop prophylaxis if the CD4 count recovers above a certain number (eg CD4 >200 in the case of co-trimoxazole for PJP) Treatment for HIV cardiomyopathy is similar to non-ischaemic cardiomyopathy with β blockers and ACE inhibitors, whereas endothelin antagonists appear to be effective in HIV-associated pulmonary hypertension

(*continued*)

Differential diagnosis	Clinical judgement and maintaining patient welfare
Skin rash/lesion	
Kaposi's sarcoma: CD4 count variable, often normal. In the HAART era this usually manifests as subtle purple patches rather than large fixed plaques Molluscum contagiosum: CD4 <50. Multiple, small, round, shiny, wart-like lumps with a depression in the centre. Facial involvement is common Erythema nodosum (often associated with immune reconstitution and CD4 >200): raised, large, red, painful nodules, typically over the shins Prurigo nodularis: itchy bumps over the arms and trunk. The itch is often maddening and unresponsive to antihistamines Photosensitivity: this is usually drug related and particularly affects those with a low CD4 count. Co-trimoxazole (PJP prophylaxis) is a common culprit	Skin biopsy is sometimes necessary to make the diagnosis (eg Kaposi's sarcoma, erythema nodosum) Most conditions associated with a low CD4 count will improve with HAART and immune reconstitution Such visible stigmata of HIV/AIDS are rarely life threatening but have a profound effect on patient's level of social interaction and general wellbeing and should be treated aggressively Skin lesions are often indicative of advanced disease and should instigate a thorough screen for other AIDS-defining illnesses which may be initially asymptomatic (eg CMV retinitis, oral candidiasis)
Chest pain	
Stable/unstable angina: protease inhibitors, a main component of HAART, induce atherogenic metabolic effects such as dyslipidaemia and insulin resistance. Premature IHD is an increasing problem in the HAART era	Ensure adequate primary and secondary prevention by early treatment of dyslipidaemia. IHD may compound other HIV-related cardiac disease (eg cardiomyopathy)
Arthralgia/myalgia	
Myositis and/or rhabdomyolysis Painful muscles (often proximal groups) with associated weakness. Dark urine Causes • Zidovudine • Infection (eg toxoplasmosis) • HIV-related polymyositis HIV-associated arthritis: an oligoarticular, asymmetrical and peripheral arthritis predominantly affecting the knees and ankles. It is usually self-limiting (1–5 weeks) Septic arthritis: fever, pain and markedly reduced range of movement. Atypical organisms include *Staphylococcus aureus*, *Neisseria gonorrhoeae*, *Candida albicans* and *M. tuberculosis*	Need to exclude emergencies (eg rhabdomyolysis or destructive arthritis) and triage investigation and treatment accordingly Cessation of a putative causative HAART agent should always be discussed with an HIV specialist

(*continued*)

Differential diagnosis	Clinical judgement and maintaining patient welfare
Visual disturbance	
CMV retinitis: CD4 <100. Patients describe floaters, photopsia or visual loss, without a red or painful eye. On the whole, visual acuity is usually good at the time of diagnosis HIV retinopathy: insidious loss of visual acuity with loss of colour and/or peripheral vision Toxoplasma choroidoretinitis: insidious bilateral loss of visual acuity which may occur many months or years after the initial infection	Need to exclude systemic manifestations of the causative organism Early treatment and regular monitoring are crucial to preserve vision

Clinical guideline: British HIV Association (BHIVA) 2012

Primary HAART for HIV-1

Two nucleoside reverse transcriptase inhibitors (NRTIs)

Plus either

- A ritonavir-boosted protease inhibitor or
- A non-nucleoside reverse transcriptase inhibitor (NNRTI) or
- An integrase inhibitor

REFERENCES

1. Scirica BM *et al* (1999). Differences between men and women in the management of unstable angina pectoris (The GUARANTEE Registry). The GUARANTEE Investigators. *American Journal of Cardiology*; 84(10), pp. 1145–1150.
2. Hasbun R *et al* (2001). Computed tomography of the head before lumbar puncture in adults with suspected meningitis. *New England Journal of Medicine*; 354, pp. 1727–1733.

STATION 3

The Cardiovascular and Neurological Examinations

THE CARDIOLOGY EXAMINATION

There is no one case that appears more than others within the cardiology station. Below are the top five cases that have been reported in the last few years of the examination. Mitral stenosis is perhaps being seen less frequently as the incidence of rheumatic heart disease decreases within the population.

1. Aortic valve replacement
2. Mitral valve replacement
3. Aortic stenosis
4. Mitral regurgitation
5. Congenital heart disease (mostly ventricular septal defect).

Examination

Approach to the patient

Introduce yourself to the patient and ask for permission to examine him or her, explaining that you would like to examine the pulse and listen to the heart. Wash your hands. Ask if the patient has any pain before you start. Position the patient correctly (sitting up at 45°). Ask permission to expose the chest, completely if possible.

Observation

Look at the patient and assess if he or she appears well/unwell, dyspnoeic at rest, cyanosed or with mitral facies, a dusky malar flush seen in mitral stenosis with pulmonary hypertension:

- Cyanotic congenital heart disease occurs in right-to-left shunts such as: tetralogy of Fallot, transposition of the great arteries, hypoplastic left heart syndrome, pulmonary atresia and stenosis, and patent ductus arteriosus.
- Non-cyanotic congenital heart disease with left-to-right shunts: atrial septal defect (ASD), ventricular septal defect (VSD) and aortic coarctation with patent ductus arteriosus (PDA). If long-standing, however, pulmonary hypertension can develop leading to reversal of the shunt from right to left and therefore cyanosis; this is known as Eisenmenger's syndrome.

Are there any obvious central sternotomy scars or deformity from a pacemaker or internal defibrillator? Occasionally it is possible to hear the ticking sound of a metallic heart valve from the end of the bed or when standing near the patient's chest.

Look for any obvious phenotypic features that fit with a particular syndrome associated with cardiological abnormalities:

- Down's syndrome: can be associated with VSD, atrioventricular septal defect (AVSD), PDA and tetralogy of Fallot. (Down syndrome is caused by trisomy of chromosome 21 and is the most common autosomal trisomy.) Complications of Down syndrome include: cognitive impairment, congenital heart disease, endocrine disorders and haematological malignancies. Phenotypic features include short stature with a thick short neck, low-set small ears, a flattened nasal bridge, upward slanting eyes with epicanthal folds, wide short hands with a single palmar crease, and a 'sandal gap' between the first and second toes.
- Turner's syndrome: commonly associated with left-sided heart defects including aortic coarctation, bicuspid aortic valve, aortic stenosis and hypertension. (Turner syndrome is caused by monosomy X where part or all of one of the X chromosomes is missing – 45X0.) Complications include heart defects and aortic dissection, endocrine abnormalities including hypothyroidism and diabetes, renal malformations with horse-shoe kidneys and hypogonadism. Phenotypic features include a short female, webbed neck, cubitus valgus, widely spaced nipples with a shield-like chest, hypoplastic nails and short fourth metacarpals, and occasionally hand and feet lymphoedema and multiple naevi.
- Noonan syndrome: most commonly associated with right-sided heart defects so

look for pulmonary stenosis, but may have other congenital heart defects such as ASD and VSD. (This condition is autosomal dominant and affects males and females.) Noonan syndrome shares many phenotypic features of Turner syndrome. Complications include variable hearing loss and mild cognitive impairment, male infertility, congenital heart disease and lymphoedema. Phenotypic features include short stature with a webbed neck, down-slanting eyes and low-set ears, triangular shaped facies, widely spaced nipples, cubitus valgus, and pectus excavatum or carinatum.

- Williams' syndrome: most commonly associated with aortic stenosis but may also be associated with pulmonary stenosis and mitral regurgitation. (This is a rare genetic disorder caused by a spontaneous deletion of part of chromosome 7.) Complications include cognitive impairment, anxiety, cardiac defects, diabetes and hearing loss. Phenotypic features include an elfin facies with a short nose and broad nasal tip, wide full mouth and small pointed chin, a long neck with sloping shoulders and short stature.

Hands

With the patient's hands outstretched, examine for the following:

- Tar stains (coronary heart disease (CHD))
- Clubbing (cyanotic congenital heart disease, subacute bacterial endocarditis (SBE), atrial myxoma and Eisenmenger syndrome)
- Cool peripheries with peripheral cyanosis
- Capillary pulsation in the proximal nailbed with aortic regurgitation (Quincke's sign)
- Osler's nodes (painful tender raised lesions on palms and feet)
- Janeway's lesions (non-tender small erythematous nodules on palms, fingers or feet)
- Splinter haemorrhages (infective endocarditis)
- Xanthomas (hyperlipidaemia and CHD)
- Arachnodactyly associated with Marfan

syndrome and other collagen disorders (mitral valve prolapse, aortic root dilatation and aortic dissection).

Pulse and blood pressure

When assessing the pulse, feel for rate, rhythm and character (the last can be difficult to assess in more peripheral pulses). If the pulse rhythm is irregularly irregular do not report this as atrial fibrillation, which can be diagnosed only on an ECG. Assess for the water-hammer/collapsing pulse seen in atrial regurgitation (AR): 'I would like to lift your right arm to assess the pulse further. Do you have any pain in this arm?' Wrap your right hand around the patient's right wrist so that your four finger pulps are aligned along the radial artery, then use your left hand to lift the patient's arm at the elbow. You are feeling for a collapsing pulse running along the fingers of your right hand.

Palpate the brachial pulse briefly and look for scars of previous angiography over the cubital fossa.

Feel for radioradial or radiofemoral delay if suspecting aortic arch pathology.

You can mention that you would like to measure the BP at this point, although some choose to leave it until the end.

Neck

Observe the jugular venous pressure (JVP), assessing height and waveform. The patient should be at 45° with the neck slightly turned away but relaxing the sternocleidomastoid muscles. The JVP height seen in the internal jugular vein acts as a measure of right atrial pressure, because there are no intervening valves between the internal jugular vein (IJV), superior vena cava (SVC) and right atrium. The normal right atrial pressure should be 10 cmH$_2$O – approximately 10 cm blood, which is 4 cm (four finger-breadths) above the manubriosternal joint or just above the clavicle, when lying at 45°.

- There are three waves (a, c and v) and two descents (x, y):
  - a wave: atrial contraction
  - c wave: ventricles contract causing pressure to rise in the atrium slightly as the tricuspid valve bulges up into the atrium
  - x descent: atrial relaxation and the tricuspid valve is now pulled down
  - v wave: atrial filling when the tricuspid valve is closed
  - y descent: rapid emptying of the right atrium into the right ventricle as the tricuspid valve opens.

It is really only possible to distinguish the a and v waves on inspection and these can be determined by timing against the opposite carotid pulse, where the a wave occurs just before the carotid impulse and the v wave just after.

The JVP can be distinguished from the carotid pulse by the following features:

- Double waveform
- Compressible
- Varies with respiration, falling with inspiration
- Enhanced by the hepatojugular reflex (manual pressure applied to the right upper quadrant of the abdomen).

The JVP is raised in the following conditions:

- Heart failure
- Iatrogenic fluid overload
- Constrictive pericarditis (Kussmaul's sign where the JVP rises with inspiration)
- Tamponade
- SVC obstruction (SVCO) – there are also no JVP pulsations.

There are large a waves in tricuspid stenosis, pulmonary stenosis and pulmonary hypertension. Very large 'cannon a waves' occur in complete heart block.

Large v waves occur with tricuspid regurgitation and the v wave coincides with the carotid pulse:

Rapid y descent occurs in constrictive pericarditis and tricuspid regurgitation.

Palpate the carotid artery where the character of the pulse is best assessed:

- Large-volume collapsing pulse (aortic regurgitation, persistent ductus arteriosus, thyrotoxicosis, pregnancy and sepsis)
- Judder on the upstroke with a jerky pulse (hypertrophic cardiomyopathy or HOCM)
- Slow rising (aortic stenosis)
- 'Alternans' with an alternating pulse made up of small and large pulsations consistent with very poor left ventricular (LV) function (severe ischaemic LV failure, dilated cardiomyopathy or aortic stenosis).

Face
- Conjunctival pallor (only look in one eye and ask the patient to pull his or her own eyelid down)
- Xanthelasma and corneal arcus (hyperlipidaemia and ischaemic heart disease (IHD))
- Blue tinge to lips and beneath the tongue (central cyanosis)
- Poor dentition in SBE
- High arched palate (Marfan, Turner and Noonan syndromes).

Inspect the chest
Ask the patent to lift the arms away from the sides, and now take more time to look for sternotomy scars, thoracotomy scars of mitral valve surgery in the left axilla, signs of pacemaker or defibrillator insertion, and unusual pulsations.

Palpation
Palpate for the apex beat and over the whole precordium for any heaves, thrills or palpable sounds.

The apex beat is normally located at the fifth intercostal space in the midclavicular line; measure it from the angle of Louis.

- A thrusting apex beat signifies a high volume load and it is usually laterally displaced. This is seen with mitral regurgitation, aortic regurgitation or an ASD. If the apex is lateral and diffuse, consider LV failure or dilated cardiomyopathy.
- A heaving, pressure-loaded apex beat that is usually non-displaced can be seen in aortic stenosis, hypertension or HOCM.
- A double impulse (palpable atrial systole) apex beat can be felt in HOCM.

Lay the flat of the hand along the left sternal edge to feel for the sustained pressure of a left **parasternal heave** of right ventricular hypertrophy as found in pulmonary stenosis, cor pulmonale, or an ASD or VSD.

Palpate each valve area in turn with the flat of the fingers, for palpable heart sounds and thrills. Thrills are palpable murmurs.

Palpable heart sounds occur in forceful closure:

- S1 (in mitral area) with mitral stenosis ('tapping' apex beat)
- P2 (in pulmonary area) with pulmonary hypertension.

Systolic thrills include:

- Aortic area (aortic stenosis)
- Left sternal edge (VSD or HOCM)
- Apex (mitral regurgitation, often due to ruptured chordae)
- Pulmonary area (pulmonary stenosis)
- Subclavicular area (subclavian artery stenosis or PDA).

Diastolic thrills include:

- Apex (mitral stenosis)
- Left sternal edge (AR).

Auscultation
Listen to each valve area in turn and then the carotids. If you suspect a specific murmur then follow its known radiation and perform any specific manoeuvres, such as changing the patient's posture or phase of respiration, to help accent-uate the murmur. Importantly, remember to PALPATE THE CAROTID while auscultating to help time murmurs.

Heart sounds
The second heart sound (S2) has physiological splitting with A2 occurring slightly before P2, and this splitting becomes wider in inspiration, with increased venous return to the right side of the heart, delaying pulmonary valve closure. It is only really possible to hear splitting of the second heart sound in those aged <30, using the bell in the pulmonary area during inspiration.

- **Reversed splitting** (ie separation between A2 and P2 becoming wider in *expiration* as A2 now comes after P2) occurs in instances where aortic valve closure is delayed such as in aortic stenosis, left bundle-branch block (eg IHD) or right ventricular pacing.
- **S2 is single** in a large VSD where the aortic and pulmonary valves close simultaneously, and **fixed** and wide in an ASD due to left-to-right shunt, causing delayed closure of the pulmonary valve in both phases of respiration.
- **A third heart sound**, S3, is pathological in those aged >30 years, when it is due to rapid filling of the ventricles, eg mitral regurgitation, VSD, dilated cardiomyopathy or a dilated left ventricle with a high LV end-diastolic pressure, eg after a myocardial infarction (MI).
- **A fourth heart sound**, S4, occurring at the end of diastole and representing atrial contraction, occurs in left atrium hypertrophy such as in hypertension, aortic stenosis or HCOM.
- **An ejection click** is a high-pitched sound heard shortly after S1, and represents opening of a stenosed aortic or pulmonary valve.
- **An opening snap** may be heard in diastole, representing mitral valve opening in mitral stenosis.

There may be closing sounds with metallic replacement valves.

Murmurs

Assess all murmurs based on their *timing* in the cardiac cycle, their *location* and their *radiation*. Individual murmurs are discussed in the relevant section.

The volume of murmurs is best graded as 'just audible', 'soft', 'moderate' or 'loud'.

The behaviour of murmurs with inspiration and expiration is crucial to help distinguish the source. Inspiration increases venous return from the vena cava to the right side of the heart, thus accentuating right-sided murmurs, while at the same time decreasing venous return to the left side of the heart and softening murmurs on this side. During expiration, venous return to the right side of the heart reduces and the pulmonary capacitance vessels collapse, increasing venous return to the left side of the heart and so augmenting left-sided heart murmurs. **Remember** that it is *during* the inspiratory and expiratory phases that these changes happen. A common mistake is for candidates to ask the patient to hold the breath in or out against a closed glottis, and this produces artefacts of Valsalva's manoeuvre.

Innocent murmurs are:

- Ejection systolic (crescendo–decrescendo)
- Between the left sternal edge and the pulmonary valve and occasionally apical
- No thrill, added sounds or cardiomegaly, and a normal ECG, chest radiograph and echocardiogram.

Pathological murmurs can be divided into:

- Organic: valvular, subvalvular, supravalvular
- Functional: dilated valve ring or increased flow.

Peripheral examination

Auscultate and percuss the posterior lung bases for signs of pulmonary oedema and/or pleural effusions. At the same time check for sacral oedema while the patient is leaning forward.

Check for peripheral ankle oedema by pressing on the shin above the ankle, for 3–5 seconds, while watching the patient's face for discomfort, then look down where you have been pressing and feel for an indentation.

Examine for a pulsatile enlarged liver if tricuspid regurgitation is suspected. This is a leading cause of hepatomegaly in the absence of stigmata of chronic liver disease. Palpate for splenomegaly in suspected bacterial endocarditis. Feel for an abdominal aortic aneurysm and auscultate for renal bruits. Examine the remaining peripheral pulses in the legs and feet.

To finish

- Ask to dip the urine (microscopic haematuria in SBE)
- Offer to perform fundoscopy (if suspected SBE) for Roth's spots
- Check the BP
- Ask to see a recent ECG
- Be careful not to ask patients to hold their breath for too long in inspiration/expiration during cardiac examination
- Always look at the patient's face to assess for any pain caused when feeling for peripheral oedema or a pulsatile liver
- Always thank and cover the patient and WASH YOUR HANDS before turning to the examiner

Station 3
Cardiology scenarios

1. Mitral stenosis
2. Mitral regurgitation
3. Mitral valve prolapse
4. Aortic stenosis
5. Aortic regurgitation
6. Mixed valve disease
7. Pulmonary stenosis
8. Pulmonary regurgitation
9. Aortic prosthetic valve
10. Mitral prosthetic valve
11. Ventricular septal defect
12. Atrial septal defect
13. Patent ductus arteriosus
14. Eisenmenger syndrome
15. Hypertrophic cardiomyopathy
16. Coarctation of the aorta
17. Tetralogy of Fallot

SCENARIO 1: MITRAL STENOSIS

Identifying physical signs

Functional status: the patient may be dyspnoeic and have a malar flush.

Hands, pulse, face: the patient commonly has the irregular pulse of atrial fibrillation (AF) or, if in sinus rhythm, there may be a low-volume pulse.

JVP: the JVP may be normal, but in severe mitral stenosis giving rise to pulmonary hypertension and functional tricuspid regurgitation (TR), the JVP will be raised with large systolic 'v' waves. The large 'v' waves represent transmission of the right ventricular pressure wave to the right atrium and great veins in systole. There will be no 'a' wave if the patient is in AF.

Inspection and palpation of precordium: the apex is undisplaced and tapping, representing a palpable first heart sound. If there is pulmonary hypertension causing increased right ventricular pressure, there may be a left parasternal heave. Check for a left thoracotomy scar from previous mitral valvuloplasty.

Auscultation: (see Figure 3.1) S1 is loud. There is an opening snap and a mid-diastolic rumbling murmur, heard best at the apex with the bell and in the left lateral position. The murmur is increased in expiration and does not radiate to the axilla. It is accentuated by exertion. If there are mobile mitral valve leaflets, you may be able to detect a presystolic accentuation of the murmur with atrial contraction. With rigid leaflets there will be no presystolic accentuation or opening snap, and there may be the additional pansystolic murmur of mitral regurgitation in the apex because the rigid leaflets are more prone to separating during ventricular contraction.

With increasing severity the opening snap moves closer towards S2 and the diastolic murmur extends in duration. Assess severity by listening over the lower left sternal edge in the tricuspid area for possible functional TR (a pansystolic murmur accentuated on inspiration). If this is heard, listen for a loud P2 in the pulmonary area associated with pulmonary hypertension and look back at the JVP for large 'v' waves. There may be the Graham Steell murmur of pulmonary regurgitation – a high-pitched, early diastolic murmur heard in the pulmonary area during inspiration.

Periphery: in severe disease with a low cardiac output there may be central and peripheral cyanosis with cool peripheries and signs of left heart failure with pulmonary oedema. If there are signs of TR on auscultation proceed to feel for a tender pulsatile liver (be gentle). Look for other signs of right-sided heart failure with sacral or peripheral oedema.

Severity: in summarising the findings remember to describe the presence or absence of clinical markers associated with severe mitral stenosis such as:

- Dyspnoea at rest
- Malar flush
- Low pulse pressure
- Early opening snap
- Longer duration of murmur
- Signs of pulmonary hypertension and cor pulmonale (raised JVP with 'v' waves, parasternal heave, palpable and loud P2, functional TR with parasternal thrill, bibasal crepitations, pulsatile liver and peripheral oedema)
- Graham Steell murmur of pulmonary regurgitation.

Additional: ask to measure the blood pressure if not done already; state that you would test the urine, perform fundoscopy and request to see a recent ECG.

Differential diagnosis of a mid-diastolic murmur

Atrial myxoma: this is a very rare tumour with a prevalence of 0.02%. Most are benign; 75% of sporadic forms occur in women and 75% are in the left atrium, connected by a pedicle to the interatrial septum. Atrial myxomas can give rise to constitutional symptoms such as fever, rash and weight loss from interleukin production. They can cause left-sided heart failure as the tumour obstructs the mitral valve. Tumours can destroy the mitral valve, leading to mitral regurgitation. Embolisation sequelae include peripheral organ infarcts giving rise to strokes or seizures. There will be a loud S1 as the tumour delays mitral valve closure, and instead of an opening snap a tumour 'plop' with an early diastolic sound at the apex.

Austin Flint murmur: this murmur is due to buffeting of the anterior mitral valve leaflets in AR, when jets from both the left atrium and the aorta are hitting the mitral valve. There will be no tapping apex or opening snap, but just a mid-diastolic murmur. Look for signs of AR including a collapsing pulse, volume-loaded ventricle (with possible lateral displacement of the apex) and an early diastolic murmur, heard best at the left sternal edge on leaning forward and on expiration.

Clinical judgement and maintaining patient welfare

Mitral stenosis typically presents 15–20 years after the development of valvular stenosis with

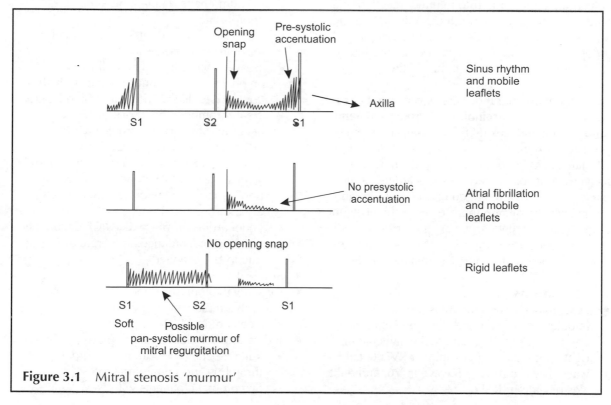

Figure 3.1 Mitral stenosis 'murmur'

the symptoms of right heart failure due to pulmonary hypertension. These are dyspnoea on exertion, orthopnoea and paroxysmal nocturnal dyspnoea (PND). The low cardiac output state can also lead to symptoms of left heart failure such as fatigue or angina. Alternatively, mitral stenosis can present with clinical deterioration associated with AF, anaemia, pregnancy or a chest infection. AF is commonly associated with mitral stenosis from left atrial dilatation and can lead to embolic phenomenon in up to 30% of patients. Rarely mitral stenosis can present with dysphagia from left atrial enlargement impinging on the oesophagus, hoarseness due to compression of the left recurrent laryngeal nerve or haemoptysis from pulmonary vein rupture in pulmonary hypertension.

Rheumatic fever is by far the most common cause. After infection with group A β-haemolytic streptococcal infection, glycoproteins of the bacterial cell wall adhere to collagen within the valve, triggering an autoimmune reaction that leads to inflammation and commissural fusion. This is reducing in incidence as most people with group A β-haemolytic streptococcal tonsillitis or scarlet fever are treated with penicillin.

Non-rheumatic mitral disease is very rare but can be caused by **carcinoid syndrome, systemic lupus erythematosus** (SLE) and **congenital mucopolysaccharoidoses**. SLE is associated with Libman–Sacks endocarditis, sometimes known as verrucous or marantic endocarditis, a non-bacterial endocarditis composed of immune complexes that attach themselves to the posterior mitral valve leaflet, and can give rise to valve incompetence or stenosis. This is seen less frequently now with improved treatment of SLE.

Investigations
- **ECG**: may show AF or sinus rhythm 'P mitrale' (broad notched P wave in leads II and III, representing left atrial enlargement), right ventricular hypertrophy or RVH (a tall R wave in V1 and deep S wave in V6) and right axis deviation (RAD).

- **Chest radiograph**: left atrial enlargement can cause splaying of the carina, a double right-sided heart border and convex upper left heart border, with bulging of the atrial appendage. Arteries may be prominent with signs of left heart failure and pulmonary congestion.
- **Echocardiogram**: calculates valve area that corresponds with severity of disease. The normal valve area is 4–6 cm^2, mild mitral stenosis corresponds with an area of >1.5 cm^2 and severe with an area <1.0 cm^2. Echocardiography can also be used to assess rigidity of valves and look for atrial thrombus.
- **Coronary angiography**: excludes other causes of symptoms such as coronary disease.

Management
- **Medical**:
  - Annual follow-up with a cardiologist
  - Avoidance of physical exercise and stress.
  - β blockers or the negatively chronotropic calcium channel antagonists may be appropriate
  - Salt restriction and intermittent diuretics for pulmonary congestion
  - Treat AF according to guidelines, with emphasis on rate control because rhythm control is unlikely with left atrial dilatation
  - Treat thromboembolic risk of AF according to guidelines (NICE Guidance 2014, www.nice.org.uk/CG180)
  - Anticoagulation is also indicated in mitral stenosis without AF if there has been a prior embolic event or evidence of left atrial thrombus
  - Endocarditis prophylaxis (NICE Guidance 2008, http://guidance.nice.org.uk/CG64 due to be reviewed).
- **Surgical**:
- Closed valvuloplasty, open commissurotomy and valve replacement (mitral valve replacement or MVR)
- Indications for closed valvuloplasty:
  - Suitable anatomy with no left atrial thrombus and no/minimal MR
  - Symptomatic patients with New York

Heart Association (NYHA) classification ≥II and mitral valve area >1.5 cm^2

- Asymptomatic patients with valve area <1.5 cm^2 and/or recurrent thromboembolic events despite anticoagulation
- Open commissurotomy is appropriate when the anatomy is not suitable for closed balloon valvuloplasty
- MVR when valvuloplasty is expected to have little benefit, has failed and/or there is coexistent MR or coronary artery disease (CAD).

Prognosis
- It can be 15–20 years before symptoms develop after rheumatic fever, so patients rarely present before their third decade.
- Symptomatic patients with NYHA >II and unsuitable for surgical intervention have a 33% 10-year survival rate.

SCENARIO 2. MITRAL REGURGITATION

Identifying physical signs

Functional status: the patient may be dyspnoeic at rest.

Hands, pulse, face: the patient is commonly in AF or if in sinus rhythm there may be the low-volume pulse of diminished cardiac output. It is important to assess for and mention the important negative finding of no signs of complicating bacterial endocarditis.

JVP: the JVP is usually normal, but in severe MR leading to pulmonary hypertension there may be functional tricuspid regurgitation with a raised JVP and large systolic 'v' waves. There will be no 'a' wave in AF.

Inspection and palpation of precordium: the left ventricle is volume loaded so the apex is thrusting and laterally displaced. There may be a palpable apical thrill. If there is pulmonary hypertension leading to RVH there will be a left parasternal heave. Look for a left thoracotomy scar indicating previous valvuloplasty that is now complicated by MR.

Auscultation: there is a soft first heart sound, softer in severe lesions. There may be a loud P2 in the pulmonary area, and wide splitting of the second heart with early closing of the aortic valve (because the left ventricle empties more rapidly due to retrograde leakage into the left atrium). There may be a third heart sound signifying rapid LV filling from the volume-loaded left atrium. The presence of S3 rules out significant concomitant mitral stenosis. There may be a fourth heart sound from atrial contraction against a stiffened left ventricle. MR gives a pansystolic murmur (PSM), heard best at the apex in expiration and radiating to the axilla. The loudness of the PSM is not proportionate to severity. In significant MR the high end-diastolic volume will also produce a flow murmur across the mitral valve, giving rise to a mid-diastolic murmur in the apical area. If there is significant tricuspid regurgitation there will be an additional PSM at the left sternal edge, louder on inspiration. Listen for the Graham Steell murmur of pulmonary regurgitation.

Periphery: in severe MR with a low cardiac output there will be central and peripheral cyanosis with cool peripheries and signs of left heart failure such as pulmonary oedema. If there are signs of TR, proceed to feel for a pulsatile liver (be gentle). Look for other signs of right-sided heart failure such as sacral and peripheral oedema.

Severity: in summarising the findings remember to describe the presence or absence of clinical markers associated with severe MR such as:

- Dyspnoea at rest
- Low pulse pressure
- Displaced and thrusting apex beat
- Soft S1
- Presence of S3 (rapid ventricular filling)
- Presence of S4 (just before S1 and signifies atrial contraction against a stiff LV wall)
- Widely split second heart sound with early A2
- Mid-diastolic flow murmur across the mitral valve
- Signs of pulmonary hypertension and cor pulmonale (raised JVP with 'v' waves, parasternal heave, palpable and loud P2, functional tricuspid regurgitation with parasternal thrill, bibasal crepitations, pulsatile liver and peripheral oedema)
- Graham Steell murmur of pulmonary regurgitation.

Additional: ask to measure the blood pressure; state that you would test the urine, perform fundoscopy and request to see a recent ECG.

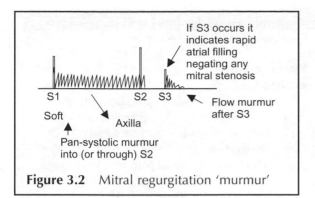

If S3 occurs it indicates rapid atrial filling negating any mitral stenosis

S1

Soft

S2   S3

Flow murmur after S3

Axilla

Pan-systolic murmur into (or through) S2

Figure 3.2   Mitral regurgitation 'murmur'

Differential diagnosis of a systolic murmur

Aortic stenosis: this gives a slow rising pulse with a small pulse pressure and a normal JVP. Precordium examination will reveal a pressure-loaded, non-displaced, heaving apex and an ejection (crescendo–decrescendo) systolic murmur best heard in the aortic area radiating to the carotids.

Mitral valve prolapse (MVP): there will be none of the peripheral stigmata of severe MR and MVP produces a mid-systolic click with a mid- to late systolic murmur. MVP is more common in well young women.

HOCM: this presents with a jerky pulse felt in the radial and carotid areas. There would be a double, forceful, heaving, pressure-loaded apex beat with an early systolic murmur (ESM) at the left sternal edge.

TR: this could be associated with MR and could complicate clinical assessment. Functional TR would be associated with a RV heave at the left sternal edge and the murmur would be loudest at the lower left sternal edge and on inspiration with no radiation to the axilla. Look for large 'v' waves in the JVP and a pulsatile liver with signs of peripheral oedema.

VSD: this produces a palpable thrill and pansystolic murmur at the left sternal edge, with no radiation to the axilla.

ASD: in an ASD right heart signs predominate. There is no murmur from the ASD itself but instead there are two flow murmurs with increased flow across the right side of the heart, leading to a pulmonary ESM and occasionally a tricuspid diastolic flow murmur. There is fixed splitting of the second heart sound as the left-to-right shunt leads to equal blood flow across the right and left atrioventricular valves, regardless of inspiration/expiration. A loud P2 signifies the development of pulmonary hypertension.

Clinical judgement and maintaining patient welfare

MR can develop acutely or indolently. Acute MR can be life threatening. Chronic MR, similar to mitral stenosis, can develop slowly over many years without symptoms, as the left atrium dilates to accommodate the extra regurgitated volume.

As the disease progresses the volume-overloaded left ventricle begins to decompensate and signs of congestive cardiac failure develop with dyspnoea, orthopnoea, PND and fatigue. Similar to mitral stenosis, AF is common. Complication with bacterial endocarditis is more common than in mitral stenosis.

Cause
Chronic MR can be functional or structural. Functional MR results from:

- A dilated MV annulus from **ischaemic injury** to the left ventricle (the most common cause in developed countries)
- A **dilated cardiomyopathy**
- A **calcified annulus** with age.

Structural chronic MR results primarily from:

- **Rheumatic heart disease** (the most common cause globally)
- **Previous valvuloplasty** for mitral stenosis
- **Floppy myxomatous degeneration** (at the severe end of the MVP spectrum and the second most common cause in developed countries after IHD)
- Connective tissue disease such as **Marfan syndrome, osteogenesis imperfecta** and **SLE**.

Acute MR is usually a medical emergency, leading to sudden-onset severe dyspnoea and pulmonary oedema. There are no compensatory changes, so the patient is usually in sinus rhythm, with an ejection systolic murmur heard at the apex. Acute MR is caused by **chordal rupture from ischaemia** or **posterior papillary muscle dysfunction**, occurring with large anterior MIs with right coronary artery involvement or, more rarely, due to **infective endocarditis.**

Investigations
- **ECG**: this may show AF or, if in sinus rhythm, 'P mitrale' (broad notched p waves in leads II and III, representing left atrial enlargement). Left ventricular hypertrophy or LVH (S in V1 + R in V6 >35 mm) may be evident. Some patients may show RVH changes instead (tall R wave in V1, deep S in V6 and RAD).
- **Chest radiograph**: left atrial enlargement can cause splaying of the carina, a double right-sided heart border and convex upper left heart border, with bulging of the atrial appendage. LV enlargement may be seen with signs of left heart failure and pulmonary congestion.
- **Echocardiogram**: this assesses the size and site of the regurgitant jet and the dimensions of the left atrium. It can help distinguish the cause of MR (functional or structural). Severity of MR is graded by measuring the LV ejection fraction and end-systolic dimension.
- **Coronary angiography**: this is used to assess the extent of any coronary disease in case bypass grafting is needed in addition to valve replacement surgery. The left atrial (LA) and pulmonary wedge pressures can provide a measure of disease severity.

Management
- **Medical**:
  - Annual follow-up with a cardiologist
  - Salt restriction, intermittent diuretics and the use of nitrates for pulmonary congestion
  - The embolic risk of MR and AF is lower than that with mitral stenosis, but still anticoagulate those with AF
  - Treat AF according to guidelines, with emphasis on rate control as rhythm control unlikely with LA dilatation
  - Treat thromboembolic risk of AF according to guidelines (NICE Guidance 2014, www.nice.org.uk/CG180)
  - In functional or ischaemic MR with LV systolic dysfunction, provide primary medical treatment with angiotensin-converting enzyme (ACE) inhibitors or β blockers and consider biventricular pacing; however, surgery should be performed ideally before LV failure develops (NICE heart failure guidelines 2010, http://guidance.nice.org.uk/CG108)
  - Endocarditis prophylaxis (NICE Guidance 2008, http://guidance.nice.org.uk/CG64 due to be reviewed)
  - In acute MR, emergency surgery is commonly indicated but acute medical treatment includes reducing the afterload on the left ventricle with nitroprusside, treating acute pulmonary oedema along standard lines and possibly bridging to surgery with an aortic balloon pump.
- **Surgical**:
  - Surgery is indicated in symptomatic patients with NYHA III or IV
  - Surgery is also indicated in asymptomatic patients with LV ejection fraction ≤60% or LV end-systolic diameter (LVESD) >45 mm (normal 20–44 mm)
  - Surgery can involve valve repair but more commonly requires mitral valve replacement.

Prognosis
- For patients who develop signs and symptoms of NYHA ≥II there is a 25% 5-year mortality rate.
- Those undergoing emergency surgery for acute MVR have a mortality rate approaching 80%.

SCENARIO 3. MITRAL VALVE PROLAPSE

Read this case together with Station 3, Scenario 2. Mitral regurgitation.

Identifying physical signs

Functional status: the patient is well, unless severe MR has developed.

Hands, pulse, face: they are in sinus rhythm unless MR and LA enlargement have led to AF. Look out for associated connective tissue disorders. It is important to assess for and mention the absence of signs of bacterial endocarditis.

JVP: this is normal.

Auscultation: (see Figure 3.3) unless MR has developed there will be no precordial scars or palpable thrills or heaves. Mitral valve prolapse (MVP) gives rise to a midsystolic click followed by a high-pitched mid- to late systolic murmur, heard best at the apex. The characteristic systolic click of MVP is dynamic because its timing within systole can be altered by manoeuvres that alter LV volume. It is possible to ask the examiner and patient if you can perform some of these man-

oeuvres, but do so only if you are confident in your clinical findings and their interpretation.

Reductions in LV volume cause the valve to prolapse earlier, and thus the click to move earlier in systole and the murmur to be more prolonged. This is because the chordae tendinae attached to the LV wall become more slack as the ventricular volume reduces, thus allowing prolapse. Manoeuvres that reduce venous return to the left heart bring the systolic click sooner and prolong the murmur of MVP. These include:

- Inspiration
- Standing
- Valsalva's manoeuvre.

Squatting increases venous return, afterload and thus LV end-diastolic volume. This delays the onset of the click and shortens the murmur.

Periphery: there will be no stigmata of heart failure in stable MVP but look for signs associated with connective tissue disorders.

Additional: ask to measure the blood pressure, test the urine, perform fundoscopy and request to see a recent ECG.

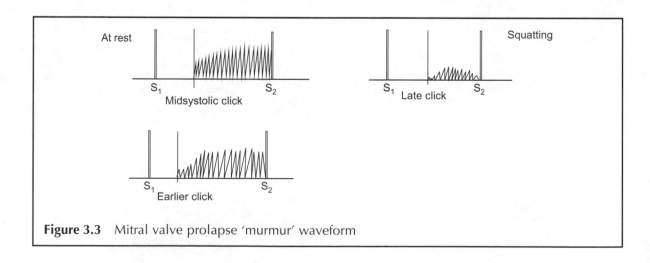

Figure 3.3   Mitral valve prolapse 'murmur' waveform

Differential diagnosis

There are several differentials for a systolic click and/or murmur. It is possible to have a systolic click from redundant parts of the mitral valve leaflets without prolapse.

Bicuspid aortic valve: the click of a bicuspid aortic valve can be heard all over the precordium; it is louder and is not dynamic.

Atrial myoxma: these are much more rare, give a low-frequency tumour 'plop' and will be associated with systemic features.

Mitral regurgitation: MVP will have none of the peripheral features of moderate-to-severe MR. Listen for the silence after S1 before the click occurs as opposed to the pansystolic murmur of MR. The murmur of MVP does not radiate into the axilla and is dynamic with different manoeuvres.

HOCM: similar to MVP, the murmur will diminish with increased end-diastolic volume such as in squatting, but will increase with reduced end-diastolic volume such as in standing or Valsalva's manoeuvre. There will be a jerky pulse and the murmur will be ejection systolic at the left sternal edge radiating all over the precordium.

Clinical judgement and maintaining patient welfare

MVP, as now defined by echocardiography criteria (see below), is equally common in men and women, with a prevalence estimated at 2–3%. Men have a higher incidence of complications such as bacterial endocarditis, severe MR and sudden cardiac death, but the vast majority of those with MVP have a very good prognosis.

A 'mitral valve prolapse syndrome' was proposed in the past, composed of: typically female, atypical chest pain, exertional dyspnoea, palpitations, syncope, anxiety, lower blood pressure and leaner body mass. Only leaner body mass and thoracic bony abnormalities such as scoliosis and pectus excavatum have remained associated with MVP in the Framingham Heart Study.

MVP is the most common cause of severe non-ischaemic MVR in developed countries.

Cause
The most common cause of MVP is **sporadic myxomatous degeneration.** Myxomatous degeneration describes the process whereby the middle of the three-layer valve structure, called the spongiosa, becomes thickened with proteoglycans, due to dysregulation of matrix protein synthesis. This degeneration also occurs within the chordae. The valve becomes thickened and flaccid and bulges out into the left atrium.

MVP is also associated with connective tissue disorders such as: **Marfan syndrome** (90% of patients have MVP), **Ehlers–Danlos syndrome**, **osteogenesis imperfecta** and **polycystic kidney disease** (PKD).

Investigations
MVP is detected either on clinical examination or as an incidental finding on echocardiography. Formal diagnosis is made with consistent echocardiography.

Echocardiography: single or bileaflet mitral valve prolapse >2 mm beyond the plane of the valve as seen in the long axis, with or without valve thickening. Prolapse with valve thickening >5 mm is termed 'classic' prolapse and has a higher risk of endocarditis, MR or sudden cardiac death.

Management
The vast majority of patients with MVP have an excellent prognosis, do not need to make any lifestyle modifications and can be followed up conservatively.

The complications of MVP are severe MR, endocarditis, sudden cardiac death and thromboembolic events.

The higher-risk patient groups include: moderate-to-severe MR, depressed LV function, AF, LA enlargement, age >50, valve thickening ⩾5 mm.

Endocarditis prophylaxis should be offered in the following cases:

- Audible click and systolic murmur
- Audible click and echocardiography evidence of prolapse *and* regurgitation
- Audible click and echocardiography changes of LA enlargement, leaflet thickening and/or ventricular dilatation
- Normal exam but echocardiography changes of myxomatous degeneration and a regurgitant jet.

The patient does *not* require prophylaxis if there is a click with echocardiography evidence of a prolapse but *no* regurgitant jet.

Patients with isolated MVP do not have an excess of atrial/ventricular arrhythmias, but those with MR do.

Treat any AF along standard lines with anticoagulant prophylaxis.

Manage severe MR with surgery: MV repair or replacement.

Prognosis

Most patients have an excellent prognosis with no complications or need for treatment, but higher-risk groups are detailed above.

SCENARIO 4. AORTIC STENOSIS

Identifying physical signs

Functional status: the patient may be dyspnoeic and/or appear pale.

Hands, pulse, face: feel for a slow-rising, low-volume pulse. Check for peripheral signs of bacterial endocarditis. There may be signs of cyanosis from LV failure and complicating pulmonary oedema in severe aortic stenosis. Comment on the presence or absence of signs of bacterial endocarditis.

JVP: severe aortic stenosis may be complicated by pulmonary hypertension and right heart failure with associated JVP changes.

Inspection and palpation of the precordium: the apex is non-displaced and heaving (pressure loaded). In severe aortic stenosis causing left-sided heart failure there is a displaced apex. There might be a systolic thrill in the aortic area.

Auscultation: (see Figure 3.4) S1 is normal and S2 is soft. There could be reversed splitting of the second heart sound in severe aortic stenosis (ie wider splitting in expiration as A2 follows P2). There might be a fourth heart sound before S1, corresponding to atrial contraction against a stiffened, hypertrophied, left ventricle. An ejection click can be heard early in systole if there is a calcified bicuspid valve. Aortic stenosis gives rise to an ejection systolic murmur (crescendo–decrescendo), loudest in the aortic area, increased with expiration and usually radiating into the carotids. Sometimes in elderly people the murmur can radiate to the apex due to reflection from the calcified aortic root (Gallavardin's phenomenon). A loud murmur does not indicate severe aortic stenosis, but rather a delayed, softer murmur can indicate increasing severity as cardiac output begins to diminish.

Periphery: in severe aortic stenosis there could be signs of congestive heart failure with bibasal

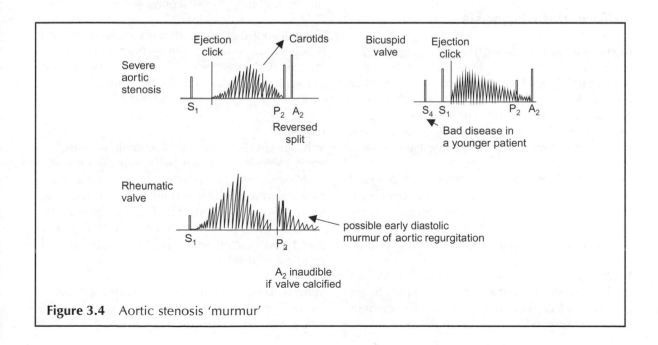

Figure 3.4   Aortic stenosis 'murmur'

crepitations and pulmonary hypertension, leading to cor pulmonale and right-sided heart failure.

Severity: in summarising the findings, remember to describe the presence or absence of clinical markers associated with severe aortic stenosis such as:

- Dyspnoea at rest
- Slow rising pulse
- Narrow pulse pressure
- Heaving or displaced apex
- Aortic thrill
- Soft S2 with reversed splitting of second heart sound
- Fourth heart sound
- Longer duration murmur with later systolic accentuation
- Signs of pulmonary hypertension
- Signs of left heart failure.

Additional: ask to measure the blood pressure if not done already, state that you would test the urine, perform fundoscopy and request to see a recent ECG.

Differential diagnosis

Aortic sclerosis is caused by calcification of the aortic valve and occurs in 25% of those aged >65 years. There is an ejection systolic murmur but no outflow obstruction, so the pulse, apex beat and heart sounds are normal. It is a progressive condition, so in time it may lead to aortic stenosis; it is a marker of cardiovascular disease.

MVP: this is a mid- to late systolic murmur heard best at the apex, with none of the peripheral stigmata of aortic stenosis and no reverse splitting of the second heart sound. The murmur of MVP will increase with Valsalva's manoeuvre.

VSD: this is a pansystolic murmur heard best at the left sternal edge with no radiation, no crescendo–decrescendo quality and the murmur passes through to S2.

HOCM: this is also an ESM but there may be a jerky pulse with a double apical sensation rather than the slow rising pulse and heaving sustained apex of aortic stenosis. The ESM will be heard best at the left sternal edge. The murmur of HOCM will increase with any manoeuvre that decreases LV volume such as standing or the straining phase of Valsalva's manoeuvre (similar to MVP), whereas these manoeuvres will decrease an aortic stenotic murmur.

Clinical judgement and maintaining patient welfare

Aortic stenosis remains clinically silent for many years until decompensation occurs and LV function beings to fail, giving rise to symptoms. With the onset of symptoms average survival is 2–3 years. Severe aortic stenosis presents with heart failure symptoms such as shortness of breath and PND/orthopnoea. Aortic stenosis can also give rise to syncope (fixed cardiac output and arrhythmias from aortic ring calcification affecting conduction pathways) and angina (increasing LV muscle mass with increasing demand but restricted coronary blood supply).

Complications of aortic stenosis include haemolytic anaemia, embolic disease from a disintegrating calcified valve, heart block from calcification of the atrioventricular conduction fibres, infective endocarditis, heart failure and sudden death.

Cause
Valvular (85%): the most common cause of aortic stenosis is senile calcification, but the 40- to 60-year age group often have a congenital bicuspid valve, which is more prone to shearing forces and subsequent calcification. Rheumatic fever is also an important cause globally, and may be associated with aortic regurgitation and mitral valve disease.

Subvalvular (15%): this type of aortic stenosis is seen in children, due to a fibromuscular ring or diffuse thickening beneath the valve.

Supravalvular (5%): this type of aortic stenosis is also seen in children, due to narrowing of the ascending aorta such as that associated with Williams syndrome.

Investigations

- **ECG**: this usually shows sinus rhythm unless there is also mitral valve disease giving rise to AF. There may be LVH on voltage criteria (S in V1 + R in V5–6 >35 mm). Conduction abnormalities include left anterior hemiblock, left bundle-branch block or LBBB (QRS >120 ms, RSR in lead V6) or complete heart block.
- **Chest radiograph**: may show LVH, calcification of the aortic valve, poststenotic dilatation of the aorta and prominent pulmonary arteries with pulmonary hypertension and pulmonary oedema.
- **Echocardiography**: this is used to diagnose and assess extent of disease. Echocardiography can be used to look for a bicuspid valve, the mobility of the valve leaflets and the extent of calcification, and to assess the aortic valve area:
  - Normal aortic valve is 3–4 cm^2.
  - Mild disease is seen with a valve area >1.5 cm^2.
  - Severe disease is seen with a valve area <1.0 cm^2.
  The gradient across the valve is also assessed with severe AS associated with a gradient of >50 mmHg (normal 2–5 mmHg). Heart failure is assessed by measuring LV volumes and ejection fraction.
- **Coronary angiography**: this is used to directly measure the gradient across the valve and assess coronary circulation as CAD usually coexists.

Management

In the asymptomatic patient management is conservative with annual follow-up and treatment of cardiovascular risk factors.

Coexistent hypertension should be treated but nitrates and ACE inhibitors should be avoided because these can reduce afterload and therefore increase the gradient across the valve.

Aortic valve replacement is indicated for those with severe aortic stenosis and:

- Symptoms
- Requiring coronary artery bypass graft (CABG) or other valve surgery
- LV systolic dysfunction (ejection fraction <0.5).

Risk algorithms, such as the EUROscore, are used to help decide on mortality risk with surgery and between surgical options.

For higher-risk patients, percutaneous options exist known as the TAVI (transcatheter aortic valve implantation), with common routes of access being transfemoral and transapical. Balloon valvotomy is rarely used for adult cases.

Mortality rate of isolated aortic valve replacement is 3–4% and 5–7% for aortic valve replacement + CABG. If LV failure (LVF) is present the mortality rate rises to 10–20%.

Prognosis

There is a long latency period with no symptoms for about 20 years.

Symptoms and prognosis reflect the progression of the disease. Initially there is LVH leading to angina symptoms (5-year 50% mortality rate), then conduction abnormalities and failing cardiac output, giving rise to syncope and finally heart failure with breathlessness (2-year 50% mortality rate).

SCENARIO 5. AORTIC REGURGITATION

Identifying physical signs

Functional status: the patient may be dyspnoeic if there is advanced aortic regurgitation.

Hands, pulse, face: look for signs of systemic disease associated with aortic regurgitation such as Marfan syndrome, ankylosing spondylitis, SLE, osteogenesis imperfecta and rheumatoid arthritis. A collapsing 'water-hammer' pulse may be felt at the radial or brachial. This represents a hyperdynamic circulation. There will be a large pulse pressure due to the low diastolic pressures associated with aortic regurgitation. Look for additional eponymous signs associated with aortic regurgitation such as:

- Quincke's sign (visible capillary pulsations in nailbed)
- De Musset's sign (head bobbing)
- Corrigan's sign (visible carotid pulsations)
- Muller's sign (uvula pulsations).

It is important to assess for and mention the important negative finding of no signs of complicating bacterial endocarditis.

JVP: this is usually normal but there may be JVP signs of pulmonary hypertension with large 'v' waves in severe AR.

Inspection and palpation of the precordium: look for any scars that could indicate previous *aortic valve replacement*. There will be a thrusting volume-loaded apical impulse, which may be displaced representing severe aortic regurgitation and ventricular dilatation. In the absence of pulmonary hypertension there will be no other heaves or thrills.

Auscultation: (see Figure 3.5) the heart sounds are normal or there may be a loud P2 if there is severe aortic regurgitation giving rise to pulmonary hypertension. The high-pitched early diastolic murmur of aortic regurgitation is heard best at the left sternal edge, with the patient leaning forward and breath held in expiration. Listen for an aortic systolic flow murmur in the aortic area due to the hyperdynamic circulation. In severe aortic regurgitation the regurgitant jet hits the anterior leaflet of the mitral valve, creating functional mitral stenosis and a low-pitched mid-

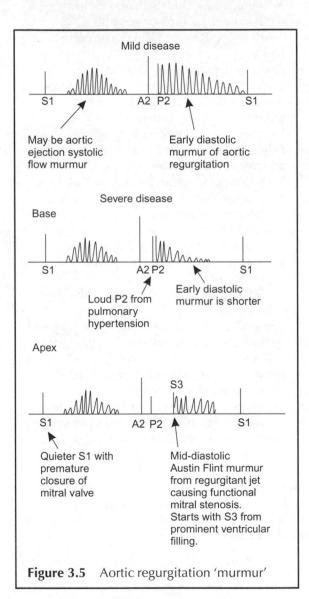

Figure 3.5   Aortic regurgitation 'murmur'

diastolic 'Austin Flint' murmur at the apex. The 'Austin Flint' murmur can be differentiated from the normal murmur of MS by the absence of a tapping apex or opening snap and signs of severe aortic regurgitation.

Periphery: if there is severe aortic regurgitation, there may be signs of pulmonary hypertension or heart failure including bibasal crepitations and ankle oedema. Other peripheral signs of a hyperdynamic circulation can be sought such as Traube's sign (a 'pistol shot' sound heard over the femoral artery) or Duroziez's sign (diastolic murmur heard over the femoral artery when it is compressed distally to the stethoscope).

Severity: in summarising the findings, remember to describe the presence or absence of clinical markers associated with severe aortic regurgitation such as:

- Dyspnoea at rest
- Wide pulse pressure
- Displaced and thrusting apex beat
- Presence of S3 (rapid ventricular filling)
- Shorter early diastolic murmur of AR
- 'Austin Flint' murmur of functional mitral stenosis
- Signs of pulmonary hypertension (raised JVP with 'v' waves, parasternal heave, palpable and loud P2, functional TR with parasternal thrill, pulsatile liver and peripheral oedema)
- Signs of left heart failure.

Additional: ask to measure the blood pressure if not done already, state that you would test the urine, perform fundoscopy and request to see a recent ECG.

Differential diagnosis

Collapsing pulse: a collapsing pulse can also be felt in other conditions with a hyperdynamic circulation such as pregnancy, anaemia, thyrotoxicosis and fever. None of the other signs of aortic regurgitation will be present.

Pulmonary regurgitation: in a patient with corrected tetralogy of Fallot or as a complication of pulmonary valvuloplasty, the murmur of pulmonary regurgitation may be heard. This will be heard in the pulmonary area, loudest in inspiration, and will not have a collapsing pulse or other peripheral signs associated with aortic regurgitation.

Clinical judgement and maintaining patient welfare

Causes of chronic aortic regurgitation:

- Valvular: bicuspid valve, rheumatic fever, rheumatoid arthritis, ankylosing spondylitis, SLE
- Non-valvular: systemic hypertension, Marfan syndrome, Ehler–Danlos syndrome, osteogenesis imperfect, syphilitic aortitis, Takayasu's arteritis.

Causes of acute aortic regurgitation:

- Valvular (endocarditis)
- Non-valvular (dissecting aortic aneurysm type A).

In developed countries congenital bicuspid aortic valve and aortic root dilatation account for most cases of aortic regurgitation but in the developing world rheumatic fever still predominates. Non-valvular (aortic root dilatation) causes account for just over 50% of the cases requiring aortic valve replacement.

Similar to aortic stenosis, there is a long asymptomatic compensated stage in chronic aortic regurgitation. Initially the left ventricle accommodates to the increased end-diastolic volume from the regurgitant jet by increasing stroke volume through ventricular hypertrophy. With disease progression the ventricle begins to fail and again the LV end-diastolic volume increases, giving rise to a dilated ventricle. In the later stages, symptoms develop such as angina (the large pulse pressure lowers diastolic coronary artery perfusion, reducing supply, and the ventricular hypertrophy increases demand) and breathlessness from heart failure as cardiac output falls.

Investigations
- **ECG**: may be normal or show voltage criteria for LVH.
- **Chest radiograph**: may reveal a calcified aortic valve or aortic root, signs of heart failure with cardiomegaly and/or pulmonary oedema.
- **Echocardiogram**: this is used to determine aortic valve morphology and the aetiology of aortic regurgitation, measure aortic root size, severity of aortic regurgitation, LV size and LV systolic function with ejection fraction.
- **Chest CT/MRI**: this is needed to visualise the ascending aorta.
- **Coronary angiography**: assesses coexistent CAD, which may provide an alternative explanation for angina symptoms and the need for bypass grafting if considering aortic valve replacement surgery.

Management
The strategy for compensated aortic regurgitation is watchful waiting.

Severe asymptomatic aortic regurgitation with LV dilatation can be treated with vasodilators such as ACE inhibitors/angiotensin receptor blockers (ARBs) and calcium channel antagonists to reduce afterload.

Aortic valve replacement is indicated for acute aortic regurgitation due to aortic dissection or endocarditis not responding to medical management.

Aortic valve replacement for chronic aortic regurgitation is indicated in the presence of:

- Symptoms
- Ejection fraction <50%
- Chronic severe aortic regurgitation and requiring CABG or other valve surgery
- LV end-diastolic volume >75 mm or end-systolic volume >55 mm
- Pulse pressure >100 mmHg.

Prognosis
Aortic regurgitation has a long period of asymptomatic compensated disease. Predictors of poor prognosis include advanced age, increased LV end-diastolic volume and reduced ejection fraction.

It is not uncommon to get mixed valve disease, which can make diagnosis difficult, but usually the clinical signs for either stenosis or regurgitation predominate. It is the nature of the peripheral signs that can help distinguish which is clinically more significant when both murmurs are heard.

Mixed aortic valve disease

Identifying physical signs
If regurgitation predominates you may see the peripheral stigmata of the large pulse volume, such as De Musset's and Corrigan's signs. There will be a large-volume, collapsing 'water-hammer' pulse, or the large-volume bisferiens pulse of mixed aortic disease. A bisferiens pulse describes a double pulsation for each systole, in which the percussion and tidal waves can be felt at appreciably separate times due to mixed aortic disease. If stenosis predominates, the pulse may have a slow rising or bisferiens character. The pulse pressure is a useful discriminator of which predominates – narrow in aortic stenosis and wide in regurgitation.

Remember to comment on the severity of disease (as determined by the same measures described above) and the functional status of the patient.

Mixed mitral valve disease

Identifying clinical signs
There are a number of useful discriminators to determine whether regurgitation or stenosis predominates. In regurgitation, the apex is laterally displaced, energetic and thrusting, but undisplaced in mitral stenosis. There may be a left thoracotomy scar if the patient has had previous valvuloplasty for mitral stenosis that has been complicated by MR. There may be a third heart sound in diastole from rapid LV filling from the volume-loaded left atrium. If this is present then there cannot be clinically significant stenosis because this would prevent rapid ventricular filling. The presence of AF suggests atrial enlargement and thus a clinically significant stenosis, although this has low specificity. A narrow pulse pressure suggests poor filling of the left ventricle in diastole and thus clinically significant mitral stenosis. Note that a malar flush may indicate the presence of mitral stenosis but does not mean that this is the dominant lesion when both mitral regurgitation and stenosis murmurs are heard.

SCENARIO 7. PULMONARY STENOSIS

Identifying physical signs

Functional status: the patient appears comfortable at rest.

Hands, pulse, face: pulmonary stenosis is associated with Noonan and Williams syndromes so be careful to look for their typical phenotypic features (see pages 170–171). The patient may be in AF if pulmonary stenosis has caused right atrial dilatation.

JVP: the JVP may be raised if there is right heart failure. If the patient is in sinus rhythm there will be large 'a' waves from atrial contraction against a stiffened right ventricle.

Inspection and palpation of precordium: there are usually no mediastinal scars, unless the pulmonary stenosis is associated with other congenital cardiac defects that have been repaired. There is a normal apex beat. There is a left parasternal heave caused by RVH and a thrill felt in the pulmonary area.

Auscultation: there is a normal S1 and widely split S2 with a quiet P2. This is due to the later closure of the stenosed pulmonary valve. There may be a fourth heart sound in diastole heard in the tricuspid region, associated with RA contraction against a stiffened right ventricle. There is an ejection click heard early in systole. The ESM that follows is in the pulmonary area, heard best during inspiration and radiating up to the suprasternal notch and occasionally into the axilla and right posterior chest wall. With increasing severity of the stenosis, the ejection click comes earlier and the murmur extends in duration and peaks later. The murmur can extend into diastole through the second heart sound. Listen carefully for additional pulmonary regurgitation from previous balloon valvuloplasty, which will be a quiet early diastolic murmur in the pulmonary area radiating to the left sternal edge. Listen for functional tricuspid regurgitation: a pansystolic murmur at the left sternal edge heard best in inspiration (this will have associated large 'v' waves in the JVP).

Periphery: with severe pulmonary stenosis there will be signs of right heart failure with peripheral oedema. *There should be no signs in the lung fields in the absence of left-sided heart lesions.*

Severity: in summarising the findings remember to describe the presence or absence of clinical markers associated with severe pulmonary stenosis such as:

* Large 'a' waves in the JVP
* Right ventricular heave from volume-loaded ventricle
* Widely split S2 with a quiet P2
* Fourth heart sound
* Early ejection systolic click
* Longer ejection systolic murmur extending into diastole
* Pansystolic murmur from functional tricuspid regurgitation.

Additional: ask to measure the blood pressure, state that you would test the urine and perform fundoscopy to exclude. Request to see a recent ECG.

Differential diagnosis

Aortic stenosis: the ESM is heard loudest in the aortic area in expiration and radiates up to the carotids. The murmur occurs between S1 and S2 whereas the ESM murmur of pulmonary stenosis can extend through the second heart sound. There is no wide splitting of the second heart sound as heard with pulmonary stenosis, although there may be reversed splitting. There are no JVP changes with AS unless there is advanced congestive cardiac failure and associated lung signs.

Ventricular septal defect: this will give a pansystolic murmur heard best at the left sternal edge with no change with respiration. A haemodynamically significant VSD will be quieter and there will be a loud P2 with the development of pulmonary hypertension.

Atrial septal defect: the cardinal sign is a fixed splitting of the heart sounds. A haemodynamically significant ASD may be inaudible itself but result in a pulmonary flow murmur. This can be distinguished from pulmonary stenosis by a loud P2, signs of pulmonary hypertension and a thrusting, displaced apex beat from LV volume overload.

Clinical judgement and maintaining patient welfare

Pulmonary stenosis usually occurs as a result of congenital heart disease and it comprises 10% of all congenital heart disease seen in adults. The obstruction can occur at different levels:

- Valvular: congenital, carcinoid, rheumatic heart disease, Noonan syndrome and Alagille syndrome. Alagille syndrome is a rare (1 per 100 000) autosomal dominant disorder characterised by cardiac, liver, kidney, eye and skeletal abnormalities, with a typical facial appearance of broad forehead, deep-set eyes and pointy chin. The main clinical presentations are cholestatic jaundice (from intrahepatic duct hypoplasia) or heart failure from congenital heart disease
- Subvalvular: tetralogy of Fallot
- Supravalvular ('peripheral pulmonary stenosis'): congenital rubella syndrome and Williams syndrome.

Patients can present with exertional dyspnoea and fatigue from poor cardiac output and cyanosis if they have a right-to-left shunt via a patent foramen ovale, or ASD or VSD.

Investigations
- **ECG**: there may be right axis deviation ($>90°$), RVH (tall R wave in V5–6, deep S wave in V1–2) and right atrial hypertrophy (P pulmonale).
- **Chest radiograph**: there may be prominent right or left main pulmonary arteries due to poststenotic dilatation. Usually there are normal lung markings. There could be a prominent right heart border if RA enlargement has occurred.
- **Echocardiogram**: this will show thickening of the pulmonary valves and enable assessment of the gradient across the valve. Echocardiography is also used to assess RA and ventricular size and systolic function. Severe stenosis is defined as a pulmonary valve area <0.5 cm^2 (normal valve area is 2.5 cm^2) and pressure gradient >75 mmHg.
- **Coronary catheterisation**: can be useful to diagnose supravalvular stenosis and other congenital heart defects.

Management
- Pulmonary stenosis requires endocarditis prophylaxis (NICE Guidelines 2008, http://guidance.nice.org.uk/CG64, due to be reviewed).
- Mild-to-moderate pulmonary stenosis requires no specific treatment but annual follow-up.
- Consider first-line balloon valvuloplasty in any patient with a pressure gradient >50 mmHg, unless there is complicated anatomy or other associated congenital heart defects, in which case open surgical repair is indicated.

Prognosis
Patients with mild-to-moderate pulmonary stenosis have the same prognosis as the general population. Those with treated severe pulmonary stenosis also have an excellent prognosis.

SCENARIO 8. PULMONARY REGURGITATION

Pulmonary regurgitation is commonly secondary to pulmonary hypertension and its attendant causes, and is rarely a primary valvular lesion. This epidemiology is reflected in the examination setting, so on finding clinical signs consistent with pulmonary regurgitation look for other cardiac or pulmonary disease that could cause pulmonary hypertension.

Identifying physical signs

Functional status: the patient appears comfortable at rest.

Hands, pulse, face: the pulse is regular and of normal volume, unless there is associated aortic stenosis (slow rising) or aortic regurgitation (collapsing 'water hammer'). Look for signs consistent with cyanotic congenital heart disease (such as peripheral and central cyanosis and clubbing) or lung disease (tar staining, clubbing with interstitial lung disease) which could both cause pulmonary hypertension. There may be a malar flush in the presence of pulmonary hypertension.

JVP: the JVP may be raised if there is right heart failure from pulmonary hypertension with large 'v' waves associated with tricuspid regurgitation.

Inspection and palpation of precordium: there may be mediastinal scars associated with previous repair of lone pulmonary stenosis, tetralogy of Fallot or pulmonary atresia. The apex beat is usually normal but there may be findings associated with other underlying disease such as: tapping, non-displaced apex beat (mitral stenosis), heaving apex beat (aortic stenosis or HOCM) or thrusting displaced apex beat (aortic regurgitation and VSD).

If the pulmonary regurgitation is secondary to pulmonary hypertension, there will be a left sternal heave from a pressure-loaded right ventricle. There may be a palpable thrill near the sternal edge from associated tricuspid regurgitation.

Auscultation: the heart sounds are usually normal but with a split second heart sound due to the delayed closure of P2 from the larger RV regurgitant volume. If the PR is secondary to pulmonary hypertension, there will be a loud P2. If there is associated mitral stenosis, S1 is loud and with aortic stenosis A2 is quiet.

The murmur of pulmonary regurgitation is an early diastolic murmur heard best in the pulmonary area and in inspiration, radiating down the left sternal edge. Listen for other left-sided murmurs that could be associated with pulmonary hypertension or the high-pitched pansystolic murmur of tricuspid regurgitation in the fourth intercostal space near the sternal edge.

Periphery: with advanced pulmonary hypertension leading to pulmonary regurgitation, there will be signs of right heart failure with peripheral oedema. In the lung fields listen for changes associated with primary lung diseases such as chronic obstructive pulmonary disease or COPD (coarse prolonged expiratory sounds with wheeze) and interstitial lung disease (fine end-inspiratory crackles).

In primary pulmonary regurgitation there may be no peripheral signs or those associated with carcinoid syndrome (facial flushing, tachycardia and hepatomegaly) or intravenous drug use (emaciation and needle-track marks).

Additional: ask to measure the blood pressure and state that you would test the urine and perform fundoscopy to exclude bacterial endocarditis. Request to see a recent ECG.

Differential diagnosis

In presenting the case the candidate should try to differentiate between primary pulmonary regurgitation due to intrinsic valvular disease and that secondary to pulmonary hypertension and its attendant causes.

Other cardiac lesions that present with diastolic murmurs include the following.

Mitral stenosis: there will be a tapping, undisplaced apex beat with a loud S1 and a rumbling mid-diastolic murmur, best heard at the apex in expiration in the left lateral position.

Aortic regurgitation: in aortic regurgitation there is an early diastolic murmur, best heard at the left sternal edge when the patient is leaning forward and during expiration. There may be a systolic flow murmur in the aortic area. There will be other peripheral signs associated with aortic regurgitation.

Clinical judgement and maintaining patient welfare

Primary pulmonary regurgitation:

- Complication of surgical repair of pulmonary stenosis or tetralogy of Fallot
- Endocarditis
- Carcinoid syndrome
- Pulmonary root dilatation (Marfan syndrome, syphilis).

Secondary pulmonary regurgitation:

- Primary pulmonary hypertension
- Secondary pulmonary hypertension:
  - COPD
  - interstitial lung disease

- Obstructive sleep apnoea (OSA)
- Mitral valve disease
- Aortic valve disease
- Systemic sclerosis
- Vasculitis
- Rheumatoid arthritis.

Investigations
- **ECG**: RV dilatation can produce right bundle-branch block (RBBB) and RAD. Pulmonary regurgitation associated with repair of tetralogy of Fallot is associated with a prolonged QRS.
- **Chest radiograph**: if associated with pulmonary hypertension there may be large central pulmonary arteries, with reduction of peripheral lung markings, known as 'pruning'. The right heart border may be enlarged.
- **Echocardiography**: this is used to determine the severity and aetiology of the pulmonary regurgitation, looking for other valvular lesions. It can be used to assess RV volume and systolic pressure gradient.

Management
- Pulmonary regurgitation of itself does not usually require treatment unless it is acute or causing heart failure symptoms (NYHA ≥II). Treatment is usually indicated by and directed at the underlying diseases causing pulmonary hypertension.
- When there is acute pulmonary regurgitation (caused by balloon valvuloplasty for pulmonary stenosis or correction of tetralogy of Fallot), then usually pulmonary valve replacement is required.

Prognosis
In general the presence of pulmonary hypertension and the underlying disease tends to determine the prognosis.

Patients with prosthetic valves are common in the PACES examination. The candidate needs to be able to identify:

- The valve that has been replaced
- Signs of valve dysfunction
- Complications such as endocarditis and anaemia.

Identifying physical signs

Functional status: the patient appears comfortable at rest.

Hands, pulse, face: it is important to assess carefully for any peripheral stigmata of endocarditis, an important complication in those with prosthetic valves. The pulse rate and character are usually normal, but if there is a malfunctioning valve with either stenosis (slow rising) or regurgitation (collapsing) then it is important to note this. Look for signs of anaemia, a complication of physical haemolysis from the prosthetic valve, bleeding from anticoagulation therapy or anaemia of chronic disease, seen with ongoing SBE (this will not be seen in the examination but is an important differential). Look for purpura from anticoagulation therapy.

JVP: the JVP is usually normal. A raised JVP and systolic 'v' waves may be seen in those patients who had long-standing pulmonary hypertension before their valve replacement surgery in which the pulmonary vascular resistance does not fully normalise.

Inspection and palpation of precordium: it might be possible to hear the prosthetic valve sounds from the end of the bed. The older Starr–Edwards ball-and-cage valves make opening and closing sounds, whereas the more modern single/double tilting disc valves make only closing sounds. Closing sounds are always louder. There will be a midline sternotomy scar, but look carefully for a pacemaker scar in the left infraclavicular area (this can be very subtle and easily missed) and look/feel for the implanted pacemaker beneath this scar. Pacemakers are common in aortic valve replacement because aortic valve disease or the surgery itself can damage the conduction pathways. The apex beat should be normal but if there has been longstanding aortic stenosis the apex beat may still be heaving. If the valve is failing, there may be a displaced thrusting apex beat signifying regurgitation. It might be possible to feel a thrill in the aortic area because there will be a flow murmur across the prosthetic valve and the opening/closing of the valve might also be palpable.

Auscultation: the first heart sound is normal, followed by the click of the prosthetic valve opening (Starr–Edwards). This is followed by an ejection systolic flow murmur across the valve, and then a click at the second heart sound as the valve closes. Time these events by palpating the carotid pulse. There should be no sounds in diastole. Check for any signs of aortic regurgitation, leaning the patient forward and listening in expiration, because this indicates a failing valve.

Periphery: check for any signs of left heart failure indicating valve dysfunction. State that you would examine for splenomegaly; check the toenails for splinter haemorrhages. Ask to dip the urine and check the temperature chart, thoroughly searching for signs of endocarditis. Look for the peripheral scars of venous grafting from the radial or long saphenous veins, indicating a concomitant CABG procedure.

Clinical judgement and maintaining patient welfare

Indications for aortic valve replacement for aortic stenosis and regurgitation are described above.

Other indications for aortic valve replacement

- Infective endocarditis affecting the aortic valve and not responding to medical therapy
- Acute (dissection) or chronic (idiopathic, Marfan syndrome) dilatation of aortic root.

Complications of a prosthetic heart valve

- Infective endocarditis:
  - Early (<2 months post-surgery)
  - Late (>2 months post-surgery)
  - Staphylococci (especially coagulase negative), HACEK (*Haemophilus*, *Aggregatibacter* (previously *Actinobacillus*), *Cardiobacterium* sp., *Eikenella corrodens*, *Kingella* sp.) organisms and fungi occur much more frequently in prosthetic valve endocarditis, compared with more streptococci and enterococci in native valve disease
  - Ring abscesses are common and vegetations tend to be larger than native valve endocarditis

- It may present as a new AV block, acute heart failure or embolic phenomenon
- Mortality rates depend on complications and the organism, but can be as high as 50%, particularly with *Staphylococcus aureus* or fungal vegetations
- Thromboembolism (calcification or thrombus formation)
- Anticoagulation complications (bleeding, interaction with many medications)
- Anaemia (haemolysis, endocarditis or bleeding)
- Valve failure (heart failure from dehiscence, leaking, calcification or stiffening of valve leaflets).

Replacement valve types

Tissue valves include xenografts (porcine or bovine) and homografts (cadaveric). Tissue valves are indicated in older patients whose life expectancy is shorter than that of the valve (approximately 10–15 years compared with a prosthetic valve duration of 20–30 years), or in those in whom anticoagulation is contraindicated (pregnancy) or considered in infective endocarditis (tissue valves are more resistant to infection).

Mechanical prosthetic valves have a longer lifespan (and thus are usually indicated in younger patients) but require anticoagulation.

SCENARIO 10. MITRAL PROSTHETIC VALVE

The candidate should look for signs of endo-carditis or valve failure and comment on the presence/absence of these in their summary of examination findings.

Read this section together with aortic valve replacement because they share the same complications.

Identifying physical signs

Functional status: the patient usually appears comfortable at rest.

Hands, pulse, face: look carefully for peripheral stigmata of endocarditis. The patient might be in AF. There may be a malar flush from persistent pulmonary hypertension. Look for signs of anae-mia, a complication of physical haemolysis from the prosthetic valve or anticoagulation therapy. Look for purpura from anticoagulation therapy.

JVP: the JVP may be normal or missing 'a' waves if there is AF. A raised JVP and systolic 'v' waves may be seen in those patients who had long-standing pulmonary hypertension (more common with mitral valve replacement patients) before their valve replacement surgery when the pul-monary vascular resistance remains high.

Inspection and palpation of precordium: it might be possible to hear the prosthetic valve sounds from the end of the bed. The older Starr–Edwards ball-and-cage valves make opening and closing sounds, whereas the more modern single/double tilting disc valves make only closing sounds. Closing sounds are always louder. There will be a midline sternotomy scar, but also look carefully for a pacemaker scar (much less common than in aortic valve replacement patients) in the left infraclavicular area, and look/feel for the im-planted pacemaker beneath this scar. Look for a subtle left lateral thoracotomy scar from previous mitral valvuloplasty. If there were changes to the JVP look again for supporting evidence of pul-monary hypertension, feeling for the left paraster-nal heave of a pressure-loaded right ventricle and a thrill at the left sternal edge with functional tricuspid regurgitation. The closing click of the first heart sound might be palpable at the apex and feel for any lateral displacement or thrusting quality of the apex signifying mitral regurgitation from valve dysfunction.

Auscultation: the first heart sound will be the closing click of the prosthetic valve. In the case of the older Starr–Edwards valves you might also hear an opening click in diastole after the second heart sound. The second heart sound may be normal or there may be a loud P2 in the case of pulmonary hypertension. There might be a mid-diastolic flow murmur across the prosthetic mitral valve, heard best at the apex in expiration and with the patient in the left lateral position. If there are signs of pulmonary hypertension, listen care-fully at the left sternal edge for the pansystolic murmur of functional tricuspid regurgitation, heard best in inspiration. Listen carefully for any signs of mitral regurgitation signifying prosthesis failure. Mitral regurgitation will give a pansystolic murmur heard best at the apex in expiration and radiating to the axilla. Be careful to correctly differentiate the murmur of valve dysfunction from that of tricuspid regurgitation with pulmon-ary hypertension.

Periphery: there are no signs of heart failure except where there is valve failure or right heart failure from advanced pulmonary hypertension. Indicate that you would like to examine for splenomegaly, check the toenails for splinter hae-morrhages, and ask to dip the urine and check the temperature chart, carefully searching for signs of endocarditis. Look for the peripheral scars of venous grafting from the radial or long saphenous veins with any concomitant CABG procedure.

Clinical judgement and maintaining patient welfare

Indications for mitral valve replacement in stenosis or regurgitation are described above. Other indications for mitral valve replacement include:

- Infective endocarditis not responding to medical therapy
- Acute mitral valve regurgitation from papillary muscle infarction or chordal rupture following an MI and where valve repair is not possible.

SCENARIO 11. VENTRICULAR SEPTAL DEFECT

When examining a patient with a VSD the candidate is expected to determine if the defect is haemodynamically significant, thus causing pulmonary hypertension and its attendant signs. In more severe cases there may even be progression to shunt reversal (right-to-left ventricular flow) termed 'Eisenmenger syndrome', causing cyanosis.

Identifying physical signs

Functional status: the patient is usually well at rest but if pulmonary hypertension has developed then the patient may be dyspnoeic and using supplemental oxygen.

Hands, pulse, face: there is usually a normal pulse in sinus rhythm. Look for phenotypic features of congenital syndromes that are associated with VSD such as Down, Edwards or DiGeorge syndrome (hypertelorism and low-set ears).

In a haemodynamically significant defect with shunt reversal there will be cyanosis and clubbing.

JVP: the JVP is usually normal. In a haemodynamically significant defect with pulmonary hypertension, there will be an elevated JVP and functional tricuspid regurgitation will give rise to large systolic 'v' waves.

Inspection and palpation of precordium: in a small VSD there are no scars, the apex is normal and there are no thrills.

In larger VSDs pulmonary hypertension develops, leading to right heart signs. There may be a parasternal heave from the pressure-loaded right ventricle and a thrill at the left sternal edge from functional tricuspid regurgitation. It is unlikely that there will be a parasternal thrill from the VSD (irrespective of shunt direction) because, in adults, VSDs have usually been surgically corrected, and clinically insignificant defects have little flow across them and thus generate no thrill.

Auscultation: (see Figure 3.6) with small defects the heart sounds are normal, but S2 may be obscured because the loud pansystolic murmur is heard till the end of systole and radiates all over the precordium.

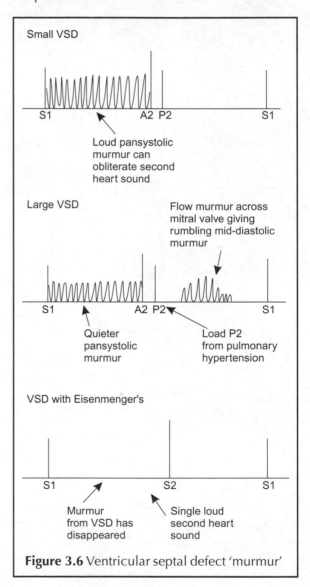

Figure 3.6 Ventricular septal defect 'murmur'

In larger defects with significant left-to-right shunting, the development of pulmonary hypertension leads to a loud P2 and the pansystolic murmur of the VSD will become quieter. With the increased blood volume returning to the left heart (due to blood re-entering the pulmonary circulation) there may be a flow murmur across the mitral valve, giving rise to a rumbling mid-diastolic murmur at the apex.

As pulmonary hypertension increases there will be shunt reversal right to left and the development of Eisenmenger's syndrome. Ventricular pressures will equalise; there will be a single loud second heart sound and the murmur from the VSD will disappear. Any systolic murmur heard at the left sternal edge will represent functional tricuspid regurgitation.

Be careful to examine for other cardiovascular lesions that can be associated with a VSD such as a bicuspid aortic valve leading to aortic stenosis, or aortic regurgitation associated with membranous VSDs in which the aortic leaflet can prolapse through the defect.

Periphery: there will be no peripheral signs in small ventricular defects. With larger haemodynamically significant defects, there will be signs of right-sided (peripheral oedema) and left-sided heart failure (pulmonary oedema).

Additional: ask to measure the blood pressure, state that you would test the urine and perform fundoscopy if suspecting bacterial endocarditis. Request to see a recent ECG.

Differential diagnosis

Atrial septal defect: there is a fixed and widely split second heart sound. The murmur is usually higher up the left sternal edge and represents greater flow across the pulmonary valve (it is not a murmur associated with the septal defect itself), so it is quieter and more ejection systolic in character.

Mitral regurgitation: a pansystolic murmur heard in the apex, radiating to the axilla and heard best during expiration.

Tricuspid regurgitation: a pansystolic murmur heard at the lower left sternal edge, heard best in inspiration. In lone tricuspid regurgitation there may be signs of right heart failure but not pulmonary hypertension seen with the functional tricuspid regurgitation associated with VSDs.

Pulmonary stenosis: this gives rise to an ejection systolic murmur in the pulmonary area heard best during inspiration and will not have the associated signs of pulmonary hypertension.

Clinical judgement and maintaining patient welfare

Broadly, there are two types of VSDs: membranous and muscular (which is further subdivided depending on location). Membranous defects are the most common form, accounting for 80%, and these are sited adjacent to the aortic ring.

Isolated VSDs are the most common congenital cardiac defect at a rate of 2 per 1000 live births, with equal sex incidence. About 50% of small defects close spontaneously in the first few years of life and have no sequelae. Historically small VSDs were called maladie de Roger. In up to 30% of those with congenital VSDs there may also be other congenital heart defects such as a bicuspid aortic valve, coarctation of the aorta, ASD or PDA. Alternatively, it might be part of the tetralogy of Fallot.

Causes
Congenital
- Spontaneous
  - Genetic: Down, Edwards, DiGeorge syndromes
  - Antenatal: maternal diabetes, fetal alcohol syndrome.

Acquired
- MI with septal necrosis
- Iatrogenic puncture of the septum from a right ventricle pacing wire or as a complication of septal ablation for HOCM.

Complications of a VSD include:

- Pulmonary hypertension
- Recurrent bronchopneumonia
- Eisenmenger syndrome and paradoxical embolus
- Endocarditis
- LVH or RVH and failure
- Aortic regurgitation with large membranous defects.

Investigations
- **ECG**: this is normal in small defects. In moderate/large defects there may be markers of left atrial enlargement and hypertrophy (P mitrale in lead II and biphasic P waves) and LVH (deep S in V1 + R in V6 >35 mm). In RVH there will be right axis deviation and tall R waves in V1 and deep S waves in V6.
- **Chest radiograph**: this is normal with small defects. In moderate/large defects with left-to-right shunts anteroposterior (AP) images will show an enlarged left atrium and ventricle with increased pulmonary vasculature. In Eisenmenger syndrome with large right-to-left shunts, there will be an enlarged right ventricle with a prominent pulmonary artery and reduced pulmonary vascular markings in the periphery ('pruning').
- **Echocardiography**: this is used to show the location and size of the defect and direction of the shunt. It is used to assess right and left ventricular sizes and function. It can assess the ratio of pulmonary:systemic blood flows.
- **Cardiac catheterisation**: used for further assessment of shunt magnitude and extent and reversibility of pulmonary hypertension.

Management
Most VSDs are small and need no other medical treatment other than endocarditis prophylaxis

(NICE Guidelines 2008: http://guidance.nice.org. uk/CG64 due to be reviewed).

Heart failure symptoms can be managed along standard lines with diuretics.

Medical management of pulmonary hypertension and Eisenmenger syndrome includes the use of pulmonary vasculature vasodilator medications:

- Endothelin antagonist (bosentan)
- Phosphodiesterase-5 inhibitor (sildenafil)
- Prostanoid infusions (epoprostenol).

Indications for surgery for VSD
- Pulmonary:systemic blood flow ⩾2.0 and LV dysfunction
- History of endocarditis
- Aortic regurgitation from prolapse of aortic leaflet through membranous defect
- Acute defect from rupture of septum post-MI (significant defects are unlikely to result from iatrogenic puncture of the septum).

Contraindications for surgery
- Irreversible pulmonary hypertension with development of Eisenmenger syndrome.

Prognosis
Most VSDs will close spontaneously or are small and require only endocarditis prophylaxis. Larger defects with significant shunts will require early surgical intervention to prevent ventricular dysfunction and pulmonary hypertension.

Maintaining patient welfare
- If your patient with a congenital heart defect has signs of an associated learning difficulty, take extra care to explain clearly what you would like to do during your examination.
- Patients with haemodynamically significant defects may fatigue easily or be breathless, so keep patient movement and breathing instructions to a minimum.

SCENARIO 12: ATRIAL SEPTAL DEFECT

ASDs come in two main forms – ostium primum and ostium secundum – depending on the defect location. Ostium secundum ASDs are more centrally placed, whereas ostium primum ASDs occur near the AV junction. Ostium secundum is the most common form comprising approximately 75% of all ASDs. Initially there is left-to-right shunting between the atria, but with the development of pulmonary hypertension there may be reversal of the shunt and Eisenmenger syndrome.

In the examination of the ASD case, the clinician should determine whether it is a haemodynamically significant ASD and if there has been shunt reversal.

Identifying physical signs

Functional status: the patient usually appears comfortable at rest, unless there is pulmonary hypertension and shunt reversal causing cyanosis and breathlessness.

Hands, pulse, face: the patient is usually in sinus rhythm unless a haemodynamically significant ASD has given rise to right atrial enlargement and AF. In large ASDs leading to Eisenmenger's syndrome there will be cyanosis and clubbing.

JVP: the JVP is usually normal. If the patient is in AF the 'a' wave will be missing.

With the development of pulmonary hypertension there will be an elevated JVP, and if present functional tricuspid regurgitation will give rise to large systolic 'v' waves.

Inspection and palpation of precordium: with a small ASD there will be no scars, heaves or thrills. An ASD might arise as a complication of atrial perforation for balloon valvotomy for mitral stenosis. If this is followed by a subsequent open mitral valve replacement there will be a lateral thoracotomy scar. There is a normal apex beat.

In a haemodynamically significant ASD there will initially be a left-to-right shunt, causing increased flow across the pulmonary valve. This will be detected as a thrill at the upper left sternal edge. This might be accompanied by a right ventricular heave.

As the condition progresses, Eisenmenger syndrome develops with a right-to-left shunt and LV dilatation and failure. There may be a thrill of functional tricuspid regurgitation at the lower left sternal edge and the apex will be displaced and thrusting with associated left heart failure.

Auscultation: *there will be fixed splitting of the second heart sound, a cardinal feature of an ASD.* This describes the phenomenon of P2 delayed behind A2 in all phases of respiration, due to the delayed closure of the pulmonary valve from the greater volume of blood flowing across it. In larger ASDs with increased blood flow across the pulmonary valve there will be a loud P2.

The ASD itself has no murmur associated with it. There may be an ejection systolic pulmonary flow murmur in the upper left sternal edge. Occasionally there is a mid-diastolic tricuspid flow murmur at the lower left sternal edge. Both these murmurs will disappear as the shunt reverses, with the development of pulmonary hypertension, to be replaced by a loud single second heart sound and the murmurs of pulmonary (Graham Steell) and tricuspid regurgitation.

Periphery: usually there are no peripheral signs unless there is a haemodynamically significant ASD that has led to pulmonary hypertension and right-sided heart failure with peripheral oedema. With further disease progression there will be signs of left heart failure and bibasal crepitations.

Differential diagnosis

VSD: the murmur is usually lower down the left sternal edge and harsher/louder.

Pulmonary stenosis: there will be an ejection systolic murmur at the upper left sternal edge and pulmonary area with a quiet P2.

Widely split S2: this phenomenon can occur in ASD, pulmonary stenosis (both delayed P2) and mitral regurgitation (early A2).

Clinical judgement and maintaining patient welfare

Investigations
- **ECG**: the most common finding is incomplete RBBB (same QRS morphology as RBBB but shorter QRS duration at 0.10–0.12 s). There may also be prolongation of the PR interval, atrial arrhythmias, and left axis deviation in ostium primum defects and right axis deviation in ostium secundum defects.
- **Chest radiograph**: this is normal in small ASDs. In Eisenmenger syndrome there will be an enlarged right ventricle with a prominent pulmonary artery but reduced peripheral pulmonary vascular markings.
- **Echocardiography**: this can show the type and size of the defect and the direction of the shunt. It can be used to calculate pulmonary:systemic flow.
- **Cardiac catheterisation** can measure the extent and reversibility of pulmonary hypertension.

Management
Unlike VSDs, ASDs are very rarely associated with bacterial endocarditis and thus patients are not advised to take endocarditis prophylaxis, unless they have had a previous episode of endocarditis.

Small ASDs with normal pulmonary pressures require no treatment.

With larger haemodynamically significant ASDs:

- Management of heart failure symptoms with diuretics
- Management of pulmonary hypertension and Eisenmenger's syndrome with pulmonary vasculature vasodilator medications (see Scenario 11. VSD).

Indications for surgery for ASD:

- Increasing pulmonary:systemic flow.

Contraindications to ASD surgery

- Development of Eisenmenger syndrome, unless there is evidence of reversible pulmonary hypertension.

Closure can include open surgical repair or, more commonly, percutaneous procedures using a septal occlusion placed across the defect under screening.

Prognosis
Small ASDs usually have no clinical sequelae. Complications can include:

- Atrial arrhythmias
- Paradoxical embolus
- Pulmonary hypertension
- Right and left heart failure
- Eisenmenger syndrome
- Infective endocarditis.

A PDA is a persistent fetal remnant of the communication between the descending aorta and the pulmonary artery. The ductus usually exits the thoracic aorta distal to the left subclavian artery. The ductus arteriosus normally closes within the first 24 hours of life in a term baby.

Identifying physical signs

Functional status: the patient usually appears comfortable at rest, unless there is pulmonary hypertension and shunt reversal when the patient may be cyanosed and breathless.

Hands, pulse, face: the pulse may be bounding and collapsing with a wide pulse pressure.

JVP: the JVP is usually normal, but elevated with large systolic 'v' waves if the patient has developed pulmonary hypertension with functional tricuspid regurgitation.

Inspection and palpation of precordium: in a haemodynamically significant PDA with pulmonary hypertension, a volume-loaded right ventricle will give rise to a heave at the left sternal edge. There may be the palpable thrill of functional tricuspid regurgitation at the lower left sternal edge. The PDA itself will give a thrill in the upper left sternal edge below the left clavicle.

With a large PDA, the greater volume of blood returning through the pulmonary system gives rise to a volume-overloaded left ventricle, which in time will dilate, leading to a thrusting displaced apex beat.

Auscultation: S1 is normal and there is a continuous 'machinery' murmur (Gibson's murmur) from the PDA in the left infraclavicular area. It is called a continuous murmur because it can carry on through to diastole after a systolic peak. The murmur can also be heard posteriorly above the left scapula.

With a large shunt there may be mid-diastolic and systolic murmurs from the increased flow across the mitral and aortic valves, respectively. There may be a third heart sound due to rapid ventricular filling. With the development of pulmonary hypertension, P2 becomes loud and the machinery murmur can grow quieter and shorten as the shunt begins to reverse and Eisenmenger syndrome develops. There may be the murmurs of pulmonary (Graham Steell) and mitral regurgitation in these latter cases.

Periphery: usually there are no peripheral signs unless there is right-sided heart failure with the development of pulmonary hypertension; then there will be peripheral oedema. The chronically overloaded left ventricle begins to fail and there will be bibasal crepitations with pulmonary oedema.

As the PDA occurs between the pulmonary artery and the descending aorta after the origins for both the innominate and left subclavian arteries, with the development of pulmonary hypertension deoxygenated blood from the pulmonary artery enters the descending aorta destined for the lower limbs. The upper limbs remain unaffected because they receive oxygenated blood from the proximal aorta before the ductus and this gives rise to the phenomenon of differential cyanosis and clubbing in the lower limbs only.

Differential diagnosis of a continuous murmur

Venous hum: this can occur in young children with kinking of the large veins in the neck, but the murmur will be heard loudest in the neck, the patient will be young, and the continuous murmur will disappear on lying supine or obliterating the cervical venous circulation with gentle pressure.

VSD with aortic regurgitation: similar to a PDA, aortic regurgitation will give a collapsing pulse and wide pulse pressure. The combination of a VSD with aortic regurgitation will give the impression of a continuous murmur starting in systole and merging across the second heart sound into early diastole.

Causes of a collapsing bounding pulse from a hyperdynamic circulation include: aortic regurgitation, PDA, pregnancy, anaemia, thyrotoxicosis and fever.

Clinical judgement and maintaining patient welfare

Cause
- Prematurity (prolonged low pulmonary oxygenation and increased pulmonary resistance delay PDA closure)
- Maternal rubella infection in the first trimester (PDA is the most common congenital cardiac lesion after maternal rubella)
- Maternal use of prostaglandins
- Down syndrome
- High altitude (low oxygen tensions give rise to similar mechanisms operating in prematurity).

Complications of PDA
- Respiratory problems, heart failure and failure to thrive in infants with large PDAs
- Infective endocarditis
- Pulmonary hypertension
- Right and left heart failure

- Eisenmenger syndrome.

Investigations
- **ECG**: this is not reliable in the diagnosis of PDA but may show LVH or LVH changes in adults.
- **Chest radiograph**: this is normal in small PDAs. In large defects with pulmonary hypertension there will be an enlarged right ventricle, with a prominent pulmonary artery but reduced pulmonary vascular markings in the periphery. There may be typical signs of left heart failure in advanced disease.
- **Echocardiography** can show the turbulent retrograde jet within the pulmonary artery and the size of the defect. It is also used to look for any other associated congenital defects.
- **Cardiac catheterisation** can reveal the extent and reversibility of pulmonary hypertension.

Management
- Endocarditis prophylaxis (NICE Guidelines 2008: http://guidance.nice.org.uk/CG64 due to be reviewed)
- Spontaneous closure in infants is as high as 75% in the first 3 months of life and others can be treated with prostaglandin inhibitors such as indometacin to increase the rate of closure
- In adults it is advisable to close the PDA because the percutaneous procedure of transcatheter closure has a lower surgical risk than that of endocarditis
- Medical management of heart failure symptoms with diuretics
- Medical management of pulmonary hypertension and Eisenmenger syndrome with pulmonary vasculature vasodilators
- PDA closure is contraindicated with the development of Eisenmenger syndrome
- In some neonates with other congenital heart defects such as transposition of the great arteries, it is necessary to maintain the PDA with administration of prostaglandins, until corrective surgery is performed.

Prognosis

- Small PDAs usually have a very good prognosis and are easily repaired with a transcatheter approach.
- More than half of all deaths from PDA are from complications of endocarditis.

- Large PDAs have an associated mortality rate as high as 60% at age 60, due to a volume-overloaded left ventricle, leading to left heart failure and the development of Eisenmenger syndrome.

SCENARIO 14. EISENMENGER SYNDROME

Eisenmenger syndrome occurs when a congenital cardiac defect leads to the development of pulmonary hypertension with shunt reversal from right to left, giving rise to central cyanosis. The causes of Eisenmenger syndrome include those conditions with shunt defects: ASD, VSD and PDA. The underlying cardiac defect that gave rise to Eisenmenger syndrome can be very difficult to diagnose clinically because the features of the original shunt are obliterated with the onset of the syndrome itself. The candidate is expected to be able to diagnose Eisenmenger syndrome from the clinical presentation of pulmonary hypertension with cyanosis and then present a differential diagnosis.

Identifying physical signs

Functional status: the patient may appear pale and breathless at rest and may be using supplemental oxygen.

Hands, pulse, face: the patient is usually in sinus rhythm but may also present in AF if an ASD has given rise to right atrial enlargement. Eisenmenger syndrome will give rise to cyanosis (differential cyanosis if there is a PDA) and clubbing.

JVP: the JVP is raised with RV heart failure and there may be large 'a' waves from forceful atrial contraction against a stiff pressure-loaded right ventricle, and large systolic 'v' waves from functional tricuspid regurgitation. If the patient is in AF the 'a' wave will be missing.

Inspection and palpation of precordium: there are no scars. There will be a left parasternal heave from a pressure-loaded right ventricle, and there may be a thrill at the lower left sternal edge, signifying functional tricuspid regurgitation and a palpable pulmonary component to the second heart sound – best felt in the pulmonary area.

The apex beat will be displaced and thrusting with associated left heart failure.

Auscultation: there is a single and loud second heart sound, from P2. The second heart sound is usually single from equalisation of the ventricular volumes with shunt reversal. Thus it is usually not possible to identify a widely split second heart sound from an associated ASD after Eisenmenger syndrome has developed.

There is an ejection systolic click heard in the pulmonic area from pulmonary artery dilatation.

There may a high-pitched early diastolic murmur at the upper left sternal edge radiating down the sternal edge, constituting the Graham Steell murmur of pulmonary regurgitation.

There is a pansystolic murmur along the lower left sternal edge, associated with functional tricuspid regurgitation.

The original murmurs associated with the instigating cardiac defect (pansystolic murmur of the VSD, pulmonary and tricuspid flow murmurs of an associated ASD, continuous 'machinery' murmur of a PDA) disappear after Eisenmenger syndrome has developed.

Periphery: there are signs of cyanosis and clubbing (which may be differential, affecting only lower limbs if the original cardiac defect was a PDA) and signs of right heart failure with peripheral oedema. The lung fields are usually clear (differentiating this from cor pulmonale).

Clinical judgement and maintaining patient welfare

Any congenital cardiac defect or palliative surgical correction that causes a large left-to-right shunt can lead to increased pulmonary blood flow. This increases pulmonary arterial pressures, which over time increases pulmonary vascular resistance, pulmonary artery pressure and eventual shunt reversal.

Complications
- RV failure
- Angina
- Arrhythmias (AF and flutter)
- Infective endocarditis
- Haemoptysis
- Recurrent pneumonia
- Paradoxical embolism (transient ischaemic attack (TIA) or stroke)
- Brain abscess
- Polycythaemia and hyperviscosity syndrome
- Bleeding disorders
- Hyperuricaemia and gout.

Management
- Endocarditis prophylaxis
- Advise avoidance of smoking, alcohol, dehydration and hot conditions which can increase the right-to-left shunt
- Contraceptive advice: maternal mortality rate approaches 50% with pregnancy in Eisenmenger syndrome. Tubal ligation or the intrauterine system of contraception (IUS) is usually advised
- Treat heart failure symptomatically with cautious use of diuretics
- Polycythaemia with a haematocrit >65% can be treated by venesection and volume replacement (rule out dehydration as a cause of increased haematocrit)
- Supplemental oxygen is used for cyanosis
- Surgical repair of the primary cardiac defect is indicated only where the pulmonary hypertension is shown to be reversible
- Heart–lung transplantation is indicated in certain cases with Eisenmenger syndrome.

Prognosis
Eisenmenger syndrome has a poor prognosis with a survival rate <50% beyond age 25 years.

SCENARIO 15: HYPERTROPHIC CARDIOMYOPATHY

Hypertrophic cardiomyopathy (HOCM) is a genetic condition and describes a usually asymmetrical form of LVH that occurs without any cause (such as hypertension or aortic stenosis). It commonly affects the interventricular septum and rarely can also affect the right ventricle. Most cases of HOCM are non-obstructive, but in 25% of cases the interventricular asymmetrical thickening, together with the systolic anterior motion (SAM) of the mitral valve leaflet, leads to left ventricular outflow tract (LVOT) obstruction and the characteristic clinical signs described below.

Identifying physical signs

Functional status: the patient usually appears comfortable at rest. The patient may be young.

Hands, pulse, face: the patient with HOCM is usually in sinus rhythm and may have a jerky double pulse felt at the radial or carotid. Alternatively the patient may be in AF. The double pulse comes from initial rapid ventricular emptying (first upstroke of the pulse) followed by a dip (obstruction of the outflow tract) and then a slower phase of ventricular emptying (second peak).

Look for typical phenotypic features seen with disorders associated with HOCM such as Friedreich's ataxia or myotonic dystrophy (see Scenarios 12 and 8).

JVP: the JVP is usually normal but may show large 'a' waves due to atrial contraction against a non-compliant right ventricle, or there may be absent 'a' waves if the patient is in AF.

Inspection and palpation of precordium: a non-displaced, double apical impulse can be felt that

is pressure loaded and heaving. The double apical impulse comes from a palpable presystolic atrial contraction against a stiff left ventricle, followed by ventricular contraction. In late-stage disease with LV systolic dysfunction there may be lateral displacement of the apex.

There will be a left parasternal thrill from the LVOT obstruction, and there may be a thrill palpable at the apex from mitral regurgitation associated with SAM of the mitral valve leaflets.

Auscultation: S1 is normal followed by a harsh ejection systolic murmur at the lower left sternal edge, radiating up the sternal edge but not as far as the carotids. There may be reverse splitting of S2 (splitting on expiration with A2 *after* P2) due to prolonged LV contraction from the large systolic pressure gradient and delayed relaxation. There may be a fourth heart sound in diastole from atrial contraction against a stiffened ventricle and this will be associated with the equivalent large 'a' waves in the JVP.

If there is SAM of the mitral valve leaflets causing mitral regurgitation, there will be a pansystolic murmur at the apex radiating up to the axilla and loudest on expiration. Some patients have *dynamic* LVOT obstruction and clinical signs evident only after certain manoeuvres that reduce the LV volume before systole (reduce preload), and hence increase the obstruction, such as standing from squatting and Valsalva's manoeuvre. The opposite is true with an increase in preload and ventricular volume before systole, decreasing LVOT flow (and the murmur), such as squatting.

Periphery: in late-stage disease LV systolic dysfunction may occur with signs of left heart failure:

Differential diagnosis

Aortic stenosis: there is a smooth, slow-rising pulse with a narrow pulse pressure. The ejection systolic murmur is heard loudest in the aortic area with radiation up to the carotids. The murmur does not usually change with manoeuvres unlike that of HOCM, and aortic stenosis may diminish with the strain phase of Valsalva's manoeuvre.

VSD: a pansystolic murmur that radiates more widely may have associated features of pulmonary hypertension and does not change with manoeuvres.

Clinical judgement and maintaining patient welfare

HOCM is present in all racial types, has an average prevalence of 0.5% and shows no sex preference. It can be associated with Friedreich's ataxia or myotonic dystrophy. At least 60% of HOCM cases have identified mutations in sarcomere genes and typically have autosomal dominant inheritance with variable penetrance.

Many patients with HOCM are asymptomatic but it is the most common cause of sudden cardiac death in adolescents, thought to result from ventricular tachyarrhythmias. Symptoms and complications include:

- Dyspnoea
- Angina (from increased myocardial demand and disruption and abnormal thickening of intramural coronary arteries)
- Syncope
- Arrhythmia (AF, ventricular ectopics, ventricular fibrillation and ventricular tachycardia)
- Endocarditis
- Diastolic heart failure
- Systolic heart failure (late stages)
- Sudden death.

Investigations

- **ECG**: there may be left axis deviation with voltage criteria for LVH, ventricular ectopic beats and Q waves in the leads facing the ventricular septum (V2–4, II, III and aVF).
- **Chest radiograph**: this is usually normal but will show left atrial dilatation and cardiomegaly in late stages with pulmonary changes of left heart failure.
- **Echocardiography**: this will show the area of hypertrophy with ventricular/interventricular septal thickening and allow measurement of the septal thickness if considering surgical correction. SAM of the anterior mitral leaflet on 'M' mode and LVOT obstruction can both be measured. Echocardiography will also assess diastolic and systolic ventricular function.
- **Treadmill testing**: this is important to assess for any exercise-induced outflow tract obstruction changes.
- **Cardiac catheterisation**: will assess coronary artery anatomy and any concomitant pathology that might explain angina symptoms. Rarely biopsy is needed if HOCM diagnosis is in doubt and other specific causes of hypertrophy are being sought.
- **Genetic testing**: this will be needed for individuals with HOCM and their relatives.

Management

Management should include patient and family education with appropriate genetic testing and cardiopulmonary resuscitation (CPR) training for family members.

Advise patients to avoid strenuous sports or activities and seek prompt medical review for symptoms that include syncope, palpitations, chest pain or breathlessness.

Endocarditis prophylaxis is indicated (NICE Guidelines 2008: http://guidance.nice.org.uk/CG64 due to be reviewed).

Manage symptomatic HOCM with:

- β blockers
- Treatment of AF by rhythm control and anticoagulation
- Amiodarone for any ventricular arrhythmias
- Implantable cardiac defibrillator (ICD) for any ventricular arrhythmias or other risks for sudden death (see later)
- Diuretics for any congestive cardiac failure
- Spironolactone, ACE inhibitor and digoxin for those with end-stage heart failure.

If there is evidence of LVOT obstruction consider alcohol or surgical septal ablation.

Prognosis
- HOCM is a progressive disease so patients should receive long-term follow-up.
- Factors indicating high risk for sudden death include: from the history – younger patients, syncope and presyncope, sudden death in family members; from investigations – blood pressure changes during treadmill testing, any arrhythmias, septal thickness >30 mm (normal <12 mm) and certain genetic mutations.

SCENARIO 16. COARCTATION OF THE AORTA

Coarctation of the aorta describes a narrowing of the aorta. This is usually the thoracic aorta either at the level of the ductus arteriosus or just after. It accounts for 5–8% of congenital heart defects and has a female:male ratio of 2:1. Adult patients in the PACES examination usually present with aortic coarctation as part of a syndrome such as Turner's, together with other heart defects, or with corrected coarctation with residual signs.

Identifying physical signs

Functional status: the patient usually appears comfortable at rest. The patient may be young. Look for signs of Turner's syndrome (approximately a third have aortic coarctation).

Hands, pulse, face: feel for radioradial delay and radiofemoral delay with differential temperature and colour in the limbs. The most common form of coarctation occurs after the origin of the left subclavian artery, so a common finding is equal radial pulses but radiofemoral delay. There may also be differential cyanosis and lower BP readings in the lower limbs compared with the upper limbs. The BP reading in the upper limbs is usually high. If the coarctation is proximal to the origin of the subclavian artery, there will be a diminished left radial artery pulse.

Coarctation of the aorta is commonly associated with a bicuspid aortic valve, so there may be a high pulse pressure if there is concomitant aortic regurgitation or a slow rising pulse in aortic stenosis.

Look for scars of the left radial artery harvesting sometimes used for repair of the coarctation.

There may be visible pulsations in the neck from the collateral circulation.

JVP: this is usually normal.

Inspection and palpation of precordium: look for any scars such as a left thoracotomy scar of open surgical repair of the aortic coarctation. There may be visible pulsations and palpable thrills corresponding to the development of a collateral circulation. These might be felt over the anterior abdominal and chest wall, in the anterior axillary line, and over the left scapula and up to the neck. The apex will be undisplaced but heaving.

Auscultation: there will be a normal S1 and S2 unless there is associated severe aortic stenosis, which will give a quiet S2, or severe aortic regurgitation, which will give a loud P2. There may be the systolic ejection click and ejection systolic murmur associated with a stenosed bicuspid aortic valve. The coarctation itself might give rise to a pansystolic murmur, heard below the left clavicle and around the thoracic spine and left scapula posteriorly. In severe coarctations the murmur will be ejection systolic and also heard over the collaterals. In addition to listening for an associated bicuspid aortic valve, listen specifically for aortic stenosis and/or regurgitation that can be associated with this and other defects such as a VSD or PDA.

Periphery: continue to look for signs of underlying Turner syndrome (small stature, wide carrying angle and peripheral oedema), or evidence of cyanosis and stunted growth of the lower limbs. In late-stage disease LV systolic dysfunction may occur with signs of left-sided heart failure.

Differential diagnosis

Aortic stenosis: will also give rise to an ejection systolic murmur, but loudest in the aortic area, a quiet S2 and equal pulses in the limbs.

Repair of tetralogy of Fallot: there will also be a diminished or absent left radial pulse with a left thoracotomy scar. However, there will be no signs of a collateral circulation or palpable thrills over the precordium and posteriorly, and no signs of an associated bicuspid aortic valve.

Clinical judgement and maintaining patient welfare

There are two main types of coarctation of the aorta:

1. **Preductal/infantile type** which presents early with tachypnoea, severe heart failure and failure to thrive (especially after ductal closure). It is commonly associated with other heart defects.
2. **Ductal/postductal/adult type** presents from adolescence to adulthood, usually with hypertension, lower limb claudication and chest pain.

It is important to consider other associated conditions such as Turner syndrome (aortic coarctation is the most commonly associated cardiac defect), berry aneurysms and renal abnormalities including autosomal dominant polycystic kidney disease (ADPKD).

Investigations

* **ECG**: it may be associated with left axis deviation (LAD) with voltage criteria for LVH, and left atrial dilatation shown by bifid or inverted P waves in V1–3.
* **Chest radiograph**: the classic sign is rib notching (coarctation is the most common cause of this; other causes include superior vena cava obstruction (SVCO) syndrome, neurofibromatosis and Blalock–Taussig shunt repair). Rib notching is seen in the posterior

ribs only between the third and eighth ribs. (The upper two ribs are spared because their intercostal supply comes off the superior intercostal from the subclavian, usually proximal to the coarctation. The anterior ribs are not notched because the main blood flow to the intercostal muscles comes from the lateral and dorsal branches and the anterior intercostal branches arising from the internal mammary are insignificant in comparison.) There may be the figure '3' sign in the left superior mediastinum, attributed variously to: a dilated left subclavian artery, aortic knob, the 'tuck' of the coarctation or a poststenotic dilatation. In late stages there may be signs of left heart failure with pulmonary oedema.
* **Echocardiography**: can assess the extent of the coarctation; check for other associated cardiac defects and measure LV diastolic and systolic function.
* **MRI**: this offers very detailed views of the coarctation, collaterals and any post-repair aneurysms or restenosis.
* **Cardiac catheterisation**: this is used as an adjunct if echocardiography is indeterminate, and for planning percutaneous angioplasty and stenting.

Management
* Endocarditis prophylaxis is indicated if there is associated valvular disease (NICE Guidelines 2008: http://guidance.nice.org.uk/CG64 due to be reviewed)
* Medical bridging therapy involves treating hypertension with β blockers, but these are used cautiously due to the risk of reducing renal or lower limb perfusion
* Definitive treatment is surgical repair of the coarctation to prevent the complications of hypertension, including stroke and heart failure:
  * **Percutaneous repair** involves balloon angioplasty and stenting
  * **Open surgical repair** involves resection and end-to-end reanastomosis, Dacron patch repair, radial artery graft repair or subclavian artery flap repair

- There may be still a need for treatment of hypertension after repair due to long-term humoral effects of renin–angiotensin changes and continued follow-up to screen for recurrent obstruction.

Prognosis
Complications include LV failure, endocarditis, intracranial haemorrhage from berry aneurysms, aortic dissection and recurrent obstruction.

SCENARIO 17. TETRALOGY OF FALLOT

This is the most common cause of cyanotic congenital heart disease and occurs in 4 per 10 000 live births. It is composed of four defects but the pathology that dictates the clinical presentation and prognosis is the degree of right ventricular outflow tract (RVOT) obstruction. The four components are:

1. RVOT (infundibular stenosis)
2. VSD (non-restrictive)
3. Rightward overarching aorta (displaced over the VSD)
4. RVH (as a result of the above three).

Other cardiac defects can occur in addition, such as an ASD (pentalogy of Fallot) or a PDA, and these should be looked for on examination and investigation. Depending on the degree of RVOT obstruction a collateral pulmonary circulation of bronchopulmonary vessels can develop and a PDA can also maintain pulmonary blood flow. The patients are cyanotic due to the RVOT obstruction and the right-to-left shunt through the large VSD. Adult patients seen in the PACES examination would have received either palliative or corrective surgery.

Identifying physical signs

Functional status: the patient usually appears comfortable at rest but may appear cyanosed if he or she has had only a palliative shunt procedure.

Hands, pulse, face: there is digital clubbing signifying cyanotic heart disease. If there has been a Blalock–Taussig shunt procedure between either subclavian and a pulmonary artery, the right or left radial pulse may be diminished.

JVP: this is usually of normal height but with absent 'a' waves due to atrial contraction occurring against a non-restrictive VSD.

Inspection and palpation of precordium: there may be a midline (total repair) or a left/right thoracotomy scar (palliative shunt procedure). The apex beat is normal and there may be a RV heave felt at the left sternal edge. A systolic thrill may be felt at the upper left sternal edge (representing flow across the obstructed RVOT). There may be subclavicular thrills felt over surgical shunts.

Auscultation: there is a normal first heart sound and single louder second heart sound, heard best in the aortic area, because P2 is very quiet. There is an ejection systolic murmur heard in the pulmonary area or mid left sternal edge, heard louder in inspiration, representing the RVOT obstruction and NOT the VSD (which is non-restrictive so has no associated murmur). The more severe the RVOT obstruction the quieter and shorter the murmur. There may be a quiet early diastolic murmur heard in the aortic area with the patient leaning forward in expiration, representing aortic regurgitation (from prolapse of the overriding aortic cusp). If the patient has had a palliative shunt procedure there may be a continuous systolic murmur through to diastole, heard below either clavicle or posteriorly, representing flow throughout the surgical shunt.

Periphery: look for signs of right heart failure with peripheral oedema and any peripheral signs of endocarditis.

Differential diagnosis

- **Pulmonary stenosis**: the patient tends to be older and has no mediastinal scars, cyanosis or finger clubbing. The JVP has large 'a' waves in pulmonary stenosis from right atrial contraction against a non-compliant ventricle, whereas the 'a' waves are absent in tetralogy of Fallot. The second heart sound can be widely split with a quiet but present P2, and there may be a fourth heart sound of atrial contraction against a stiffened right ventricle, not heard in tetralogy of Fallot due to the VSD. The ejection systolic murmur in the pulmonary area radiates up to the suprasternal notch.
- **PDA**: these patients are unlikely to have clubbing or a mediastinal scar. There may be a volume-loaded collapsing pulse, with an elevated JVP and large 'v' waves (if pulmonary hypertension and TR have developed). There is a displaced, heaving apex. The PDA can give rise to a 'machinery' murmur beneath the left clavicle, but this murmur disappears because there is shunt reversal of right-to-left and the development of Eisenmenger syndrome. Thus a murmur beneath the left clavicle and posteriorly, together with signs of RVH, cyanosis and clubbing, must be from a Blalock–Taussig shunt (because the murmur of PDA would have diminished).

Clinical judgement and maintaining patient welfare

Cause

The aetiology of tetralogy of Fallot is thought to be multifactorial with interplay of environmental factors and genetics. Associated factors include:

- Maternal rubella
- Maternal carbamazepine use
- Maternal diabetes
- Down syndrome

- DiGeorge syndrome with phenotype summarised by CATCH-22 (**c**ardiac defects, **a**bnormal facies, **t**hymic hypoplasia, **c**left palate and **h**ypocalcaemia), which is an acronym describing the phenotypic features associated with deletions in chromosome 22
- Scoliosis.

Tetralogy of Fallot usually presents soon after birth with cyanosis and signs of heart failure, timing depending on the degree of RVOT obstruction. Children have 'tet spells' of sudden cyanosis, thought to be due to infundibular spasm causing a sudden fall in pulmonary blood flow. Older children do adaptive manoeuvres such as squatting which increases systemic vascular resistance, thus reducing or reversing the right-to-left shunt across the VSD and causing more blood to pass through the RVOT into the lungs, improving oxygenation. In addition squatting reduces systemic venous return of acidotic deoxygenated blood, which reduces infundibular spasm.

Cyanosis can also be worsened with:

- Fever
- Acidosis
- Hypoxia
- Infection
- Dehydration
- Stress.

Complications include:

- Endocarditis
- Polycythaemia leading to hyperviscosity complications
- Bleeding disorders
- Paradoxical emboli (right-to-left shunt)
- Brain abscess
- Right heart failure.

Investigations
- **ECG**: this will show right axis deviation (>90°) and RVH (tall R wave in V5–6, deep S wave in V1–2). There may be partial or complete RBBB after repair.

- **Chest radiograph**: this shows a boot-shaped heart (RVH leading to an upturned apex), reduced pulmonary vascular markings and 25% have a right-sided aortic arch.
- **Echocardiography**: this can delineate the anatomy and extent of the RVOT obstruction and degree of aortic override with aortic regurgitation. It is also used to assess for any associated PDA and ASD.
- **Cardiac catheterisation**: this is used in the assessment for anomalous coronary artery anatomy when planning surgical correction.

Management
- Most children have total corrective surgery under cardiopulmonary bypass at around 12 months of age, with pulmonary blood flow maintained until then by maintaining the patency of the ductus arteriosus with prostaglandins.
- Rarely, palliative systemic-to-pulmonary shunt procedures are performed now, including the Blalock–Taussig procedure and Waterston's anastomosis (anastomosing the back of the ascending aorta to the right pulmonary artery).

Prognosis
- Before surgical correction, prognosis was very poor with most patients dying in childhood and only a 10% survival rate up to the age of 20 years.
- After corrective surgery survival rates are up to 95% at 20 years.

THE NEUROLOGICAL EXAMINATION

Unlike the cardiology, respiratory and abdominal examinations, there is no standard approach to the neurological examination. The examination has to be prompted by the instructions and then adapted as the most likely pathology becomes apparent. Your examination is geared towards answering two questions:

1. Where in the nervous system is the lesion?
2. What are the likely causes of that lesion?

You are commonly asked to examine one or more of the following:

- Upper limbs
- Lower limbs
- Motor or sensory system
- Cranial nerves
- Cerebellar system
- Speech
- Eyes
- Gait.

Remember, as part of your examination, to look out for signs of systemic diseases that could be associated with the neurological findings. If time permits, be ready with a request to examine other systems if you feel that this is appropriate to help you form your differential diagnosis.

Examination routine

Approach to the patient
Introduce yourself to the patient, wash your hands and ask for permission to examine them which may require exposing part of the body. Check the patient has no pain before you start.

Observation and introduction
After introducing yourself you could ask the patient for his or her name and whether he or she is right or left handed. The answers may reveal a dysarthria or dysphasia.

General observation of the patient is likely to reveal important clues, so stand back and take a few moments for this part of the examination. While doing this you can alleviate any awkwardness by describing what you are doing to the patient and examiner: 'I am going to start my examination by taking a few moments for general first impressions.'

Specifically look for:

- Asymmetry in the face or limbs or any deformity
- Reduced, exaggerated and abnormal movements
- Posture of the patient at rest
- Muscle wasting, fasciculation or a resting tremor
- Walking aids and wheelchairs.

Cranial nerve examination

Position the patient opposite you, ideally on the edge of the bed or at a chair so that you can access him or her easily from both sides.

General inspection of the face

Look for:

- Asymmetry or facial droop
- Ptosis
- Scars (some look for scars at the end of the cranial nerve examination)
- Neurofibromas
- Naevi (eg a port-wine stain in the Sturge–Weber syndrome)

Inspect the back of the head and neck for scars or shunts.

Olfactory (I)

It is very unlikely that you would be asked to formally test smell but instead you can screen for any abnormality by asking: 'Have you noticed any change or difficulty with your sense of smell?' If you were to test olfaction formally you would be supplied with bottles of substances such as coffee and peppermint. Initially you would need to check the patency of each nostril then ask the patient to close their eyes and smell with each nostril separately while you occlude the other. The patient would be asked to try to identify the scent and describe whether it is weaker in either nostril.

Causes of anosmia/reduced olfaction include:

- Upper respiratory tract infection
- Smoking

- Nasal polyps
- Older age
- Tumours: ethmoid sinus, meningioma of the olfactory groove, frontal lobe tumours
- Trauma: basal or frontal skull fracture
- Congenital: Kallman syndrome
- Degenerative: Parkinson's and Alzheimer's dementia.

Ophthalmic (II)

In testing the ophthalmic nerve you need to examine visual acuity, visual fields and fundoscopy.

Visual acuity

You can start by asking whether the patient has any difficulty with vision and to wear his or her spectacles if he or she has them. Visual acuity should be tested in each eye separately and formally with a Snellen chart. This should be held 6 m from the patient.

Visual acuity is recorded as:

Distance at which the chart is held/Line number of smallest letters the patient can read.

For example, 6/6 is the smallest line a person with normal visual acuity can read at 6 m. A person with 6/20 acuity in the right eye can read from 6 m only letters from the line '20' which a person with normal visual acuity could read from 20 m. If the person cannot read the top letter at 6 m then move the chart forward until the patient can identify the top letter and change the top number of the ratio accordingly, eg 1/60 if the chart is moved forward to 1 m. If the person cannot read letters at 1 m then assess at what shorter distance they can correctly count fingers. If this is not possible then assess their perception for light in the affected eye(s).

Sites of lesions causing reduced visual acuity:
- Cornea, eg *Chlamydia trachomatis*
- Aqueous humour, eg aberrant drainage in glaucoma
- Lens, eg cataract

- Vitreous, eg preretinal haemorrhage
- Retina, eg retinitis pigmentosa or macular degeneration
- Optic nerve, eg optic neuritis
- Intracerebral, eg tumour or stroke.

Visual fields

Sit yourself opposite the patient about 1 m away, so that his or her fields can be tested against your own. You will be testing the patient's left visual field against your right visual field, and vice versa, by asking him or her to cover the appropriate eye while you mirror this by covering the opposite eye. Peripheral visual fields can be tested with a red- or white-headed hat pin (or

moving fingers if not available) but detection and measurement of central scotomata can be done only with a hat pin. Make sure that you hold your fingers or the hat pin half-way between yourself and the patient, such that it subtends the same angle and you are truly testing the patient's visual field against your own.

An initial **general inspection** may reveal a condition associated with visual field defects such as hemiparesis or acromegaly.

Test for **visual inattention** that could be associated with a parietal lesion from a stroke. Ask the patient to leave both eyes uncovered and

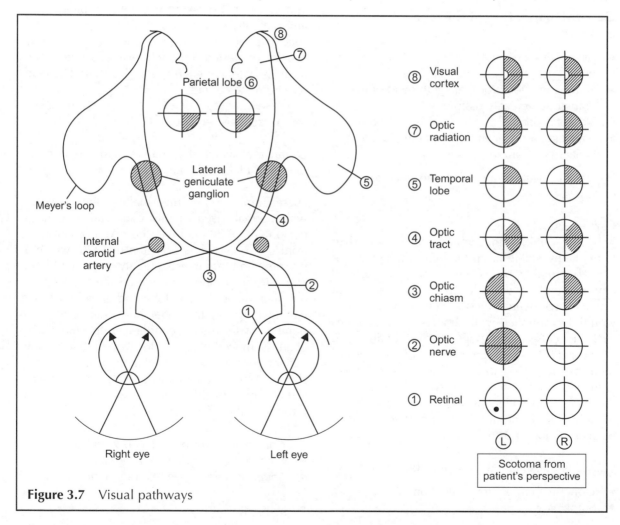

Figure 3.7　Visual pathways

look straight ahead, fixating on your nose; then holding your index fingers at the limits of your temporal fields wiggle them in turn and together, and ask the patient to report which finger he or she sees moving. A patient with visual inattention will identify only one finger moving at the times you are moving both.

Examine the **peripheral visual fields** of each eye in turn, reminding the patient to keep fixated on your nose while bringing in your object from each 45° angle of the periphery. In this manner work your way around eight angles within a 360° visual field including the vertical and horizontal axes (see Figure 3.7).

Map out any **scotomata** by bringing in the red-headed hat pin from the temporal field across the centre and to the nasal field, asking the patient to tell you whether it disappears or changes colour. If a scotoma is found, move the hat pin in the vertical axis as well to delineate its full size. **Peripheral scotomata** are caused by pathology within the retina, eg toxic effects of methanol, nutritional deficiencies or vascular changes with hypertension.

Next, test for the **blind spot,** which is a special type of **central scotoma** corresponding to the optic disc. Still with the patient covering one eye and fixating on your nose, move a red-headed hat pin between you, moving it slowly along the horizontal from the temporal to the nasal field. Ask the patient to say when the red pinhead disappears and reappears. The size of the blind spot should match your own. The blind spot can become enlarged and form a true central scotoma in papilloedema or optic atrophy.

Common field lesions in the context of the neurological examination would include a homonymous hemianopia or quadrantanopia indicating disease behind the optic chiasma, eg a left-sided middle cerebral infarct would cause a right homonymous hemianopia – the more posterior the lesion, the more congruent the visual field loss.

Fundoscopy
There is no substitute for practise. Repeat this examination on your colleagues and friends, making sure that you are comfortable with the different refractive settings on your ophthalmoscope. Some candidates prefer to leave this until the end of the examination and, if you do, state this to the examiner or patient: 'I will be performing fundoscopy at the end.' It can be very hard performing fundoscopy in a lit room with no pupil dilatation – make sure that the conditions are optimal.

Ask the patient to look straight ahead at a fixed point, but blink as needed, then place your left thumb against the right eyebrow and, with the ophthalmoscope close to your eye and at arm's length from the patient, check the red reflex in both eyes. This may reveal cataracts, which may make the fundoscopic examination more challenging. Then move in closer at an angle of roughly 45° to the visual axis, resting your left thumb against the patient's right brow to steady you. In this manner you will use your right eye to examine his or her right eye, and vice versa when you move to the left side. Remind the patient that he or she can blink but to keep looking straight ahead. Move through the lens settings until you can clearly see the retina by focusing on a vessel, then move along it until you find the disc. In the neurological examination you are looking for signs of papilloedema, papillitis, optic atrophy or retinitis pigmentosa (see Figure 3.8).

Oculomotor (III), trochlear (IV) and abducens (VI)
Remember the third nerve controls pupil constriction, maintains an open eye through innervating the levator palepbrae superioris and controls four out of six extraocular muscles.

Pupil examination, light reflex and accommodation
Initially perform a general inspection of both pupils for:

• Size

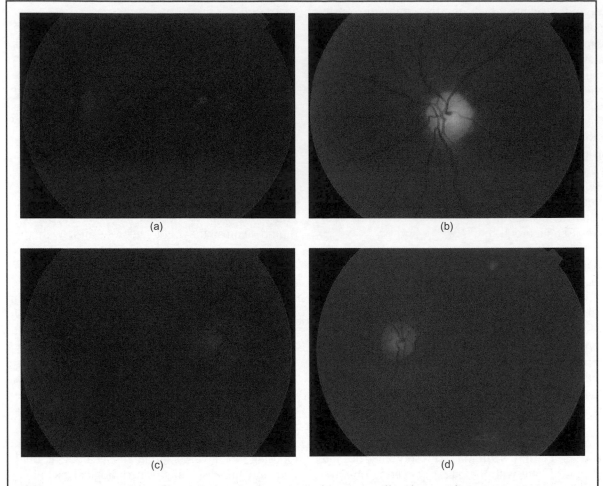

Figure 3.8   (a) Diabetic retinopathy, (b) Optic atrophy, (c) Papilloedema, (d) Retinitis pigmentosa

- Shape
- Equality
- Regularity.

Pupil findings in the neurological station include:

- Small pupil:
  - Horner's syndrome: includes meiosis, ptosis, anhidrosis and enophthalmos
  - Argyll–Robertson pupil: a small irregular pupil which **a**ccommodates but does *not* **r**eact to light
- Large pupil
  - Third nerve palsy: pupil fixed and dilated, eye in down and out position and ptosis

- Holmes–Adie pupil: the pupil is large and irregular and accommodates but reacts only slowly to light. It is a tonic pupil because, once constricted, it is slow to dilate. If associated with absent deep tendon reflexes, it is known as Holmes–Adie syndrome. This is a normal variant.

Test the pupillary light reflex from an angle to avoid shining the light directly onto the fovea. The afferent limb of the light reflex is through the ophthalmic nerve (II) and the efferent limb is through the oculomotor nerve (III). Look for the direct and consensual reflexes on both sides with use of the swinging light test by moving the torch in an arc from pupil to pupil. Look for a relative afferent pupillary defect (RAPD or Marcus Gunn pupil), which indicates a defective afferent limb of the light reflex in the affected eye. Shining light in the normal eye will produce normal and equal constriction in both eyes due to an intact afferent limb in the normal eye and an intact consensual reflex in the affected eye. Now, swinging the light to the affected eye will cause relative pupil dilatation in the affected eye (and normal eye) because the afferent limb is defective. Causes of a RAPD include optic neuritis, optic atrophy and retinal detachment.

Test the accommodation–convergence reflex by asking the patient to focus on your finger held in the central axis at arm's length distance, and then bring your finger forward towards the nose; the eyes should adduct and intort and the pupils constrict. This reflex is a coordination of cranial nerves II and III and higher centres including the Edinger–Westphal nucleus.

Extraocular eye movements

There are six cardinal directions of gaze (Figure 3.9). Initially inspect the patient's straight-ahead gaze for any obvious gaze paresis or ptosis that may provide clues. The patient may be holding the head in a certain posture to try to overcome any diplopia. With the patient now using both eyes, move your finger making a letter 'H', thus isolating the action of each extraocular muscle in turn. Ask the patient to report if he or she sees double at any point. If the patient does see double, there are three rules:

1. If the images are side by side, only the lateral or medial recti can be responsible.
2. Separation of the two images is greatest in the direction of movement of the affected muscle (or direction in which it has its purest action).
3. Using the cover test, the eye that gives the outer or most peripheral image is the affected eye.

If the pattern of ophthalmoplegia is complex, then always consider Graves' disease or myasthe-

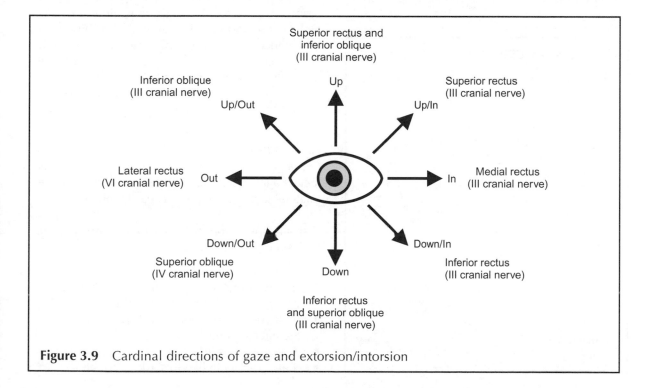

Figure 3.9   Cardinal directions of gaze and extorsion/intorsion

nia. Look for fatigability of eye movements, particularly sustained upward gaze.

Look for **internuclear ophthalmoplegia** (INO) when examining eye movements. A left-sided INO from a lesion affecting the left medial longitudinal fasciculus will give failure of left eye adduction on gaze to the right, but intact adduction with accommodation. All other eye movements will be normal.

Also look for **nystagmus** during the eye movement examination.

Trigeminal (V)

The motor root runs with the mandibular division of nerve V. Inspect for **wasting of the temporalis or masseters**. Loss of bulk is best appreciated on palpation while the patient clenches the teeth. If there is unilateral weakness on opening the jaw, it will deviate to the affected side, pushed by the intact pterygoid. Another way to test for power is to ask the patient to close the mouth against resistance as you try to keep the mouth open, resting your index finger on the patient's chin.

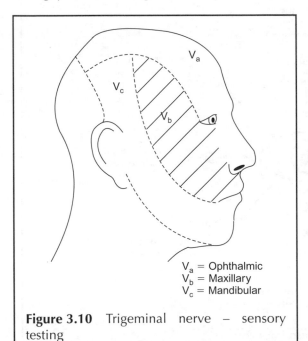

V_a = Ophthalmic
V_b = Maxillary
V_c = Mandibular

Figure 3.10 Trigeminal nerve – sensory testing

Look for the jaw jerk by using the tendon hammer on your index finger held against his or her chin. The jaw jerk may be absent/reduced (bulbar palsy) or exaggerated (pseudobulbar palsy).

Test for **sensation in each division** of the trigeminal nerve: **ophthalmic, maxillary** and **mandibular** (see Figure 3.10). The mandibular division is not affected in cavernous sinus syndrome because it leaves through the foramen ovale in the middle cranial fossa before reaching the cavernous sinus.

Test for the **corneal reflex** made up of an afferent (V) and efferent (VII) limb. Touch the cornea lightly at the edge of the eye with a wisp of cottonwool coming from the side while the patient looks straight ahead. Loss of the corneal reflex may be one of the first signs of pathology, eg acoustic neuroma. In herpes zoster ophthalmicus affecting one or more branches of the ophthalmic division (supraorbital, lacrimal and nasociliary), corneal involvement is thought more likely if the nasociliary branch is affected because this innervates the globe. (The unique dermatomal distribution of this branch is the tip of the nose and when this is affected (Hutchinson's disease) it is thought to predict ocular involvement. However, up to a third of those without this sign have ocular involvement.)

Facial (VII)

On general inspection you may detect unilateral facial sagging with loss of the nasolabial fold. A bilateral facial nerve palsy is easily missed.

Test all movements of facial expression and the platysma:

- 'Raise your eyebrows'
- 'Screw your eyes tight shut' (show that you can easily open the affected eye)
- 'Puff your cheeks out' (you can easily 'pop' the affected cheek)
- 'Can you whistle?'
- 'Bare your teeth like this' (demonstrate)

- 'Evert your bottom lip' (demonstrate loss of platysma function).

Some candidates choose to test the motor function of the trigeminal nerve with the facial nerve.

You can assess the sensory component of the facial nerve by asking to test taste on the anterior two-thirds of the tongue (chorda tympani), enquiring about hypersensitivity to certain sounds (nerve to stapedius) and pain in the outer ear (intermedius branch to external meatus).

Upper motor neuron lesion

This implies a lesion between the motor cortex and the facial nucleus in the pons (Figure 3.11). There is bilateral cortical representation of the upper facial muscles (frontalis and orbicularis oculi), so in an UMN lesion there is **contralateral lower** facial weakness.

- Sagging is less prominent because there is no loss of tone as with LMN lesions
- Sparing of frontalis and orbicularis oculi
- Flattened nasolabial fold

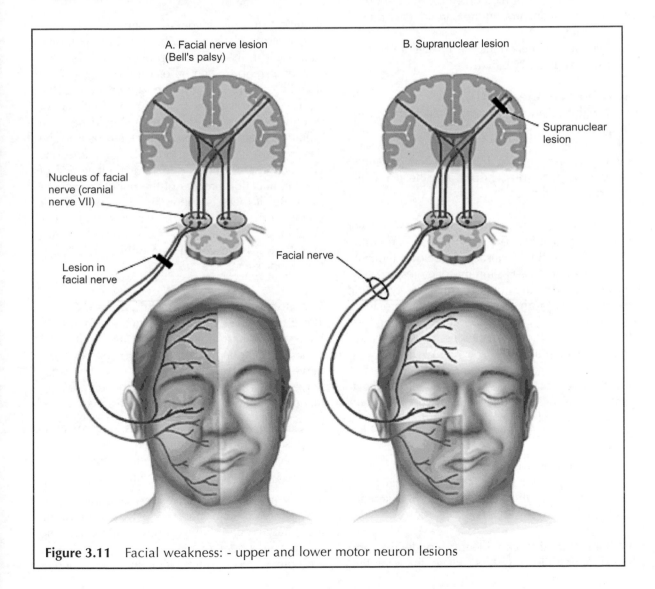

Figure 3.11   Facial weakness: - upper and lower motor neuron lesions

- Flattened mouth on smiling or bearing teeth
- There may be an associated ipsilateral limb weakness.

Lower motor neuron lesion
The facial weakness is more pronounced due to loss of tone and upper and lower facial muscles being affected:

- Paralysis of all ipsilateral facial muscles
- Bell's phenomenon (on attempted eye closure, the orbit rolls upwards)
- Look for scars around the parotid, ear and mastoid
- Look for lesions on the hard palate and external auditory canal.

Vestibulocochlear (VIII)

Start with the query: 'Any problem with hearing in either ear?'

Informally test hearing by asking the patient to repeat numbers you whisper into the ear while covering the other ear.

If there is any hearing loss then assess whether this is conductive or sensory by performing Weber's and Rinne's tests (see below) typically with 256- and 512-Hz tuning forks, respectively. First of all check the auditory canal and tympanic membrane with an otoscope, if this is provided, to exclude causes of any conductive hearing loss. If there is bilateral hearing loss these tests are much less helpful.

Conductive hearing loss is due to lesions affecting the external auditory canal, tympanic membrane, bones of the middle ear (incus, malleus and stapes) and eustachian tube.

Sensorineural hearing loss is of most interest in the neurological station setting and reflects lesions affecting the cochlear and vestibulocochlear nerves.

Weber's test: this can identify conductive and sensorineural hearing loss. Place the vibrating 256-Hz tuning fork in the centre of the patient's forehead and ask whether it sounds equally loud in each ear or louder on one side. Weber's test relies on the vibration being transmitted through the bones of the skull to functioning sensorineural pathways. In a normal Weber's test it is heard equally. If heard louder in one ear then this signifies either a conductive deafness in this ear or sensorineural defect on the opposite side.

Proceed to the Rinne's test to help distinguish.

Rinne's test: this identifies conductive hearing loss. Hold the base of a vibrating 512-Hz tuning fork against the mastoid process and ask the patient to report when he or she no longer hears it and then hold it next to the same ear and ask if he or she now hears it again. In a normal or 'positive' Rinne's test the patient should hear the vibration again when the fork is held next to the ear, because air conduction is better than bone conduction (AC > BC) due to the efficiency of the amplification process of the middle-ear apparatus. But if there is conductive hearing loss, air conduction is no longer better than bone conduction – rather the reverse is true (BC > AC) and the test is described as an abnormal, 'negative' Rinne's test.

Glossopharyngeal (IX) and vagus (X)

These two nerves are tested together. They both have sensory and motor components but it is the sensory component of the glossopharyngeal nerve and the motor component of the vagus nerve that are tested in the cranial nerve examination. The glossopharyngeal nerve serves:

- General sensation in the tonsils, pharynx and posterior third of the tongue
- Taste to the posterior third of the tongue
- Parasympathetic fibres to the parotid gland.

Its only motor branch serves the stylopharyngeus muscle, a very slim muscle involved in elevating the pharynx and larynx and swallowing. The motor component of the vagus nerve tested in the cranial nerve examination includes innervations of the muscles of the soft palate, larynx and pharynx.

Inspect the palate with the torch. Is the uvula central? Now ask the patient to say 'ah' and, if there is an LMN unilateral vagal nerve pathology, the palate will not lift on the ipsilateral side of the lesion, hence the contralateral intact palatal movement will pull the uvula up and towards the contralateral side. In a unilateral UMN lesion, the palate will not lift on the *contralateral* side to the lesion and the uvula will now be pulled up and towards the same side as the UMN lesion.

It is usual to tell the examiner that you would normally test the gag reflex but this is an unpleasant test for the patient undergoing multiple examinations. The sensory afferent limb is transmitted by the glossopharyngeal nerve and the motor efferent limb by the vagus nerve. Each side of the pharynx is supposed to be tested separately with an orange stick or swab. An intact gag reflex does not reflect the ability to coordinate swallowing, but instead the latter should be tested formally by the speech and language team (SALT).

Accessory (XI)
In practice this is usually tested last.

Test trapezius by asking the patient to shrug the shoulders keeping them up as you try to push down. Test sternocleidomastoid by asking the patient to turn the head and then try to return it straight against the palm of your hand. Both these muscles are innervated by the spinal branch of the accessory nerve.

Hypoglossal (XII)
This is a purely motor nerve serving the muscle of the tongue. Inspect the tongue resting in the mouth for wasting or fasciculation. Then ask the patient to put the tongue out. More subtle weak-

ness can be tested for by asking the patient to put the tongue in the cheek and push against your hand. The tongue is controlled by the contralateral cortex. Each half of the tongue pushes the tongue to the opposite side.

In a LMN lesion (eg syringobulbia), the most affected side shows ipsilateral weakness and fasciculations and on protrusion the tongue will point towards the affected side.

In an UMN lesion (eg pseudobulbar palsy), which tends to be bilateral, there will be a stiff spastic tongue.

Peripheral nervous system examination

General inspection
In your introduction shake hands with the patient and specifically consider:

* Which hand do they shake with?
* Is there weakness and wasting of the hand muscles?
* Is there myotonia?
* Is there tremor?
* Are there any speech changes or diminished facial expression?

Look around the bed: is there a wheelchair or any walking aids or can you see adapted orthoses, such as callipers or built-up heels on their shoes?

Lower limbs
Gait
Ask the patient if he or she is able to demonstrate walking unaided or with a frame. Note the posture, width of the base, stride length, arm swing and any involuntary movements.

Types of gait

- Parkinsonian
- Hemiparetic
- Ataxic
- Paraparetic
- Spastic
- Choreoathetoid
- High stepping
- Waddling
- Shuffling (*marche à petit pas*)

Ask the patient to **stand on his or her toes**, which is a quick test of the strength of the ankle plantar flexors, gastrocnemius and soleus, served by nerve roots S1–2.

Similarly ask the patient to **stand on his or her heels** – failure to do so indicates foot drop. This is a screen of the ankle dorsiflexor, tibialis anterior, served by the deep peroneal nerve from roots L4–5. Foot drop may be bilateral, suggesting Charcot–Marie–Tooth disease (CMT or hereditary sensory motor neuropathy/HSMN) or unilateral, as with a localised common peroneal nerve palsy.

Perform **Romberg's test** to assess the integrity of proprioception and the presence of dorsal column disease. Romberg's test is based on the premise that, to maintain balance, there must be input from two of the three senses: proprioception, vestibular function and vision. Ask the patient to stand with the feet together and arms by the side with eyes open. Ask the patient now to close the eyes and observe him or her for up to 1 minute as you put your arms out near the patient ready to catch him or her. If the patient has poor balance with the eyes open you cannot proceed with Romberg's test; this suggests that the patient may have cerebellar ataxia. If the patient maintains balance with the eyes open but on closing them begins to sway or tilt, this is a **positive Romberg's test**, indicating lack of proprioception and disease of the dorsal column.

Note that it can also indicate vestibular disease (but the history and examination would help distinguish these in practice).

Inspection of the lower limbs

Adequately expose the patient and perform a visual inspection of the lower limbs looking for:

- Discrepancy in leg length: old polio and infantile hemiplegia may cause shortening of one limb.
- Pes cavus: describes a high-arched foot with fixed plantar flexion that does not flatten on weight bearing. There may be a degree of toe clawing and metatarsal heads will be callused with the uneven pressure distribution. It is thought to arise from an imbalance between the stronger plantar flexors, posterior tibialis and peroneus longus, and the weaker dorsiflexor, anterior tibialis:
  - Unilateral: poliomyelitis, spinal cord tumour, spinal trauma
  - Bilateral: idiopathic (20%), cerebral palsy, CMT/HMSN, Friedreich's ataxia, muscular dystrophies, syringomyelia.
- Neuropathic/Charcot's joints: reduction/loss of peripheral sensation and proprioception leads to recurrent microtrauma and progressive inflammatory changes. The joint becomes swollen and deformed, with an abnormal range of movement and marked crepitus. It is more common in weight-bearing joints such as the ankle.
- Posture: pyramidal disease will give a flexed upper limb and extended and adducted lower limb.
- Muscle bulk: is there any wasting of particular muscle groups such as distal wasting in CMT/HMSN or more proximal wasting with a primary myopathy?
- Look for fasciculations, which are small involuntary muscle contractions resulting from spontaneous firing of motor units. They can be benign or occur normally after exercise. They can also signify LMN pathology such as motor neuron disease,

cervical spondylosis, syringomyelia or HMSN/CMT. They may be elicited by tapping a muscle.

- Skin: look for any surgical or traumatic scars, particularly around the neck of the fibula, and neurofibromas.
- Last, palpate any visible thickened nerves such as the common peroneal around the fibular neck or posterior tibial near the medial malleolus associated with HMSN, neurofibromatosis and leprosy.

Tone

Roll the legs gently at the knees or thighs watching that the feet flop side to side symmetrically. Lift the legs gently at the knees in turn, allowing the foot to slide up and down the bed. With increased tone the foot will lift off the bed as you lift the knee.

Hypertonia

- **Spasticity (clasp knife):** this is velocity-dependent increased tone, where resistance can suddenly be overcome. This is characteristic of UMN disease and seen in stroke, cerebral palsy and spinal cord injury.
- **Rigidity (lead pipe):** this is tone that is increased all the way through the range of movement and is not velocity-dependent. If tremor is superimposed this gives 'cogwheel' rigidity. This sort of hypertonia is common with basal ganglia pathology such as Parkinson's disease.

Power

Grade power using the MRC (Medical Research Council) scale. Remember to ask about any pain beforehand.

MRC scale for muscle power

5   Normal power
4   Active movement against gravity and some resistance
3   Active movement against gravity but not resistance
2   Active movement with gravity eliminated
1   Flicker of contraction but cannot move joint
0   No contraction visible

Medical Research Council. *Aids to the Examination of the Peripheral Nervous System.* Memorandum no. 45. London: The Stationery Office, 1981.

Test each muscle group comparing sides as you go:

- 'Lift your leg off the bed, stop me pushing it down' (pushing down on their thigh)
- 'Relax your leg on the bed, now push my hand down into the bed' (placing your hand under the thigh)
- 'Bend your knees, resting your heels on the bed, now don't let me straighten your knee' (pulling forward on their ankle)
- 'Bend your knee now try and straighten the leg' (pushing in on the ankle, maybe steadying the knee)
- 'Relax your legs down and point your toes to the sky' (demonstrate by dorsiflexing your wrists), 'Now don't let me push the feet down' (push down against each foot in turn with border of your hand)
- 'Now push your feet down against my hand like a car pedal' (border of hand against the metatarsal heads)
- 'Point your large toe to the sky, don't let me push it down' (pushing edge of index finger down against the large toe)

- 'Point your toe down, don't let me push it up' (pushing up against the large toe with the edge of your index finger).

Muscles tested are listed in Table 3.1, together with their peripheral nerve and root level.

When presenting the neurological findings, it is best to summarise the motor assessment rather than listing all muscle groups and nerve roots tested, eg it might be better to say, 'there is proximal weakness' or 'there is weakness in the left lower limb in a pyramidal distribution' as appropriate.

Reflexes

Make sure that the patient is relaxed and the muscles involved in the reflex arc can be seen. Strike the tendon of the muscle being tested with a tendon hammer, and compare sides. Do not accept that reflexes are absent until you have tried reinforcement with Jendrassik's manoeuvre. In Jendrassik's manoeuvre the patient interlocks the fingers, one hand palm up, the other palm

down, then tries to pull the hands apart while gripping the fingers when you say 'pull' as you strike the tendon.

Reflexes can be hyperactive (UMN lesions), normal, or reduced/absent (LMN lesions or sometimes with cerebellar disease).

Knee jerk (L3, L4)
Placing your hand beneath the knee and lifting it slightly, ask the patient to allow the leg to go floppy as you take the weight, look at the thigh and strike the patellar tendon. You should see the thigh muscles contract and the lower leg will extend. Do not try to support both knees at once because the weight of two legs together is too heavy and you will be leaning over the patient unable to properly observe both thigh muscles simultaneously.

Ankle jerk (S1, S2)
With the patient's leg laterally rotated at the hip (ask about pain first), bend the patient's knee, and maintain dorsiflexion of the ankle with the

Table 3.1 Muscles tested

Action	Muscle	Nerve	Root level
Hip flexion	Iliopsoas	Femoral	**L1,L2,** L3
Hip extension	Gluteus maximus	Inferior gluteal	**L5, S1,** S2
Hip adduction	Adductors[a]	Obturator	**L2, L3,** L4
Hip abduction	Abductors[b]	Superficial guteal	**L4, L5,** S1
Knee flexion	Hamstrings[c]	Sciatic	L5, **S1,** S2
Knee extension	Quadriceps[d]	Femoral	L2, **L3, L4**
Ankle dorsiflexion	Tibialis anterior	Deep peroneal	**L4,** L5
Ankle plantar flexion	Gastrocnemius and soleus	Tibial	**S1,** S2
Ankle inversion	Tibialis posterior	Tibial	L5, S1
Ankle eversion	Peroneus longus and brevis	Superficial peroneal	L5, **S1**
Great toe extension	Extensor hallucis longus	Deep peroneal	**L5,** S1
Great toe flexion	Flexor hallucis longus	Tibial nerve	L5, **S1, S2**

[a]Obturator externus, adductor longus, magnus, and brevis and gracilis.
[b]Gluteus medius, gluteus minimus and tensor fasciae latae.
[c]Semitendinosus, semimembranosus and biceps femoris.
[d]Rectus femoris, vastus lateralis, vastus medialis and vastus intermedius.

palm of your hand on the sole of the foot, so stretching the Achilles tendon. Tap the Achilles tendon just above the heel and observe the calf muscles contract; the ankle will flex against the palm of your hand.

Plantar response
With the foot relaxed over the side of the bed, use a single-use blunt orange stick or your thumb nail and firmly run this along the lateral side of the sole of the foot from the heel to the base of the fifth toe, and then medially across the base of the toes. Look at the reaction of the first metatarsophalangeal joint. In a normal response the large toe plantarflexes. An abnormal extensor plantar response (Babinski's sign) describes the great toe dorsiflexing and the other toes fanning out, as occurs with UMN lesions from damage to the corticospinal tracts. As the degree of damage to the corticospinal tracts increases, the area from which an extensor plantar response can be elicited spreads until an extensor plantar response can be achieved with pressure against the medial tibia (Oppenheimer's sign).

Clonus
Some candidates prefer to test this with tone but, if you are at the feet having tested the plantar response, then clonus can be easily tested. With the foot relaxed gently flex and extend the ankle joint (to encourage relaxation of the joint) and then rapidly dorsiflex the foot and sustain upward pressure. Look for rhythmic beats of the foot against your hand. In a healthy individual there may be up to three to four beats of clonus and this should be symmetrical in the other ankle; any more and this indicates an UMN lesion.

Coordination
Testing gait is a good initial screen for coordination or you could ask the patient to perform heel-to-toe walking. To test coordination in the lower limbs specifically, ask the patient to put the heel on the opposite knee, run the heel down the shin to the ankle, lift it off, make an arc in the air and place the heel back down on the knee again, repeating this process several times. In the face

of weakness it is difficult to assess coordination. You could ask the patient to tap the foot against the sole of your hand quickly and repeatedly, testing for dysdiadochokinesia.

Sensation
Test all five modalities of sensation if possible and in dermatomes L1–S1 (Figure 3.12). In the examination if there is any concern about cauda equina pathology then inform the examiner you would also test perianal sensation, anal tone and palpate for an enlarged bladder.

Compare left with right and abnormal to normal, starting by asking the patient to identify what normal is, usually on the anterior chest. Ask the patient to close his or her eyes and report when he or she feels a sensation and if each side feels

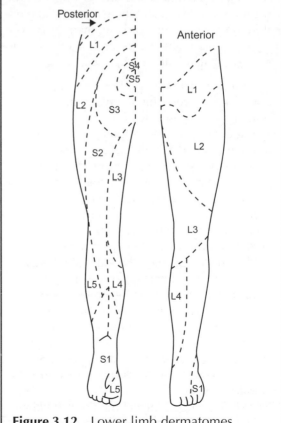

Figure 3.12   Lower limb dermatomes

the same. How you proceed with the sensory examination might be dictated by what you found so far in the motor and reflex assessments, eg if you suspect a unilateral loss of sensation in the lower limb associated with a hemiparesis and unilateral UMN signs, you can start testing sensation at the thigh and work your way down comparing dermatomes between the two legs. If you suspect a more peripheral neuropathy associated with distal weakness, you could start at the toes and move upwards, asking the patient to identify when sensation first becomes normal. If there is loss of sensation in both limbs then look for a sensory level.

Remember that light touch, vibration and proprioception are transmitted by the dorsal columns, and pain (pinprick) and temperature by the lateral spinothalamic tracts. The dorsal columns remain uncrossed in the periphery and decussate in the medulla, whereas pain and temperature fibres enter the cord and then cross over a few segments higher to ascend in the contralateral spinothalamic tracts (Figure 3.13).

- **Light touch**: dab a wisp of cottonwool. Do not stroke because this stimulates the spinothalamic pathway.
- **Vibration**: use a 128-Hz tuning fork first on the sternum and ask the patient to identify when the vibration stops as you deaden it. Now compare this with vibration in the first metatarsophalangeal head, asking the patient to identify when it stops vibrating. If it is normal there is no need to proceed, but if vibration sense is lost then proceed to the medial malleolus, then the anterior tuberosity followed by the anterosuperior iliac spine.
- **Proprioception**: holding the patient's toe by the sides and bending it at the phalangeal joint identifies what represents 'up' and 'down' with the patient's eyes closed. Then ask the patient to identify varying positions. Move proximally as necessary, similar to vibration sense.
- **Pain**: using a neurological pin ask the patient to identify if it is sharp on the sternum, then

test pinprick sensation in the lower limbs, asking him or her to report if it feels sharp or blunt. Remember to look for patterns of dissociated sensory loss between the spinothalamic and dorsal column tracts, as seen in syringomyelia.
- **Temperature**: this is usually not tested but you could state that you would proceed to test for this with test tubes of hot and cold water.

Upper limbs
Inspection of the upper limbs
- Deformity or Charcot joints: there may be clawing of a hand or a deformed, swollen elbow joint.
- Posture: pyramidal disease will result in a flexed upper limb.
- Muscle bulk: is there any wasting of particular muscle groups, such as the small muscles of the hands or proximal limb-girdle, or winging of the scapulae visible above the shoulders?
- Look for fasciculations or any tremors.
- Skin: look for any surgical or traumatic scars, particularly around the wrist and elbow, or any digital ulceration or amputation (eg as seen in syringomyelia).
- Last palpate any visible thickened nerves such as the median and radial cutaneous nerves at the wrist, or the ulnar nerve at the medial elbow.

Observe outstretched hands
Ask the patient to stand with the arms out, palms upwards and eyes closed, and look for:

- **Pronator drift**: in pyramidal lesions the arm on the affected side might begin to fall while the forearm pronates.
- **Dysmetria**: in cerebellar disease the arms may drift upwards, but when pushed down against resistance they overcorrect/rebound before finding the correct starting position.
- **Pseudoathetosis**: in severe sensory ataxia with loss of joint position sense the fingers can writhe.

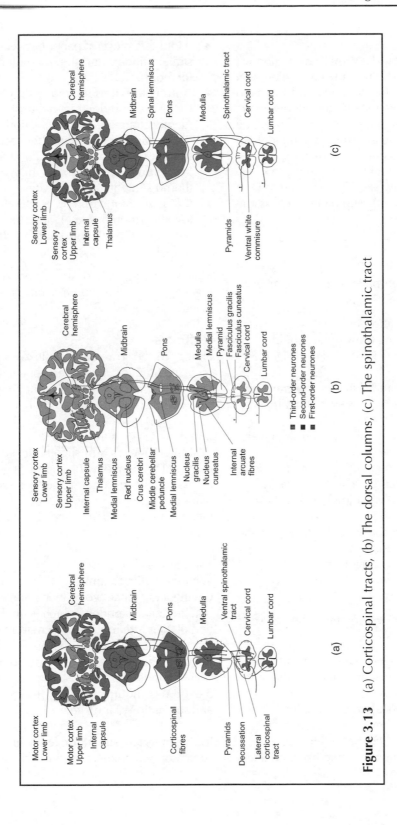

Figure 3.13   (a) Corticospinal tracts, (b) The dorsal columns, (c) The spinothalamic tract

Tone

Ask the patient to relax the arms and 'go floppy', then enquire if he or she has any pain before you start. Hold the elbow in one hand and the hand in the other; flex and extend the elbow while rotating around the wrist, testing tone over the two joints. Also pronate and supinate the forearm repeatedly. Compare sides and look for spastic or rigid tone with cogwheeling. In early UMN disease there may be only slightly increased tone in pronation compared with supination, felt as the 'pronator catch'.

Power

Grade power using the MRC scale as described for the lower limb (see page 231). Remember to ask about any pain beforehand.

- 'Put your arms up and out like this' (demonstrate holding arms up at shoulder level, elbows fully flexed) 'and don't let me push them down'
- 'Bend your elbow and don't let me straighten it' (demonstrate bent elbow with forearm supinated)
- 'Now push against me and try and straighten the elbow'
- 'Put your arms out straight with fist clenched, now try and push your wrist down' (make sure you isolate the wrist joint as you resist wrist flexion)
- 'Now try to cock the wrist back' (compare the two sides against resistance)
- 'Squeeze both of my fingers to stop me pulling them out of your grip' (offer two fingers to both sides).

More specific instructions for the small muscles of the hands:

- 'Now hold your fingers out straight and stop me bending them' (use the side of your hand to resist finger extension)
- 'Spread your fingers apart and stop me pushing them together' (use your index finger against their index finger and fifth finger against their fifth finger, testing like with like)

- 'Hold this piece of paper between your straight fingers and stop me pulling it out' (demonstrate)
- 'Turn your palms up and point your thumbs to the sky and don't let me push them down' (demonstrate the thumb position)
- 'Hold this piece of paper between your straight thumb and side of hand and do not let me pull the paper out while keeping your thumb straight' (demonstrate)
- 'Put your thumb and tip of little finger together' (demonstrate) 'and stop me pulling them apart' (with your thumb and little finger).

Muscles being tested are listed in Table 3.2, together with their peripheral nerve and root level.

Reflexes

Similar to the lower limb reflexes, use reinforcement techniques if reflexes appear to be absent at first; commonly this is clenching the jaw or making a fist with the opposite hand.

Biceps jerk (C5, C6)

With the patient's arm slightly flexed and relaxed on the lap, place your index finger or thumb across the biceps tendon and then tap your finger with the tendon hammer. You should see the bicep muscle contract, and the forearm will lift slightly.

Supinator jerk (C5, C6)

With the patient's arm slightly flexed and relaxed on the lap, place your index finger across the brachioradialis tendon, which is on the radial portion of their forearm about 7 cm from the wrist. Do not strike straight on to the bone because this is uncomfortable and the tendon should be placed slightly under tension as in other reflex assessments. You should see slight flexion at the elbow and supination of the forearm.

In the **inverted supinator jerk**, when testing the supinator reflex there is no activity in brachio-

Table 3.2 Muscles tested, their action, the nerve and root level

Action	Muscle	Nerve	Root level
Shoulder abduction	Deltoid	Axillary	C5, C6
Elbow flexion (forearm fully supinated)	Biceps	Musculocutaneous	C5, C6
Elbow flexion (forearm midway between supination and pronation)	Brachioradialis	Radial	C5, C6
Elbow extension	Triceps	Radial	**C6, C7**, C8
Wrist flexion	Flexor carpi ulnaris and radialis	Median and ulnar nerves	C6, C7, C8, T1
Wrist extension	Extensor carpi ulnaris and radialis	Radial	C5, **C6, C7**
Hand grip	Finger and thumb flexors and thenar and hypothenar eminence[a]	Median and ulnar nerves	C8, T1
Finger extension	Extensor digitorum	Radial	C7, C8
Finger abduction	Dorsal interossei and abductor digiti minimi	Ulnar	C8. T1
Finger adduction	Palmar interossei	Ulnar	C8, T1
Thumb adduction	Adductor pollicis	Ulnar	C8, T1
Thumb abduction	Abductor pollicis brevis	Median	C8, T1
Thumb opposition	Opponens pollicis	Median	C8, T1

Assessing hand grip (sometimes known as power grip) is a crude screening test of C8–T1 and hand function. A normal hand grip involves intact finger and thumb flexors, and thenar and hypothenar eminence. Flexor digitorum superficialis is innervated by the median nerve and flexes the four fingers at the middle phalanx. Flexor digitorum profundus inserts distally, causing flexion at the distal phalanx of the four fingers, with the median nerve serving the index and middle finger part of the muscle, and the ulnar serving the middle, ring and little fingers (thus dual innervation to the middle finger). The muscles of the thenar eminence include abductor pollicis brevis, flexor pollicis brevis and opponens pollicis all served by the median nerve. Adductor pollicis is also part of the thenar eminence but served by the ulnar nerve. The muscles of the hypothenar eminence include abductor, flexor and opponens digiti minimi, and are all served by the ulnar nerve.

radialis (C5, C6) but instead there is finger flexion (C8), and occasionally triceps contraction with elbow extension (C6, C7). This is thought to occur from cord pathology at C5–6 causing LMN signs at the tested reflex level (absent brachioradialis) and UMN pyramidal tract signs at the lower levels (finger flexion), resulting from spread of the receptive fields for these lower reflexes.

Triceps jerk (C6, C7)
Bringing the forearm across the body to expose the triceps tendon, place it under tension and tap with the hammer just above the elbow. There will be contraction of triceps with slight extension at the elbow joint.

Finger jerk (C8)
Ask the patient to rest his or her fingers on your fingers and then tap the tendon hammer on the back of your own fingers; the patient's fingers will flex with a positive response. The finger reflex is not usually present (due to cortical downward inhibition) unless it is pathologically brisk.

Hoffmann's reflex
This can be tested in one of two ways. Some candidates hold the middle finger of the patient at the sides of the proximal interphalangeal joint and then flick the nail of this finger, flexing the distal interphalangeal joint, whereas others choose to rest the terminal phalanx of the patient's middle finger against the candidate's own index finger and flick the nail. In a positive Hoffman's reflex, the interphalangeal joint of the thumb will flex. This is not always a pathological sign because some patients are naturally more hyperreflexive, although it is pathological if it is unilateral or of recent onset.

Coordination
Dysdiadochokinesis: describes impaired ability to perform rapid alternating movements and is the hallmark of cerebellar ataxia. Ask the patient to tap one hand alternately palm down then dorsum down on the palm of the other hand as quickly as possible. Demonstrate this activity. Patients with cerebellar disease will perform this activity poorly with a slowed rate and irregular rhythm. It is normal for the non-dominant hand to be a little less coordinated.

Finger-to-nose testing: this can demonstrate dysmetria in which there is incoordination when reaching for an object, leading to either past-pointing/over-shooting (hypermetria) or under-shooting (hypometria). Ask the patient to touch your index finger with his or her index finger just inside arm's reach, and then to touch the nose with the same index finger and repeat this activity as quickly and accurately as possible. In cerebellar disease you can see an intention tremor that increases in amplitude as the patient reaches the target and he or she may over- or under-shoot the target index finger.

Sensation
Test all five modalities of sensation if possible and in dermatomes C2–T1 (Figure 3.14). Remember to think specifically if there is dissociated loss between the spinothalamic and dorsal column tracts as seen in intrinsic cord lesions.

When testing vibration sense, again ask the patient to identify normal vibration sense at the sternum, then start your upper limb examination vibration assessment by touching the tuning fork to the distal interphalangeal joint. Work your way proximally through to the proximal interphalangeal, metacarpophalangeal, wrist and elbow joints until normal vibration is perceived.

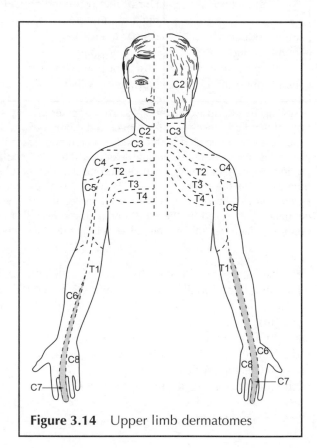

Figure 3.14   Upper limb dermatomes

If suspecting a sensory level with cord disease, then remember the landmarks on the trunk:

- Nipple – T4
- Umbilicus – T10.

Assessment of speech
Dysarthria
Dysarthria is usually encountered in the PACES examination as part of the assessment of another main diagnosis, such as cerebellar disease or pseudobulbar palsy. Rarely, the examination rubric can ask you to start with an assessment of speech and then you will be expected to move fluently on to examining other relevant parts of the nervous system to make a unifying diagnosis.

Dysarthria is a motor speech disorder secondary to damage in the motor system that can affect all components of speech including: phonation, articulation, prosody, resonance and respiration.

We can imagine these components as building blocks, starting with the basics of speech and becoming more sophisticated:

- **Phonation**: describes the process of creating sound through modulating the passage of air through the vocal folds and larynx.
- **Articulation**: in this context refers to the use of the muscles of the face, lips, tongue and jaw in making words or syllables.
- **Resonance**: describes the change in speech quality from the vibration of the sound waves within the nasal, oral and pharyngeal cavities and through movement of the soft palate.
- **Prosody**: provides speech with meaning over and above that just contained in the words, eg sarcasm or whether the speaker is asking a question or giving a command. The tools of prosody include emphasis and modulating pitch and rhythm, and require coordination.

The main groups of dysarthria seen in the PACES examination include the following.

Ataxic dysarthria
Characteristics: due to impaired coordination in phonation, speech can be **loud** and **explosive**, sometimes described as **staccato/scanning** and e**qual stress** is given to all syllables. This can be heard when the patient repeats 'Bri-tish con-sti-tut-ion' and 'ba-by hipp-o-pot-a-mus'. Prosody can be lost due to equal stress and **poor rhythm**. Poor coordination of all muscles involved in speech production affects articulation, producing **marked slurring** of words, with particular difficulty with consonants.

Site of the pathology: cerebellar disease or its connections.

Causes: toxins (including alcohol), stroke, posterior fossa tumour, trauma and multiple sclerosis.

Additional: examine the cranial nerves, limbs and gait to find other cerebellar signs and form a differential diagnosis.

Spastic dysarthria
Characteristics: the voice can sound harsh and **strangled**. Spasticity in the soft palate affects resonance, causing the voice to sound **nasal**, and in the tongue and facial muscles can affect articulation, causing **indistinct slurred speech**. Stiffness in the muscles of phonation can cause explosive **speech** with **short phrases**.

Site of the pathology: there is bilateral cortical innervation to all motor cranial nerve nuclei except the cranial nerve VII nucleus innervating the lower half of the face and cranial nerve XII nucleus. Instead these receive contralateral unilateral corticobulbar innervation. Thus there has to be bilateral damage to the UMN corticobulbar tracts to cause a spastic dysarthria, also known as a pseudobulbar palsy.

Causes: congenital lesions, eg cerebral palsy, bilateral hemispherical infarction or neurodegenerative diseases, eg amyotrophic lateral sclerosis, progressive supranuclear palsy and motor neuron disease (MND).

Additional: examine the cranial nerves for other signs of pseudobulbar palsy and the remaining peripheral nervous system to form a differential diagnosis.

Flaccid dysarthria

Characteristics: weakness and wasting in the soft palate and pharyngeal muscles can cause hypernasality. Weakness in the muscles of phonation can cause a quiet, breathy voice. The weak wasted tongue has particular difficulty articulating lingual and labial consonants.

Site of the pathology: for striking effects on speech there is usually a bilateral LMN lesion affecting the lower cranial nerves such as pathology in the brain stem causing bulbar palsy. Neuromuscular junction disease and myopathies can also cause a flaccid dysarthria.

Causes: MND, syringobulbia, brain-stem tumour or stroke.

Additional: look for cranial nerve signs consistent with bulbar palsy and examine the remainder of the PNS considering the above differential.

Station 3
Neurological scenarios

1. Multiple sclerosis
2. Parkinson's disease
3. Motor neuron disease
4. Hemiparesis
5. Spastic paraparesis
6. Cervical myelopathy
7. Syringomyelia/Syringobulbia
8. Myotonic dystrophy
9. Myasthenia gravis
10. Muscular dystrophy
11. Charcot–Marie–Tooth disease
12. Friedreich's ataxia
13. Cerebellar syndrome
14. Peripheral neuropathy
15. Facial nerve palsy
16. Wasting of the small muscles of the hand
17. Median nerve palsy
18. Ulnar nerve palsy
19. Radial nerve palsy
20. Common peroneal nerve palsy and L4–5 root lesions
21. Nystagmus
22. Ophthalmoplegia
23. Visual field defect
24. Dysphasia
25. Bulbar and pseudobulbar palsy
26. Brain-stem syndromes
27. Cerebellopontine angle lesion
28. Jugular foramen syndrome
29. Old polio
30. Involuntary movements and Huntington's disease

SCENARIO 1. MULTIPLE SCLEROSIS

Identifying physical signs

Multiple sclerosis (MS) is an inflammatory de-myelinating condition characterised by central nervous system (CNS) dysfunction caused by CNS lesions separated in time and space. Thus, there must be at least two distinct episodes of neurological dysfunction to support a diagnosis of MS.

The areas of the CNS most affected in MS include the **optic nerve, brain stem, cerebellum, dorsal columns, corticospinal tracts** and, rarely, **spinothalamic tracts**. Thus, in the examination setting a patient may present with a myriad of signs and the examiner may direct you to any of these areas. Identifying the location of the lesion(s) is a highly discriminatory test of candidates' understanding of neuroanatomy, which is why MS appears frequently in PACES.

Look for clues in the examination prompt, eg 'This patient presented with painful blurred vision and incoordination; please examine her lower limbs'. The patient tends to be aged 20–40 years and female.

General appearance
There may be a wheelchair or walking aids. The patient may be seated, maintaining a **pyramidal posture** with a flexed upper limb and lower limbs crossed at the ankle, with **wasting from disuse atrophy** (not lower motor neuron (LMN) wasting) if they have had MS for several years. Depending on the examiner's instruction it is reasonable before assessing gait to ask patients *how* their walking is (rather than the closed question 'Can you walk?'), which elicits a longer reply and allows assessment of speech, perhaps detecting **ataxic dysarthria**. The speech might be **slurred** from difficulty articulating consonants and 'explosives', from the increased effort of articulation and stressed delivery of all syllables.

Gait
Check that the patient is safe to walk unaided. He or she may have a broad-based **ataxic gait** with difficulty in heel-to-toe walking. Alternatively he or she may have the **scissored** leg-crossing gait of bilateral pyramidal tract disease, with increased tone in the leg extensors. Patients might exhibit a **sensory ataxic gait** with slow, deliberate, uncertain steps as they watch their feet to compensate for lack of proprioceptive feedback.

Cranial nerve examination
Eye signs are the most common finding and up to 50% of MS patients will develop an episode of optic neuritis. Look for **intranuclear ophthalmoplegia** (INO) on conjugate gaze testing (see the neurological examination) as a sign of brain-stem disease; this is usually bilateral. There may be a **relative afferent pupillary defect** (RAPD, see the neurological examination) from optic neuritis, or frank optic atrophy which may also give a **central scotoma** on visual field testing, **reduced visual acuity** or **changes of colour vision** perception if formally tested, particularly loss of red discrimination.

Fundoscopy may reveal the signs of **optic neuritis** with early stage hyperaemia and swelling of the disc or the well-demarcated pale disc of **optic atrophy** (or no signs at all if the disease is retrobulbar). With cerebellar disease there may be ipsilateral **nystagmus** with or without INO signs. Occasionally patients can experience trigeminal neuralgia symptoms and may have reduced facial sensation and corneal reflex. Rarely a patient will present with a supranuclear (upper motor neuron or UMN) facial nerve palsy with unilateral paralysis of the lower half of the face. An unusual finding on conjugate gaze testing is that of Fisher's 'one-and-a-half syndrome', so called because there is no functioning conjugate gaze to the side of the lesion and only half a functional horizontal gaze away from the side of the lesion. (One-and-a-half syndrome occurs from simultaneous pathology to the paramedian pontine reticular formation (PMRF) controlling conjugate gaze and the ipsilateral adjacent medial longitudinal fasciculus (MLF) which connects the cranial nerve III and VI nuclei, or from ipsilateral nerve VI disease with adjacent MLF pathology. In simpler terms, there is paralysis of all conjugate horizontal gaze movements except for abduction on the contralateral side to the lesion. Similar to an INO, there is preservation of nerve III function and so bilateral adduction in accommodation is normal.)

Upper and lower limb examination

This may reveal pyramidal, cerebellar, dorsal column signs or a combination of these. Signs will tend to be asymmetrical or unilateral:

- Pyramidal signs include increased clasp-knife tone with weakness and brisk reflexes. There may be ankle clonus and an extensor plantar response.
- **Cerebellar signs** include **dysdiadochokinesis** with pronation/supination hand tapping and dysmetria as shown by **impaired finger–nose pointing** with an **intention tremor** or **impaired heel–shin coordination** and possibly **hypotonia**.
- **Dorsal column disease** includes **reduced vibration** and **joint position sense** including **positive Romberg's sign** and **pseudoathetosis** of the fingers with eyes closed (see the neurological exam).

Additional

If you suspect MS then move on to examine the other limbs, cerebellar system or cranial/visual systems if time allows.

When presenting your findings describe the consistency of the features with a **CNS demyelinating condition** and state that you would go on to test or enquire about autonomic and sphincter dysfunction.

Differential diagnosis

Neuromyelitis optica (NMO; Devic's disease): presents acutely with optic neuritis and spinal cord myelitis with spastic paraparesis/tetraparesis. It is very rare to get brain-stem or cerebellar involvement (see below). (NMO is thought to be quite distinct from MS due to its different epidemiology, pathology and presentation. There is a non-white preponderance of disease, particularly among Asians. It is an antibody-mediated autoimmune pathology, with IgG antibodies (NMO antibodies) against the aquaporin-4 water channel in astrocytes surrounding the blood–brain barrier. It is not known how this leads to the demyelination process that follows. It is diagnosed using the Mayo Clinic criteria. Acute attacks are treated with methylprednisolone or plasmapheresis if unresponsive. Secondary prevention includes treatment with intravenous immunoglobulin (IVIG), azathioprine, cyclophosphamide or rituximab.)

Myelopathy from cervical spondylosis: signs and symptoms are all below the neck with no cranial/optic nerve involvement and the patient would describe a gradual onset with no separated episodes in time or space. MRI of the cervical spine would aid diagnosis.

Vitamin B_{12} deficiency with subacute combined degeneration of the cord (SACD): the dorsal columns and lateral corticospinal tracts are affected and there may be a peripheral neuropathy. Signs tend to be more symmetrical than in MS. Rarely there can be cranial nerve and cerebellar involvement. There will be low serum vitamin B_{12} and high serum levels of methylmalonic acid and homocysteine without the characteristic MRI findings of MS.

Ischaemic stroke: this may present with unilateral symptoms and homonymous hemianopia, with no retinal signs. The clinical course is very different with an acute onset of signs and symptoms.

Peripheral neuropathy: there are distal signs with loss of sensation and reflexes, and no pyramidal or cerebellar signs.

Guillain–Barré syndrome: this affects the myelin sheaths of peripheral nerves so it has a very different course with progressive bilateral flaccid paralysis and hypo-/areflexia with distal sensory symptoms (sensory signs are unusual). Neuroimaging is normal and there are no oligoclonal IgG bands in the CSF with lumbar puncture testing.

Amyotrophic lateral sclerosis (ALS): there will be UMN and LMN signs in the same muscle groups with no sensory signs or visual changes. There are bulbar/pseudobulbar speech changes in ALS and not the ataxic dysarthria that can occur in MS.

Differential diagnosis of optic neuritis
- **Ischaemic optic neuropathy** has no other cranial nerve, peripheral nervous system (PNS) or cerebellar signs and has a hyperacute onset.
- **Rhinogenous optic neuritis**, from extension of disease from the paranasal, sphenoid or ethmoidal sinus, causes exophthalmos, ophthalmoplegia and optic neuritis/atrophy. Often there are surprisingly few rhinological symptoms. There will be no other cranial nerve, PNS or cerebellar signs.
- **Lyme borreliosis optic neuropathy** can also present with LMN signs of cranial or peripheral nerves but with signs of arthritis, lymphadenopathy, constitutional upset and the pathognomonic erythema migrans rash.
- **HIV-associated optic neuropathy** is bilateral and tends to present late in disease, so there will be other manifestations of HIV infection.
- **Syphilis** can present with a unilateral optic neuritis – often with other neurological manifestations, lymphadenopathy and a maculopapular rash of the torso or palms and soles.

Differential diagnosis of INO or lateral gaze palsy
- The two most common causes are **MS** and **stroke**.

- Other causes include: trauma, herniation, infection (including HIV, meningitis and cysticercosis), tumours (including pontine gliomas and metastases), aneurysms, vasculitides and systemic lupus erythematosus (SLE).

Clinical judgement and maintaining patient welfare

Tell the examiners that you would like to take a history to establish the likely clinical category of MS:

- **Relapsing–remitting MS (RR-MS)**: the majority of patients (80–85%). Acute short exacerbations followed by partial or complete recovery with no disease progression between attacks.
- **Secondary progressive MS (SP-MS)**: >50% of patients with RRMS may secondarily evolve into a progressive course without acute relapses.
- **Primary progressive MS (PP-MS)**: presents with gradually progressive symptoms from the onset without acute episodes (15–20%). Tends to occur in older-aged patients and the F:M ratio is even (unlike in RRMS where females predominate).
- **Relapsing–progressive MS (RP-MS)**: progressive disease with occasional marked deteriorations (5%).

Investigations
The diagnosis of MS is a clinical one with supportive evidence from cross-sectional imaging. The key feature is multiple lesions at different sites at different times. The revised 2010 McDonald criteria cover clinical and MRI diagnosis (Polman CH, Reingold SC, Banwell B, *et al.* Diagnostic criteria for multiple sclerosis: 2010 Revisions to the McDonald criteria. *Annals of Neurology* 2011;69(2): 292–302).

MRI T2 imaging is used for gadolinium-enhancing and non-enhancing lesions at the same time and in at least two of the four main areas affected by MS (periventricular, juxta-cortical, infratentorial or spinal cord).

Other diagnostic tests are used only when MRI is contraindicated such as in patients with a pace-maker, to rule out alternative diagnoses or where diagnosis is still unclear.

MRI of the cervical cord can help differentiate MS from a cervical spondylosis.

Visual evoked potentials (VEPs) reveal asymmetrical and prolonged conduction.

Lumbar puncture with CSF analysis will show IgG oligoclonal bands in greater concentrations than in the serum, in 80% of those with MS. CSF analysis is needed only if there is suspicion of CNS infection.

Blood tests including full blood count (FBC), biochemistry, thyroid function tests (TFTs) and vitamin B_{12} should all be normal.

Anti-NMO antibodies can be requested if Devic's disease is suspected.

Relapsing patients should be quickly and thoroughly assessed for intercurrent infection that can unmask or provoke MS symptoms.

Management
General points
- The main goals of treatment are prevention of disability and improvement in quality of life.
- The patient and carers should have a central role in management decisions, preserving autonomy and self-management.
- Patients and carers should be directed to support organisations, eg Multiple Sclerosis Society.

Treatment can be divided into three main areas:

1. Treatment of the acute attacks

2. Secondary prevention of future attacks with disease-modifying agents
3. Management of pain, reduced mobility, bladder and bowel disturbance, and cognitive effects.

Acute attacks
These are managed with 3–5 days of high-dose IV/oral methylprednisolone or second-line with IVIG. Plasma exchange can be beneficial in severe cases. Patients benefit from early neuro-rehabilitation after acute episodes.

Secondary prevention (disease-modifying agents)
RR-MS and RP-MS may benefit from starting secondary prevention with either interferon-β or glatiramer (immunomodulatory treatments) and then second line with natalizumab (Tysabri, a monoclonal antibody treatment) if this is unsuccessful.

SP-MS can be treated with mitoxantrone (antineoplastic, type II topoisomerase inhibitor) but this can be poorly tolerated due to fatigue and gastrointestinal side effects, and the potential for serious adverse effects including cardiotoxicity and myelogenous leukaemia.

There are currently no recommended treatments for PP-MS, although the above medications and cyclophosphamide, azathioprine and methotrexate have been tried with uncertain benefit.

Managing symptoms of neurological impairment
Early involvement of the multidisciplinary team (MDT) helps to mitigate many symptoms, and preserve function and independence, but specific management of several key areas is described in Table 3.3.

Prognosis
The prognosis for MS sufferers can vary from a benign slow-course disease that responds well to treatment, to rapidly disabling disease within several years.

Table 3.3 Management of the symptoms of multiple sclerosis

Symptom	Management
Fatigue	Graded exercise, sleep hygiene, stimulants (amantadine, modafinil)
Urinary symptoms	Investigate for infection and urinary retention, bladder stabilisers (oxybutynin, solifenacin, tolteridone), botulinum toxin injection, intermittent self-catheterisation, long-term suprapubic catheter
Bowel dysfunction	Pre-empt constipation, laxatives, enemas
Neuralgia	Low-dose anticonvulsants (gabapentin, pregabalin, carbamazepine)
Dystonia and contractures	Physiotherapy, oral baclofen, tizanadine, dantrolene, clonazepam, gabapentin or botulinum toxin, supportive casts, corrective surgery
Gait impairment	Physiotherapy, dalfampridine (Ampyra, a potassium channel blocker that may improve nerve conduction)
Osteoporosis	Higher incidence than in the general population due to reduced mobility, poor intake of calcium and vitamin D, and exposure to high-dose corticosteroids. Osteoporosis should be screened for and treated along standard lines
Cognitive symptoms	Over half the patients with MS have changes in their memory, and their ability to concentrate or plan. Patients should be appropriately screened for these symptoms
Mood changes	Hyper-emotionality and depression should be enquired about and treated with tricyclic antidepressants or SSRIs along with psychological therapies

SSRI, selective serotonin reuptake inhibitor.

Epidemiological studies suggest female sex, sensory symptoms and optic neuritis incur a more favourable prognosis, whereas frequent relapses, and motor and cerebellar symptoms, indicate a poorer prognosis.

SCENARIO 2: PARKINSON'S DISEASE

Identifying physical signs

The key signs are tremor, bradykinesia, rigidity and postural instability.

General appearance

The patient may have a 'mask-like facies' with little spontaneous facial expression, paucity of blinking and a slight tremor of the chin. In advanced disease the patient may be drooling (**sialorrhoea**). There may be an **asymmetrical pill-rolling tremor of 4–6 Hz** (ask the patient to rest the hands on his or her lap to see this fully), or there may be an asymmetrical foot-tapping tremor. If you cannot clearly see a tremor but you suspect that the patient has Parkinson's disease (PD), ask him or her to tap the knee with one hand or count backwards from 20, and this may elicit the tremor on the most affected side.

Gait

Ask the patient if he or she is safe to walk unaided. The patient may **freeze**, finding it difficult to initiate standing or walking. Once started he or she will have a **stooped posture**, leaning forward slightly with the head low, flexed at the hips, knees and elbows (simian-like posture). The patient may have a **narrow-based festinant gait**, taking small shuffling and quickening steps as if falling forward. There is typically **little arm swing**. It is sometimes easier to see the tremor when the patient is walking. In advanced disease there can be postural instability with **propulsion** (a tendency to fall forward) and **retropulsion** (falling backward). If you ask the patient to turn around this may reveal postural instability, bradykinesia and axial rigidity as the patient **moves en bloc**.

Speech

Ask the patient if he or she could describe how he or she got to the examination centre. Patients with PD have **quiet, monotonous speech**.

Rigidity

At the elbow feel for **lead-pipe rigidity** with resistance to passive movement all the way through movement (unlike 'clasp-knife' pyramidal hypertonia, which is stiffness that suddenly releases). Rotate a supported wrist slowly feeling for **cog-wheeling**, which is tremor superimposed on lead-pipe rigidity.

Additional

Ask the patient to write his or her address, which may reveal **micrographia** with smaller and more bunched letters as the sentence progresses. **Bradykinesia** can be further elicited by asking the patient to tap the thumb against opposing fingers as quickly as possible, or to play pretend piano keys on the palm of the opposite hand; movements may become slower and smaller with repetition.

Parkinson-plus syndromes
It is important to show the examiner that you are trying to differentiate idiopathic PD from the rarer Parkinson-plus syndromes:

* Ask to measure a **lying and standing blood pressure** (autonomic dysfunction)
* Fully assess eye movements for any **supranuclear gaze palsy**
* Examine for **pyramidal tract** or **cerebellar signs**
* Ask to assess **cognition** with a simple screening tool
* Request a **drug history** to rule out parkinsonism secondary to medications, although this would commonly give rise to symmetrical symptoms.

Differential diagnosis

Differential diagnosis of tremor

Tremor can be divided into rest, postural and action tremors (Table 3.4).

Table 3.4 Types of tremor

Tremor type	Features	Examples
Rest tremor	Seen when body part is fully supported, such as resting the arm and hand on a bed Exacerbated by movement in other body parts Suppressed by voluntary movement of the affected part Usually low frequency, 4–6 Hz	Parkinson's disease Parkinsonian disorders Severe essential tremor Wilson's disease
Postural tremor	Seen when the body part has to maintain a fixed posture against gravity Can be seen when holding arms outstretched Usually high frequency, 10–12 Hz	Essential tremor[a] Physiological tremor[b]
Action tremor (includes intention tremor)	Seen in a body part during voluntary action, eg finger–nose pointing, speaking, writing, eating	Essential tremor Cerebellar disease Midbrain stroke/trauma Multiple sclerosis

[a]Essential tremor (ET): the tremor can vary from a low-amplitude/high-frequency tremor of the hands to a larger-amplitude tremor exacerbated by particular postures. Tremor is seen typically in the hands or arms, but can occur in any of the head, chin, voice, trunk or limbs. ET is the most common cause of postural or action tremors, and up to 50% have an autosomal dominant pattern of inheritance. There should be no other neurological signs that, in addition to the pattern of tremor, help to distinguish it from Parkinson's disease. Alcohol can relieve symptoms. If treatment is indicated the most commonly used drugs are propranolol and primidone (an anticonvulsant).

[b]Physiological tremor: this is a high-frequency tremor of 10–12 Hz that is not normally visible but can be enhanced in certain conditions:

- Anxiety
- Muscle fatigue
- Thyrotoxicosis
- Phaeochromocytoma
- Drugs: salbutamol, adrenaline, SSRIs, tricyclic antidepressants, levodopa, lithium, steroids, alcohol and opioid withdrawal
- Toxins: mercury, lead, arsenic.

Differential diagnosis of parkinsonism

Parkinson's disease is the most common cause. PD is a neurodegenerative disease of unknown cause with increasing age being a recognised risk factor. Mean age of onset is 65 years. There is selective loss of the dopaminergic neurons in the substantia nigra of the basal ganglia with intracytoplasmic eosinophilic inclusions (Lewy bodies) composed of the protein synuclein.

Drug-induced parkinsonism is the second most common cause. Frequently implicated drugs are neuroleptics with anti-dopaminergic action, metoclopramide and sodium valproate.

Cerebral anoxia: this can cause bilateral basal ganglia infarction, eg after resuscitation from cardiac arrest.

Normal pressure hydrocephalus: this classically presents with a triad of dementia, urinary incontinence and gait abnormalities, although in reality only one or two of these signs may be prominent.

Infections: post-encephalitis, AIDS and prion disease.

Toxicity: MPTP, carbon monoxide, manganese, Paraquat and mercury poisoning. (MPTP is 1-methyl-4-phenyl-1,2,3,6-tetrahydropyridine, an impurity in a narcotic recreational drug produced in the 1980s that gave a rapid onset of PD symptoms and is now used in experimental animal models.)

Dementias: Lewy body dementia (characterised by visual hallucinations and fluctuating mental state) and Alzheimer's dementia with parkinsonism.

Parkinson-plus syndromes: these syndromes share a characteristic lack of response to levodopa, early onset of dementia, and postural instability and symmetry of signs unlike PD. The group includes:

- Progressive supranuclear palsy (Steele–Richardson–Olzewski syndrome)
- Multiple-system atrophy (MSA):
  - MSA-A, formerly Shy–Drager syndrome
  - MSA-P, striatonigral degeneration
  - MSA-C, olivopontocerebellar atrophy
- Corticobasal ganglionic degeneration
- Diffuse Lewy body disease.

Clinical judgement and maintaining patient welfare

Investigations
There are no specific diagnostic tests for idiopathic PD, which is based predominantly on history and clinical examination. Improvement on treatment (see below) often confirms the diagnosis.

MRI of the brain with or without contrast would be indicated if there were atypical features such as rapid onset, early dementia, symmetrical features, UMN signs or additional signs of a vascular aetiology.

Functional neuroimaging with $[^{123}I]\beta CIT$ and SPECT (single photon emission computed tomography) is not in routine use but can be helpful in distinguishing cerebrovascular disease, essential tremor and psychogenic causes. ($[^{123}I]\beta CIT$ is 2β-carbomethoxy-3-β(4-iodophenyl)-tropane. DaTSCAN is a tradename for a form of radioactive iodine compound also used with SPECT.)

Formal psychometric testing is indicated if any symptoms of cognitive impairment are present.

Management
Initiation of pharmacological treatment is based on severity of symptoms and should be given alongside early access to occupational therapy, physiotherapy, speech and language therapy, and dietician services to maintain independent living. Patients should be signposted to local and national support groups such as Parkinson's UK.

Patients with PD should inform the DVLA and insurance company at the time of diagnosis.

There is no universal consensus on first-line drug therapy for early PD.

Dopamine agonists (pramipexole, ropinirole, cabergoline, pergolide, lisuride): can be used as first line in younger patients who are more susceptible to dyskinesias with early use of levodopa/carbidopa. Side effects include nausea, constipation, hypotension, drowsiness, confusion and hallucinations.

MAO-B inhibitors (monoamine oxidase-B inhibitor, such as rasagiline): can be used as monotherapy in early mild disease by preventing the breakdown of the endogenous dopamine. Selegiline is not approved for monotherapy and is used only as an adjunctive treatment. Side effects can include constipation, depression and hallucinations.

Levodopa: this treatment is preferred in older patients who are more likely to have orthostasis or hallucinations with dopamine agonists. They are combined with decarboxylase inhibitors to prevent peripheral breakdown to dopamine, which can cause severe nausea and vomiting. Common preparations are co-careldopa (combined with carbidopa) and co-beneldopa (combined with benserazide). Side effects can include nausea and vomiting, arrhythmias, postural hypotension, depression, insomnia, psychosis and cognitive impairment.

Anticholinergics (benzhexol, benzatropine, procyclidine): can be used for refractory tremor but worsening of cognitive function may preclude their use.

As disease progresses dopaminergic agonists and levodopa are usually combined to prevent fluctuating symptoms. Alternatively, the dosing frequency of the dopamine agonists can be increased, or levodopa can be combined with catechol-*O*-methyl transferase (COMT) inhibitors to prolong its half-life.

COMT inhibitors (entacapone, tolcapone): these should be avoided in hepatic impairment or ischaemic heart disease. They inhibit the gastrointestinal breakdown of levodopa. Side effects include confusion, dizziness, insomnia, hallucinations and dyskinesias.

Apomorphine: this is an injectable form of dopamine delivered subcutaneously. It can be useful in the mornings, for freezing or dysphagia in advanced PD, or when oral preparations cannot be taken (eg pre- or post-surgically). Continuous subcutaneous infusions can be used to reduce 'off-times' and dyskinesias.

Amantadine: this may improve dyskinesias associated with increasing doses of levodopa. Side effects may include gastrointestinal disturbance, mood changes, postural instability, confusion and hallucinations.

Deep brain stimulation: can be used in patients refractory to standard medical therapy. The aim is to create a continuous 'on state'. The main target is the subthalamic nucleus (STN), although other areas such as the thalamus and globus pallidus interna are occasionally targeted. It involves delivering electrical pulses via a lead from a pulse generator which is usually implanted beneath the clavicle.

Non-motor symptoms: side effects of nausea and vomiting with dopamine agonists can be treated with domperidone and constipation with laxatives. Dementia symptoms can be treated with cholinesterase inhibitors. Careful use of clozapine and quetiapine can help in the treatment of psychotic symptoms, but typical antipsychotics must be avoided because these worsen motor symptoms. Patients should be reviewed regularly for symptoms of depression, which can be treated with cognitive–behavioural therapy (CBT) and selective serotonin reuptake inhibitors (SSRIs).

Palliative care needs of the patient should be considered early. End-of-life considerations should be discussed with patients and their family and carers so that they can make appropriate decisions and provisions.

SCENARIO 3. MOTOR NEURON DISEASE

Identifying physical signs

Motor neuron disease (MND) is characterised by both UMN and LMN signs in the same muscle groups, without sensory involvement.

General appearance

There may be a wheelchair, walking aids or foot supports for foot drop. **Wasting** and contractures are characteristics of advanced disease. Look very carefully at the upper and lower limbs for **fasciculation**, asking the patient if you can observe the limbs carefully for a moment while he or she remains at rest. There may be drooling with advanced disease with bulbar/pseudobulbar involvement.

Cranial nerve examination

Wasting of temporalis and masseters may be present. The motor function of cranial nerves V, VII, IX, X, XI and XII might be affected *but note that the oculomotor muscles are spared.*

Bulbar palsy (LMNs of nerves IX, X, XI and XII) signs:

- Weakness of the muscles of mastication
- Absent jaw reflex
- Upper and lower facial muscle weakness
- Palatal weakness
- Reduced gag reflex
- Flaccid and wasted tongue with fasciculation
- Weak sternocleidomastoid and trapezius.

Speech can be tested by asking the patient to repeat the phrases 'British constitution', 'statistical analysis' and 'baby hippopotamus', which test all the phonetic components of speech. The patient may have **slurred, quiet** and **nasal speech** with difficulty with consonants.

Pseudobulbar (UMN) pathology:

- Emotional lability, with spontaneous laughing or crying

- Pronounced gag reflex
- Small stiff tongue that is difficult to protrude and has slowed rotational or sideways movements
- Brisk jaw reflex
- Speech is slow, thick and indistinct, and due to the tongue moving little (sometimes described as 'hot potato' speech).

Upper and lower limbs

Again, look for a combination of UMN and LMN signs. There may be LMN signs of **wasting, fasciculation**, **reduced tone** and **weakness** in the upper and lower limbs, usually starting distally and slightly asymmetrically in early disease but then progressing proximally and bilaterally. Thus, in early disease there may be foot drop or reduced strength in the hand muscles. Look at the hands for dorsal guttering from muscle wasting, which when advanced can lead to claw hand deformity. In the lower limbs, look for foot drop and wasting of the anterior tibialis.

UMN signs will include increased clasp-knife spastic tone, weakness and brisk reflexes, ankle clonus and extensor plantars. Look for combinations of UMN and LMN signs, such as absence of knee reflexes but upgoing plantars. There are no sensory signs.

Additional

State to the examiner that you would like to assess respiratory function with a respiratory system examination, specifically looking for an increased respiratory rate, abdominal paradox and reduced chest expansion and performing pulse oximetry. Diaphragmatic strength could be tested at the bedside with forced vital capacity (FVC) both standing and supine. State that you would request a formal speech, language and swallowing assessment, and would like to test cognition with a Mini-Mental State Examination (MMSE).

Differential diagnosis

Differentiating types of MND

Amyotrophic lateral sclerosis (ALS): the most common form that presents with UMN and LMN signs.

Primary lateral sclerosis: presents initially with UMN signs but eventually progresses to include LMN signs and is known as 'UMN-dominant ALS'.

Progressive muscular atrophy: presents initially with LMN signs, but most progress to develop UMN signs, and is known as 'LMN-dominant ALS'.

Progressive bulbar palsy: presents with LMN (bulbar) or UMN (pseudobulbar) signs involving bulbar muscles.

There is a group of diseases called 'MND-mimic disorders', some of these affecting LMNs, UMNs or both, and others affecting muscles alone.

Cervical spondylosis with myelopathy and radiculopathy: this presents with UMN and LMN signs but the former occur only below the level of the lesion. There will be no bulbar/cranial nerve involvement and there are usually sensory signs and symptoms of pain. There may be bladder and bowel involvement. MRI of the cervical spine would show spinal cord and nerve root compression.

Dual pathology: a cervical myelopathy with a coexistent peripheral neuropathy can present with mixed UMN and LMN signs. There would be dermatomal sensory symptoms and the weakness would be in a peripheral nerve pattern. There would not be any cranial or bulbar signs. Cervical imaging would differentiate this from MND.

Syringomyelia/Syringobulbia: this will give a mixture of UMN and LMN signs (see Scenario 7). At the level of the lesion (typically in the cervical or high thoracic spine) there will be UMN signs and a dissociated sensory loss. Below the level of the lesion there will be LMN signs. Dissociated sensory loss results from damage to decussating spinothalamic pathways, which give loss of pain and temperature at the level of the lesion but preserve the dorsal columns, leaving normal pressure, proprioception and vibration sense. Sensory signs help differentiate this from MND.

Multifocal motor neuropathy (MMN) with conduction block: this is a rare disease usually presenting in young or middle-aged men and its onset and progression are slower than that of MND. It is an acquired autoimmune demyelinating disease that is progressive and gives rise to LMN signs, such as weakness, wasting and fasciculations, with little or no sensory involvement. Clinically it can be difficult to distinguish from MND in the initial stages, except that there are only LMN signs and weakness with little atrophy until much later. Nerve conduction studies (NCS) can show multiple sites of conduction block and CSF analysis might be positive for anti-GM1 ganglioside antibody. The patient's condition may improve with IVIG.

Benign cramp fasciculation syndrome: this presents only with cramps and fasciculations, usually of large limb muscles, made worse after exercise or sleep deprivation. There are no other LMN or any UMN signs and no disease progression.

Inclusion body myositis: this is an inflammatory myopathy that presents with slowly progressive weakness and wasting in distal and proximal muscle groups in the limbs without sensory symptoms. There are no UMN signs. It tends to affect older age groups. Diagnosis is by electromyography (EMG) and muscle biopsy, and it tends to have a more benign course than MND.

Monomelic amyotrophy (benign focal amyotrophy): this is a focal LMN disease characterised by weakness and wasting of a single limb, usually a hand or arm rather than foot or leg. There will be no UMN or sensory signs. Typically it affects young Asiatic males (aged 15–25 years), most commonly in India or Japan. It plateaus after 2–5 years without improvement or progression. There is no treatment other than physiotherapy.

Chronic inflammatory demyelinating polyneuropathy (CIDP): this is an autoimmune chronic demyelinating condition that can be relapsing and remitting. It can present with predominant motor symptoms affecting both proximal and distal muscle groups or with mixed motor–sensory symptoms. Differentiating signs from MND include LMN and sensory symptoms and occasional autonomic features. CSF analysis shows a raised protein and there can be good response to IVIG and plasmapheresis.

Spinal muscular atrophy: these are a group of autosomal recessive diseases in which there is loss of the *SMN1* gene causing motor neuron cell death and subsequent widespread muscle wasting. It is usually diagnosed in infancy and rarely in early adulthood. There are only LMN signs and symptoms, with markedly reduced tone and muscle fasciculation. EMG and genetic testing are diagnostic.

Myasthenia gravis: an autoimmune neuromuscular disorder leading to fluctuating symptoms of skeletal muscle weakness (see Scenario 9). Fatigability and involvement of extraocular muscles differentiate this from MND. Diagnosis is through detecting acetylcholine receptor antibodies and treatment is with acetylcholinesterase inhibitors and removal of any thymoma if present.

Post-poliomyelitis syndrome: this can occur 20–30 years after the initial viral infection and presents with progressive fatigue, muscle weakness and pain in the muscle groups initially affected by the infection. There are only LMN signs. The diagnosis is made through exclusion of other possible neurological disorders and management is supportive.

Clinical judgement and maintaining patient welfare

Investigations
MND is a clinical diagnosis, based on the coexistence of LMN and UMN signs with no sensory signs and a progressive course. However, tests such as MRI or CSF analysis may be required to exclude other causes as described above.

Management
The condition is progressive and treatment is aimed at preventing complications and palliating symptoms.

The only disease-modifying treatment supported by NICE guidance is riluzole which can prolong life by approximately 3–4 months and should be offered to all patients at diagnosis.

Involvement of a multidisciplinary team is essential, including a neurologist, physiotherapist, dietician, respiratory therapist, speech and language specialist, occupational therapist, social worker and primary care team.

Patient-centred care is paramount and should promote patient and carers' autonomy, decision-making and independence.

Discussions surrounding prognosis, ongoing needs, advanced directives and end-of-life care should be stage appropriate and guided by patients' primary concerns.

Specific symptoms requiring treatment include the following.

Respiratory: difficulty with mucus or coughing can be helped with cough augmentation devices, physiotherapy and suction. As the disease progresses, non-invasive ventilatory (NIV) methods can be used as described in specific NICE guidance. (NICE Guidelines 2010, http://www.nice.org/uk/guidance/cCG105, due to be reviewed)

Pharyngeal and gastrointestinal: dysphagia and weight loss can be treated with dietary changes, supplementation and percutaneous endoscopic gastrostomy (PEG) feeding. Drooling can be treated with anticholinergics or radiotherapy of salivary glands.

Musculoskeletal: physiotherapy and occupational therapy can support and maintain function. Spasticity can be treated with baclofen and tizanidine. Muscle cramps can be treated with quinine or diazepam.

Psychological: anxiety and depression can be treated with SSRIs and counselling. Emotional lability/pseudobulbar affect may be helped by amitriptyline or dextromethorphan.

Complications: include respiratory failure, aspiration pneumonia, nutritional deficiencies and occasionally side effects from riluzole treatment.

The last includes hepatotoxicity and rarely neutropenia, so it is necessary to monitor liver function tests (LFTs) and full blood count (FBC) in the first few months of treatment.

Prognosis

MND progresses without relapses, remission or any stabilisation. The clinical time course varies, with a median life expectancy of 3–5 years. Of patients 10% may survive >10 years.

Good prognostic indicators include: younger age at onset, onset of disease in limbs and FVC >75% at baseline.

Poor prognostic factors include older age at onset, bulbar symptoms at onset, co-morbidity, frontotemporal dementia and FVC <75% at baseline.

SCENARIO 4. HEMIPARESIS

Identifying physical signs

General appearance
There may be a wheelchair or other walking aids nearby.

The patient may sit with the typical **dystonic pose** of unilateral pyramidal tract pathology, with adducted shoulder and flexed elbow and wrist, extension of the fingers, and a relatively extended and adducted ipsilateral leg (which is easier to see when examining the gait).

There may be a characteristic **circumducting unilateral scissor gait** and more prominent pyramidal signs in the ipsilateral arm without arm swing.

At the start of your examination remember to check for **pronator drift**, preferably with the patient's eyes closed, because this is a very specific sign of pyramidal weakness.

Cranial nerve examination
The key signs are:

- A **visual field defect** such as a homonymous quadrant/hemianopia
- **UMN facial weakness**
- **Palatal and tongue** weakness.

A conjugate horizontal gaze palsy may also be elicited.

Upper and lower limb examination
The key signs are:

- **Clasp-knife spasticity** felt particularly with the **supinator catch** in the upper limbs
- **Ankle clonus**
- Increased tone in the lower limbs
- **Pyramidal weakness** where flexors in the upper limb and extensors in the lower limbs are relatively stronger, although in a dense

hemiparesis all muscle groups are affected equally
- **Hyperreflexia** compared with the unaffected side
- **Extensor plantar** response
- **Sensory loss** to light touch, proprioception and joint position sense. A dissociated sensory loss with loss of pinprick/temperature on the contralateral side to the hemiparesis and numbness to light touch would suggest a cervical cord hemisection lesion/pathology giving rise to a Brown–Séquard syndrome.

Additional signs for UMN lesions include **Hoffman's reflex** (see page 238) in the upper limbs and **Oppenheimer's sign** (see page 233) in the lower limbs.

Testing for coordination can be difficult when there is limb weakness and/or increased tone. Gait and eye movements may be more helpful in detecting cerebellar signs that may point toward additional/other pathology rather than a typical presentation of hemiparesis from an acute cerebrovascular cause (stroke).

Note: if asked to examine the upper limbs, then complete your examination by asking to examine the gait and lower limbs, and vice versa.

Speech
There may be a motor/non-fluent/**expressive dysphasia** where there may be sparse, hesitant, stuttering speech with normal comprehension (and often great patient effort and frustration). Alternatively you may elicit a sensory/fluent/**receptive dysphasia** where there is fluent, plentiful but incomprehensible speech with little or no patient insight (see Scenario 24).

You would expect speech to be affected by pathology in the 'dominant' hemisphere, which in 95% of right-handed patients (and 60% of left-handed patients) is in the left hemisphere (and so associated with a right hemiparesis).

Additional

Tell the examiner that, to complete your examination, you would like to assess cardiovascular risk factors with measurement of BP, blood sugar, auscultation for carotid bruits, assessing pulse for atrial fibrillation and listening for any additional heart sounds including murmurs.

Differential diagnosis

The aim of examination is to locate the lesion. Although you should mention that the most common cause of hemiparesis is a cerebrovascular event, say that you would like to take a full history to determine the timing and pattern of onset to rule out a demyelinating process, space-occupying lesion (tumour, abscess, cyst), post-ictal state (Todd's paresis) or a conversion/somatisation disorder.

Transient ischaemic attack (TIA): describes acute focal neurological symptoms from transient brain, retinal or spinal cord ischaemia, with symptoms lasting <24 hours and no evidence of acute infarction on brain imaging.

Demyelinating conditions such as MS would be likely to give rise to symptoms and signs disseminated in time and space, so a protracted history with worsening of symptoms over days including sensory, cerebellar and cranial nerve signs, is inconsistent with a cerebrovascular cause.

Space-occupying lesions would give rise to slowly developing symptoms and signs, possibly with a history of early morning headache and signs of raised intracranial pressure including ocular palsies and papilloedema. There may be signs of malignancy elsewhere because intracranial tumours are more likely to be secondary than primary cancers.

Post-ictal hemiparesis would follow a seizure and would usually resolve within minutes to hours; it commonly affects only one limb rather than a whole side. There can be gaze palsies with 'wrong-way' eye deviation toward the hemiparetic side, unlike strokes, which tend to deviate gaze away from the hemiparetic side and towards the side of the lesion.

Complex migraines can give rise to neurological symptoms that mimic an ischaemic/haemorrhagic cerebrovascular event. There is often a history of recurrent, fully resolving events, preceded by an aura, headache and positive symptoms such as paraesthesias, visual hallucinations and confused speech (rather than the negative symptoms associated with stroke such as visual loss, weakness and numbness).

Somatisation/conversion disorders: neurological signs will be inconsistent and not correspond to a vascular territory. There are no cranial nerve signs. Tone is usually reduced rather than increased with even reflexes bilaterally. Power 'fades off' at the end of movement rather than being consistently low from initiation onwards, and weakness is not in a pyramidal distribution.

Ischaemic stroke/intracerebral haemorrhage

The vast majority of strokes are subdivided into ischaemic (thrombotic or embolic) or haemorrhagic stroke. Ischaemic stroke accounts for approximately 85% of cases and haemorrhagic stroke for the remaining 15%. Rarely a central venous sinus thrombosis can be a cause of stroke.

It is not possible to reliably distinguish between ischaemic and haemorrhagic stroke clinically, although haemorrhagic strokes are more often associated with reduced consciousness and signs of increased intracranial pressure.

Localisation of a vascular deficit giving rise to stroke syndromes is not always accurate from clinical signs alone but the combination of clinicoradiological findings can best localise stroke, which is important for ongoing management and secondary prevention.

The anterior cerebral artery syndromes
- The anterior cerebral artery (ACA) supplies the medial frontal and parietal lobes.
- Infarction of this territory causes a contralateral hemiplegia and sensory loss affecting the leg more than the arm or face. There may be behavioural effects resulting from damage to the frontal lobes.

The middle cerebral artery syndromes
- The middle cerebral artery (MCA) supplies the rest of the frontal and parietal lobes as well as the superior part of the temporal lobe.
- Infarction of the complete territory causes contralateral hemiparesis and sensory loss and hemianopia. The arm and the face may be more affected. In dominant-lobe MCA lesions there will be language impairment with an expressive, receptive or mixed dysphasia. Damage to the corresponding areas in the non-dominant hemisphere may cause hemi-neglect syndromes and/or subtle language defects such as aprosodia (an inability to interpret emotional intonations of speech). If more distal lesions of the MCA are present then medial brain structures will be spared, resulting in incomplete sensory and motor deficits.

The posterior cerebral artery syndromes
- The posterior cerebral artery (PCA) supplies the inferior temporal lobe and the occipital lobes.
- Distal lesions not affecting the deeper branches can cause contralateral hemianopia. Bilateral occipital lobe damage can lead to cortical blindness often with denial of any deficit.

Lacunar syndromes
- Subcortical strokes (lacunar or striatocapsular) arise from occlusion of one of the smaller deep penetrating arteries that arise from the main circle of Willis, cerebellar arteries or basilar artery. These vessels feed the posterior part of the internal capsule, the thalamus and the anterior part of the pons. Discrete lacunar syndromes typically solely affect face, arms and legs due to infarction of motor or sensory tracts, while sparing cortical functions:
  - Pure motor hemiparesis – posterior internal capsule infarction
  - Pure hemianaesthesia – thalamus infarction
  - Hemi-sensorimotor loss – posterior internal capsule and thalamus infarction
  - Ataxic hemiparesis – posterior internal capsule and anterior pons infarction
  - Dysarthria/clumsy hand – anterior pons infarction
  - Extrapyramidal movement disorders – infarction to the basal ganglia.

Brain-stem syndromes (includes cerebellar syndromes)
- The brain stem is supplied by penetrating arteries from the vertebrobasilar system (VBS) and proximal portions from the cerebellar arteries. The cerebellum is supplied by the posteroinferior, anteroinferior and superior cerebellar arteries.
- Infarction of the cerebellar hemispheres can cause ipsilateral limb ataxia and nystagmus.
- The brain stem contains many compact neural tracts and cranial nerve nuclei, so slight variations in infarction site can cause significantly varied symptoms.
- The corticospinal motor tracts decussate at the base of the medulla serving contralateral limbs, whereas brain-stem cranial nerve nuclei (nerves III–XII, except for the trochlear nerve) serve ipsilateral structures. Thus we see the classic 'crossed signs' in brain-stem strokes, such as LMN weakness in the right face with UMN weakness in the left arm and leg.
- There are several recognised eponymous brain-stem syndromes (see Scenario 26).

Clinical judgement and maintaining patient welfare

Investigations

Brain and cervical spine imaging: this will help differentiate a vascular, demyelinating or space-occupying lesion.

In the case of suspected stroke, which is treated as a medical emergency, brain CT/MRI is used to rule out haemorrhagic stroke so that thrombolysis can be started as soon as possible, with guidance recommending imaging within 25 minutes of arrival at the accident and emergency department (A&E).

In the initial stages infarction will not clearly show on non-contrast brain CT but will reveal the high-intensity signal of haemorrhage. MRI is the imaging of choice for suspected brain-stem strokes due to its superior imaging of the posterior fossa compared with CT. Contrast CT/MRI is requested if cerebral venous sinus thrombosis is suspected (headache, depressed level of consciousness, seizures, signs of raised intracranial pressure).

Blood tests: glucose, FBC, urea and electrolytes (U&Es), clotting/international normalised ratio (INR) and cardiac enzymes, erythrocyte sedimentation rate (ESR) (to exclude giant cell arteritis).

Non-urgent investigations for ischaemic stroke aetiology include chest radiograph/CT of the chest, ECG, echocardiography and carotid artery ultrasonography.

Management

Management of ischaemic stroke:

- Patients should be managed in specialist stroke units.
- Thrombolysis with tPA (tissue plasminogen activator) is advised within 4.5 hours of symptom onset, preferably within 60 min of arrival at A&E.
- Contraindications to tPA include: recent history of head trauma, myocardial infarction

(MI), gastrointestinal (GI) or urinary tract haemorrhage, recent surgery, previous history of intracranial haemorrhage and seizures. Patients must have BP <185/110, and normal platelet count, INR and glucose levels.
- Aspirin 300 mg, started >24 hours after tPA but <48 hours after stroke, is continued for 14 days.
- Active physiological management and supportive care, including blood glucose control and appropriate hydration, and nutrition including assessment of swallow (with nasogastric feeding if necessary), supplemental oxygen (if oxygen saturation <92%), thromboembolic prophylaxis, prevention of pressure sores and early mobilisation.

Management of haemorrhagic stroke:

- Urgent neurosurgical evaluation is required because surgery may be required for a decompensating or extending stroke.
- Early airway intubation (if there is depressed conscious level) and invasive BP and intracranial pressure monitoring may be required.
- Active physiological management and supportive care as above.

Management of cerebral venous sinus thrombosis:

- Anticoagulation with IV heparin
- Active physiological management and supportive care as above.

Secondary prevention in ischaemic stroke:

- Patients with anterior circulation strokes/TIA and without severe disability may have carotid artery disease as a suspected cause of their stroke. Endarterectomy should be considered for men with >50% and women >70% carotid artery stenosis.
- Anticoagulation should be started (usually after 2 weeks when stable) for those with an identified cardioembolic cause such as atrial fibrillation or mural thrombus.
- Low-dose aspirin 75 mg and M/R dipyridamole 200 mg.

- Statins (irrespective of cholesterol level).
- Consider treatment with angiotensin-converting enzyme (ACE) inhibitor and thiazide (usually perindopril and indapamide), irrespective of BP (but not in the acute stage).

Complications of stroke can include haemorrhagic transformation of ischaemic stroke, cerebral oedema and raised intracranial pressure, deep vein thrombosis (DVT)/pulmonary embolism (PE), aspiration pneumonia and depression. Rarely, orolingual oedema may be a side effect of tPA infusion.

Prognosis for ischaemic stroke

The mortality rate from stroke can be up to 15%. Long-term significant disability is seen in a further 15–30%. Patients who have lacunar strokes have a greater chance of surviving beyond 30 days (96%) than those with other types of stroke (85%). Between 70% and 80% of patients with lacunar strokes are functionally independent at 1 year.

Only thrombolysis and dedicated stroke units are associated with improved outcome. There is a 6% risk of intracranial haemorrhage with tPA; the number needed to treat (NNT) is 8 to prevent one case of stroke-related disability.

SCENARIO 5: SPASTIC PARAPARESIS

Identifying physical signs

The cardinal signs include a pyramidal pattern of weakness in the lower limbs and a sensory level representing spinal cord pathology. The instruction is usually to examine the gait and/or lower limbs.

General appearance
There may be a wheel chair or other walking aids and foot supports for any foot drop. In long-standing disease, there will be muscle wasting from disuse atrophy and possibly the appearance of contractures.

Cranial nerve examination
If time permits try to examine eye movements, perform fundoscopy and visual field testing, and examine speech to help illicit any cerebellar signs, papilloedema or visual field defects that may help in the diagnosis of MS as a cause of the spastic paraparesis.

Peripheral nerve examination
Ask the patient if he or she is able to show you the gait, which shows typical pyramidal weakness with scissoring of the legs, caused by relative weakness in the flexors and abductors compared with the extensors and adductors. This imbalance in muscle group strength leads to stiffly extended legs with pronated feet, which causes a tiptoe circumduction gait. The gait can be made more unsteady by foot fall stimulating ankle clonus. There will be increased tone shown by rocking the legs gently at the knees or gently raising the leg off the bed at the knee. Power is reduced globally but more so in the flexor and abductor groups. Deep tendon reflexes are brisk and plantar responses upgoing with ankle clonus. Weakness and increased tone can make it difficult to study coordination, but it may be possible to illicit an intention tremor with the foot–shin test or dysdiadochokinesis with repeated foot tapping against your palm; alternatively look for the equivalent signs in the upper limb or eye movements. With clearly bilateral signs, look for a spinal cord sensory level, starting with light-touch examination at the sternum and moving downwards. Before starting light-touch testing now is a good time to ask/help the patient to sit forward so that you can examine the thoracic and lumbar spine for any signs of deformity or surgery.

Additional
Tell the examiner that you would like to assess perianal sensation and tone, and enquire about bladder and bowel dysfunction. Ask to examine the upper limbs to help diagnose the level and possible aetiology of the lesion, and the cranial nerves.

Differential diagnosis

A diagnosis of spastic paraparesis describes only the presence of UMN signs in the lower limbs, so a full diagnosis involves examination of the cranial nerves and upper limbs to help describe the pattern and level of pathology, and thus its potential aetiology.

Causes of spastic paraparesis can be broadly divided into compressive and non-compressive. A further dichotomy can include whether onset of signs was (sub-)acute or chronic. Patients with compressive lesions will mostly be spared signs above the level of the lesion.

Compressive disease
Trauma: a primary fracture–dislocation of a vertebra (road traffic accidents account for almost half of these) or secondary/pathological fracture from osteoporosis or Pott's disease. Consider also degenerative diseases such as spondylosis and intervertebral disc prolapse.

Clues are the age of the patient (older with degenerative disease), the sensory level and surgical scars or deformity. There are no signs above the lesion.

Tumours: primary spinal tumours are rare but include osteosarcomas, osteochondromas, multiple myeloma and primary bone lymphoma. Secondary tumours from metastatic disease are much more common and include metastases from prostate, breast, lung, renal and gastric cancers.

Clues are mainly from the history and physical signs are similar to those of trauma.

Tubercular disease: consider other infective abscesses in this group.

Clues include patients possibly being systemically unwell (unlikely to come to examination in the acute stage) and exhibiting signs of other organ disease such as pulmonary TB.

Non-compressive disease

MS (see Scenario 1): look for sensory and cerebellar signs with upper limb and cranial nerve pathology.

MND (see Scenario 3): there will be LMN and UMN signs together and no sensory signs. Look for bulbar involvement.

Parasagittal tumour: meningiomas arising from the middle third of the parasagittal sinus and involving the frontal motor cortex can initially present with spastic paraparesis. There may be additional sensory signs of cortical sensory loss if the parietal lobes are also involved such as loss of both stereognosis (ability to identify an object by touch with eyes closed) and graphaesthesia (ability to recognise simple numbers/letters drawn on the body without visual cues).

Hereditary spastic paraparesis: hereditary spastic paraparesis, sometimes referred to as the Strumpell–Lorrain syndrome, is usually dominantly inherited (X-linked and recessive forms also exist), and leads to progressive stiffness and UMN weakness of the lower limbs from axonal degeneration. It can be associated with other neurological features such as cerebellar signs, peripheral neuropathy, epilepsy and cognitive changes. It may be associated with cataracts and optic neuropathy. Diagnosis is usually from typical presentation with a family history and after genetic testing. There are no sensory signs and upper limbs tend not to be involved.

Friedreich's ataxia (see Scenario 12): this is an autosomal recessive condition leading to degeneration of the nerve cells in the dorsal route ganglions, lateral corticospinal tracts, spinocerebellar tracts and posterior columns, thus leading to cerebellar, pyramidal and dorsal column signs. Patients develop symptoms in their teens or early adulthood with difficulties walking from spasticity, pes cavus, ataxia, and loss of vibration and position sense; they also develop slurred speech. The disease is associated with cardiomyopathy and diabetes.

Syringomyelia (see Scenario 7): this involves the development of a fluid-filled syrinx within the spinal canal, most commonly in the cervical spine. It may be congenital or secondary to lesions disrupting normal CSF flow. Most commonly there is damage to the decussating spinothalamic tracts, but preservation of the dorsal columns leading to a dissociated sensory loss of pain and temperature, and relative preservation of vibration and position sense. There can be UMN signs in the lower limbs with LMN signs in the upper limbs. With extension of the syrinx into the brain stem there may be cerebellar or cranial nerve signs.

Transverse myelitis: this can have many causes including MS (most common), SLE, sarcoid, paraneoplastic syndromes, antecedent viral infection including HSV, VZV, HIV, HTLV-1 (tropical spastic paraparesis), CMV and EBV, or antecedent bacterial infection including syphilis and Lyme borreliosis. Transverse myelitis is a heterogeneous inflammatory disorder of the spinal cord that can give rise to acute or subacute symptoms, including motor weakness, sensory symptoms, and bladder and autonomic dysfunction depending on the level of the lesion. The motor deficit is usually pyramidal with symptoms predominantly in the lower limbs and patients develop an ascending tingling or numbness below the level of the lesion.

Vascular: the anterior spinal artery syndrome (also known as Beck's syndrome) is the most common form of spinal cord infarction and it can be caused by embolic, thrombotic, dissection, vasculitic or hypotensive/low-flow causes or arteriovenous malformations. The anterior spinal artery serves the anterior two-thirds of the spinal cord so presentation includes acute-onset spastic paresis (quadraparesis in higher lesions) with loss of pain and temperature at or below the level of the lesion but preservation of the dorsal columns.

Subacute combined degeneration of the cord: this is caused by nutritional deficiencies (vitamin B_{12} deficiency is by far the most common) and results in dysfunctional myelination preferentially affecting the dorsal and lateral columns of the cord and affecting longer fibres first. Patients can present with spastic paraparesis associated with loss of vibration and joint position sense, which may also be associated with a peripheral neuropathy, and as the disease progresses there is loss of light touch, pin-prick and temperature. Associated features may include a beefy red smooth tongue and pale or lemon-tinged skin.

Clinical judgement and maintaining patient welfare

Investigations

With (sub-)acute onset it is very important to rule out remediable spinal cord compression, because, once sphincter dysfunction has been present for >24 hours, it is irreversible.

Urgent investigations in this case would include FBC, ESR, chest radiograph and MRI of the spine or a CT myelogram.

In a non-acute presentation other tests would include:

- **Blood tests**: ESR/CRP, autoantibody screening, vitamin B_{12} and folate
- **Infection screen**: serological testing for HIV, HTLV-1 and syphilis; blood culture, sputum culture and early morning urine
- **Lumbar puncture with CSF analysis**: oligoclonal bands, bacterial culture, acid-fast bacilli and mycobacterial culture, ACE and cell count
- **MRI of the CNS**
- **Biopsy** of any identified spinal cord masses
- **Electrophysiology studies**: EMG and nerve conduction studies.

Management

In cases of (sub-)acute spinal cord compression an urgent neurosurgical opinion is needed.

With acute onset and (pending) sphincter involvement, treatment may include urgent surgical decompression or, in the case of malignant compression, the use of intravenous dexamethasone ± spinal radiotherapy.

With non-compressive spastic paraparesis, therapy is targeted at the underlying cause such as treatment of ongoing infectious causes, correction of deficiencies, treatment of MS and anticoagulation for underlying thromboembolic disease.

A multidisciplinary team approach is needed for the maintenance and improvement of independent living and management of symptoms, and will include physiotherapy, occupational therapy, and specialist bladder and bowel services as required. Physiotherapy is needed to maintain remaining muscle strength, prevent contractures and help with transfers and mobility.

Medical therapies include baclofen, tizanidine and dantrolene to help treat contractures.

Contractures may be treated with local botulinum toxin injections.

Treatments for neuropathic pain include amitriptyline and gabapentin.

Surgical treatments include neurosurgical removal of compressive lesions or placing of shunts for syringomyelia.

Orthopaedic surgery may be needed to treat contractures with tendon release or transfer.

Depending on the severity of the paresis, potential complications that require preventive strategies or treatment include pressure sores, dependent oedema and DVT.

Prognosis
The prognosis is very dependent on the severity and level of the spinal cord pathology and the effectiveness of the treatment. Patients with spinal cord injury have a reduced life expectancy compared with the general population.

Identifying physical signs

Pathology affecting the cervical cord will cause a pattern of UMN and LMN (radiculopathy) signs in the upper limbs and UMN and dorsal column signs in the lower limbs. Candidates are usually asked to examine the upper limbs, but remember cervical myelopathy as a differential diagnosis if asked to examine the lower limbs.

General appearance
There may be a wheelchair or other walking aids nearby. Look for general signs of osteoarthritis (OA) or rheumatoid arthritis (RA) in the hands that could be associated with cervical joint disease.

Cranial nerve examination
Normal (there is usually insufficient time to include this but it may help you rule out other diagnoses).

Upper and lower limb examination
There will be a **mixture of LMN and UMN signs** in the upper limbs depending on the degree of myelopathy and radiculopathy. The most common nerve roots affected are **C5–7** where the spinal canal is narrowest and even mild spondylosis can cause symptoms/signs.

Thus there may be LMN signs in a C5–7 distribution, with **fasciculations, weakness and wasting with loss of reflexes** and **UMN signs beneath this level**. There might be weakness of the deltoid and shoulder abduction (C5–6), biceps and elbow flexion in supination (C5–6), brachioradialis and elbow flexion midway between supination/pronation (C5–6) and triceps with elbow extension (C6, C7, C8). The small muscles of the hand are less likely to be involved (C8–T1) unless there have been vascular changes to the cord below the lesion. Reflexes may be absent, brisk or inverted.

The **midcervical reflex pattern** describes the loss of biceps and supinator reflexes (C5 and C6) and a brisk triceps reflex (C7) and is almost pathognomonic of a cord lesion due to pathology at C5–6. **Inverted reflexes** describe contraction of the triceps with bicep reflex testing and finger flexion with supinator testing (the mechanism is uncertain).

Sensory loss will be dermatomal and reflect dorsal column pathology. Pay particular attention to the areas served by C5 (lateral upper arm), C6 (lateral forearm and thumb), C7 (middle finger) and C8 (ring and little fingers). The lateral spinothalamic pathways are relatively spared because degenerative disease causing cervical myelopathy tends to cause compression in the anteroposterior axis.

There are a number of further specific signs that may be elicited in cervical myelopathy:

- **Pseudoathetosis**: damage to cervical dorsal columns causes loss of joint position sense, so with eyes closed and arms held out the fingers writhe unconsciously.
- **Hoffman's reflex**: this is the equivalent of the plantar response for the fingers and demonstrates a UMN lesion of the hands. Holding the patient's middle finger loosely, resting on your index finger and then flicking downwards on the nail with your thumb, produces a reflex flexion of the index finger and thumb. In very early cervical myelopathy, dynamic testing may be needed to elicit this sign, by repeating the test with the neck in extension (less commonly flexion).
- '**Myelopathy hand sign**' which has two components:
  1. **'Finger escape sign'**: with the patient holding the forearms out and hands pronated, the little finger can be seen to abduct ('escape') and there may be

difficulty with full finger extension. This phenomenon can spread to the ring and middle fingers with more severe cervical lesions. The little finger can abduct and flex normally, differentiating this from an ulnar nerve lesion.

2. **Grip and release testing**: the patient remains in the same position as above and is asked to grip and then fully extend the hand and fingers as fast as possible for 10 seconds. There is a slowed response with difficulty in fully extending fingers on release with fewer than the 20 repetitions seen in healthy individuals.

Additional

Ask the examiner for permission to examine the lower limbs for a spastic paraparesis if you suspect cervical myelopathy. Cervical myelopathy might also give a positive Romberg's sign from damage to dorsal columns, giving rise to both a spastic and an ataxic gait. Request examination of the neck for deformity and scars, and areas of tenderness, and test the range of neck movements. State that you would also like to assess perianal sensation and tone, and enquire about bladder and bowel dysfunction.

Differential diagnosis

MND: would present with UMN and LMN signs in the upper limbs but there is neither a clear level nor sensory disturbance.

MS: a demyelinating cervical cord lesion can mimic cervical myelopathy, but the presence of bulbar, cerebellar and cranial nerve signs and symptoms distributed in time indicate that MS is more likely. There would usually be a disturbance of spinothalamic as well as dorsal column tracts on sensory testing.

Friedreich's ataxia (see Scenario 12): weakness and wasting in the arms are a late feature compared with signs in the lower limbs. There would be the mixture of pyramidal weakness with dorsal column signs seen in cervical myelopathy, but

also signs of peripheral neuropathy leading to reduced reflexes. Marked cerebellar signs would be present. Look for the typical associated features of younger age, scoliosis and pes cavus.

Syringomyelia (see Scenario 7): there would be preferential loss of spinothalamic pathways rather than dorsal columns. Diffuse LMN weakness in the upper limbs starts distally with wasting of the small muscles of the hands and absence of reflexes.

Subacute combined degeneration of the cord: LMN signs predominate over UMN signs without a clear cervical level demarcation.

Transverse myelitis: (see Scenario 5).

Clinical judgement and maintaining patient welfare

Investigations

These are focused on determining the underlying cause:

- Trauma
- Tumour
- Tubercular (and other causes of spinal abscess)
- 'Wear and tear'.

The most common cause of cervical myelopathy is degenerative disease (spondylosis) in the facet joints and/or intervertebral discs in either a normal or a congenitally stenosed cervical canal.

Plain cervical radiograph: may show loss of the normal curvature of the C-spine and loss of vertebral height with osteophyte formation. Oblique views are better for showing facet joint pathology. A fracture with atlantoaxial instability may also be revealed.

MRI of the cervical cord: this is the preferred investigation when cervical myelopathy is suspected because it will show spinal cord or nerve compression.

Cervical CT myelogram: this is invasive because it requires intrathecal injection of radio-opaque dye but it is the test of choice when MRI is contraindicated.

Management

For axial neck pain: first-line therapies include physiotherapy and oral analgesia/non-steroidal anti-inflammatory drugs (NSAIDs). Non-responsive symptoms may require the additional use of muscle relaxants (tizanadine or diazepam), or facet and trigger point injections using a combination of a long-acting corticosteroid with a local anaesthetic.

Cervical spondylotic radiculopathy: first-line therapies include physiotherapy, oral analgesia/ NSAIDs. Recalcitrant symptoms may require cervical nerve root blocks or cervical nerve decompression.

Cervical spondylotic myelopathy: in addition to **conservative** treatment with oral analgesia, patients with moderate-to-severe signs and symptoms should proceed to **surgical** decompression and those who are not good surgical candidates should have cervical immobilisation with a hard collar.

Prognosis

Typically, degenerative cervical changes worsen with age. However, cervical radiculopathies tend to resolve with appropriate treatment after 1–2 years. Spinal cord decompression for cervical myelopathy usually stabilises or improves neurological function but may increase neck pain symptoms.

SCENARIO 7. SYRINGOMYELIA/SYRINGOBULBIA

Identifying physical signs

Cervical syringomyelia is characterised by LMN signs in the upper limbs (and more rarely bulbar muscles) with dissociated sensory loss affecting pain and temperature, but preserving vibration, proprioception and light touch in the upper limbs. This is occasionally associated with autonomic signs including Horner's syndrome and/or long-tract signs in the lower limbs with UMN weakness.

General appearance

There may be walking aids or a wheelchair nearby if the patient has an advanced spastic paraparesis. A kyphoscoliosis may be present as a consequence of asymmetrical weakening of the thoracic paraspinal muscles.

Cranial nerve examination

Involvement of the cranial nerves will depend on the rostral extent of the syrinx.

Inclusion of medullary **cranial nerve nuclei IX– XII (syringobulbia)** would give the signs of **palatal weakness**, **reduced gag reflex**, and a **hoarse and nasal voice** with a weak, wasted and fasciculating tongue. Bilateral weakness of the sternocleidomastoid and trapezius muscles would also be observed.

The long trigeminal nerve V sensory nucleus may be affected because it extends from the midbrain as far down as the upper cervical cord. The segmental distribution of the trigeminal nerve in the cord corresponds to a concentric 'onion skin' distribution on the face. The more rostral part of the trigeminal nucleus near the pons receives sensory fibres from the central portion of the face, and the more caudal part of the trigeminal nucleus within the upper cervical cord receives sensory fibres from the outer parts of the face. Thus, as the syrinx extends upwards it may initially cause anaesthesia around the outer part

of the face (the 'balaclava helmet'), which then slowly progresses inwards as the syrinx ascends (see Figure 3.15).

The vestibular nerve VIII nucleus may also be affected along with its connections with the medial longitudinal fasciculus. There may be **nystagmus** which is usually bilateral and may be torsional (seen best with lateral downward gaze), horizontal (lateral gaze) or downbeat (lateral downward gaze). In general, torsional nystagmus is seen in more caudal lesions, but may develop into a horizontal nystagmus and then vertical nystagmus with rostral extension. This is usually seen in the higher brain-stem lesions, especially in association with the Arnold–Chiari malformation.

Involvement of the **medial longitudinal fasciculus** may result in an **intranuclear ophthalmoplegia**. Demonstration of INO means that the syrinx is at least at the level of C5, the caudal limit of extension of the MLF from the midbrain.

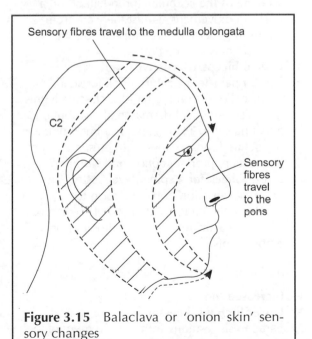

Sensory fibres travel to the medulla oblongata

C2

Sensory fibres travel to the pons

Figure 3.15 Balaclava or 'onion skin' sensory changes

Horner syndrome (see Station 5) may result from involvement of the descending sympathetic outflow from the hypothalamus, which travels in the intermediolateral column of the spinal cord, exiting at C8–T2 spinal cord levels. This is often bilateral.

Upper and lower limb examination

There may be an **ataxic broad-based gait** with failure of heel–toe walking and a **negative Romberg's sign**, pointing towards cerebellar pathology. This indicates involvement of the cerebellar peduncles with a syringobulbia or a concomitant Arnold–Chiari malformation.

Upper limb:

- **Flaccidity or reduced tone.**
- **Reduced power which is more marked distally, with hyperextension of the metacarpophalangeal (MCP) and flexion of the proximal interphalangeal (PIP) and distal interphalangeal (DIP) joints,** distal wasting with dorsal guttering and fasciculations.
- If C5–7 are involved there may be **bilateral winging of the scapulae** (pronounced on a push-up movement against the wall) from paralysis of serratus anterior due to long thoracic nerve involvement.
- **Loss of biceps/triceps/wrist reflexes**.
- **Loss of pain/temperature** (look for scars/burns/callouses on the hands): classically this is in a symmetrical dermatomal distribution, affecting C4 to T1–2 (cape distribution); it is a dissociated sensory loss, with preservation of light touch, proprioception and vibration sense. **Check for a spinal level**, testing pinprick sensation down the torso to delineate the caudal extension of the syrinx. **Charcot's arthropathy** of the shoulder or elbow joints.

Lower limb:

- **Increased tone.**
- **Lower limb weakness** if there is a spastic paraparesis resulting from involvement of the descending lateral corticospinal tracts.

- **Hyperreflexia** with up-going plantars.
- **Ataxic broad-based gait** with failure of heel–toe walking may result from involvement of the cerebellar peduncles from either syringobulbia or a concomitant Arnold–Chiari malformation.

Lumbar syringomyelia is much less common, presenting with bilateral LMN weakness, wasting in the legs, hypo-/areflexia and dissociated sensory loss in the lumbar and sacral dermatomes. There is usually early sphincter disturbance so the patient may have a **suprapubic catheter** and/or be wearing incontinence pads. There would be no upper limb or cranial nerve signs.

Differential diagnosis

CIDP: can present with a subacute symmetrical weakness in all four limbs and distal > proximal weakness, but unlike syringomyelia affects the lower limbs more than the upper. There will be hypo-/areflexia. Sensory loss usually affects all modalities and is in a glove-and-stocking distribution. Nerve conduction studies are consistent with demyelination.

Peripheral neuropathy: a dissociated sensory loss affecting only spinothalamic pathways can be seen with small-fibre peripheral neuropathies (see Scenario 14) such as diabetes or amyloidosis. These will not typically present with upper limb LMN and lower limb UMN signs unless there is additional pathology, such as a cervical myelopathy, and signs are usually asymmetrical.

Amyotrophic lateral sclerosis (MND): there may be solely LMN or UMN signs but these usually affect the same muscle groups rather than occurring in a segmental manner. There will be marked fasciculations and no sensory findings.

Multiple sclerosis: there are usually sensory symptoms, but no demonstrable sensory signs, and segmental dissociated sensory loss does not occur. Sensory symptoms may occur in contiguous dermatomal bands and there may be the Brown–Séquard phenomenon. There may be pyramidal weakness and hyperreflexia in the lower limbs, but without the LMN weakness in the upper limbs seen in syringomyelia. Both syrinx and MS may present as INO or with cerebellar signs. There can be isolated cranial nerve lesions such as nerve VI palsy and signs of optic atrophy that won't be present with syringomyelia. The history will describe relapses and remissions.

Cervical spondylosis: degenerative change may cause myelopathy ± radiculopathy signs. There may be weakness and decreased reflexes in upper limb radiculopathy but this will not be symmetrical. There may be brisk reflexes and pyramidal weakness in the lower limbs with a compressive cervical myelopathy, but again this is usually asymmetrical. There will not be disso-ciated sensory loss in pure cervical spondylosis but, instead, posterior columns may be affected, particularly where there is ossification of the posterior ligamentum flavum and osteophyte en-croachment.

Anterior spinal artery syndrome: the single, mid-line, anterior spinal artery supplies the anterior two-thirds of the cord including the corticospinal and spinothalamic tracts. Anterior spinal artery syndrome is an acute vascular event caused by infarction or haemorrhage, presenting with severe back pain. It can present with a quadra-/parapar-esis, depending on the level of the injury, with loss of pain and temperature sensation but pre-servation of proprioceptive and vibration sense below the lesion.

Clinical judgement and maintaining patient welfare

Investigations
Syringomyelia is the development of a fluid-filled cavity (syrinx) within the central substance of the spinal cord which can slowly progress and expand over time. Investigations should establish underlying cause and anatomical extent.

There are several causes, including:

- **CSF blockage**: this is the most common cause (>50%) and can be due to the Arnold–Chiari malformation, other hindbrain malformations, spina bifida, tumours near the foramen magnum, and scarring of the meninges from basal arachnoiditis or meningeal carcinomatosis.
- **Spinal cord injury**: this can include traumatic injury, haemorrhage, infection or infarction.
- **Intramedullary tumours**: these produce secretions or can give rise to haemorrhage. The most commonly associated are ependymomas and haemangioblastomas.
- Idiopathic.

Neuroimaging: MRI best visualises the posterior fossa to look for Arnold–Chiari malformations and assess brain-stem involvement. Gadolinium enhancement may be required for assessment of associated spinal cord tumours.

Management
Surgery is advised to prevent progression of any neurological deficit from the syrinx, to ameliorate any CSF blockage and for removal of spinal cord tumours. There are several options including cer-vical decompression with laminectomy.

Shunts can be placed to drain the syrinx or any associated hydrocephalus, and these include syr-ingoperitoneal and ventriculoperitoneal shunts respectively.

Physiotherapy will improve recovery and main-tain function postoperatively.

Permanent loss of spinothalamic pathways will require patient advice with regard to care, with daily activities and frequent careful inspection of hands and feet for prompt treatment of ulcera-tion/wounds.

SCENARIO 8: MYOTONIC DYSTROPHY

Identifying physical signs

Myotonic dystrophy is the most common adult-onset form of muscular dystrophy and is a multisystem disorder characterised by slowly progressive muscle wasting, myotonia (slow relaxation of muscle after voluntary/reflex contraction), cataracts, cardiac conduction defects, and endocrine, respiratory and CNS effects.

General appearance
They may have a **myopathic facies** with a long, thin face and neck from weakness and wasting of the temporalis, masseter, facial and sternocleidomastoid muscle groups. There may be **bilateral ptosis** and **cataracts**, and the mouth might hang slightly open. In male patients there might be **frontal balding**. If, from first glance, you suspect myotonic dystrophy you could introduce yourself with a firm handshake and assess for **myotonia** on attempted release. You may see walking aids, orthoses or adapted footwear.

Gait
There may be **bilateral foot drop** with a **high-steppage gait** or, as disease progresses, a **waddling gait** from weakness of the proximal hip flexors. Romberg's test is negative.

Upper and lower limb examination
* **Tone is normal**.
* **Symmetrical distal wasting and weakness** in the limbs that advance proximally with disease progression.
* **Wasting of the small muscles of the hands**.
* **Myotonia** can be demonstrated by tapping on the thenar eminence, which will cause dimpling and adduction of the thumb with slow relaxation. Alternatively you could ask the patient to grip your hand tightly for 5 seconds and let go quickly, and there will be delayed release.

* On repeating the hand-grip exercise several times the myotonia phenomenon can reduce, described as the 'warm-up' effect in myotonia (contrast this with the fatigability seen in myasthenia gravis). The phenomenon of myotonia can disappear with disease progression as muscle weakness increases.
* **Deep tendon reflexes will be reduced** and plantar reflexes will be downward.
* **Coordination will be normal** within the limits of muscle weakness.
* **No sensory impairment**.

Cranial nerve examination
The patient may have **difficulty opening the eyes after tight closure** and you will feel reduced muscle bulk of temporalis and masseters with jaw closure, and reduced power of the sternocleidomastoid muscles on attempted lateral turn of the head or flexion of the neck against resistance. Testing the **red reflex will demonstrate cataracts**. It is rare to see any ophthalmoplegia (contrast this with myasthenia gravis). In assessing speech the weakness and myotonia of oropharyngeal muscles may give patients a **nasal quality to speech**, with hoarseness, slowed, indistinct or quieter speech.

Additional
You could end the examination by stating that you would like to test **blood glucose**, perform a **cardiovascular examination** for any signs of arrhythmias or presence of a pacemaker, examine for any **thyroid nodules**, perform a genital examination for **testicular atrophy** in male patients and perform a **Mini-Mental State Examination**.

Note
Do not test for percussion myotonia on the tongue because this is painful for the patient. Be sensitive when describing any possible cognitive effects associated with the disease, describing them as 'cognitive impairment'.

Differential diagnosis

The differential diagnosis of myotonia

Myotonia congenita: this is a chloride ion channelopathy affecting skeletal muscle. Thomsen's disease (autosomal dominant) presents in the first few years of life with non-progressive muscle stiffness and hypertrophy. Becker's disease (autosomal recessive) presents a bit later but with more severe stiffness.

Paramyotonia (PM/Eulenberg's disease): a sodium channelopathy (autosomal dominant). This presents in the first decade of life with paradoxical myotonia that is worse after exercise and triggered by cold.

Hyperkalaemic periodic paralysis (HPP): a sodium channelopathy (autosomal dominant) affecting the same sodium channel gene (*SCN4A*) as PM, but thought to be clinically distinct. It is characterised by transient but frequent episodes of paralysis starting in infancy, associated with raised serum potassium and triggered by fasting or rest after exercise.

Mild tetanus: this is caused by the neurotoxin from Gram-positive *Clostridium tetani*. Local or mild tetanus can occur in the area local to the initial injury causing spasms and stiffness, although severe generalised tetanus is the most common presentation.

Stiff person syndrome: a rare syndrome of unknown cause associated with autoimmune anti-GAD (anti-glutamic acid decarboxylase) antibodies and diabetes. The syndrome can occur at any age and in both sexes. It starts as axial muscle spasms and progresses to generalised proximal stiffness that can cause skeletal fracture and muscle rupture. It is either self-limiting or progressive.

The differential diagnosis of symmetrical LMN muscle weakness

Distal spinal muscular atrophy: a variant of spinal muscular atrophy, presenting similarly to Charcot–Marie–Tooth disease (see Scenario 11) but with no sensory involvement.

Peripheral neuropathies: these tend to cause wasting, and include sensory signs, reduced reflexes and distal–proximal progression.

Neuromuscular junction pathology: this manifests as diffuse weakness in the absence of wasting, sensory signs or abnormal reflexes. There is fatigability, and ocular, bulbar and respiratory muscles are involved. Diseases include myasthenia gravis and Lambert–Eaton myasthenic syndrome.

Myopathies: these manifest as wasting with no sensory signs, normal or reduced reflexes and no fatigability. The myotonic phenomenon may occur in a proximal pattern. Myopathies can be inherited or acquired.

Inherited:

- **Muscular dystrophies**: Duchenne, Becker, scapuloperoneal (Emery–Dreifuss), distal, facioscapulohumeral, limb–girdle, oculopharyngeal
- **Congenital myopathies**: includes nemaline, myotubular, central core and hyaline body myopathy
- **Mitochondrial myopathies**: Kearns–Sayre syndrome
- **Metabolic myopathies**: includes glycogen storage diseases (eg McArdle's disease), lipid storage disease and disorders of purine nucleotide metabolism.

Acquired:

- **Drug induced**: corticosteroids, fibrates, statins, colchicine, D-penicillamine, zidovudine, β blockers, ciclosporin
- **Toxins**: alcohol, organophosphates, snake venom
- **Endocrine**: diabetes, hypo-/hyperthyroidism, Cushing syndrome, hypo-/hyperparathyroidism, pituitary dysfunction

- **Inflammatory**: polymyositis, dermatomyositis, inclusion body myositis.

Clinical judgement and maintaining patient welfare

Investigations
These focus on confirming the diagnosis, classifying the type of disease and identifying multisystem involvement.

Genetic testing
MD type 1 is caused by an autosomal dominant gene mutation in the *DMPK* (dystrophia myotonica protein kinase) gene on chromosome 19. The mutation is an expansion of a CTG trinucleotide repeat sequence, above its normal upper limit of 35.

It is a 'dynamic' mutation showing an increase in the number of repeats with successive generations and hence earlier onset ('anticipation') and disease severity.

Type 1 disease can be divided into three overlapping types:

1. **Congenital MD**: >2000 repeats; presents at birth with hypotonia, respiratory deficits and intellectual impairment. Life expectancy 30–40 years.
2. **Classic MD**: 100–1500 repeats; presents at age 10–30 years. Life expectancy 45–55 years. This is the typical case that presents at MRCP.
3. **Mild MD**: 50–150 repeats; presents at age 20–70 years with mild hypotonia and cataracts; normal life span.

MD type 2 (proximal myotonic myopathy, PROMM) is also an autosomal dominant condition but involves a tetranucleotide repeat sequence, CCTG, in the *ZNF9* (zinc finger protein 9) gene on chromosome 2. MD type 2 shares many of the clinical features of MD type 1 such as progressive weakness, myotonia, cardiac defects, cataracts, male hypogonadism and insulin resistance/diabetes mellitus, but shows less distal limb, facial and bulbar weakness, no cognitive impairment and does not have a severe congenital form.

Other tests
- **Blood tests**: γ-glutamyl transferase (GGT) and creatine kinase (CK) (may be raised by 2–10 times normal range), IgG, follicle-stimulating hormone (FSH) (raised), testosterone (low/normal), fasting glucose and glycated haemoglobin (HbA1c)
- **EMG**: shows myotonic discharges if present
- **ECG**: conduction defects or arrhythmias
- **Echocardiography**: look for cardiomyopathy
- **Genetic testing**
- **Muscle biopsy**: infrequently used in diagnosis now.

Management
There is no cure so treatment is aimed at symptom control, maintaining function and preventing complications (see below). Patients should be signposted to patient groups such as the Myotonic Dystrophy Support Group.

Muscle weakness is managed with physiotherapy and orthoses such as foot and wrist splints.

Myotonia, if symptomatic, may be helped by procainamide or phenytoin.

Speech and language therapy can help with any communication and swallowing difficulties.

Management of GI symptoms is along standard lines using metoclopramide for delayed gastric emptying and antibiotics for bacterial overgrowth.

Ophthalmology referral for cataracts.

Cardiology referral with ECG (24-hour ECG) surveillance is made at least annually or prompted by symptoms. There may be the need to insert a pacemaker.

Avoid:

- Statins, which may worsen myopathy
- Opiates, which may reduce respiratory drive
- Care with anaesthetic agents that may trigger malignant hyperthermia.

A 'MedicAlert' bracelet should be provided.

Genetic counselling for patients and family members is key. This is a common scenario in the communication skills station of PACES.

Specific complications

Cardiac complications with classic MD

- Cardiomyopathy does not correlate with the extent of muscle weakness or size of CTG repeat expansion.
- Sudden cardiac death occurs in 10–30%.
- Up to 90% of individuals have conduction defects.
- Approximately 65% have an abnormal resting ECG including prolonged PR interval, prolonged QTc interval and QRS widening.
- Mitral valve prolapse.
- Arrhythmias including: supraventricular tachycardia (SVT), ventricular tachycardia (VT) and atrial fibrillation (AF).

Respiratory complications with classic MD

- Account for 30–40% of deaths in MD.
- Reduced central drive and muscle weakness lead to nocturnal hypoventilation and hypersomnolence, and increased risk of anaesthesia.
- Increased incidence of pneumonia.

Endocrine complications with classic MD

- Increased incidence of diabetes and insulin resistance
- Testicular atrophy and male impotence
- Thyroid nodules but normal circulating thyroid hormone levels.

GI complications with classic MD

- Delayed gastric emptying with reflux and dysphagia
- Smooth muscle dysfunction with bacterial overgrowth, diarrhoea, malabsorption or megacolon.

Immune complications with classic MD

- Hypogammaglobuinaemia from increased catabolism.

Identifying physical signs

This is a chronic autoimmune disorder targeting the postsynaptic nicotinic acetylcholine receptor (nAChR) in skeletal muscle. Typical features include fluctuating muscle weakness with diurnal variation, fatigability that improves with rest and ophthalmoplegia.

General appearance

Patients may have an **expressionless face** with **asymmetrical ptosis**. They may be holding their head back or furrowing their brow to overcome the eyelid weakness.

Gait

Patients will usually have a normal gait but they may have difficulty getting in and out of a chair due to **proximal muscle weakness**.

Upper and lower limb examination

- Normal appearance with **normal muscle bulk and tone**
- There may be **proximal muscle weakness** usually affecting the upper more than the lower limbs
- Test for **fatigability** by assessing power before and after performed repeated shoulder abduction
- **Normal deep tendon reflexes and plantars**
- **Normal sensation**.

Cranial nerve examination

There may be **bilateral facial weakness** and **asymmetrical ptosis** with reduced ability to bury the eyelashes when asked to close the eyes tight. Eye closure can be easily overcome by the examiner.

Look for poor cheek-puff and a flat smile ('myasthenic snarl'); muscles of mastication are weak as evidenced by **weak jaw opening/closing** against resistance. The patient may sit **supporting the chin** to overcome a weak sagging jaw. There

may be a **complex ophthalmoplegia** due to ocular muscle weakness with no single dominant nerve lesion. **Diplopia** is usually reported on lateral gaze and there are no pupillary signs.

Fatigability can be demonstrated by asking the patient to sustain upward gaze; eventually the eyes will begin to close. Sustaining lateral gaze in either direction could produce a **pseudo-internuclear ophthalmoplegia** with the medial rectus of the adducting eye growing weak and slowly moving to the midline position, with coarse nystagmus in the abducting eye. Unlike a classic INO, covering the abducting eye does not return the adducting eye back to full adduction because the muscles are now fatigued. There may be **weakness in the bulbar muscles** with direct testing, or evident only as nasal and quiet speech with frequent throat clearing from palatal and pharyngeal weakness. Asking the patient to count upwards from zero will also demonstrate **voice weakness** with fatigability because the voice will grow quieter. Sternocleidomastoid muscles may be weaker with **reduced strength of lateral or forward neck flexion**.

Additional

End the examination by stating that you would like to look for other associated features such as a **thymectomy scar** (**sternotomy**) and for evidence of associated **autoimmune diseases** such as diabetes mellitus (finger-prick testing, peripheral neuropathy), rheumatoid arthritis (deforming arthropathy of hands and feet most commonly), thyroid dysfunction (goitre, thyroidectomy scar, Graves' disease proptosis, tachy- or bradycardia and hypo-/hyperreflexia) and systemic lupus erythematosus or SLE (malar rash). Look for evidence of **steroid treatment** (cushingoid appearance, thin skin, bruising, striae). State that you would also like to assess for respiratory muscle compromise by measuring the **FVC** and take a **drug history**.

Differential diagnosis

Lambert–Eaton myasthenic syndrome

This can present in a very similar fashion to myasthenia gravis, but with some important differences. The syndrome occurs as a result of presynaptic anti-voltage-gated calcium channel antibodies. There is prominent proximal leg and arm weakness, which can improve with exercise, unlike myasthenia gravis. Deep tendon reflexes are reduced but can become normal after exercise. Ptosis and weakness of extraocular muscles are less prominent and respiratory failure is less common. There can be autonomic symptoms and signs such as postural hypotension and pupil abnormalities which are not seen in patients with myasthenia gravis. Similar to myasthenia gravis, there are no sensory changes.

Lambert–Eaton myasthenic syndrome (LEMS) is associated with small cell lung cancer in 70% of patients, but other associations include malignant thymoma, and carcinoma of the breast, colon and prostate. LEMS precedes the cancer diagnosis in most cases. It can be associated with autoimmune diseases such as thyroid disease and type 1 diabetes. There is an equal sex ratio and LEMS tends to occur in older adults in the sixth and seventh decades. Repetitive nerve stimulation shows increasing amplitudes, compared with myasthenia gravis which shows decreasing amplitudes. Management includes treating the underlying cancer and immunomodulation with steroids or plasmapheresis.

Primary myopathies

These include inflammatory, mitochondrial myopathies ± external ophthalmoplegias or oculopharyngeal muscular dystrophy. These patients have a proximal muscle weakness that neither is fatigable nor improves after exercise. Deep tendon reflexes will be reduced. Patients will usually give a positive family history.

Miller–Fisher syndrome

This is one of the subtypes of Guillain–Barré syndrome/acute inflammatory demyelinating polyneuropathy that presents with a descending paralysis and the classic triad of ataxia, areflexia and ophthalmoplegia.

Thyroid disease

Hypothyroidism can give a mild symmetrical proximal myopathy, but without the classic fatigability and recovery after rest of myasthenia gravis. Deep tendon reflexes will be normal or delayed. There may be other signs of hypothyroidism such as bradycardia, cold peripheries, periorbital puffiness, croaky voice, hair thinning and slow-relaxing reflexes. Hyperthyroidism may also give a proximal myopathy, but again without fatigability, and reflexes tend to be brisk. Thyrotoxicosis can also present with bulbar weakness with oropharyngeal dysphagia mimicking myasthenia gravis, but other thyroid signs such as tremor and tachycardia will also be prominent. The common ocular signs include unilateral/bilateral proptosis, eyelid retraction and lid lag, periorbital oedema, chemosis and restrictive ophthalmoplegia which affects the inferior and medial rectus muscles most commonly, but can give complex ophthalmoplegias similar to myasthenia gravis. Unilateral lid retraction can cause a pseudoptosis in the contralateral eye and levator dehiscence may cause true ptosis. The important differentiating signs will include no fatigability and other signs of thyroid disease such as goitre, tachycardia, sweating, tremor and weight loss. Remember that thyroid disease may occur in association with myasthenia gravis.

Multiple sclerosis

The weakness, unlike myasthenia gravis, will be pyramidal, not fatigable and there will by hypertonia and hyperreflexia.

Amyotrophic lateral sclerosis

The most common form of MND may present initially with just LMN signs in the upper and lower limbs, with reduced tone, reduced reflexes, and no fatigability or improvement after rest. LMN signs usually include loss of muscle bulk and fasciculations which are not seen in myasthenia gravis.

Drug-induced myasthenia-like syndrome

Certain drugs have been implicated in worsening myasthenia gravis, unmasking subclinical cases of myasthenia gravis or causing a myasthenia-like syndrome that recovers on withdrawal of the medicine. In most drugs the mechanism that produces the myasthenic syndrome is unknown (with the notable exceptions of D-penicillamine, interferon-α and the neuromuscular-blocking anaesthetic agents).

- **D-Penicillamine**: used in the treatment of rheumatoid arthritis, scleroderma or Wilson's disease. This produces an autoimmune-mediated myasthenic syndrome clinically identical to sporadic myasthenia gravis. The symptoms and signs can develop months to years after initiation of the drug. Most patients will have raised anti-nAChR autoantibodies but lower titres than sporadic myasthenia gravis. The condition improves/resolves on removal of the drug and responds to cholinesterase inhibitors
- **Interferon-α**: similar to above; used in the treatment of leukaemia or chronic active hepatitis C
- **Antibiotics/antimicrobials**: including aminoglycosides (gentamicin, streptomycin), fluoroquinolones (ciprofloxacin), macrolides (erythromycin, clarithromycin), penicillins and sulfonamides
- **β Blockers**: propranolol, atenolol, timolol
- **Calcium-channel blockers**: verapamil
- **Anticonvulsants**: phenytoin, carbamazepine, benzodiazepines
- **Psychiatric drugs**: lithium, phenothiazines
- **Anaesthetic agents**: propanediol ether, methoxyflurane, lidocaine, procainamide, vecuronium.

Toxins:

- **Snake venom toxins**: eg α-bungarotoxin of krait and α-toxin of cobras bind to the acetylcholine receptor
- **Botulinum toxin**: produced by the *Clostridium botulinum* bacterium. The toxin stops the release of acetylcholine from the presynaptic membrane. Botulism poisoning is most commonly caused by eating home-preserved foods, fermented uncooked foodstuffs or wound contamination. The symptoms include acute onset of dry mouth and blurred vision, quickly progressing to diplopia, pupillary dilatation (unlike myasthenia gravis), ophthalmoplegia, bulbar, respiratory and limb weakness with preserved reflexes and normal sensation. There may be a relative bradycardia with hypotension. It is a medical emergency and treated by botulinum anti-toxin and supportive care.

Clinical judgement and maintaining patient welfare

Approximately 80–90% of those with myasthenia gravis have detectable nAChR autoantibodies and 3–7% have antibodies directed against muscle-specific tyrosine kinase (MuSK), another neuromuscular junction protein. There is a remaining group that has seronegative disease clinically indistinguishable from the anti-AChR group. The MuSK subset is predominantly women (90%), with disease at an earlier age, a higher incidence in black women, and more severe generalised or prominent bulbar and respiratory symptoms with frequent myasthenic crises.

There are several classifications but disease can be broadly divided into two clinical groups: generalised disease (85%) and ocular disease (15%).

Investigations

Tensilon test: this involves the IV administration of edrophonium, a short-acting acetylcholinesterase inhibitor, which will increase the amplitude and duration of the action potential. After administration the patient is observed for improvement in muscle strength; the results are most reliable when assessing resolution of ptosis or extraocular palsy. As the acetylcholinesterase inhibitor causes acetylcholine to remain around the neuromuscular junction (NMJ) for longer there are several conditions that can give false-positive results such as ALS, LEMS, botulism and poliomyelitis.

Ice-pack test: this is mainly used for those with a contraindication to the Tensilon test. An ice-pack is placed over the eye for 2–5 min and then assessed for improvement in ptosis.

Serology: test for anti-AChR and, if negative, test for anti-MuSK antibodies. False-positive tests for anti-AChR with low titre can be seen in: D-penicillamine therapy, LEMS, MND and auto-immune liver disease including primary biliary cirrhosis. False-negative tests for anti-AChR may occur early in disease or with the use of steroids.

Electrophysiology studies: these include repetitive nerve stimulation (RNS) and single-fibre electromyography (SF-EMG). RNS shows a decrement in the amplitude of the compound muscle action potential (CMAP). SF-EMG is more sensitive and will show 'jitter' in the face of normal fibre density.

CT of the chest: should be performed in all newly diagnosed patients to look for thymoma or evidence of thymic hyperplasia. The origin of the autoantibodies is uncertain but thymic dysfunction may be involved because myasthenia gravis is associated with thymic hyperplasia in 70% and thymoma in 10% of patients. Those with thymomas tend to be older, have higher titres of anti-AChR and more severe disease.

Management
Complications include:

- **Myasthenic crisis**: defined as weakness in a myasthenia gravis patient that is severe enough to affect respiratory function and require intubation and ventilatory support. It is usually associated with worsening bulbar weakness. It can occur spontaneously with no obvious trigger or is more usually triggered by infection, weaning of immunosuppression, surgical intervention, pregnancy or childbirth, or by certain medications detailed above.

- **Cholinergic crisis** (from excessive treatment with cholinesterase inhibitors) can also cause weakness which might sometimes be mistaken for a myasthenic crisis.
- **Pneumonia**: more common due to reduced respiratory reserve and weak oropharyngeal muscles, leading to higher aspiration rates and an inability to increase respiratory rate for long periods.

Cholinesterase inhibitors
Patients with frequent symptoms should be treated with cholinesterase inhibitors. The most commonly used is pyridostigmine. Muscarinic side effects may include bradycardia, hypotension, bronchoconstriction, salivation and increased respiratory secretions, lacrimation and diaphoresis, increased GI peristalsis leading to nausea and vomiting, abdominal cramps, diarrhoea and urinary frequency. Patients with MuSK myasthenia gravis tend to respond less well to cholinesterase inhibitors.

Immunosuppressants
Corticosteroids are used in patients with moderate disease that is not responsive to cholinesterase inhibitors alone. Low-dose therapy is started and then gradually increased until there is clinical improvement. Starting high-dose steroids can precipitate a myasthenic crisis so treatment is started at low doses, increasing slowly. For those in whom symptoms are uncontrolled on steroids or who require steroid-sparing agents, azathioprine, mycophenolate mofetil, ciclosporin or tacrolimus is used.

Plasmapheresis and intravenous immunoglobulin
In acute myasthenia gravis crises, IVIG or plasmapheresis is used in the short term to quickly improve symptoms, and steroid treatment is started, increasing to a maintenance dose. Intubation and supportive care are needed. Cholinesterase inhibitors are usually stopped due to their troublesome side effect of increased bronchial secretions impeding intubation care. Plasmapheresis can bring about clinical improvement slightly

faster than IVIG but may not be possible if venous access is difficult and has concomitant increased risks of infection, thrombosis and bleeding diathesis.

Thymectomy
The only absolute indication for thymectomy is the presence of thymoma but all myasthenia gravis patients aged <55 years are usually treated with thymectomy, regardless of thymoma disease. There is far less evidence of benefit to those aged >55 years and decisions are made on a case-by-case basis. Benefits of surgery may not be evident for several years.

Patient education and support
Patients should be pointed towards support groups and advised to seek medical attention early with worsening symptoms, when suffering with infection or fever or when considering new medications or surgery. Patients can be supplied with MedicAlert bracelets, particularly if taking steroids or if they have previously had myasthenic crises. Choice of treatments should be made in discussion with the patient, explaining all the potential side effects. Acetylcholine receptor antibody levels should be checked annually and also the adverse effects of immunosuppressant therapy should be monitored.

Prognosis
Myasthenia gravis often requires long-term drug maintenance and exacerbations can occur secondary to new medications, surgery, infection, pregnancy and malignancy. Patients with myasthenia gravis have a normal life span.

Muscular dystrophies comprise a group of progressive, non-inflammatory muscle diseases characterised by ongoing degeneration and aberrant regeneration of damaged muscle tissue. They typically affect proximal muscle groups, and then progress distally, such as Duchenne muscular dystrophy (DMD) and Becker muscular dystrophy (BMD). Alternatively they can affect more specific muscle groups such as facioscapulohumeral dystrophy (FSHD) or oculopharyngodistal myopathy.

DMD is the most common and severe form but least likely to be seen in the MRCP PACES examination due to its early onset and reduced life expectancy. FSHD is most commonly seen in the PACES examination due to the later onset and benign course.

FACIOSCAPULOHUMERAL DYSTROPHY

Identifying physical signs

General appearance
Look for walking aids, a wheelchair or adapted footwear. The patient will have an expressionless **myopathic facies**, which may appear thin and long and the jaw may be hanging open slightly. There is **no frontotemporal balding or cataracts** as seen in myotonic dystrophy.

Gait
Patients may well have a normal gait because the upper body is preferentially affected, but lower limb girdle, back muscles and ankle dorsiflexors can be affected so the patient could have an **exaggerated lumbar lordosis** with a **myopathic/ waddling gait** and **foot slapping/drag/circumduction** if there is foot drop. Assess for proximal

lower limb weakness, watching how the patient gets up from the chair.

Upper and lower limb examination
- Tone will be normal.
- **Weakness of the shoulder girdle muscles** results in **winging of the scapulae** where the upper part of the scapulae appears above the clavicles when looking at the patient head on. Asking the patient to press against a wall may reveal more subtle winging of the scapulae.
- There will be loss of muscle bulk around the pectoral, humerus and triceps muscles with relative preservation of the forearm muscles, which can give the arms a 'Popeye' appearance.
- There is **weakness in proximal muscle groups** but the deltoid muscle may be spared.
- The lower limbs may show no abnormality, or minor wasting of anterior tibialis with weak ankle dorsiflexion and foot drop.
- **Deep tendon reflexes may be reduced or absent**.
- Plantar reflexes will be normal.
- Coordination is normal within the confines of reduced power.
- Sensation will be normal.

Cranial nerve examination
- There is **no ptosis or ophthalmoplegia**, in contrast with myotonic dystrophy or myasthenia gravis which may give a similar facial appearance on first impression.
- Weakness typically occurs first in the facial muscles, making it difficult for the patient to close the eyes or mouth tightly, with wasting of the masseters and difficulty whistling or smiling.
- Look for **hearing aids** because the condition can be associated with high-frequency sensorineural deafness.

- On fundoscopy there may be **retinal telangiectasias** which can be associated with FSHD.

Additional

Very rarely there is an association with **atrial arrhythmias**, **conduction defects** and **dilated cardiomyopathy**, so feel the pulse, look for a pacemaker insertion, and perform a cardiovascular examination for functional valve defects from a dilated cardiomyopathy.

Differential diagnosis

DMD and BMD: the patient will tend to be much younger and the muscle weakness more severe, and lower limbs are more affected with a clearly waddling gait, if still ambulant, and calf hypertrophy. Importantly, there is no facial muscle weakness as seen with FSHD.

Limb–girdle muscular dystrophy: presents similarly to DMD or BMD with similar cardiomyopathy and calf hypertrophy, but tends to have a later onset. Again muscle weakness of the lower limb girdle is more pronounced and there is no facial muscle weakness.

Emery–Dreifuss muscular dystrophy: similar to FSHD there is winging of the scapulae but, unlike the other dystrophies, it presents early with contractures, even before muscle weakness, in the Achilles tendon, elbows and posterior neck muscles; forward flexion of the entire spine may become restricted. The weakness is in a humero-peroneal distribution, proximal in the upper limbs and distal in the lower limbs. There are X-linked recessive and autosomal dominant forms. There is no facial muscle weakness.

Clinical judgement and maintaining patient welfare

Investigations
- CK levels are raised.
- EMG shows myopathic potentials.

- Genetic testing: FSHD is an autosomal dominant condition in up to 90% and sporadic in the remainder with the mutations localised to chromosome 4, but the related genes remain unidentified.
- Muscle biopsy.

Management
- Physiotherapy to delay/prevent contractures
- Surgery to the scapulothoracic area to fixate the scapulae and improve shoulder girdle function
- Eye protection and lubrication for incomplete eye closure.

Prognosis

Approximately 20% will require wheelchair assistance in their lifetime and life expectancy is normal.

DUCHENNE AND BECKER MUSCULAR DYSTROPHIES

Identifying physical signs

General appearance

This will be a younger patient (most likely male) and there will be **walking aids**, adapted footwear or a **wheelchair nearby**. The patient will have a normal facies in contrast to FSHD, myotonic dystrophy or myasthenia gravis. Patients may have a **kyphoscoliosis** from weakness of paraspinal and abdominal muscles.

Gait

If the patient is not wheelchair bound he or she may well require assistance getting up from the chair due to marked proximal lower limb weakness. There is a **myopathic/waddling gait** and foot slapping/drag/circumduction to accommodate for gluteal weakness and possible foot drop. With the myopathic gait the upper body swings to either side over the current weight-bearing limb. In children there is hyperlordosis and consequent abdominal protuberance as the patient shifts the centre of gravity as much as possible over the weight-bearing limb.

Upper and lower limb examination

- Tone is normal.
- Look and feel for any contractures.
- There is **wasting and weakness of the proximal upper and lower limbs and neck muscles**.
- There may be **pseudohypertrophy** of the calf muscles.
- There is **preferential weakness of the extensor muscle groups** in the neck, wrist, hip, knee and ankle.
- **Deep tendon reflexes are reduced or absent** and plantar reflexes are normal.
- Coordination and sensation are normal.

Additional

A cardiovascular examination may show features consistent with associated **cardiomyopathy** and **pulmonary hypertension** such as a laterally displaced apex with right ventricular heave, loud P2 and a systolic murmur of functional mitral regurgitation. State that you would request **spirometry** to assess vital capacity.

Differential diagnosis

DMD and BMD: these forms of muscular dystrophy affect the same muscle groups but the age of onset is younger and disease progression is more rapid in DMD. Adult patients presenting to the examination with DMD may be younger and wheelchair dependent, with severe weakness, contractures and kyphoscoliosis, and marked calf muscle hypertrophy.

Clinical judgement and maintaining patient welfare

Investigations

- **CK levels**: these are very high (later on these levels will fall with muscle wasting).
- **EMG**: myopathic picture.

- **Muscle biopsy**: muscle cell proteins become replaced by adipose and connective tissue.
- **Genetic testing**: both DMD and BMD are X-linked recessive disorders caused by mutations in the dystrophin gene on the short arm of the X chromosome at Xp21. Thus in the vast majority of cases males are affected (the very rare females with the disease have mutations on both X chromosomes or an inactive X chromosome). The dystrophin gene is the largest known human gene and has the highest spontaneous mutation rate. In DMD the dystrophin protein is absent and in BMD there is 10–40% of the normal amount. The dystrophin gene is a cytoskeletal protein that helps maintain membrane stability, preventing calcium influx and degeneration of muscle fibres.
- **Echocardiography**: dilated cardiomyopathy.

Management

- Referral to the MDT for appropriate counselling, education and follow-up.
- Genetic diagnosis and counselling for the family.
- Pneumococcal and influenza immunisations.
- Early disease management when the patient is ambulant: regular physiotherapy to prevent contractures and orthopaedic review for casting or release of any contractures.
- Corticosteroid therapy can delay wheelchair dependence by up to 3 years and may have some effects on cardiomyopathy, but this must be balanced against serious side effects, including bone density loss, and treatment should include calcium and vitamin D supplementation ± bisphosphonates.
- Physiotherapy to help with pulmonary function and assessment for walking aids.
- Occupational therapy review for home adaptations.
- Regular respiratory review, measuring FVC and pulse oximetry and nocturnal oximetry. Prompt treatment of any chest infections and consideration for NIV.

- Regular cardiology review with frequent ECGs and assessment of left ventricular ejection fraction (LVEF): instigating treatment with cardioprotective ACE inhibitor, β blocker and spironolactone when LVEF falls to <50%.

Prognosis

Patients with DMD become wheelchair dependent between the ages of 7 and 12 years and those with BMD can have a very varied prognosis, with onset of wheelchair dependence ranging from 30 years to 50 years.

Survival in DMD is now much improved with the advent of NIV support and 10–40% of patients are surviving to age 40 years.

SCENARIO 11. CHARCOT–MARIE–TOOTH DISEASE

Identifying physical signs

Charcot–Marie–Tooth disease (CMT; aka hereditary motor and sensory neuropathy [HMSN] or peroneal muscular atrophy) is the most common inherited neurological disorder affecting 1 in 2500 people. The term CMT encompasses most of the inherited peripheral neuropathies and represents a genetically heterogeneous group of diseases.

General appearance
The patient may be younger with orthotic supports or adapted footwear.

Gait
The patient may have a **high-steppage gait** to ensure clearance of the toes with a **bilateral foot drop**. The patient may have an **ataxic gait** and look down at the feet due to **reduced proprioception**. If there is no obvious foot drop but an appearance of **distal muscle wasting**, a sensitive test is to ask the patient to try heel walking. The patient has a **positive Romberg's test**.

Upper and lower limb examination
- Tone is normal.
- There may be fasciculations.
- There is **marked symmetrical distal wasting** with preserved proximal musculature leading to the classic 'inverted champagne bottle' appearance of the lower limbs.
- Distal wasting leads to prominent extensor tendons in the feet and possible hammer toes, or the classic **pes cavus** with a shortened forefoot and high arch.
- There is **symmetrically reduced power in distal muscle groups.**
- In late disease ankle plantar flexion is reduced.
- Feel for **thickened peripheral nerves** particularly at the medial malleolus. There is **deep tendon hypo/areflexia** and **reduced/absent plantar responses**.

- Sensory examination will show loss of vibration and proprioception, but all sensory modalities can be affected.
- If the upper limbs have become affected there could be finger pseudoathetosis testing with eyes shut.
- There may be **wasting of the small muscles of the hands**, a claw hand appearance and a palpable ulnar nerve around the elbow.
- Similar to the lower limbs there will be a symmetrical distal weakness with hypo-/areflexia and reduced sensation, mainly to proprioception and vibration sense.

Additional
There may be an **associated scoliosis** and a **resting or postural tremor** in the upper limbs.

Differential diagnosis

Peripheral neuropathy of other causes: in HMSN/CMT motor signs predominate over sensory signs. As the neuropathy of CMT is long-standing, pes cavus and scoliosis are more common features in this sort of neuropathy.

Mononeuropathy: diabetes and vasculitides can give rise to a mononeuropathy. Common peroneal nerve palsy with foot drop can be caused by trauma, as a complication of knee surgery or compression to the neck of the fibula, but these conditions do not present with the symmetrical distal motor and sensory neuropathy of CMT.

L4–5 nerve root lesion: this is most commonly unilateral, caused by lumbar disc herniation; ankle inversion is also reduced. Reflexes tend to be normal and sensory impairment is dermatomal.

Cauda equina lesions: caused by lumbar stenosis, trauma or infiltrative processes resulting in bilateral lower limb LMN weakness with bilateral foot drop and dermatomal sensory impairment, including saddle anaesthesia and sphincter disturbance.

Clinical judgement and maintaining patient welfare

Investigations

Nerve conduction tests: reduced conduction velocity or reduced amplitudes.

Genetic testing: using family pedigree and the speculated form of inheritance to focus testing.

CMT is a genetically heterogeneous group of conditions with >40 different gene mutations and classification systems change frequently. The classification below describes the main mode of inheritance and pathology:

- CMT1: autosomal dominant inheritance; most common form of CMT, underlying pathology is hypertrophic demyelination, leading to reduced nerve conduction velocities and palpable nerves.
- CMT2: autosomal dominant; underlying pathology is axonal degeneration so normal conduction velocity but reduced amplitude.

- CMT4: autosomal recessive; underlying demyelination, incorporates the old CMT3/Dejerine–Sottas disease (a severe form of CMT with onset in infancy).
- CMTX: X-linked, mixed axonal or demyelination pathology; can be associated with sensorineural deafness.

Management

- MDT includes physiotherapy with exercise and orthotic appliances and review by occupational therapy.
- Surgical correction of foot deformity or straightening of hammer toes and tendon transfer.
- Pharmacological treatment of associated neuropathic pain or restless legs syndrome.
- Treat other systemic disorders that could exacerbate neuropathy such as diabetes.
- Avoid drugs that can exacerbate neuropathy such as vincristine and isoniazid.

Prognosis

Prognosis depends on the subtype of CMT. Those with CMT1 have a very good prognosis, with 95% remaining ambulatory. Those with CMT2 have a worse prognosis with earlier onset and many are non-ambulatory by 20 years of age.

SCENARIO 12. FRIEDREICH'S ATAXIA

Identifying physical signs

Friedreich's ataxia is the most common inherited ataxia. It is a neurodegenerative disease causing demyelination and axonal loss that affects the peripheral large myelinated fibres, posterior columns, and corticospinal and spinocerebellar tracts.

General appearance
The patient may be younger with orthotic supports, adapted footwear or a wheelchair. There may be **kyphoscoliosis**.

Gait
The **gait ataxia** is of both cerebellar and sensory origin. The cerebellar component causes a wide-based gait with difficulties in standing and sitting due to truncal ataxia. The sensory component causes the patient to look down at the feet with a stomping gait due to lack of proprioceptive feedback. There is a **positive Romberg's test**.

Upper and lower limb examination
- Tone may be normal or reduced.
- There is **distal wasting and weakness** in the lower limbs and **pes cavus**.
- **Weakness will be pyramidal** due to disease affecting the corticospinal tracts, so there are relatively weaker flexor groups in the lower limbs and weaker extensors in the upper limbs.
- **Deep tendon reflexes are reduced or absent**, particularly at the knee and ankle.
- There are **extensor plantar responses** from corticospinal tract degeneration.
- There is **impaired vibration and position sense**.
- With advanced disease, pinprick and temperature sensation may be impaired.

- There is limb ataxia with **impaired heel–shin testing** in the lower limbs, and **dysdiadochokinesis** and **impaired finger–nose testing** in the upper limbs.
- Look for **an intention tremor**.

Cranial nerve examination
- There will be **bilateral gaze-evoked nystagmus** when the patient is asked to look in an eccentric position and **jerky saccadic movement** with loss of smooth pursuit.
- There will be no pupillary abnormalities.
- There may be weakness of the facial muscles and impaired speech and swallowing due to effects on cranial nerve VII, X and XII nuclei.
- There may be associated sensorineural deafness, so look for the presence of **hearing aids**.
- Fundoscopy may reveal some degree of optic **atrophy**.
- There may be dysarthria with **staccato speech**.

Additional
Look specifically for the **high-arched palate**, **kyphoscoliosis** and **pes cavus** deformities that can be associated with Friedreich's ataxia. Finish your examination by requesting to examine the cardiovascular system for signs of hypertrophic cardiomyopathy and perform BM testing for any associated diabetes.

Differential diagnosis

Other causes of reduced/absent ankle jerks with extensor plantar reflex
- Subacute combined degeneration of the cord
- Conus medullaris lesion
- MND

- Tabes dorsalis
- Combined pathology: diabetic neuropathy plus stroke, peripheral neuropathy with a central myopathy.

Clinical judgement and maintaining patient welfare

Investigations

Nerve conduction tests: these show mildly reduced conduction velocity and reduced amplitudes.

Visual evoked potentials: abnormal in up to two-thirds of patients.

Brain-stem auditory-evoked potentials: may show involvement of central auditory processing pathways.

ECG: inferolateral T-wave inversion, conduction defects, voltage criteria for left ventricular hypertrophy.

Echocardiography: concentric ventricular hypertrophy and dilated cardiomyopathy.

Blood tests: perform a fasting glucose and HbA1c (10% have frank diabetes and up to a further 40% have impaired glucose intolerance) and rule out abnormalities of vitamin E or copper metabolism, which could cause similar syndromes.

Genetic testing: Friedreich's ataxia is an autosomal recessive ataxia arising from defects of the *FXN* gene on chromosome 9. It is a trinucleotide repeat disease with an excessive number of GAA repeats in the *FXN* gene, leading to reduced frataxin production. Increasing number of repeats leads to earlier onset and more severe disease. Cells expressing a large amount of frataxin, such as the dorsal root ganglion, cerebellar nuclei and myocardial cells, are more sensitive to the deficiency. Frataxin is essential for normal mitochondrial function and iron homeostasis pathways. Iron toxicity and oxidative damage lead to neuronal cell death.

Brain and spinal cord imaging: MRI will show atrophy of the cervical spinal cord and signs of degeneration within the cerebellar hemispheres and vermis.

Management

Management occurs within an MDT:

- Physiotherapy is needed to maintain function and reduce contractures, and supply appropriate orthoses and mobility aids.
- Occupational therapy input is for environmental adaptation.
- Speech and language therapy is to help with communication and swallowing difficulties.
- Patients may require surgical correction of foot deformity/pes cavus and advanced kyphoscolisis that is causing pain or cardiorespiratory compromise.
- Screen for and treat associated diabetes.
- Visual and hearing aids as appropriate.
- Cardiology review and management of any cardiomyopathy, arrhythmias or heart failure.

Prognosis

The disease is progressive with nearly all patients wheelchair bound by age 45 years. There is reduced life expectancy, which ranges from 30 years to 70 years, particularly for those patients with cardiac and diabetic complications.

SCENARIO 13: CEREBELLAR SYNDROME

Identifying physical signs

The cerebellum functions to regulate balance, muscle tone and coordination of voluntary movement. Cerebellar disease causes ipsilateral signs, with vermal lesions resulting in truncal instability and cerebellar hemisphere lesions in limb ataxia.

General appearance

The patient may appear well until asked to stand and then a **truncal** or **limb ataxia** may be revealed. It may be possible to see signs associated with the cause of the cerebellar syndrome. A younger patient may have one of the inherited cerebellar syndromes/ataxias such as Friedreich's ataxia or ataxia telangiectasia, or one of the spinocerebellar ataxias. There may be signs of jaundice, rosacea, seborrhoeic dermatitis, rhinophyma and parotid swelling in a patient with chronic alcoholism.

Gait

There is an **unsteady/ataxic** and **broad-based gait** with a tendency to fall toward the side of the lesion. If this is not evident, then it can be sought by asking the patient to perform heel–toe walking. In a pure cerebellar syndrome, Romberg's test will be negative (ie not worsen with eye closure, although there may be poor stability in truncal ataxia). If there is a positive Romberg's test, this suggests that the ataxia has a sensory component, due to a lack of proprioceptive input from damage to the dorsal columns as seen in alcoholic ataxia, Friedreich's ataxia and MS.

Upper and lower limb examination

- Tone may be reduced on the side of the lesion; however, in long-standing cerebellar disease corticospinal tracts compensate and return tone to normal.
- Tone may be increased with spasticity if cerebellar disease is secondary to MS.

- Power should be normal, unless the cause of the cerebellar syndrome is MS, when there might be additional pyramidal weakness.
- In the upper limbs there will be poor coordination with **impaired finger–nose testing** and **intention tremor** that worsens as the target is approached and with past pointing (**dysmetria**).
- There is **dysdiadochokinesis**.
- In the lower limbs there is poor coordination with the **heel–shin test**.
- Deep tendon reflexes may be normal, reduced or pendular at the knee. Pendular knee reflexes can be seen if the knee is hanging freely for reflex examination, eg hanging over the edge of the bed. Knee reflex testing will cause several swings of the leg after the initial stretch reflex which are thought to be due to general hypotonia.

Cranial nerve examination

- On testing eye movements, there is **horizontal nystagmus** with the fast component toward the side of the lesion and maximal in this direction.
- There may be **loss of smooth pursuit** with jerky eye movements.
- Look for an intranuclear ophthalmoplegia and optic atrophy, indicating that a demyelinating disease such as MS may be present.

If there is bilateral cerebellar disease there will be **dysarthria** in the form of slurred and **staccato/scanning speech** so words become disjointed and syllables stressed equally such as 'Bri-tish con-sti-tut-ion' and 'ba-by hipp-o-pot-a-mus'.

Look for signs that may give clues to the underlying cause of the cerebellar syndrome (see differential diagnosis, below) such as:

- **Alcoholic cerebellar degeneration**: jaundice, parotid swelling, peripheral neuropathy, peripheral cerebellar signs.

- **Multiple sclerosis**: pyramidal signs with spastic tone, reduced sensation, INO, optic atrophy and signs of sphincter disturbance such as a urinary catheter.
- **Ischaemic/haemorrhagic stroke**: posterior circulation or brain-stem strokes may produce unilateral or bilateral cerebellar signs. Look for contralateral hemiparesis and brain-stem features such as crossed signs.
- **Posterior fossa space-occupying lesion**: raised intracranial pressure (ICP) gives rise to papilloedema and the classic false localising signs of unilateral/bilateral nerve VI palsy because the nerve is stretched as it exits between the pons and medulla from the downward pressure of the brain stem.
- **Friedreich's ataxia**: younger age, pes cavus, scoliosis, bilateral pyramidal dorsal column and cerebellar signs with depressed ankle jerks and extensor plantars.
- **Paraneoplastic cerebellar degeneration**: bilateral signs of severe ataxia, dysarthria, nystagmus with cachexia and possible Horner's syndrome.

Differential diagnosis

Sensory ataxia is the other differential diagnosis for an ataxic gait, but of course sensory and cerebellar ataxia may coexist in alcoholic cerebellar degeneration, MS and Friedreich's ataxia. Sensory ataxia describes the lack of coordination that arises from the loss of proprioception. It can be mostly overcome by visual input, so tests for coordination such as finger–nose pointing and heel–shin may be normal. The patient tends to have a stomping gait, watching the feet/floor to provide visual cues. Romberg's sign will be positive and there may be pseudoathetosis, with unconscious writhing of the fingers in outstretched hands when the eyes are closed. There is loss of vibration sense as well as joint position sense on peripheral nerve examination and deep tendon reflexes are often absent. In a pure sensory ataxia there will be no dysarthria, nystagmus or other oculomotor signs or intention tremor. Causes of a sensory ataxia include damage to the dorsal columns from injury, vascular or demyelinating insults, or peripheral neuropathy.

Common causes of cerebellar syndrome
- Alcoholic cerebellar degeneration
- Ischaemic or haemorrhagic stroke
- MS.

Less common causes of cerebellar syndrome
- Friedreich's ataxia: see Scenario 12.
- Drug-induced ataxia: more common in children and seen after phenytoin, carbamazepine, vigabatrin, gabapentin, phenobarbital, fluorouracil, intrathecal methotrexate, lithium.
- Secondary to hypoxic encephalopathy or heat stroke: the Purkinje cells of the cerebellum are selectively vulnerable to heat-induced injury; a recognised clinical sign is palatal myoclonus.
- Acute cerebellitis: more common in children; seen after viral illness, eg chickenpox or Coxsackievirus.
- Posterior fossa space-occupying lesions:
  - Tumours: cerebellar astrocytomas and medulloblastomas
  - Abscess: local spread of otitis media or mastoiditis, or more rarely haematogenous spread.
- Paraneoplastic cerebellar degeneration (PCD):
  - Results from an abnormal immune response to underlying malignancy and approximately 60% occur before underlying malignancy is detected
  - Associated with uterine, ovarian, breast, small-cell lung cancer and Hodgkin's lymphoma
  - Associated autoantibodies include:
    - anti-Yo (anti-Purkinje cell) associated with ovarian or breast malignancy
    - anti-Hu (anti-neuronal mRNA) associated with lung malignancy
    - 40% with PCD have no known autoantibodies.

- Hypothyroidism:
  - Postulated to be an immune-mediated phenomenon
  - Can be associated with raised anti-thyroid antibodies in the absence of hypothyroidism
  - Usually responds to thyroid replacement.
- Hypoparathyroidism including: Kearns–Sayre syndrome is a rare mitochondrial disorder presenting as the triad of onset before age 20 years, progressive external ophthalmoplegia and retinitis pigmentosa. It can also include: complete heart block, cerebellar dysfunction, CSF protein >100 mg/dL, ptosis, cataracts and diabetes.
- Vitamin B_1 (thiamine) deficiency:
  - Underlying cause of several syndromes including Wernicke–Korsakoff and wet and dry beri-beri syndromes
  - Caused by chronic alcohol abuse because alcohol blocks the active transport of thiamine in the GI tract, nutritional deficiencies such as eating polished rice in Asian populations or poor absorption post-GI resection
  - Wernicke–Korsakoff syndrome presents with acute confusion, amnesia with confabulation, oculomotor palsies, nystagmus and ataxia ('CONA').
- Vitamin E deficiency: can be caused by malabsorption states such as cystic fibrosis, biliary atresia, GI resection, and more rarely in genetic disorders such as abetalipoproteinaemia and ataxia with isolated vitamin E deficiency (AVED), which are both rare metabolic autosomal recessive conditions presenting in childhood.
- Telangiectasia ataxia:
  - A rare autosomal recessive ataxia, caused by a mutation of the *ATM* gene, used in DNA repair
  - Characterised by early onset cerebellar ataxia, telangiectasia in the eyes and skin, reduced immunoglobulins leading to more frequent sinopulmonary infections, and increased incidence of malignancies particularly lymphomas and leukaemia.
- The von Hippel–Lindau syndrome (VHL):
  - Rare autosomal dominant disease from mutation in the VHL tumour-suppressor gene
  - Associated with haemangioblastomas in the cerebellum, spinal cord, retina and kidney, and associated with clear cell renal carcinoma and phaeochromocytomas.
- Spinocerebellar ataxias:
  - A group of inherited degenerative conditions with many subtypes
  - Many subtypes are polyglutamine diseases from expanded expression of the amino acid glutamine (codon CAG), hence their other name of 'CAG triple repeat' diseases.
- Arnold–Chiari malformation: describes a malformation of the brain leading to herniation of the cerebellar tonsils through the foramen magnum; can cause a non-communicating hydrocephalus. There are subtypes I–IV depending on the degree of herniation.
- Multiple system atrophy: this is a degenerative condition comprising one of the Parkinson-plus syndromes (see Scenario 12).
- Wilson's disease:
  - An autosomal recessive condition causing an inability to degrade phytanic acid which accumulates and causes a neurocutaneous syndrome including retinitis pigmentosa, peripheral neuropathy and cerebellar atassia.
  - This is important to mention because it can present with ataxia and is treatable.
- Refsum's disease:
  - See page 547
  - This is important to mention because it can present with ataxia and is treatable.

Clinical judgement and maintaining patient welfare

Investigations

Cerebellar syndrome has many different possible causes so investigations will be tailored to the most likely diagnosis.

Blood tests: LFTs, GGT, TFTs, bone profile with parathyroid hormone (PTH), vitamins E and B_{12}, and thiamine levels.

Serum ceruloplasmin levels (will be low) and 24-hour urinary copper excretion (will be high) should be measured if Wilson's disease is suspected.

Serum phytanic acid level is measured if suspect Refsum's disease is suspected.

Should screen for implicated drug levels.

Autoantibody screen if paraneoplastic cerebellar degeneration is suspected.

Neuroimaging is indicated as a first-line investigation if a stroke, space-occupying lesion or MS is suspected. Imaging is best performed with diffusion-weighted MRI.

Further investigations for suspected paraneoplastic phenomena would be tailored to the most likely primary malignancy and in women would include mammography and imaging of the pelvis, and in both sexes CT of the chest for evidence of small cell lung cancer or lymphoma, and possibly lymph node or bone marrow biopsy.

Management

Management will be tailored to the specific cause. Conditions giving rise to acute cerebellar syndrome that require urgent treatment include the following.

Ischaemic cerebellar stroke: urgent dedicated stroke and neurosurgical teams' input with regard to safe administration of thrombolysis due to the attendant risk of brain-stem compression if there is secondary intracranial haemorrhage.

Cerebellar haemorrhage: urgent neurosurgical review because there may be a need for ventriculostomy or decompressive surgery.

Acute cerebellitis: this may rarely cause oedema and raised ICP risking brain-stem compression, so patients suspected to be at risk of oedema will require careful monitoring in case of the need for urgent decompressive surgery.

Wernicke–Korsakoff syndrome: this needs to be recognised quickly and treated with IV thiamine.

Acute drug toxicity: management involves discontinuing the offending drug.

SCENARIO 14. PERIPHERAL NEUROPATHY

Identifying physical signs

Peripheral neuropathies are divided into primarily motor, sensory or sensorimotor with additional autonomic effects.

Sensory peripheral neuropathies are further subdivided into small- and large-fibre neuropathies.

The vast majority of peripheral neuropathies show length-dependent signs due to their underlying axonal and/or demyelinating pathology, so most cases will involve examination of the lower limbs. Asymmetrical neuropathies or signs presenting in the upper limbs should make you consider alternative diagnoses such as a focal entrapment neuropathy or a multifocal neuropathy that can arise with vasculitides.

General appearance

Look for signs of systemic diseases associated with neuropathies such as typical rashes associated with systemic lupus erythematosus (SLE) or vasculitic disease. Patients may have signs of chronic alcoholism such as rhinophyma, seborrhoeic dermatitis or parotid swelling. There may be foot supports or adapted shoes for foot drop in motor neuropathies, or the appearance of the limbs in a younger patient with pes cavus and scoliosis may point towards a hereditary neuropathy.

Gait

A sensory neuropathy gives a **wide-based ataxic gait** with a stamping quality and the patient looks down at the floor/feet for visual cues. A motor neuropathy giving rise to weaker distal muscle groups may give a bilateral foot drop, with the forefoot catching along the floor or the patient compensating with a **high stepping gait** and a slapping quality. Watching the gait gives you time to note the appearance of the lower limbs and feet, looking for **pes cavus**, which suggests

long-standing neuropathy, or the **inverted champagne bottle** appearance with preserved proximal muscles and wasted distal leg muscles. There may be a **positive Romberg's test** in a large-fibre sensory neuropathy with loss of dorsal column proprioception.

Upper and lower limb examination

- In the lower limbs look for **distal muscle wasting** of tibialis anterior and small muscles of the feet, with dorsal guttering of the tendons of the foot, hammer toes or overriding toes from the imbalance between the dorsiflexor and plantarflexor muscle groups.
- There may be **nerve thickening**, most commonly affecting the common peroneal nerve in the upper lateral calf and posterior tibial behind the medial malleolus.
- Look for **Charcot's joints**, which in the lower limb are swollen, deformed ankles or forefeet, representing a neuropathic arthropathy. They are usually warm and red, and there may be marked crepitus and abnormal range of movement within the joint.
- There may be **trophic changes** to the skin, leading to hair loss and dry shiny skin, and loss of sensation may lead to the accumulation of unrecognised trauma in vulnerable areas, giving rise to **ulceration** and **callosities** and, in severe cases, **amputation**.
- Tone is normal.
- Test for power, vibration, proprioception, temperature and pinprick, and make a note of which modalities are affected and to what level.
- In motor or sensorimotor neuropathy there is an **LMN weakness**, **deep tendon reflexes are depressed** and **plantars are downward**.
- Classically in a sensory neuropathy the pattern of loss is described as **glove and stocking**.

- The upper limb examination is similar but instead Charcot's joint changes may be seen in the shoulder or elbow, and thickened median, ulnar and radial nerves palpated in the wrist, elbow and triceps areas.

Additional

If there is a sensory neuropathy try to:

- Delineate large fibre (vibration and proprioceptive sense) conducted by Aα- and Aβ-fibres making up the spinal dorsal columns from small fibre (pain and temperature sense) conducted by myelinated Aδ(III)- and unmyelinated group C-fibres, which form the spinal lateral spinothalamic tracts
- Assess autonomic function by measuring postural blood pressure and standing heart rate
- Request a full drug history.

Differential diagnosis

Types of neuropathies and their underlying causes are summarised in Table 3.5.

Clinical judgement and maintaining patient welfare

Investigations

These focus on confirming the type of peripheral neuropathy, the underlying cause and additional effects of systemic disease.

- **Blood tests**: FBC, renal, bone profile, liver profile and GGT, ESR, fasting glucose, TFTs, vitamin B_{12}, folate and thiamine levels, serum ACE (sarcoidosis)
- **Infection panel**: HIV, Lyme disease and syphilis serology
- **Serum protein electrophoresis** for multiple myeloma and monoclonal gammopathy of unknown significance (MGUS)
- **Urinalysis 24-hour collection**: porphyrias, Bence Jones protein

- **Lumbar puncture with CSF analysis** for Guillain–Barré syndrome/CIDP
- **Genetic testing** for HMSN
- **Autonomic function tests**
- **Nerve conduction tests and EMG studies**: NCTs assess large myelinated fibres. Axonal loss is shown by reduced amplitude and demyelination is shown by prolonged latency and slowed conduction velocity
- **Skin tests** for small-fibre neuropathy.
- **Nerve biopsy.**

Management

Treatment is aimed at controlling the underlying disease process and managing symptoms:

- Neuropathies developing over hours must be managed as an inpatient because there is a risk of respiratory or autonomic failure with cardiac arrhythmias. Diseases in this group include: Guillain–Barré syndrome, acute porphyrias and toxicities (botulism and heavy metal poisoning).
- Diagnosis should be established as soon as possible so that appropriate specific treatment can be started such as IVIG for Guillain–Barré syndrome.
- Diabetic neuropathy is the most common chronic complication in types 1 and 2 diabetes mellitus as a result of prolonged exposure to hyperglycaemia.
- Tight glycaemic control has been shown to reduce the incidence of neuropathy in types 1 and 2 diabetes mellitus.
- Good foot care is essential to reduce the risk of neuropathic ulcers and the development of Charcot's joints.
- Pregabalin, gabapentin or duloxetine is a first-line choice for treating painful neuropathy, with tricyclic antidepressants or SSRIs for second-line management.
- Autonomic neuropathies are managed symptomatically:
  - Orthostatic hypotension: fludrocortisone, avoiding medications that aggravate hypotension and sudden changes in posture, raising head of the bed by 45°

Table 3.5 Types of neuropathies and their causes

Cause		Mixed sensory/ motor	Motor pre-dominant	Sensory pre-dominant	Small fibre (pain and temperature)	Autonomic	Cranial nerve	Mono-neuritis multiplex
Endocrine	Diabetes	■	■	■	■	■	■	■
	Hypothyroidism	■	■	■	■			
	Acromegaly	■	■	■				
Autoimmune	Rheumatoid arthritis	■	■	■				■
	SLE	■	■	■				■
	Sjögren's syndrome	■	■	■	■			
	PAN	■	■					■
	Wegener's granulomatosis	■	■					■
	Churg–Strauss syndrome	■	■					■
	Guillain–Barré syndrome	■	■			■	■	
	Sarcoid	■	■	■			■	

(continued)

Table 3.5 (continued)

Cause		Mixed sensory/ motor	Motor pre-dominant	Sensory pre-dominant	Small fibre (pain and temperature)	Autonomic	Cranial nerve	Mono-neuritis multiplex
Infections	HIV	✓	✓	✓	✓	✓	✓	✓
	Lyme disease	✓	✓	✓	✓		✓	✓
	Leprosy					✓		✓
	Chagas' disease					✓		
	Diphtheria		✓			✓	✓	
	Botulism		✓			✓	✓	
Metabolic	Porphyrias		✓			✓		
	Amyloidosis	✓	✓	✓	✓	✓		
Drug/Toxin	Alcohol	✓	✓	✓	✓			
	Nitrofurantoin	✓	✓	✓				
	Amiodarone	✓	✓	✓				
	Gold	✓	✓	✓				
	Cisplatin	✓	✓	✓		✓		
	Vincristine	✓	✓	✓		✓		

(continued)

Table 3.5 (*continued*)

Cause		Mixed sensory/ motor	Motor pre-dominant	Sensory pre-dominant	Small fibre (pain and temperature)	Autonomic	Cranial nerve	Mono-neuritis multiplex
Drug/Toxin	Isoniazid			■				
	Pyridoxine			■				
	Metronidazole			■				
	Chloroquine			■				
	Arsenic			■				
	Thallium			■				
	Lead		■					
	Dapsone		■					
Nutritional	Vitamin B$_{12}$	■	■	■				
	Folate	■	■	■				
	Thiamine	■	■	■				
Paraneo-plastic	Myeloma	■	■	■		■		■
	Lymphoma	■	■	■		■		■
	MGUS	■	■	■				

(*continued*)

Table 3.5 (*continued*)

Cause		Mixed sensory/motor	Motor pre-dominant	Sensory pre-dominant	Small fibre (pain and temperature)	Autonomic	Cranial nerve	Mono-neuritis multiplex
Hereditary	HMSN	▓	▓					
	HSAN	▓		▓				

HMSN, hereditary motor and sensory neuropathy; HSAN, hereditary sensory and autonomic neuropathy; MGUS, monoclonal gammopathy of unknown significance; PAN, polyarteritis nodosa; SLE, systemic lupus erythematosus.

- Gastric paresis: metoclopramide or erythromycin and frequent small meals
- Bladder dysfunction: bethanecol, bladder training or catheterisation if dysfunction is severe
- Erectile dysfunction: phosphodiesterase-5 (PDE-5) inhibitors, intracavernosal injections, vacuum devices or prostheses.

SCENARIO 15. FACIAL NERVE PALSY

Identifying physical signs

General appearance
There is a **unilateral facial weakness affecting all facial muscles** and this is evidenced by a unilaterally smooth face with relaxed expression lines.

Cranial nerve examination
- In an LMN weakness there will be failure to fully crease the forehead and raise the eyebrows, close the eyes tightly (**Bell's phenomenon** may be seen where the orbit rolls upward on attempted closure of the eye), puff the cheeks out, smile and show the teeth.
- On sticking the tongue out it may deviate toward the opposite side of the facial palsy. The tongue appears deviated only as a result of the ipsilateral lax mouth muscles. This could be confused with a contralateral LMN nerve XII palsy but tongue waggling will be normal with no wasting.
- Look for any scars around the parotid or ear/mastoid that could signify trauma or iatrogenic damage to the facial nerve, and look for any parotid enlargement.
- Check the other cranial nerves, particularly noting if there are associated palsies in nerves V, VI and VIII, which could point towards a cerebellopontine angle tumour as a cause for the LMN nerve VII palsy.
- When checking cranial nerve V, also test the corneal reflex where the afferent arm is nerve V and the efferent arm (blink) nerve VII. Look for a subtle rash while checking nerve V, which may be consistent with Ramsay Hunt syndrome (RHS).
- When checking nerve VI, look for any other ophthalmoplegia. This will help diagnose myasthenia gravis, which may give complex ophthalmoplegia and facial muscle weakness (though usually bilateral).
- Test nerve VIII with Weber's and Rinne's tests, but also look in the external auditory canal for any rashes consistent with RHS or signs of

otitis media or mastoid infection. Ask the patient about any hyperacusis, which can occur with lesions affecting the chorda tympani branch of the facial nerve.
- On testing the gag reflex, look carefully at the palate for any lesions that may be consistent with RHS.

Additional
- Ask to test taste on the anterior two-thirds of the tongue (carried by the chorda tympani) and also enquire about tear and salivary production (parasympathetic innervation via the greater petrosal nerve serving the lacrimal glands and parasympathetic branch of the chorda tympani which serves the submandibular and sublingual glands).
- Ask about symptoms of hyperacusis, which occurs when the nerve to stapedius is affected (this is the first branch of the facial nerve as it leaves the facial canal and before the branch of the chorda tympani).

Differential diagnosis

LMN facial weakness
- **Bell's palsy:**
  - This is an idiopathic LMN facial nerve palsy
  - Some degree of recovery is expected within 4–6 months (which is diagnostic); 70% make a full recovery, 15% have slight impairment and 15% have permanent significant dysfunction of the facial nerve
  - Risk factors include: hypertension, diabetes, pregnancy and a positive family history.
- **Ramsay Hunt syndrome:** this is the association of facial nerve palsy and loss of taste on the anterior two-thirds of the tongue, with herpes zoster reactivation in the trigeminal nerve causing a rash around/in the

auricle or on the oropharynx/palate. There may be associated tinnitus, deafness, vertigo, peripheral nystagmus and ataxia. It is usually preceded or accompanied by facial and deep ear pain.

- **Demyelination**: brain-stem MS.
- **Trauma**: base-of-skull fracture, petrous/temporal bone fracture.
- **Surgery**: middle-ear, mastoid or parotid surgery.
- **Tumour**: meningioma, parotid tumour, cerebellopontine tumour (includes nerves V, VI, VII, VIII and cerebellar signs, (see Scenario 27).
- **Vascular**: brain-stem stroke (see Scenario 26).
- **Mononeuritis multiplex**.

Bilateral facial weakness

- **Bilateral Bell's palsy**.
- **Miller–Fisher** variant of Guillain–Barré syndrome causes descending paralysis, ophthalmoplegia and areflexia.
- **Myasthenia gravis** is an NMJ cause of weakness rather than a nerve palsy with fatigable weakness and variable ptosis, complex ophthalmoplegia and peripheral proximal weakness.
- **Facioscapulohumeral dystrophy** causes myopathic weakness rather than nerve palsy, winged scapulae and proximal upper limb wasting with reduced/absent reflexes.
- **Myotonic dystrophy** is a myopathic weakness rather than nerve palsy, with frontotemporal balding, cataracts, weak neck muscles and myotonic handshake.
- **Motor neuron disease** can present with mixed features of LMN and UMN facial weakness.
- **Mononeuritis multiplex**.

Clinical judgement and maintaining patient welfare

Investigations

If the history is acute with no associated features such as other cranial nerve involvement, gradual onset or significant pain, then no other investigations are required other than a fasting glucose and BP measurement.

If there are any unusual features, it is important to rule out malignancy with imaging and tailor the remaining tests to the most likely diagnosis.

Blood tests: FBC, CRP, ESR, Blood glucose/HbA1c, serum ACE, autoantibodies, infection screen.

Nerve conduction studies and EMG if Guillain–Barré syndrome or NMJ disease suspected.

Imaging: MRI with contrast if there is facial or nerve VIII involvement (schwannomas, cerebellopontine angle tumours, temporal bone tumours or parotid tumours).

Management

Steroids: high-dose oral prednisolone should be started as soon as possible.

Antivirals: there is little evidence for their use in Bell's palsy. They should be used in suspected RHS and started within 72 hours. Valaciclovir is the first choice.

Eye protection against corneal injury and dryness: use artificial tears hourly in the day and lubricants at night, taping the eye closed. If there is suspected involvement of the ophthalmic branch of nerve V, ophthalmological review is mandatory.

Surgery: with severe paralysis and no improvement after the first 4 weeks, decompression or reconstruction may be of benefit.

Prognosis

Complications include corneal drying and ulceration, ectropion (may need tarsorrhaphy), contracture and synkinesis, eg 'crocodile tears' with gustatory hyperlacrimation from aberrant regeneration of salivary fibres to lacrimal branches.

The extent of facial paralysis at presentation is an independent predictor of outcome. On average, 70% have near normal recovery. Predictors of poor outcome include older age, diabetes, pregnancy and association with RHS.

SCENARIO 16. WASTING OF THE SMALL MUSCLES OF THE HAND

The instruction may be 'examine the upper limbs' or 'examine this patient's hands'. The latter instruction can confuse a candidate who has learned a good upper limb exam but not thought about an approach to specific examination of the hands in a neurological case.

Read this case together with Scenarios 17–19 of this chapter for a thorough grounding in upper limb neurological assessment.

Revision of intrinsic muscles of the hand

Intrinsic muscles of the hand are composed of five groups:

1. **Thenar muscles (four)** (Figure 3.16)
   • Abductor pollicis brevis
   • Flexor pollicis brevis
   • Opponens pollicis
   • Adductor pollicis.
2. **Hypothenar muscles (three)** (Figure 3.16)
   • Abductor digiti minimi
   • Flexor digiti minimi brevis
   • Opponens digiti minimi.
3. **Dorsal interossei**: flex the MCP, extend the PIP and abduct the four ulnar digits (DAB).
4. **Palmar interossei**: adduct the four ulnar digits together (PAD).
5. **Lumbricals**: extend the IP joints in any position of the MCPs.

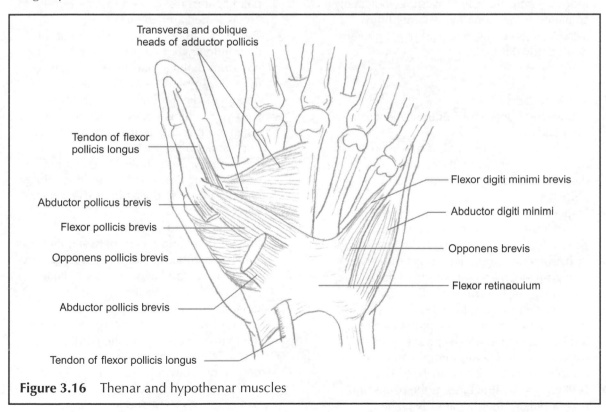

Figure 3.16 Thenar and hypothenar muscles

Innervation of the small muscles of the hand

The ulnar nerve innervates most of the intrinsic muscles of the hand except for the two radial **l**umbricals, **o**pponens pollicis, **a**bductor pollicis brevis and **f**lexor pollicis brevis (LOAF), which are served by the median nerve. The nerve roots serving the small muscles of the hand are from C8 and T1, and form the lower part of the brachial plexus.

Examining the hand at the neurological station

General appearance

- Survey the face for ptosis with Horner's syndrome, general facial wasting, ptosis and frontotemporal balding with myotonic dystrophy.
- Look for any obvious signs of lower limb involvement with walking aids, adapted footwear and lower limb wasting, indicating spinal cord (myelopathy), anterior horn (MND) or generalised causes of peripheral neuropathy (HMSN).

Hand examination

- Expose the upper limbs of the patient, not just the hands.
- Start by asking if the patient has any pains in the arms or hands and to let you know during the examination if he or she starts to feel pain.
- **Inspection**: ask the patient to hold the hands out in front, palms upwards, and look for any general deformity, wasting of the thenar and/or hypothenar eminences, scars (surgery or syringomyelia), and ulceration or damage to the finger pulps (syringomyelia). Look for scars or deformity at the elbow and shoulder joint (high ulnar nerve lesion or Charcot's joints with syringomyelia), fasciculations (MND) and any neurofibromas and nerve thickening (neurofibromatosis, CMT).
- Feel for any contractures in the palms and loss of bulk of the thenar or hypothenar eminences.

- Ask the patient to turn the hands over palms down and look for signs of clubbing (Pancoast's tumour), wasting with dorsal guttering, deformity with claw hand (see Scenario 18), joint, and skin or nail changes consistent with deforming arthropathy (RA or psoriatic) that could cause disuse atrophy (less likely at neurology station). At this point radial nerve lesions (not intrinsic to the hand) can be seen if the patient is asked to keep the hands up from the lap because there will be wrist drop and finger flexion.
- Note if there is **unilateral or bilateral** wasting of the hand muscles.
- **Testing tone**: if MND is the cause for wasting of the muscles of the hand, the patient may have increased spastic tone.
- **Testing motor function**: ask patients to do the following:
  - Point the thumb upwards away from the palm against resistance (abductor pollicis brevis – median nerve).
  - Touch the tip of the thumb to the tip of their little finger in a pincer grip and stop you from pulling your finger through (opponens pollicis – median nerve; opponens digiti minimi – ulnar nerve).
  - Stop you pulling a card from between adjacent fingers (adductors of the palmar interossei – ulnar nerve).
  - Abduct their index finger as you apply resistance against it with your index finger (abductors of the dorsal interossei – ulnar nerve).
  - Place their hand sideways, thumb upwards and grip a card between their straight thumb and index finger as you try to pull it out (adductor pollicis – ulnar nerve). If there is weakness just in the ulnar nerve the patient will use flexor pollicis brevis (median nerve) by bending the thumb and gripping the card.
  - Test for finger and wrist extension (radial nerve), which will be normal if there is only median and/or ulnar nerve pathology. Fix the hand and test MCP joint extension against resistance, and fix

the forearm and test wrist extension against resistance.

- If you feel that patients are able, you can ask them to make a fist and relax the hand several times quickly, looking for the 'warm-up' effect, or lightly tap on the thenar eminence looking for myotonia.
- **Testing for sensory loss**:
  - Differentiate a dermatomal pattern (spinal or nerve root pathology), a single peripheral nerve lesion, dissociated loss (syringomyelia) or a peripheral neuropathy giving a glove-and-stocking distribution.
  - Test light touch along the lateral border of the index finger (median nerve), medial border of the little finger (ulnar nerve) and first dorsal interosseus between first and second metacarpals (radial nerve).
  - To identify a dermatomal pattern of sensory loss, test sensation further up the arm. Loss of sensation of the lateral border of the index finger could represent median nerve or C6 dermatomal pathology, so check further along the C6 dermatome up the lateral lower arm (see neurological exam) and adjacent C5 and C4 dermatomes, which would usually be affected in nerve root or cord lesions. Similarly loss of sensation along the medial border of the little finger could represent ulnar nerve pathology or C8 dermatomal loss, so test sensation further up the wrist (continuation of C8 dermatome) and the medial border of the lower arm (T1).
  - Test for pinprick sensation in the same way but concentrate on dermatomal patterns because here you are looking for segmental dissociated sensory loss, particularly around the cape area, that would signify syringomyelia.
  - If there is weakness in all hand muscle groups, suspect length-dependent peripheral neuropathy at this point and

look for a glove pattern of sensory loss including joint position sense.

- **Deep tendon reflexes**:
  - In anterior horn cell (MND) or central cord disease, reflexes may be reduced, increased or inverted (in cord disease).
  - In nerve root lesions reflexes will be reduced/absent (biceps reflex C5–6, supinator C5–6, triceps C7–8 and finger C8–T1).
  - Reflexes will be normal in single or combined median and ulnar nerve lesions
  - In generalised peripheral motor neuropathies causing wasting of the hand muscles, reflexes may be reduced.
  - With NMJ diseases such as myasthenia gravis, reflexes tend to be normal
  - In myopathies such as muscular dystrophy or myotonic dystrophy, reflexes may be reduced or absent due to muscle weakness.
- **Testing coordination**:
  - This is usually normal but peripheral causes of muscle wasting may give reduced coordination through general muscle weakness
  - If there are central causes of wasting of the small muscles of the hand such as syringobulbia or Friedreich's ataxia, look for cerebellar signs.

Differential diagnosis

See Table 3.6.

Clinical judgement and maintaining patient welfare

Investigations, management and prognosis are discussed under the relevant scenarios that follow.

Table 3.6 Differential diagnosis for wasting of the small muscles of the hand(s)

Level of lesion	Disorder	Distribution	Motor exam	Sensory exam	Additional signs
Cervical cord/ anterior horn cells C8–T1	Cervical cord tumour	Bilateral	LMN signs at level of lesion	Sensory level at C8–T1	UMN signs below the lesion
	Syringomyelia	Bilateral	LMN signs at level of lesion	Dissociated sensory loss with loss of pain and temperature in cape distribution	UMN signs below lesion Ulceration and callosities on finger pulps Horner's syndrome
	MND	Bilateral	Mixture of LMN and UMN signs	Normal	Fasciculations Bulbar signs
	Friedreich's ataxia	Bilateral	UMN signs but reduced reflexes	Reduced vibration and proprioception (dorsal columns)	Cerebellar signs Pes cavus Kyphoscoliosis High arched palate
	HMSN	Bilateral	LMN signs	Glove-and-stocking loss	Inverted champagne bottle appearance of legs
	Old polio	Unilateral	LMN signs	Normal	Smaller wasted limb
Nerve roots C8–T1	Pancoast's syndrome	Unilateral	LMN signs with loss of finger reflexes	C8–T1 dermatomal sensory loss	Clubbing Horner's syndrome Chest signs Supraclavicular lymph nodes
	Cervical myelopathy	Bilateral	UMN or LMN signs depend on lesion level Inverted reflexes	C8–T1 dermatomal sensory loss	UMN signs in lower limbs Pseudoathetosis in fingers
Brachial plexus	Pancoast's syndrome	As above			
	Thoracic outlet syndrome	Unilateral	Hand wasting, normal reflexes	Dermatomal pattern	Absent radial and/or brachial pulse, palpable cervical rib
Neuropathy	Combined median and ulnar nerve palsy	Unilateral	Hand wasting, normal reflexes, normal finger and wrist extension		Scars around elbow or at wrist

(*continued*)

Table 3.6 (*continued*)

Level of lesion	Disorder	Distribution	Motor exam	Sensory exam	Additional signs
Myopathy	Myotonic dystrophy	Bilateral	Hand wasting, reduced reflexes	Normal	Myotonia, frontal balding, ptosis
	Muscular dystrophy	Bilateral	Hand wasting, reduced reflexes	Normal	Winging of scapulae, waddling gait

HMSN, hereditary motor and sensory neuropathy; LMN, lower motor neuron; MND, motor neuron disease; UMN, upper motor neuron.

SCENARIO 17: MEDIAN NERVE PALSY

Identifying clinical signs

The median nerve serves the intrinsic small muscles of the hand not served by the ulnar nerve. The median nerve also serves muscles of the volar surface of the forearm, which includes the main wrist flexors.

The most common median nerve palsy appearing in the PACES examination is a carpal tunnel syndrome. Indeed this is the most common peripheral mononeuropathy. However, there can be more proximal lesions of the median nerve that offer more objective clinical signs.

Distal median nerve lesions (carpal tunnel syndrome)

Inspection: the hand shows **thenar wasting** (a late sign) with hypothenar and first dorsal interosseous sparing. The **thumb is externally rotated and adducted** into the plain of the palm (Figure 3.18) due to weakness of opponens pollicis and abductor pollicis, and some refer to this as 'apehand' deformity (but it is best to describe the position of the thumb). The **index (first) and middle (second) fingers may also be held in extension** due to weakness of flexor digitorum

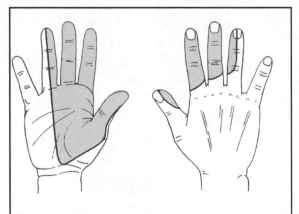

Figure 3.17   Median nerve cutaneous distribution

profundus I and II and flexor digitorum superficialis, and unopposed action of the radial nerve-innervated finger extensors. Some call this the 'papal sign'. Look for surgical or traumatic scars at the wrist, palmar crease, forearm or elbow.

Motor function: there is **weak thumb abduction** (abductor pollicis brevis), tested for by asking the patient to place the hand palm up and point the thumb up to the sky perpendicular to the plane of the palm and test against resistance of your thumb. There is **weakness of thumb opposition**, tested for by asking the patient to oppose the thumb with the little finger and stop you pulling them apart. There may be normal flexion at the thumb MCP joint due to intact ulnar nerve innervation of flexor pollicis brevis. There **is normal flexion of the thumb at the IP joint** due to intact innervation of flexor pollicis longus in the forearm. **Arm pronation and wrist flexion are also normal** if the median nerve lesion is distal.

Sensory loss: there is **sensory loss in the palmar aspect of the thumb and lateral two and a half fingers** but **normal sensation over the thenar eminence** (supplied by the palmar cutaneous branch of the median nerve which does not pass through the carpal tunnel).

Additional tests: you can ask to perform **Tinel's test** – tapping over the median nerve at the wrist may cause paraesthesia in the distal median distribution. **Phalen's test** involves flexing the wrist to 90° for at least 60 seconds, which may cause paraesthesia in the distal median distribution. The **median nerve compression test** involves pressing on the palmar aspect of the wrist for up to 60 seconds, which may cause paraesthesia in the distal median distribution.

Additional signs

Examine for signs of other diseases associated with carpal tunnel syndrome such as:

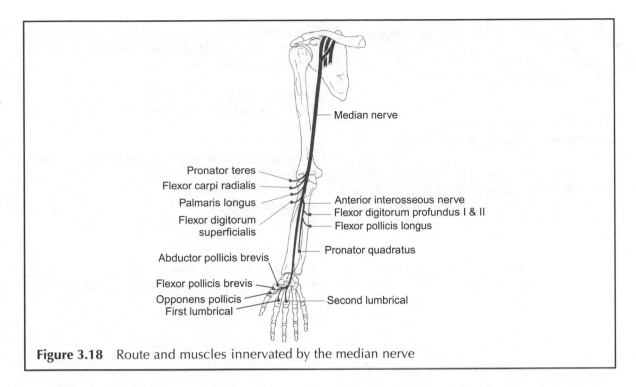

Figure 3.18   Route and muscles innervated by the median nerve

- **Hypothyroidism**: goitre, slowly relaxing reflexes, pretibial myxoedema
- **Acromegaly**: supraorbital ridge, prognathism, interdental separation, bitemporal hemianopia, large doughy hands, hypertension
- **Rheumatoid arthritis**: deforming arthropathy, elbow nodules, steroid skin changes, episcleritis/scleritis, interstitial lung disease
- **Diabetes mellitus**: finger-prick testing, peripheral neuropathy, retinopathy
- **Gout**: deforming arthropathy and gouty tophi on hands, ears and feet.

Proximal median nerve lesions

Pronator syndrome: compression of the median nerve can occur as it passes between the two heads of the pronator teres, high in the volar aspect of the forearm. It can present with **purely sensory symptoms** of pain over the volar surface of the forearm at rest or with forearm pronation. There will be sensory loss within the median distribution **including the thenar eminence** (unlike carpal tunnel syndrome).

Anterior interosseous nerve palsy

This nerve has branches to flexor digitorum profundus I and II, flexor pollicis longus and pronator quadratus. It is typically affected by a midshaft fracture of the radius, excessive exercise or penetrating injuries of the forearm. There is **weakness of the thumb and index finger flexion**, best shown with the 'okay' sign, ie flattened due to failure of distal flexion (see Figure 3.17). The thenar eminence muscles are spared. There is **no sensory loss**.

Differential diagnosis

- Elbow lesions:
  - Fracture: supracondylar fractures are most common
  - Dislocation
  - Compression: ligament of Struthers
- Forearm lesions:
  - Fracture: midshaft radial fracture causing anterior osseous nerve palsy
  - Injury: penetrating injuries of the forearm

- Compression: pronator teres syndrome
- Wrist lesions:
  - Fracture/trauma
  - Carpal tunnel syndrome (CTS).

Clinical judgement and maintaining patient welfare

CTS is caused by compression of the median nerve within the carpal tunnel, which is bound by the carpal bones below, flexor retinaculum above, radially by the scaphoid and trapezium, and medially by the pisiform and hamate.

It is most commonly idiopathic, but associated conditions include: pregnancy, menopause, hypothyroidism, diabetes, acromegaly, rheumatoid arthritis, gout, renal failure, multiple myeloma and amyloidosis.

Investigations
Electrophysiology: nerve conduction studies and EMG.

Imaging: seldom needed, but MRI might be considered.

Management
- Treat any underlying associated conditions
- Physiotherapy and splint the wrists with a degree of dorsiflexion
- Steroid injections into the carpal tunnel area
- Surgical decompression of the carpal tunnel.

SCENARIO 18. ULNAR NERVE PALSY

Identifying clinical signs

The ulnar nerve serves most of the intrinsic small muscles of the hand. However, the ulnar nerve also supplies two important extrinsic muscles of the hand: flexor carpi ulnaris and flexor digitorum profundus 4 and 5; it is important to remember this when considering a claw hand deformity. Clues pointing towards an ulnar nerve lesion include unilateral signs, clawing of the hand and wasting of the hypothenar eminence with sparing of the thenar eminence.

Distal ulnar nerve lesion (distal to the elbow)

Inspection: with the hands held prone there is **dorsal guttering** and marked **wasting of the first interosseous** between the thumb and index finger. The hand shows a claw deformity (you might want to say a **clawed appearance**) with hyperextension at the fourth and fifth MCP joints and flexion at the fourth and fifth PIP and DIP joints, due to paralysis of the medial lumbricals. There is slight ulnar deviation of the fifth finger (known as **Wartenburg's sign**) from unopposed action of extensor digiti minimi (which inserts into the ulnar side of the little finger and is innervated by

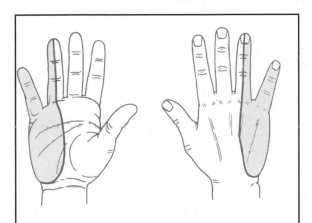

Figure 3.19   Ulnar nerve cutaneous distribution

the radial nerve). With the hands held supine, **marked hypothenar wasting** with sparing of the thenar eminence can be seen, and no wasting of the forearm muscles. Look for scars or deformity from trauma, surgery or arthritis around the forearm and wrist.

Motor function: there is **weak abduction** (dorsal interossei) and **weak adduction** (palmar interossei) of the fingers. There is **weak thumb adduction** (adductor pollicis) as demonstrated by attempting to grip a piece of paper held between the borders of the index finger and extended thumb. Grip can be maintained only using thumb flexion (intact flexor pollicis longus served by the median nerve), known as **Froment's sign**. There is **intact flexion of the fourth and fifth DIP joints**, as shown by the marked ulnar claw appearance (it is difficult to test actively when the fingers are held in fixed flexion). There is **intact medial/ulnar flexion of the wrist.**

Sensory loss: in the **ulnar distribution** over the fifth finger (see Figure 3.19), adjacent ulnar side of the fourth finger, ulnar side of the palm and dorsal aspect of the hand. (In distal ulnar nerve lesions this sensory loss may be variable or present only in the fifth finger.) Test along the radial side of the fourth finger and up the ulnar border of the wrist and forearm to check that this does not represent a C8–T1 lesion instead (muscle wasting would also be different, see Scenario 16).

Additional tests: you can ask to perform **Tinel's test** tapping along the course of the ulnar nerve from the wrist along the ulnar border of the forearm and up to the elbow, which may elicit tingling from irritation of the nerve.

Proximal ulnar nerve lesion (at the elbow)
Inspection: with the hands held prone there is **dorsal guttering** and **marked wasting of the first**

interosseous between the thumb and index finger. The hand shows a **mild/no clawed appearance** with hyperextension at the fourth and fifth MCP joints but only mild flexion at the fourth and fifth PIP joints and no flexion at the DIP joints. This is known as the **ulnar paradox**, with proximal lesions resulting in less clawing. There is slight ulnar deviation of the fifth finger known as **Wartenburg's sign** (see above). With the palms facing up, there is **marked hypothenar wasting**, with sparing of the thenar eminence. In addition, there is **wasting of the ulnar border of the forearm**. Look for scars or deformity from trauma, surgery or arthritis around the elbow.

Motor function: there is **weak abduction** (dorsal interossei) and **weak adduction** (palmar interossei) of the fingers. There is **weak thumb adduction** (adductor pollicis) with **Froment's sign** (see above). There is **loss of flexion of the fourth and fifth DIP joints** (loss of flexor digitorum profundus with high lesions) as shown by holding the fourth and fifth MCP and PIP joints extended and asking the patient to try to flex the fourth and fifth DIP joints (this takes practice to demonstrate effectively!). There is **weakness of medial/ulnar flexion of the wrist** (flexor carpi ulnaris) not found in distal lesions (see above).

Sensory loss: this occurs in the **ulnar distribution** over the fifth finger, ulnar side of the fourth finger, ulnar side of the palm and dorsal aspect of the hand (see Figure 3.19).

Additional tests: you can ask to perform **Tinel's test**, tapping along the course of the ulnar nerve from the wrist up the ulnar border of the forearm towards the elbow, which may elicit tingling from nerve irritation.

The **elbow flexion test** can be used to test for ulnar nerve compression at the elbow, particularly in cubital tunnel syndrome. The elbow is flexed fully with the forearm supinated, and within 60 seconds the patient starts to feel pain or tingling in the fourth and fifth fingers.

Differential diagnosis

Elbow lesions
- Fractures:
  - Supracondylar fractures are most common and late complications of fracture/surgery can include cubitus valgus deformity of the elbow joint.
- Dislocation:
  - Arthritis: bony spurs and narrowing of the ulnar groove
  - Compression: cubital tunnel syndrome describes constriction under the fibrous arch of the two points of insertion of flexor carpi ulnaris. Certain occupations are more at wrist such as secretaries (from leaning on elbows) and decorators (from repeated elbow flexion and extension).

Wrist lesions
- Fractures
- Ganglion
- Tumour
- Mononeuritis multiplex.

Clinical judgement and maintaining patient welfare

Investigations
Imaging: plain radiograph of elbow joint, ultrasonography of the cubital tunnel or MRI.

Nerve conduction studies localise the site of the lesion

Blood tests: FBC, CRP, ESR, anti-nuclear antibodies (ANAs), anti-DNA, pANCA (perinuclear anti-neutrophil cytoplasmic antibody or ANCA), cANCA (cytoplasmic ANCA), rheumatoid factor, hepatitis B and C serology (mononeuritis multiplex).

Management
Conservative: avoidance of aggravating factors, physiotherapy, splinting, NSAIDs.

Surgical: transposition of the ulnar nerve and/or decompression of the cubital tunnel.

SCENARIO 19. RADIAL NERVE PALSY

Identifying clinical signs

The radial nerve serves the extensors of the elbow, wrist and fingers. With knowledge of the anatomy of radial nerve innervation it is possible to describe the level of the lesion giving rise to clinical signs (see Figure 3.20).

Radial nerve lesion at the axilla

Inspection: there is wrist drop and slight finger flexion but with no wasting of the hand muscles. Look for surgical or traumatic scars anywhere along the route of the radial nerve from the axilla to the wrist.

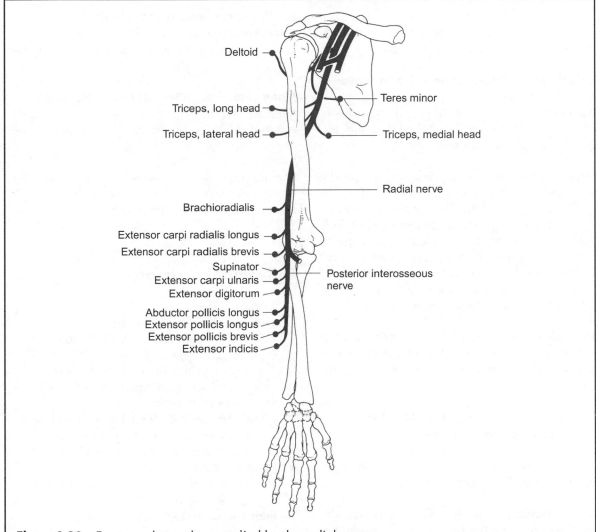

Figure 3.20   Route and muscles supplied by the radial nerve

Motor function: there is weakness of all radially innervated muscles:

- **Weakness of elbow extension and flexion** (midway between supination and pronation)
- **Forearm supination** (tested with arm by the side and attempted supination of forearm against resistance applied to the patient's hand)
- **Wrist extension and finger extension at the MCP joints**.

Both triceps and brachioradialis (biceps) deep tendon reflexes are absent.

Sensory loss: this occurs over the triceps, posterior forearm and first dorsal interosseous.

Radial nerve lesion in the spiral groove of the humerus

Inspection: there is wrist drop and slight finger flexion but with no wasting of the hand muscles. Look for surgical or traumatic scars.

Motor function: there is weakness of all radially innervated muscles below the triceps. There is weakness of elbow flexion (midway between supination and pronation) but elbow extension is intact (triceps innervation above the spiral grove). There is weakness of forearm supination, wrist extension and finger extension at the MCP joints. The triceps reflex is preserved but the brachioradialis (biceps) deep tendon reflex is absent.

Sensory loss: there is sensory loss over the posterior forearm and first dorsal interosseous. There may be variable loss of sensation over the triceps.

Radial nerve lesion confined to the posterior interosseous nerve

Inspection: there is wrist drop and slight finger flexion but with no wasting of the hand muscles. Look for surgical or traumatic scars.

Motor function: there is weakness of radially innervated muscles below the supinator (the supinator nerve comes off before the posterior inter-

osseous nerve dips beneath the fibrous arcade of Frohse ('supinator arch') which is the common entrapment area). There is intact elbow flexion (midway between supination and pronation) and intact elbow extension and forearm supination. There is weakness of wrist extension and finger extension at the MCP joints. Triceps and brachioradialis deep tendon reflexes are intact.

Sensory loss: there is no sensory loss because the posterior interosseous branch is a purely motor nerve.

Radial nerve lesion at the wrist

Inspection: the arm and hand appear normal. Look for surgical or traumatic scars around the wrist.

Motor function: there is **no motor** weakness (because the radial nerve serves only extrinsic extensor muscles of the hand from above the wrist).

Sensory loss: there is sensory loss in the first dorsal interosseous only (as the sensory branch becomes superficial at the wrist).

Differential diagnosis

- **Axillary lesions**:
  - Fracture/dislocation of humeral head
  - Compression: use of shoulder crutch or 'Saturday night palsy' from prolonged hanging of the arm over the back of a chair (when intoxicated)
- **Spiral groove lesions**:
  - Fracture: mid-shaft fracture of the humerus
  - Compression: wheelchair users resting back of their arm against the chair
- **Posterior lesions**:
  - Compression: from the arcade of Frohse/supinator arch
- **Interosseous lesions**:
  - Tumours/lipomas or ganglia near the elbow

- **Wrist lesions**:
  - Fracture: at the distal radius
  - Compression: tight bracelets/handcuffs/ plaster casts.

Clinical judgement and maintaining patient welfare

Investigations
Electrophysiology: nerve conduction studies and EMG.

Imaging: ultrasonography/MRI may rarely be considered.

Management
- Conservative management of 'Saturday night palsy' with spontaneous improvement
- Physiotherapy and splinting for mild compressive lesions
- Surgical correction of fracture/dislocations.

SCENARIO 20. COMMON PERONEAL NERVE PALSY AND L4–5 ROOT LESION

Identifying clinical signs

Common peroneal nerve palsy is the most common cause of foot drop. However, a lesion in any of the areas, including the motor cortex, spinal cord, lumbar nerve roots L4–5, lumbosacral plexus and sciatic nerve, and peripheral neuropathies or myopathies, can cause foot drop with different associated clinical signs. Knowledge of the anatomy of the common peroneal nerve will help determine the level of the lesion.

The sciatic nerve (L4, L5, S1–3) divides into its terminal branches, the tibial nerve and the common peroneal nerve, two-thirds down the posterior thigh. The tibial nerve serves the posterior compartment of the lower leg, producing plantar-flexion and inversion. The common peroneal nerve (Figure 3.21) serves the anterior part of the lower leg, winding around the neck of the fibula and dividing into the superficial peroneal nerve (foot eversion and sensation to lateral lower leg and dorsum of foot) and the deep peroneal nerve (foot and toe dorsiflexion and sensation to the dorsal web space between the hallux and second toe).

Common peroneal nerve palsy

Inspection: there is **foot drop with a high-stepping gait**. There is **wasting of the antero-lateral compartment of the lower leg**. Look for **surgical or traumatic scars** near the knee and neck of the fibula. Look for any ankle supports/adapted footwear.

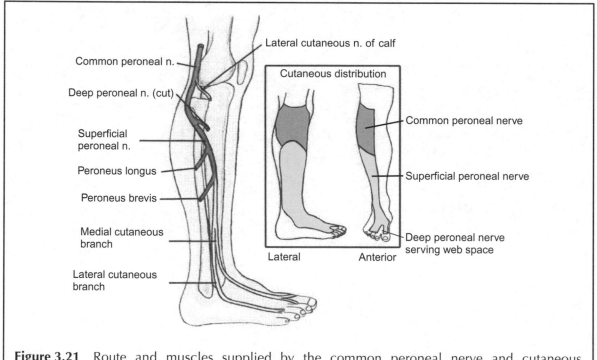

Figure 3.21 Route and muscles supplied by the common peroneal nerve and cutaneous distribution

Motor function: there is **weakness of ankle dorsiflexion**, and **hallux extension** (deep peroneal nerve) and **eversion** (superficial peroneal nerve). Test for eversion in a passively dorsiflexed foot because the everters cannot exert their action if the foot is in plantarflexion. The ankle jerk is intact and plantar reflex is downwards. There is normal plantarflexion and inversion. In mild cases, weakness may be seen only when asking the patient to walk on the heels.

Sensory loss: over the **lateral calf and dorsum of the foot, but sparing the little toe.** The little toe has sensation from the sural nerve, a branch of the tibial nerve.

Superficial peroneal nerve palsy
Inspection: there is **wasting of the lateral compartment of the lower leg but no obvious highstepping gait**. Look for **surgical or traumatic scars** near the knee and neck of the fibula. Look for any ankle supports/adapted footwear.

Motor function: there is **slight weakness of ankle dorsiflexion** which might be seen only when the patient is asked to walk on the heels. There is **no weakness in hallux extension**, but there is **weakness of eversion**. There is normal plantarflexion and inversion.

Sensory loss: over the **lower lateral calf and dorsum of the foot, but sparing the little toe**.

Deep peroneal nerve palsy
Inspection: there is **foot drop with a highstepping gait**. There is **wasting of the anterior compartment of the lower leg**. Look for **surgical or traumatic scars** near the knee and neck of the fibula, anterior lower leg. Look for any ankle supports/adapted footwear.

Motor function: there is **weakness of ankle dorsiflexion** (deep peroneal nerve) and **hallux extension** but **intact eversion** (superficial peroneal nerve).

Sensory loss: only in the **dorsal web space between the hallux and second toe.**

Differential diagnosis
Myopathy: tends to give rise to proximal weakness but there are distal variants. Signs will be bilateral. All foot movements will be weak including plantarflexion and hallux flexion. The ankle jerk may be reduced. There will be no sensory loss. There will be myopathic signs in the upper limbs and possibly the face.

Sensorimotor peripheral neuropathy: there is also weak plantarflexion and a stocking pattern of sensory loss including the little toe. Signs will be bilateral. There may be dorsal column signs and a positive Romberg's test and sensorimotor signs in the upper limbs.

Neuromuscular junction disorder: signs tend to be bilateral with upper limb and facial involvement. Weakness will affect plantarflexion and be fatigable. Reflexes and sensation will be normal.

MND: signs are bilateral, although in early disease there can be asymmetry. There will be a mixture of UMN and LMN signs with increased tone, brisk ankle jerks, possibly upgoing plantar reflexes, marked wasting and fasciculations. There tend to be signs in the upper limbs and face. There are no sensory findings.

Sciatic nerve lesion: a peripheral nerve lesion affecting the sciatic nerve can cause foot drop, but also weak plantarflexion and inversion, weak knee flexion (with preserved knee extension) and hip extension. The ankle jerk is absent with a preserved knee jerk. Sensory loss will be along the posterior thigh, lower leg and foot, sparing the medial side of the lower leg. Injury to the sciatic nerve can occur through hip surgery, misplaced gluteal injections and pelvic pathology, such as trauma, haematoma, abscess or tumours.

Lumbosacral plexus lesion: presents similarly to a sciatic nerve lesion but with femoral nerve involvement. This will cause additional weakness in hip flexion, abduction and adduction, and knee extension. The knee and ankle jerks are lost. There will be more extensive sensory loss including the anterior thigh and medial lower leg.

L4–5 radiculopathy: leads to similar findings as a common peroneal nerve lesion. In addition there will be weak hip abduction and adduction and variable effects on knee flexion and extension. The knee jerk (L3–4) may be lost but ankle jerks (S1–2) preserved. Sensory loss will include the medial part of the lower leg (L5). The patient often has back pain because nerve root compression usually arises from lumbar disc herniation (less commonly a tumour). Straight leg raise, stimulating nerve root irritation from stretching, will reproduce symptoms.

Spinal cord lesion: this can cause weakness in foot dorsiflexion but will also cause weakness in other muscle groups of the leg depending on the level of the lesion. Foot drop is not so obvious due to the UMN spasticity. Lesions can be unilateral or bilateral. Sensory signs will depend on the location of the lesion in the cord and there may be dissociated sensory loss, giving rise to the Brown–Séquard syndrome if the lesion is unilateral.

Cortical lesion: a tumour or stroke affecting the motor cortex, such as a lacunar infarct or parasagittal meningioma, can rarely cause localised lower limb weakness and foot drop. There will be UMN signs.

Causes of common peroneal nerve palsy
- Trauma
- Fibular fracture
- Knee surgery
- Compression: plaster cast, leg crossing, weight loss.

Clinical judgement and maintaining patient welfare

Investigations
Electrophysiology: nerve conduction studies and EMG.

Imaging: MRI might be considered.

Management
- Avoidance of aggravating factors such as leg crossing or squatting
- Physiotherapy and splinting of the ankle/foot
- Surgical repair or release if there has been transection or tethering.

SCENARIO 21. NYSTAGMUS

Nystagmus will usually be a sign as part of another disorder such as cerebellar syndrome or MS, but rarely it can form the full case in the PACES neurology station.

Nystagmus is an involuntary rhythmic oscillation of the eye(s) that may be physiological, congenital or acquired. It represents a problem with the neural mechanisms/centres involved in maintaining image fixation on the fovea for optimal visual acuity.

Identifying clinical signs

Nystagmus is usually described with reference to:

- Monocular or binocular/conjugate
- Position: primary (looking forward) or only gaze related
- Type: pendular (equal velocity in either direction) or jerk: a slow drift then fast corrective phase – the direction of nystagmus refers to the fast phase
- Plane: horizontal, vertical or rotatory/torsional (sometimes it is easier to tell by looking at the pull on the conjunctival vessels).

Cerebellar nystagmus

This is a **binocular/conjugate**, **primary** and **gaze-related jerk nystagmus** which is in the **horizontal plane**, and the direction of the nystagmus (**fast phase**) is **towards** the same side as the cerebellar lesion and **maximal on looking towards this side**. The nystagmus **does not fatigue** with continued gaze to the affected side. There is also loss of smooth saccades.

Further cerebellar testing will show homolateral **poor finger–nose pointing** with dysmetria and **intention tremor, dysdiadochokinesis,** poor heel–shin coordination and an **ataxic gait** falling to-wards the side of the lesion. There may be **dysarthric speech**.

Additional

Finish your exam by asking to test the cranial nerves, particularly looking for any abnormality of cranial nerve V (corneal and facial sensation) or cranial nerve VIII which may suggest a lesion at the cerebellopontine angle (see Scenario 27). Ask to examine the fundus for optic atrophy which may be present in MS.

Ask to examine the upper and lower limbs, which may show pyramidal weakness consistent with MS, or dorsal column signs in alcohol misuse or vitamin B_{12} deficiency.

Romberg's test is not a test of cerebellar function, but rather of dorsal column/proprioceptive function. A patient with a cerebellar lesion cannot usually stand steady, feet together with arms by the sides even with the eyes open, so Romberg's test cannot be performed.

Differential diagnosis

Unilateral cerebellar pathology and nystagmus will tend to be caused by structural lesions:

- Cerebrovascular events, eg lateral medullary syndrome
- Demyelination, eg MS
- Cerebellar/posterior fossa tumours, eg astrocytomas, haemangioblastomas, medulloblastomas and metastatic disease (breast, lung, skin, kidney).

Bilateral cerebellar nystagmus will be caused by systemic pathology:

- Toxins (alcohol, chemotherapy and anticonvulsants)
- Autoimmune and paraneoplastic processes
- Inherited disorders involving cerebellar degeneration, eg olivopontocerebellar

degeneration and Friedreich's ataxia (see Scenario 12).

Vestibular nystagmus

Peripheral vestibular nystagmus: this is a binocular/conjugate horizontal or rotatory/torsional nystagmus which is a primary and gaze-related unidirectional jerk nystagmus with the fast component maximal to the opposite side of the vestibular lesion. With upward or downward gaze the nystagmus remains horizontal and in the same direction. With continued gaze away from the side of the lesion the nystagmus fatigues. There are no cerebellar signs. The gait may be unsteady, falling towards the side of the lesion, and the patient may describe vertigo symptoms. These are often worse when testing gait. Tinnitus and deafness may be found on the side of the lesion.

Differential diagnosis
The peripheral vestibular system includes the semicircular canals, otoliths and the vestibular portion of cranial nerve VIII.

The causes of peripheral vestibular nystagmus include labyrinthitis, acoustic neuroma, Ménière's disease, benign paroxysmal positional vertigo (BPPV), autoimmune inner ear disease (AIED) and degenerative middle-ear disease such as otosclerosis.

Central vestibular nystagmus

This is a **binocular/conjugate horizontal/vertical/rotatory** or **mixed** (may appear chaotic) nystagmus, which is a **primary and gaze-related nystagmus**. It is **multidirectional** so that on looking to the left it is leftward (fast component to the left), looking to the right it is rightward and looking up it is upward. There is **no fatigue** of the nystagmus on sustained gaze in any direction. The patient may have a tendency to fall in any direction on testing gait; vertigo is unusual. There

are no peripheral symptoms such as tinnitus or deafness and no cerebellar signs.

Differential diagnosis
The central vestibular system includes the vestibular nerve nuclei and their projections to the cerebellum, extraocular nuclei via the medial longitudinal fasciculus, the spinal cord via the vestibulospinal tract and projections to the cortex.

Causes of central vestibular nystagmus include brain-stem stroke and vertebrobasilar insufficiency, brain-stem tumours, demyelination such as MS, syringobulbia (see Scenario 7) and basilar-type migraine (some classify this as a cause of peripheral vestibular nystagmus when it is associated with benign paroxysmal positional vertigo).

Pendular nystagmus

This is a conjugate or monocular **multidirectional nystagmus** that can appear chaotic. The **oscillation has equal velocity in all directions**. It is present in all positions including the primary position.

Additional: look around the bed for clues of visual aids used by the blind patient and a general appearance that might suggest albinism. Ask to perform fundoscopy to look for optic atrophy, signs of retinitis pigmentosa and cataracts with disruption of the red reflex.

Differential diagnosis
Monocular or binocular visual deprivation is the most common cause of pendular nystagmus, but other causes include demyelinating disease such as MS and brain-stem dysfunction.

Internuclear ophthalmoplegia (INO or ataxic nystagmus)

There is **failure of conjugate eye movements on lateral gaze**. In the primary position there may be a divergent strabismus. In a left-sided INO (lesion in the ipsilateral MLF) there is **partial or total failure of adduction** of the left eye on looking right, but normal abduction of the right eye, with **jerk horizontal nystagmus in the abducting eye** with fast corrective phase towards the right side (opposite side to the lesion). The nystagmus of the abducting eye is not necessary for the diagnosis of INO. The patient may describe diplopia when looking to the right (contralateral) side. It can be shown that this is not a left medial rectus palsy by the fact that, by covering the right abducting eye, the left eye adducts normally with convergence. Sometimes convergence can be affected if the lesion extends into the midbrain. In a bilateral INO there will be failure of adduction of either eye with lateral gaze in the opposite direction.

Additional
State that you would like to look for additional eye signs supportive of MS such as optic atrophy, visual field defects, optic disc pallor on fundoscopy and/or a relative afferent pupillary defect (RAPD). Look for cerebellar signs in support of MS or brain-stem infarction.

Differential diagnosis
INO is due to a lesion in the MLF within the pons and midbrain, which connects the contralateral nerve VI nucleus to the ipsilateral oculomotor (nerve III) nucleus.

MS is the most common cause in a younger person, and brain-stem infarction causing unilateral INO is the most common cause in an older person. Other causes include brain-stem tumours, viral infection, syphilis infection, Lyme disease, trauma, Arnold–Chiari malformation, syringobulbia, and drug (phenothiazines, phenytoin, tricyclic antidepressants) and alcohol intoxication.

Downbeat nystagmus

There is a **bilateral downbeat nystagmus in the primary gaze**, which remains downbeat in all directions of gaze. Lateral gaze may accentuate the nystagmus.

Additional
Look for signs of syringobulbia and syringomyelia which may occur together with an Arnold–Chiari malformation, eg bulbar palsy, INO, balaclava-helmet loss of facial sensation, a dissociated sensory loss usually in a cape distribution, LMN signs in the upper limbs and UMN signs in the lower limbs. Look for cerebellar signs that may also suggest syringobulbia or a posterior fossa tumour.

Differential diagnosis
Downbeat nystagmus usually signifies pathology at the craniocervical junction. Arnold–Chiari malformation is the most common cause. Downbeat nystagmus may also be seen with brain-stem stroke, syringobulbia, spinocerebellar degeneration, MS and drug (phenytoin, lithium) and alcohol toxicity.

Upbeat nystagmus

There is a **bilateral vertical nystagmus** in the primary position with the fast phase beating in the upward position.

If the nystagmus increases on upward gaze, this suggests pathology in the anterior vermis of the cerebellum. There may be other cerebellar signs such as loss of smooth saccades, slurred speech and truncal ataxia.

If the nystagmus increases on downward gaze, this suggests pathology in the medulla. There may be associated brain-stem signs such as palatal weakness with nasal speech.

Physiological nystagmus

This is a gaze-evoked jerk nystagmus occurring at the extremes of gaze and absent in the primary position. The elastic pull of the extraocular muscles and tendons exerts a force that tends to bring the eye back to the midline, but the neural integrator tries to overcome this with corrective quick movement (jerk nystagmus) to the desired extreme of gaze.

Clinical judgement and maintaining patient welfare

Investigations
These will be determined by the type of nystagmus and the associated differential diagnosis.

Management
- Cessation of causative medications
- Correction of refractive errors with contact lenses
- Downbeat nystagmus may be treated with base-out prisms, which induce convergence
- Botulinum toxin injection into rectus muscles can ameliorate acquired nystagmus. However, this diminishes all types of eye movement and can cause diplopia, ptosis and increased nystagmus in the uninjected eye.

SCENARIO 22. OPHTHALMOPLEGIA

The most common gaze palsies seen in the PACES examination are cranial nerve III and VI palsies. Remember to look for associated cranial nerve abnormalities or peripheral examination signs that will point towards a specific disease or help further localise the lesion.

It is worth revisiting the anatomy and function of the extraocular nerves III, IV and VI together with their muscles so that their examination becomes straightforward (see Figures 3.22 and 3.23).

Nerve III (oculomotor) palsy

See Figure 3.24. Nerve III supplies most of the extraocular muscles including superior rectus (elevation), medial rectus (adduction) and inferior

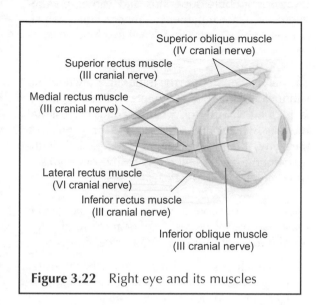

Figure 3.22   Right eye and its muscles

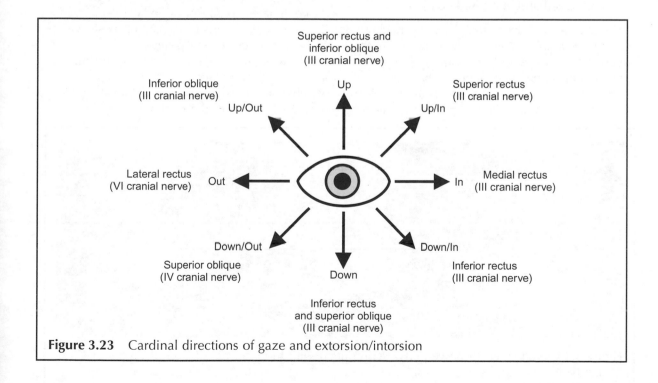

Figure 3.23   Cardinal directions of gaze and extorsion/intorsion

oblique (extorsion, elevation and abduction). It also elevates the eyelid through its innervation of levator palpebrae superioris and carries preganglionic parasympathetic innervation which causes pupil constriction via the sphincter (constrictor) pupillae.

The nerve III nucleus in the midbrain is divided into subnuclei to innervate the separate muscles, and it is partnered with the nearby Edinger–Westphal nucleus which gives rise to the preganglionic parasympathetic fibres; these lie superficially within the nerve and are therefore easily compromised by compressive lesions.

The subnuclei serve the IPSILATERAL extraocular muscles (medial rectus, inferior rectus and inferior oblique) with two important exceptions:

1. The nucleus sends fibres across to the opposite oculomotor nucleus, which then innervates the CONTRALATERAL superior rectus.
2. The nucleus supplies BOTH levator palpebrae with crossed and uncrossed fibres.

The nerve III fascicles/trunks leave the midbrain passing ventrally. Nerve III then passes in the subarachnoid space and runs close to the posterior communicating artery. It enters the lateral side of the cavernous sinus, crosses over the trochlear nerve, and exits medially as superior and inferior branches through the superior orbital fissure. The superior branch serves levator palpebrae superioris and superior rectus, which is also joined by sympathetic supply from the internal carotid artery. The inferior branch serves the other oculomotor muscles and carries the parasympathetic axons to the constrictor pupillae.

Identifying clinical signs

There is a left-sided **ptosis** (see Figure 3.24) and when the eyelid is raised the eye is in a **down and out** position (due to the unopposed combined action of lateral rectus and superior oblique), giving a **divergent strabismus/squint**. The patient cannot move the affected eye across the midline. **Diplopia** is maximal on trying to look away from the affected side and up. There is a **dilated and non-reactive pupil** (to light or attempted accommodation) from parasympathetic fibre involvement.

With a nuclear lesion there will be contralateral eye signs in addition to the ipsilateral signs. There is a contralateral partial ptosis (bilateral innervation of levator palpebrae superioris) but ptosis will be more pronounced on the ipsilateral side. There will also be a contralateral elevation palsy (the nucleus innervates the contralateral superior rectus). Remember, there is an ipsilateral elevation palsy because fibres from the contralateral subnucleus

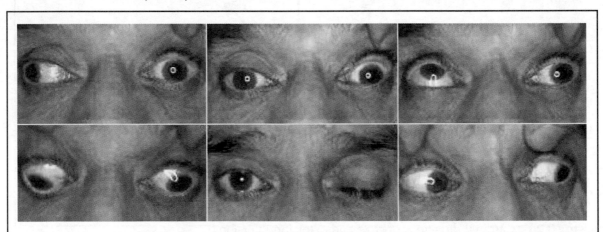

Figure 3.24   Left-sided III nerve palsy. Reproduced with the kind permission of Professor Chua Chung Nen

pass through the ipsilateral subnucleus before innervating the superior rectus.

Differential diagnosis

Nuclear lesion: infarction, haemorrhage, tumour, abscess, demyelination.

Midbrain lesion: herniation, infarction, haemorrhage, tumour, abscess, demyelination (MS).

Subarachnoid lesion: aneurysm, haemorrhage, meningitis, inflammation including vasculitides (giving rise to mononeuritis multiplex), tumour, migraine.

Cavernous sinus lesion: tumour (pituitary, craniopharyngioma), thrombosis, aneurysm, fistula, infection, inflammatory.

Orbital lesion: trauma, tumour.

Small vessel disease: diabetes, hypertension, atherosclerosis.

Infection: Lyme disease, syphilis, basilar meningitis (bacterial, mycobacterial, fungal, parasitic).

Nerve IV (trochlear) palsy

Nerve IV supplies the superior oblique muscle which intorts, depresses and abducts the globe. This combined action allows the eye to look down and in. The nerve IV nuclei lie in the midbrain where the nerves decussate and then exit dorsally. It is the only cranial nerve to exit the brain dorsally and it has a long course, making it susceptible to trauma.

A nerve IV palsy can be very subtle so a candidate must actively look for it.

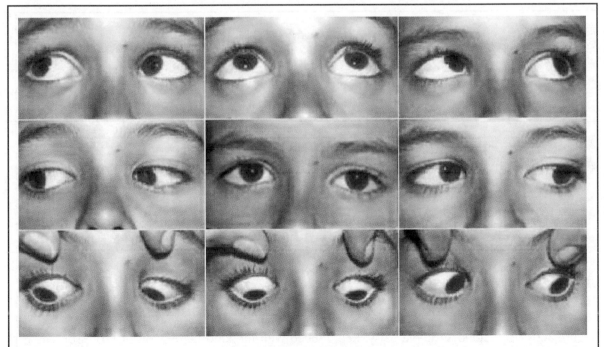

Figure 3.25   Right-sided IV nerve palsy. Reproduced with the kind permission of Professor Chua Chung Nen

Identifying clinical signs

The right eye appears slightly elevated/normal and the patient has a **head tilt** away from the side of the lesion, tucking the chin in slightly to bring the visual axis of the affected eye central again (see Figure 3.25). The affected eye **cannot look down in adduction** (towards the nose). It is in this position that the patient experiences most **vertical diplopia** (giving rise to the classic history of difficulty reading books or climbing stairs when this direction of gaze is needed). Remember that diplopia is always worse in the direction of gaze of the paretic muscle. The false outer/upper image disappears when the affected eye is covered.

Differential diagnosis

- Congenital
- Trauma (most common cause)
- Small vessel disease: diabetes, hypertension, atherosclerosis
- Inflammatory: mononeuritis multiplex, peripheral neuropathy

- Infection: Lyme disease, syphilis, basilar meningitis (bacterial, mycobacterial, fungal, parasitic)
- Midbrain/nuclear lesion: infarct, haemorrhage, tumour, abscess, demyelination (MS)
- Cavernous sinus lesion: tumour (pituitary, craniopharyngioma), thrombosis, aneurysm, fistula, haemorrhage, infection, inflammatory.

Nerve VI (abducens) palsy

Nerve VI innervates the ipsilateral lateral rectus, which abducts the eye. The nerve VI nucleus is in the caudal part of the pons. Approximately 40% of its neurons pass to the nearby MLF, to then cross over to the contralateral nerve III nucleus to innervate the contralateral medial rectus and produce conjugate lateral gaze.

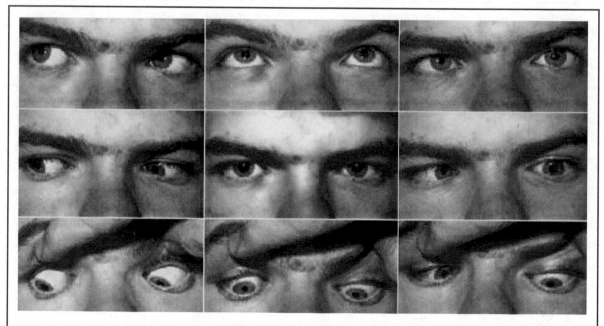

Figure 3.26   Left sided VI nerve palsy. Reproduced with the kind permission of Professor Chua Chung Nen

Identifying clinical signs

There is a **convergent strabismus** in the primary position due to the unopposed action of the intact medial rectus (see Figure 3.26). There is **horizontal diplopia** maximal on attempted gaze in the direction of the paretic muscle. The outer image disappears on covering the affected eye.

On testing the remaining cranial nerves, pay particular attention to nerves VII and VIII, and check for nystagmus and other cerebellar signs that would indicate a cerebellopontine angle lesion. There may be signs of bilateral papilloedema on fundoscopy from a space-occupying lesion or idiopathic intracranial hypertension. Here, the nerve VI palsy acts as a 'false localising sign' due to downward displacement of the brain stem causing stretching of the abducens nerve.

Differential diagnosis

- Congenital: congenital absence of nerve VI – Duane's syndrome
- Trauma
- Raised ICP: space-occupying lesion or idiopathic intracranial hypertension
- Small vessel disease: diabetes, hypertension, atherosclerosis
- Inflammatory: mononeuritis multiplex, postviral, peripheral neuropathy
- Infection: Lyme disease, syphilis, basilar meningitis (bacterial, mycobacterial, fungal, parasitic)
- Pontine/nuclear lesion: infarct, haemorrhage, tumour, abscess, demyelination (MS)
- Petrous bone pathology: in severe ongoing otitis media there can be infiltrative osteomyelitis involving the petrous temporal bone
- Cavernous sinus lesion: tumour (pituitary, craniopharyngioma), thrombosis, aneurysm, fistula, haemorrhage, infection, inflammatory.

Complex ophthalmoplegia

Identifying clinical signs

Thyroid ophthalmopathy will usually present as a complex ophthalmoplegia not attributable to any single nerve lesion. This does not represent a true ophthalmoplegia. It is due to soft-tissue inflammation and swelling within the orbit causing restriction of eye movements. There is usually proptosis, chemosis, lid lag and other thyroid signs.

Myasthenia gravis may present as a complex ophthalmoplegia not attributable to any single nerve lesion. Eye movements are fatigable and there are no pupillary signs.

The **Miller–Fisher** variant of Guillain–Barré syndrome may present initially with an ophthalmoplegia, with the descending paralysis from peripheral demyelination giving the classic triad of ophthalmoplegia, ataxia and areflexia.

Chronic progressive external ophthalmoplegia (CPEO) is the most common manifestation of mitochondrial myopathy, in itself very rare, and usually presents as a bilateral progressive ptosis, which proceeds to a bilateral ophthalmoplegia without pupillary changes. Kearns–Sayre syndrome is a mitochondrial myopathy that presents with the triad of age <20 years, CPEO and retinitis pigmentosa. Other associated features include cerebellar syndrome, cognitive impairment, Babinski's sign, hearing loss, seizures, short stature and delayed puberty, with other endocrine abnormalities and cardiac conduction defects.

Oculopharyngeal dystrophy (see Scenario 10) is an autosomal dominant trinucleotide repeat disease occurring in 60–70 year olds, with progressive ptosis and ophthalmoplegia without pupillary changes, leading to dysphagia and facial weakness, and in the latter stages of disease to proximal muscle weakness.

Cavernous sinus syndrome

Structures contained within the cavernous sinus:

- Internal carotid artery
- Sympathetic carotid plexus
- Cranial nerves: III, IV, VI and V1 and V2 branches (V3 lies outside the sinus).

Cavernous sinus syndrome signs:

- Painful ophthalmoplegia (unilateral single or usually combined nerve III, IV and VI palsies)
- Horner's syndrome (with no associated anhidrosis because the lesion occurs after the superior cervical ganglion and the pupil may be mid-position and fixed with both parasympathetic and sympathetic disruption)
- Anaesthesia of forehead, maxilla and conjunctiva (V1 and V2 branches)
- Proptosis (if pulsating suggests carotid–cavernous fistula)
- Conjunctival injection with chemosis
- Papilloedema ± visual loss
- Orbital bruit.

Differential diagnosis of cavernous sinus syndrome

- **Tumours**: meningiomas, extension of pituitary or craniopharyngiomas, metastatic disease
- **Vascular**: cavernous sinus aneurysms or fistulae
- **Thrombosis**: usually complicating infection of the ethmoid, frontal and sphenoid sinuses or extension of dental or orbital infection
- **Inflammatory**: herpes zoster, sarcoidosis and Wegener's granulomatosis
- **Idiopathic**: Tolosa–Hunt syndrome is a rare granulomatous inflammation of the cavernous sinus and superior orbital fissure. It causes a painful ophthalmoplegia ± pupillary effects.

Clinical judgement and maintaining patient welfare

Investigations

- These are urgent if an aneurysm, subarachnoid haemorrhage (SAH), uncal herniation, meningitis, stroke or trauma is suspected.
- **Imaging**: CT or MRI of the brain is indicated if suspecting aneurysmal, SAH, stroke, space-occupying lesion ± herniation, or traumatic cause. Cerebral angiography may be needed to investigate aneurysmal disease and arteriovenous (AV) malformations including fistulae.
- **Blood tests**: investigations for small-vessel disease will include fasting blood glucose/HbA1c, autoimmune profile, pANCA and cANCA, ESR and CRP if suspecting giant cell arteritis (GCA).
- **Lumbar puncture**: indicated if suspecting meningitis, and a space-occupying lesion has been ruled out.

Management

This is directed by the underlying cause.

Nerve III (oculomotor) palsies may resolve spontaneously over months if the underlying cause is ischaemia (typically in hypertensive or diabetic patients) of the vasa nervosa. This typically gives relative sparing of the pupil and is often painful for unknown reasons. NSAIDs may ameliorate this. Patching of the deviated eye can be a useful short-term measure. In the long term, surgical correction may be indicated for a non-resolving stable angle.

Nerve IV (trochlear) palsies have been treated successfully with botox injection (of other muscles), prisms and surgical correction.

Nerve VI (abducens) palsies, when isolated in children and young patients, are often benign and resolve spontaneously within 6 months. The cause is unclear. Alternate patching may be useful to prevent amblyopia. In older patients GCA should be considered and treated with steroids if appropriate.

The examiner's instruction is usually to examine the cranial nerves/visual fields and proceed as appropriate. A visual field defect will form part of a wider diagnosis and it is important to examine for associated PNS signs.

A good understanding of the anatomy of the visual field pathway will enable correct localisation of the lesion and help direct the rest of the examination for associated clinical signs (see Figure 3.27).

Visual pathway anatomy

Each **optic nerve** carries visual information from both halves of the visual field of the **ipsilateral** eye. Thus unilateral lesions in front of the optic chiasma cause **ipsilateral** visual field defects in **one** eye.

The nasal optic nerve fibres, carrying temporal visual field information, decussate at the chiasma and thus **anything behind the chiasma** (optic tract, lateral geniculate nucleus (LGN), optic radiation and visual cortex) receives fibres from **both** eyes, relating to the **contralateral** half of the visual field. These visual field defects are **homonymous**, indicating that the same side of the visual field is affected in **both eyes**. The congruity (symmetry) of homonymous visual field defect lesions increases with more posterior lesions. Thus optic tract lesions tend to give incongruous homonymous hemianopias and, after the LGN, optic radiation lesions tend to give congruous visual field defects.

Lesions *at* the optic chiasma, where fibres decussate, will cause different fields in each eye to be disrupted, so these are not homonymous. Thus, a medial compressive lesion from below (eg from an expanding pituitary tumour) will affect nasal fibres from both eyes, creating a bilateral temporal/bitemporal hemianopia. Compressive lesions from outside the optic chiasma will cause unilateral or bilateral nasal hemianopia.

The **upper** half of the visual field forms images on the lower half of the retina. Fibres from the lower part of the retina travel in the **temporal** lobes (Meyer's loop) in the optic radiations. The **lower** half of the visual field forms images on the upper half of the retina. Fibres from the upper part of the retina travel in the **parietal** lobes in the optic radiations.

Due to the importance of the macula for visual acuity it has disproportionately large representation in the LGN and visual cortex. The macula is represented in the most posterior part of the occipital pole and can be spared in occipital lesions.

Homonymous hemianopia (eg right sided)

Identifying clinical signs
On confrontation testing of the peripheral visual fields there is loss of the right visual field in both eyes, a **right homonymous hemianopia**. This indicates a left-sided lesion behind the chiasma, from the optic tracts to the occipital visual cortex. The more congruous the field loss, the more posterior the lesion.

Differential diagnosis
- Cerebrovascular event: look for a right-sided hemiparesis, UMN facial palsy, with possible dysphasia. Examine for associated signs such as AF, a pacemaker or carotid bruit, and ask to measure the BP.
- Tumour: examine for papilloedema and other cranial nerve and cerebellar signs. Ask to palpate the scalp, feeling for scars and step deformity, and look for a shunt.
- Trauma.

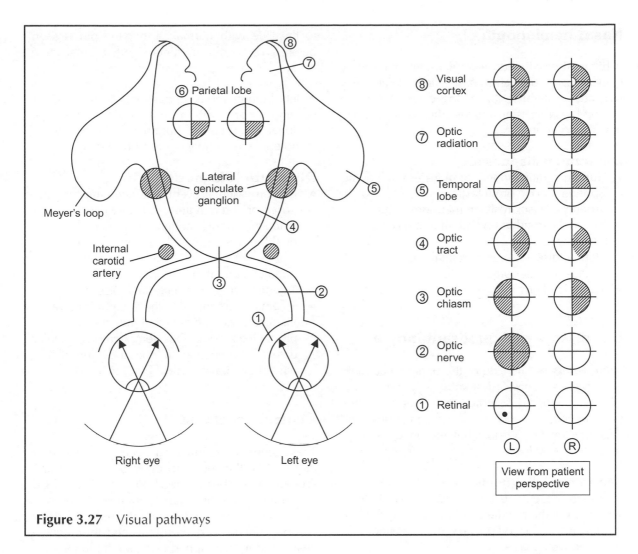

Figure 3.27 Visual pathways

Bitemporal hemianopia

There is **loss of the temporal fields** in both eyes, pointing towards a lesion at the optic chiasma. Be careful not to confuse tunnel vision with a bitemporal hemianopia by careful checking of the upper, lower and nasal fields.

Differential diagnosis
- Tumour: pituitary tumours from below initially affect nerve fibres from the lower retina serving the upper visual fields, so field loss will progress from top to bottom. In

craniopharyngiomas and suprasellar meningiomas pressing from above the field, loss progresses from bottom to top. Metastatic disease may also affect the chiasma. Look for papilloedema, cranial or nasal scars, and signs of acromegaly (see Station 5).
- Aneurysm: anterior communicating artery aneurysms can compress the optic chiasma from above, causing initially a bitemporal inferior quadrantanopia, which progresses to full bitemporal hemianopia.
- A unilateral nasal field defect

Nasal hemianopia

A bilateral nasal field defect is usually caused by glaucoma. A unilateral nasal field defect may indicate a lateral lesion at the chiasma causing bilateral compression against the flanking internal carotid artery.

Differential diagnosis
* Tumours: meningioma from lesser wing of the sphenoid bone or metastases
* Aneurysms: sclerosis or aneurysm of the internal carotid artery lateral to the optic chiasma
* Retinal disease: branch retinal artery or vein occlusion, chorioretinitis
* Chronic glaucoma.

Upper/superior quadrantanopia

There is loss of one side of the upper visual field in both eyes (sometimes known as 'pie in the sky' symptom). This indicates a lesion on one side behind the chiasm (as homonymous) and affecting Meyer's loop within the optic radiation of the temporal lobe.

Differential diagnosis
* Cerebrovascular event: ischaemia within the region of the middle cerebral artery which may also affect Wernicke's area, causing receptive aphasia
* Tumour: astrocytomas or metastases
* Trauma: accidental or iatrogenic secondary to surgery.

Homonymous hemianopia with macular sparing (eg left sided)

There is loss of the left half of the visual field in both eyes but with macular sparing.

Macular sparing is detected by careful testing of the central portion of the visual field. Moving a red pin slowly from the side with visual field loss to the side with normal vision, the pin is seen before crossing the midline, signifying that there is macular sparing.

A left homonymous hemianopia with macular sparing occurs with a lesion within the right occipital visual cortex, but anterior to the occipital pole where the macula is represented.

Differential diagnosis
* Cerebrovascular event: infarction affecting the posterior cerebral artery territory causes macular sparing, thought to be related to the dual blood supply of the occipital pole, which is also served by a branch of the middle cerebral artery
* Tumour: primary or metastatic disease
* Trauma: blunt injury to the occiput is more likely to affect the occipital **pole** thus producing a congruous homonymous macular defect. If both occipital lobes are injured the patient can have cortical blindness.

Central scotomata

These tend to be unilateral because they are at the level of the retina or optic nerve. A central scotoma describes a small loss of visual field within the centre of vision surrounded by normal vision, and visual acuity is usually reduced. They can be difficult to demonstrate and the affected area needs to be mapped using a red pin.

Differential diagnosis
* Optic neuritis: in addition to central scotoma on visual field testing, there is disc swelling on fundoscopy, RAPD and reduced visual acuity (VA). Eye movements can be painful. Causes include: MS, syphilis and vasculitic disease, so look for associated signs such as INO, cerebellar disease, joint disease, rashes and tender non-pulsatile temporal arteries indicating GCA.
* Optic atrophy: fundoscopy shows disc pallor, with severely reduced VA and a RAPD. Causes include MS, frontal tumours,

Friedreich's ataxia, advanced retinitis pigmentosa, advanced syphilis, advanced glaucoma and advanced Leber's optic atrophy. Foster Kennedy's syndrome describes the changes seen with a frontal tumour (usually olfactory groove meningioma or metastasis), which presents with ipsilateral optic atrophy, central scotomata and anosmia with contralateral papilloedema (from raised ICP).

- Age-related macular degeneration (ARMD): a major cause of blindness in older people, with pathology starting at the macula and progressing outwards. There are 'dry' and 'wet' forms. Dry ARMD describes the appearance of yellow drusen between the retina and the choroid layer behind, which can lead to retinal detachment, whereas the more severe wet form describes vessels growing up from the choroid behind the retina, leading to retinal detachment. It can be treated with laser coagulation or regular injection of anti-VEGF (anti-vascular endothelial growth factor) into the vitreous.
- Genetic: Leber's atrophy and Stargardt's disease.

Peripheral scotomata

These tend to be unilateral because they are at the level of the retina or optic nerve. A peripheral scotoma describes a small loss of visual field surrounded by normal vision. Visual acuity is usually intact in the early stages because the macula is unaffected.

Differential diagnosis

- Glaucoma: fundoscopy shows an increased cup:disc ratio. A peripheral scotoma can progress to tunnel vision with sparing of central vision until severe disease can eventually threaten sight completely.
- Branch retinal artery occlusion can produce peripheral scotoma or unilateral quadrantanopias. Central retinal artery occlusion will cause unilateral complete loss

of vision. Look for a pale area of the retina on fundoscopy.
- Branch retinal vein occlusion is similar to above, except pathology in the venous drainage will cause flame haemorrhages in the affected area.
- Retinitis pigmentosa (see Station 5): visual loss starts at the periphery and there will be fundoscopic changes.
- Chorioretinitis: causes include toxoplasmosis, cytomegalovirus, syphilis and onchocerciasis, and usually there is an underlying diagnosis of HIV.

Clinical judgement and maintaining patient welfare

Investigations are determined by the suspected location of the lesion. This is why clinical determination of the nature of the visual field defect is crucial. Bedside confrontation testing is usually adequate to determine the nature of the visual field defect, and therefore the likely site of the lesion. However, more accurate mapping of a visual defect may be useful to monitor progression/regression with treatment.

Goldman perimetry uses a static or kinetic light source on the background of a white bowl and tests the entire visual field. The **Amsler grid** tests only the central 20° of the visual field and is used predominantly to assess macular vision.

Imaging with CT or MRI of the brain forms a central part in diagnosis of lesions that are localised posterior to the orbit, eg aneurysmal, SAH, stroke, space-occupying lesion ± herniation or a traumatic cause. Cerebral angiography may be needed to investigate aneurysmal disease and AV malformations including fistulae.

Blood tests: investigations for small-vessel disease will include fasting blood glucose/HbA1c, autoimmune profile, pANCA and cANCA, ESR and CRP, if suspecting GCA.

Management

This is directed at the underlying cause. Visual field defects after stroke can be managed with compensatory scanning training (also useful for visual neglect) and/or prisms, although there is little evidence that these impact substantially on activities of daily living.

Dysphasia describes an acquired deficit with the understanding and/or production of language. It is distinct from dysarthria, which solely describes pathology in the motor production of speech.

Dysphasia could be encountered in the PACES examination as part of the assessment in a specific diagnosis such as stroke or MND, or may arise as part of the examiner's broader line of questioning.

Identifying physical signs

There are four domains of language that can be quickly screened in the PACES examination to identify the type of dysphasia:

1. **Fluency**: Does the patient's speech flow with the normal patterns of undulations and sentence length? Non-fluent speech will be halting with short phrases or single words and will lack the normal melody of speech. Ask patients to describe their journey to the examination centre or what they had for breakfast.
   Example: '... coming to the house ... and there ... inside here ... sitting ... tree sometimes ...'
2. **Comprehension**: Is the patient able to understand language, starting with simple commands that can be built up to multilevel commands? Do not ask the patient to try to do something that he or she is physically unable to do because then you will not be assessing comprehension.
   Example:
   'Can you take this piece of paper?'
   'Can you take this pen and put it on the table please?'
   'Can you take this piece of paper, put it on the floor and then put your foot on top of it?'
3. **Repetition**: Is the patient able to repeat phrases accurately? This function requires intact connections between language comprehension and production.
   Example: repeat 'seven cats are sitting on seven mats' or 'no ifs, ands or buts'.
4. **Naming**: Are patients able to name common objects shown to them? If they are unable to name them, can they agree or disagree with correct or incorrect suggestions as you propose them?
   Example: show patients a pen and ask them to name it. If they appear to understand the question but propose incorrect suggestions, then ask them: 'Is it a ball?', patient: 'no'; 'Is it a key?', patient: 'no'; 'Is it a pen?', patient: 'yes'.

Other common language patterns in the different types of dysphasia are:

- **Paraphasias**: these are substitutions of part or the whole of a word with phonemically or semantically related sounds or words.
  Example:
  'Can I have a smork [fork]?'
  'The cat [dog] likes the bone.'
- **Neologisms**: these are new words (mostly used as nouns) constructed by the patient.
  Example: 'I will have some plipper please.'
- **Agrammatism**: patients omit function words from their sentences which become shorter **telegraphic** phrases – collections of nouns, verbs and adjectives but with no structure or relationships between them.
  Example: 'two run ... house ... yes ... the man ... red car ... rain ... run ...'

Additional findings
After identifying a dysphasia it is important to proceed to examine for associated signs to determine a unifying diagnosis. Look for visual field defects and visual neglect, and associated motor and sensory dysfunction in the limbs (see below).

The language deficits can be used to determine the type of dysphasia and the neuroanatomical site of the lesion. Language centres reside in the dominant hemisphere. The left hemisphere is dominant in >95% of right-handed individuals and also in >70% of left-handed individuals. Thus you can expect to see right-sided motor weakness together with dysphasia and, when one is present, it should prompt assessment for the other.

Figure 3.28 shows the language centres in a left dominant hemisphere. Broca's area is in the inferior frontal gyrus, Wernicke's area in the superior temporal gyrus, and between the two runs the arcuate fasciculus. It is a simplification but the arcuate fasciculus can be thought of as bridging between the receptive Wernicke's area and the motor Broca's area.

Receptive/Sensory dysphasia (Wernicke's dysphasia)

Speech is **fluent** with normal length sentences but with **nonsense content** and examples of **paraphasias** and **neologisms**. The patient has **reduced comprehension**, cannot follow simple commands and has **impaired repetition**. It can be difficult to assess repetition and naming ability due to the lack of comprehension. The patient appears calm and shows **anosognosia** (lacking awareness of the language deficit).

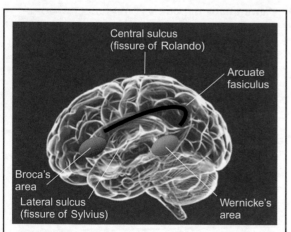

Central sulcus
(fissure of Rolando)

Arcuate
fasiculus

Broca's
area

Lateral sulcus
(fissure of Sylvius)

Wernicke's
area

Figure 3.28 The language centres in a left dominant hemisphere

The lesion is in Wernicke's area in the dominant superior temporal gyrus or its connections. This is in the area served by the inferior division of the left MCA.

Examine the cranial nerves with particular attention to the visual fields looking for a right-sided homonymous upper quadrantanopia seen with temporal lobe lesions ('pie in the sky'). Depending on the cause and extent of the lesion there may be right-sided weakness and sensory deficits.

Expressive/Motor dysphasia (Broca's dysphasia)

Speech **is non-fluent** and **halting** with **agrammatism**. The patient has mostly **intact comprehension** as shown by an ability to follow commands and correct identification of an object's suggested name; however, there may be deficits in comprehension of more complex sentence constructions. The patient is **aware** of the language deficit, which can cause great frustration when he or she tries to find the correct words. **Repetition is impaired**.

The lesion is in Broca's area in the dominant inferior frontal gyrus or its connections. This is the area served by the superior division of the left MCA.

Examine the cranial nerves and limbs looking for UMN right-sided facial and limb weakness.

Conduction dysphasia

Speech is **fluent** and there is **intact comprehension** with the patient able to follow commands. There is **impaired repetition** and the patient has **difficulty with naming** objects. The **patient is aware** of the language deficit and can become frustrated.

The lesion is in the dominant hemisphere within the arcuate fasciculus or its connections. This is an area in the left inferior parietal lobe served by the inferior division of the left MCA.

Examine the cranial nerves including the visual fields looking for a right-sided homonymous hemianopia or a right-sided inferior quadrantanopia. In the visual field examination, look for signs of visual neglect. Depending on the extent of the lesion there may be a right-sided hemiparesis.

Global dysphasia
Speech is **non-fluent** and **halting** and with **nonsense content** and **paraphasias** and **neologisms**. The patient has **impaired repetition and naming**. The patient may or may not be aware of the language deficit.

The lesion is in the dominant hemisphere affecting both Broca's and Wernicke's areas. This size of lesion is usually caused by an ischaemic or haemorrhagic stroke associated with the left MCA.

Look for right-sided homonymous hemianopia and right-sided UMN facial and limb hemiparesis and sensory loss.

Transcortical sensory dysphasia
This presents as for Wernicke's sensory dysphasia but repetition is intact.

The lesion is in the dominant hemisphere near to Wernicke's area in the inferior posterior temporal gyrus. This is in a watershed area between the left MCA and the left posterior cerebral artery.

There may be right-sided homonymous hemianopia and a right-sided hemiparesis.

Transcortical motor dysphasia
This presents as for Broca's motor dysphasia but **repetition is intact**.

The lesion is in the dominant hemisphere superior to Broca's area near the pre-motor cortex. This is in a watershed area between the left MCA and the left anterior cerebral artery.

Examine the limbs for a right-sided hemiparesis.

Differential diagnosis

- Stroke is the most likely cause of all types of dysphasia.
- Trauma: haemorrhage or contusions secondary to traumatic head injury.
- Tumour: dysphasia could occur with primary or metastatic disease.
- Infection: viral encephalitis (eg herpes encephalitis), bacterial meningitis or abscess, fungal abscess, mycobacterial meningitis, Lyme disease, toxoplasmosis could all cause various types of dysphasia along with other systemic signs of infection.
- MS (see Scenario 1): a rare cause of dysphasia and one would expect to detect additional neurological signs.

Clinical judgement and maintaining patient welfare

Investigations and management
See the related scenarios pertinent to underlying causes for more details.

Speech and language therapy provides the backbone of dysphasia management.

SCENARIO 25. BULBAR AND PSEUDOBULBAR PALSY

Bulbar and pseudobulbar palsy are most likely to be seen in the PACES examination as part of the assessment for dysarthria in the integrated clinical assessment (ICA) station (Station 5) or within the context of the assessment of stroke, MND or MS.

Bulbar palsy refers to impaired function of the lower cranial nerves IX–XII, the nuclei of which are in the medulla, leading to problems with speech production and swallowing. More broadly, bulbar palsy is now taken to mean impairment of cranial nerves V, VII and IX–XII, all of which can affect speech, swallowing and lower facial movements, from disease within the brain stem, peripheral cranial nerves, neuromuscular junction or muscles that they innervate.

In contrast, pseudobulbar palsy describes a UMN lesion within the corticobulbar tracts that synapse on these lower cranial nerves IX–XII, also producing dysarthria and difficulties with swallowing.

Identifying physical signs

Also see Station 5 for assessment of dysarthria.

Bulbar palsy
Speech
There is a **flaccid dysarthria**. The voice is **weak and quiet**. There is a **nasal quality** to speech. The weak wasted tongue has particular difficulty **articulating lingual and labial consonants**.

Cranial nerve examination
Examine the lower cranial nerves first. Look for a **weak wasted tongue** with **fasciculations**. Ask the patient to protrude the tongue, then push the tongue against your hand when inside the cheek. These tongue movements are weak. Inspect the palate with the patient saying 'ahh'; there will be **unilateral/bilateral palatal weakness**. Tell the examiner that you would test for a **reduced gag reflex**. Feel for the muscle bulk of the masseters

and note **weak jaw opening** against resistance. The **jaw jerk is absent**. There may be **weak shoulder shrug** and head turn (LMN nerve XI). There may be LMN facial weakness. Examine eye movements for an INO if considering syringobulbia. Look for ptosis and fatigue with upward gaze, which may represent myasthenia gravis as a cause of bulbar palsy.

Upper and lower limb examination
Examine for mixed UMN and LMN signs in the limbs if considering MND. Look for the association of wasting of the small muscles of the hands with UMN weakness in the upper and lower limbs, and sensory dissociation seen with syringobulbia.

Pseudobulbar palsy
Remember that there are bilateral signs with pseudobulbar palsy because there is bilateral cortical innervation of the cranial nerves except for cranial nerves VII and XII.

Speech
There is a **spastic dysarthria**. The voice is **harsh** and **sounds strangled**. There is a nasal quality to speech.

Cranial nerve examination
The **tongue is small and stiff** with attempted movements from side to side. The jaw may hang open and there is **a brisk jaw jerk**. There may be signs of a bilateral UMN facial weakness. This is difficult to ascertain because usually we think of upper facial sparing with UMN lesions, but with bilateral UMN lesions upper and lower facial movements will be affected. Examine the eyes looking for an INO, nystagmus and/or optic atrophy if considering the diagnosis of MS.

Upper and lower limb examination
Look for UMN and LMN signs in the limbs if considering MND. With bilateral cerebral vascular disease there will be bilateral UMN signs.

Look for cerebellar signs in the limbs if considering MS.

Additional
There can be **emotional lability** with pseudobulbar palsy, expressed as spontaneous and involuntary laughing or crying.

Differential diagnosis

Bulbar palsy
* Motor neuron disease
* Syringobulbia
* Brain-stem stroke
* Brain-stem tumour
* Poliomyelitis
* Guillain–Barré syndrome
* Diphtheria
* Myasthenia gravis.

Pseudobulbar palsy
* Motor neuron disease
* Multiple sclerosis
* Bilateral neurovascular disease
* Tumour of the pons.

Clinical judgement and maintaining patient welfare

Both bulbar and pseudobulbar palsies are syndromes associated with other underlying conditions. Investigation and management of these are described in the relevant scenarios.

Patients should be referred to neurologists and may require admission if there are nutritional issues related to dysphagia. Physiotherapy to modify posture may improve drooling and prevent aspiration. Input from speech and language therapists and dieticians is essential.

SCENARIO 26: BRAIN-STEM SYNDROMES

These rarely come up in the PACES examination but strike fear into most candidates. With some basic knowledge of the neuroanatomy of the brain stem and a confident neurological examination the assessment of brain-stem syndromes can become an enjoyable challenge. The candidate (and examiner) is not expected to know an exhaustive list of brain-stem syndromes, but instead should be able to demonstrate a methodological approach to illicit the physical signs and form a differential diagnosis.

P Gates* describes an excellent 'rule of four' for understanding how brain-stem anatomy relates to the vascular brain-stem syndromes. This is not a complete presentation of the neuroanatomy of the brain stem but acts as a guide to help localise lesions from the clinical presentation.

The 'rule of four' (adapted from P Gates):

1. There are four medial structures in the brain stem (**m** for **m**edial):
   motor pathways (corticospinal/pyramidal tracts)
   medial lemniscus (becomes the dorsal columns)
   medial longitudinal fasciculus (MLF)
   motor nuclei (LMN) as in (4) and their ipsilateral nerves.
2. There are four lateral structures in the brain stem (**s** for **s**ide):
   spinothalamic pathways
   spinocerebellar pathways
   sympathetic tract
   sensory nucleus of cranial nerve V (this is a large nucleus extending from the midbrain down to the upper cervical cord).
3. There are four cranial nerve nuclei in the medulla, four in the pons and four above the pons (two in the midbrain, nuclei of cranial nerves III and IV).
4. There are four motor nuclei in the midline (dividing into 12) – III, IV, VI and XII – and

the remaining nuclei with motor components – V, VII, IX and XI are situated laterally in the brain stem.

The MLF has ascending and descending fibres and these include links between the cranial nerve nuclei controlling extraocular eye movements (III, IV and VI) and the vestibular nucleus (VIII) to coordinate head and eye movements. The MLF also yokes the opposite cranial nerve III and VI nuclei to enable conjugate horizontal gaze, which is disturbed in INO.

Remember that the motor/pyramidal tracts and dorsal columns decussate at the level of the medulla, the spinothalamic tracts cross within one to two levels of entering the spinal cord, and spinocerebellar, sympathetic tracts and the cranial nerves (which are LMNs) serve ipsilateral structures. Thus lesions within the brain stem give rise to 'crossed signs' (discordance between cranial and peripheral neurology).

If we combine the above 'rule of four' mnemonic with knowledge of the anatomy of the circulation to the brain stem and upper cervical cord (Figure 3.29) then we have a sound basis for approaching brain-stem clinical syndromes.

Identifying physical signs

Lateral medullary syndrome (Wallenburg's syndrome), eg left sided
Cranial nerve examination
There is a **left-sided Horner's syndrome** with ptosis and meiosis. There are normal extraocular eye movements but there is a **horizontal nystagmus** with a fast component to the left, worse on lateral gaze to the left. There is **left-sided reduced facial sensation to pinprick** (pain and temperature), but normal sensation to light touch. There are normal facial movements. There is **left-sided palatal weakness** (LMN nerve X palsy). There is a diminished/

---

* Gates, P. (2005). The rule of 4 of the brainstem: a simplified method for understanding brainstem anatomy and brainstem vascular syndromes for the non-neurologist. *Internal Medicine Journal*, 35: 263–266 doi: 10.1111/j.1445-5994.2004.CD732

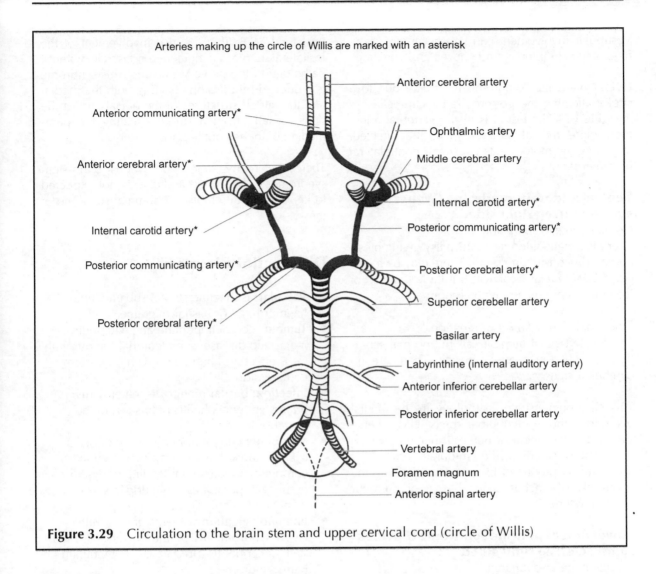

Arteries making up the circle of Willis are marked with an asterisk

- Anterior cerebral artery
- Anterior communicating artery*
- Ophthalmic artery
- Middle cerebral artery
- Anterior cerebral artery*
- Internal carotid artery*
- Internal carotid artery*
- Posterior communicating artery*
- Posterior communicating artery*
- Posterior cerebral artery*
- Superior cerebellar artery
- Posterior cerebral artery*
- Basilar artery
- Labyrinthine (internal auditory artery)
- Anterior inferior cerebellar artery
- Posterior inferior cerebellar artery
- Vertebral artery
- Foramen magnum
- Anterior spinal artery

Figure 3.29   Circulation to the brain stem and upper cervical cord (circle of Willis)

absent gag reflex (LMN nerve IX and X palsy). Tongue movements are normal (intact nerve XII). There is weakness of left sternocleidomastoid and trapezius (LMN nerve XI palsy).

Note: in the examination it is best to state that you would assess the gag reflex but this may be uncomfortable for the patient.

Upper and lower limb examination
There is **right-sided impairment of sensation to pinprick** (pain and temperature), but normal sensation to light touch. There is no motor weakness.

There are **left-sided cerebellar signs** in the upper and lower limbs.

The above case demonstrates pathology in the sympathetic, spinocerebellar, spinothalamic tracts and sensory component of cranial nerve V. Thus using the 'rule of four' we can identify this as a lateral brain-stem syndrome. Involvement of the lower cranial nerves IX–XI places this at the level of the medulla, so these signs are consistent with a left-sided lateral medullary syndrome.

Vestibular involvement can cause vertigo, dizziness, vertical diplopia, and nausea and vomiting.

Lateral medullary syndrome is usually due to a stroke affecting the posteroinferior cerebellar artery (PICA). If the lesion is in the vertebral artery then more medial structures can be affected, including the motor tracts causing a contralateral hemiparesis.

Ventral midbrain syndrome (Weber's syndrome), eg right sided

Cranial nerve examination
There is **a right-sided nerve III palsy** giving ptosis and a non-constricting pupil. There may be a **left-sided UMN facial weakness** but the remainder of the cranial nerve examination is normal.

Upper and lower limb examination
There is **left-sided hemiparesis** but normal sensation to light touch and pinprick. There are no cerebellar signs.

This case demonstrates pathology in the medial pyramidal and corticobulbar tracts (UMN nerve VII) and involvement of nerve III nucleus, and is consistent with a right-sided midbrain lesion. This syndrome is produced by a stroke affecting the paramedian branches of the basilar or posterior cerebral arteries.

Lower dorsal pontine syndrome (Foville's syndrome), eg right sided

Cranial nerve examination
There is a right-sided **nerve VI palsy** with failure to abduct the right eye looking to the right. There is a right-sided **INO** with failure to adduct the right eye when looking towards the left, but there is normal adduction on convergence. There is a right-sided **LMN nerve VII palsy** with ipsilateral facial weakness.

Upper and lower limb examination
There is contralateral left-sided hemiparesis.

This case demonstrates pathology in the right medial pyramidal tracts and involvement of the

ipsilateral MLF. There is also involvement of the ipsilateral nerve VII nucleus or fascicle without pathology in the nerve V nucleus. This syndrome is produced by a lesion affecting both the medial and the lateral structures of the dorsal part of the pons, usually from a stroke affecting the paramedian branches of the basilar artery.

There are many more eponymous brain-stem syndromes, which the candidate is not expected to know in detail; Table 3.7 summarises some of these.

Differential diagnosis

- **Vascular**: ischaemic stroke, subarachnoid haemorrhage or basilar migraine
- **Tumour**: cerebellopontine angle tumours, metastatic disease, supratentorial tumour with mass effect and herniation with brain-stem compression
- **Infection**: basilar meningitis, enterovirus brain-stem encephalitis or abscess of the posterior fossa
- **Metabolic**: central pontine myelinolysis (CPM), (caused by over-rapid correction of chronic hyponatraemia, leading to dysarthria, dysphagia, paraparesis, quadriparesis or coma) and Wernicke's encephalopathy
- **Immunological**: myasthenia gravis, Miller–Fisher syndrome (MFS) and Bickerstaff's brain-stem encephalitis (BBE) variants of Guillain–Barré syndrome
- **Demyelinating disease**: MS
- **Trauma**: vertebral artery dissection.

Clinical judgement and maintaining patient welfare

Investigations
- **Imaging**
  - **CT of the head**: can rule out haemorrhagic stroke, supratentorial tumour, brain metastases or abscess.
  - **MRI of the head**: more sensitive for the

Table 3.7 Summary of brain-stem syndromes

Eponymous syndrome	Location	Clinical signs		Vascular supply
		Ipsilateral	Contralateral	
Weber's	Midbrain (ventral)	Nerve III palsy	UMN nerve VII palsy (±) Hemiparesis	Basilar and posterior cerebral artery
Benedikt's	Midbrain (dorsal)	Nerve III palsy	Cerebellar (tremor, ataxia)	Basilar and posterior cerebral artery
Millard–Gubler	Pons (medial)	Nerve VI and VII palsies	Hemiparesis	Basilar artery paramedian branches
Raymond's	Pons (ventral medial)	Nerve VI palsy	Hemiparesis	Basilar artery paramedian branches
Foville's	Pons (dorsal)	Nerve VI and VII palsy INO	Hemiparesis	Basilar artery paramedian branches
Wallenburg's	Medulla (lateral)	Nerve V sensory (pain and temperature) Horner's syndrome Cerebellar (nystagmus, limb ataxia) Nerve IX–XI palsies	Hemisensory loss (pain and temperature) Hemiparesis (±)	Posteroinferior cerebellar artery Vertebral artery (±)
Dejerine	Medulla (medial)	Nerve XII palsy	Hemisensory loss (vibration and proprioception) Hemiparesis	Branches of anterior spinal and vertebral arteries

INO, internuclear ophthalmoplegia.

diagnosis of early ischaemic stroke, demyelination and posterior fossa pathology, including brain-stem stroke. MR angiography (MRA) may be indicated if vertebrobasilar dissection is suspected, especially in younger patients presenting with brain-stem infarction.

- **Blood test**: FBC, U&Es, LFTs, ESR, (fasting) lipids and glucose:
  - In younger patients or those without recognised cardiovascular risk factors, consider lupus anticoagulant, anticardiolipin antibodies and a thrombophilia screen.
- **Lumbar puncture**: provided that an intracranial mass has been ruled out, a lumbar puncture would be indicated for investigation of autoantibodies associated with Guillain–Barré syndrome variants, oligoclonal bands seen with demyelinating disease or CSF analysis for suspected meningitis or encephalitis.

SCENARIO 27: CEREBELLOPONTINE ANGLE LESION

This has rarely presented at the PACES examination but it is an important differential diagnosis to consider in the presence of cranial nerve palsies.

Identifying physical signs (eg left-sided lesion)

Cranial nerve examination
There is a left **lateral gaze palsy** with the patient experiencing **diplopia** on looking to the left (**nerve VI palsy**). There is **nystagmus** on trying to look to the left with the fast component towards the left. There is **reduced sensation to light touch and pinprick on the right side of the face** (**nerve V palsy**). The patient has **upper and lower facial weakness** on the left (**LMN nerve VII**) and there is reduced muscle bulk of the masseters and temporalis on the left side with attempted jaw clench, and on opening the mouth the **jaw deviates towards the left side** (pushed over by the intact right pterygoid) (**LMN nerve V**). There is a **reduced/absent jaw jerk**. The patient may be wearing a hearing aid and there is reduced hearing on the left side to whispered numbers (**nerve VIII palsy**). The remainder of the cranial nerve examination is normal.

Upper and lower limb examination
The patient has an **ataxic gait** falling towards the left. Examination of the upper and lower limbs reveals normal tone, power, sensation and reflexes, but left-sided **dysdiadochokinesis with past pointing** and **uncoordinated heel–shin testing** on the left (**cerebellar disease**).

Additional
Inform the examiner that you would test the **corneal reflex** and expect it to be reduced on the left. Ask to examine with an auroscope to check for any vesicles in the outer ear and the patency of the external auditory canal. Also check that there are no vesicles on the soft palate (considering Ramsay Hunt syndrome). Perform **Weber's test**, which would **lateralise to the right** (sensorineural hearing loss on the left) and perform **Rinne's test** which would show **air conduction better than bone conduction (AC > BC) bilaterally**. Ask to perform a visual survey of the skin looking for café-au-lait spots and neurofibromas, and take a family history (association with neurofibromatosis type II).

Advanced disease: as the cerebellopontine angle (CPO) lesion expands there is involvement of the lower cranial nerves. There is a unilateral palatal palsy, reduced gag reflex and a hoarse voice (nerve IX and X palsies), unilateral weakness of the tongue (nerve XII), and weakness in trapezius and sternocleidomastoid (nerve XI) on the affected side. The patient may have bilateral papilloedema as drainage for the fourth ventricle becomes obstructed and hydrocephalus develops.

Differential diagnosis

- **Tumour**: the vast majority of CPO lesions are caused by vestibular nerve schwannomas (thus the alternative name acoustic neuroma is a misnomer). Other tumours include: meningiomas, epidermoid tumours, facial nerve schwannomas, medulloblastomas, brain metastases. Benign bilateral vestibular nerve schwannomas are associated with neurofibromatosis type II (NFII, see Station 5), an autosomal dominant disease caused by mutations in the tumour-suppressor merlin gene on chromosome 22.
- **Brain-stem syndromes**: a brain-stem syndrome would present with crossed long tract signs and there would be a history of acute onset typical of a vascular event.

- **Ramsay Hunt syndrome**: reactivation of dormant varicella-zoster virus infection affecting the geniculate ganglion within the facial nerve canal causes Ramsay Hunt syndrome. Typical features include pain within the auditory canal associated with a zoster rash around the external auditory canal and/or soft palate. There is ipsilateral LMN facial weakness; there may be an associated trigeminal neuralgia and reduced hearing with tinnitus and balance problems.
- **Sensorineural deafness**: the most common cause is presbycusis of advancing age. Other acquired causes include infections such as mumps, measles and meningitis, ototoxic drug use including aminoglycosides (eg gentamicin), loop diuretics or amphotericin, and trauma to the temporal bone.

Clinical judgement and maintaining patient welfare

Investigations
- **Gadolinium-enhanced MRI**: MRI is the best form of imaging for the posterior cranial fossa.
- **Audiogram**: will show sensorineural hearing loss.

Management
- Vestibular nerve schwannomas can be very slow growing and the neurosurgical team along with the patient may choose a watch-and-wait approach.
- Stereotactic surgery ± radiotherapy is a definitive treatment option depending on the tumour size, type of deficit, patient choice and local neurosurgical expertise.
- Patients with a diagnosis of NFII will require genetic counselling and family screening.

SCENARIO 28: JUGULAR FORAMEN SYNDROME

Jugular foramen syndrome (JFS) has rarely presented at the PACES examination, but it is an important differential diagnosis to consider in the presence of lower cranial nerve palsies.

Knowledge of the basic anatomy helps in understanding the physical signs. As shown by Figure 3.30, cranial nerves IX–XI, along with the posterior meningeal artery and sigmoid sinus, which becomes the internal jugular vein, exit from the jugular foramen. The jugular foramen tends to be larger on the right due to the greater venous sinus drainage on the right, so lesions from compressive disease are more common on the left. Nearby, cranial nerve XII exits from the hypoglossal canal and the facial and vestibulocochlear nerves (nerves VII and VIII) enter the internal acoustic meatus.

Identifying physical signs (eg right-sided lesion)

Cranial nerve examination

There is a right **palatal palsy**, the **uvula is deviated** towards the left side on saying 'ahhh' and the **gag reflex is reduced/absent**, consistent with **right-sided nerve IX and X palsies**. There is reduced taste on the posterior third of the tongue if formally tested. There is a **flattened shoulder** on the right side with **weakness in trapezius** on attempted shoulder shrug. **Weak sternocleidomastoid muscles** are seen on the right when trying to turn the head to the left side against resistance, consistent with a right-sided **nerve XI palsy**. The tongue has a normal appearance and movements. The remainder of the cranial nerve examination is normal.

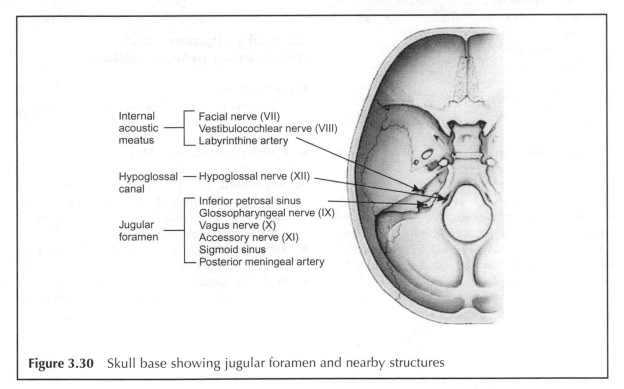

Internal acoustic meatus — Facial nerve (VII) / Vestibulocochlear nerve (VIII) / Labyrinthine artery

Hypoglossal canal — Hypoglossal nerve (XII)

Jugular foramen — Inferior petrosal sinus / Glossopharyngeal nerve (IX) / Vagus nerve (X) / Accessory nerve (XI) / Sigmoid sinus / Posterior meningeal artery

Figure 3.30   Skull base showing jugular foramen and nearby structures

Upper and lower limb examination

There are no peripheral signs.

Additional

Look specifically for involvement of the hypoglossal nerve XII, other brain-stem structures such as the sympathetic tracts with an ipsilateral Horner's syndrome, involvement of the trigeminal sensory nucleus with ipsilateral facial numbness and 'crossed signs' in the PNS.

Differential diagnosis

There are several eponymous syndromes associated with lower cranial nerve involvement from pathology in the skull base foramina; sometimes JFS is used as a broad term to describe any pattern of involvement of the lower four cranial nerves:

- **Vernet's syndrome**: this is jugular foramen syndrome proper involving cranial nerves IX–XI.
- **Collet–Sicard syndrome**: involvement of cranial nerves IX–XI and XII, usually from an extracranial lesion.
- **Villaret's syndrome**: involvement of cranial nerves IX–XII and the cervical sympathetic chain.

Glomus jugulare tumour: this is the most common cause of JFS and is a rare form of vascular tumour called a paraganglioma, which is composed of neural tissue and arises within the temporal bone. These tumours can produce catecholamines and thus present with symptoms similar to phaeochromocytoma. Most commonly they present with tinnitus and hearing loss followed by lower cranial nerve involvement. These can be hereditary with an autosomal dominant pattern.

Other tumours include meningiomas or neurofibromas of the lower cranial nerves, metastatic disease or extension of a locally destructive cholesteatoma.

Trauma: basal skull or temporal bone fracture.

Infection: otitis media spreading to the posterior fossa and temporal bone, retroparotid abscess or cephalic herpes zoster.

Vascular: thrombosis of the sinus–jugular junction, aneurysm of the internal carotid artery.

Brain-stem syndromes: a brain-stem syndrome would present with crossed long tract signs and there would be a history of acute onset typical of a vascular event.

CPO lesions: extending CPO lesions can involve the lower cranial nerves.

Clinical judgement and maintaining patient welfare

Investigations

- **Skull radiography** may show erosion of the temporal bone or enlargement of the jugular foramen.
- **Gadolinium-enhanced MRI**.

Management

- This depends on the cause of the JFS but in the case of glomus tumours surgical excision is the definitive treatment.
- Radiotherapy can be used in larger tumours or in frailer patients.
- In glomus tumours, a course of α- and β-blocker medication may be required before surgery to prevent catecholamine surge.

This occasionally presents at the PACES examination and it is an important differential diagnosis to consider in the presence of lower motor neuron signs in the limbs.

Poliomyelitis is caused by poliovirus types 1–3, which are RNA enteroviruses. Type 1 is responsible for 85% of polio cases. It is spread through faeco-oral transmission. The virus replicates in the nasopharynx and GI tract. It can initially present with a viral prodrome with diarrhoea and signs of upper respiratory tract infection. Spread to the CNS leads to destruction of the motor neurons within the spinal cord and brain stem.

Identifying physical signs (eg right lower limb)

General observation
Look around the bed for **walking aids**, **adapted shoes** or a **wheelchair**. Note the age of the patient because cases of old polio in the UK will be seen among older generations who became infected in the pre-immunisation era. Polio most commonly affects the lower limbs in an asymmetrical fashion.

Upper and lower limb examination
The right **leg is severely wasted** with evidence of **contractures** at the knees and ankles and **pes cavus**. There are scars around the ankle joint (from tendon transfer or arthrodesis). There are **no fasciculations**. There is **reduced tone** in the right leg and **weakness** in all muscle groups. The **knee and ankle reflexes are absent** and there is **no plantar response**. Coordination cannot be tested in the right limb in the context of marked weakness. **Sensation to all modalities is normal** in the right leg. Examination of the left leg and upper limbs is normal.

Differential diagnosis

There are several polio clinical syndromes (Table 3.8).

Post-polio syndrome (PPS) can occur up to 40 years after initial polio infection and is estimated to affect 30–60% of those who have had acute infection. The underlying mechanisms are not known but patients present with new-onset muscle weakness and atrophy, pain and fatigue.

Table 3.8 Polio clinical syndromes

Group	Poliomyelitis syndrome	Clinical features
Minor	Abortive	90% are asymptomatic or minor self-limiting viral symptoms
Major	Non-paralytic	Fever, pharyngitis, gastrointestinal symptoms or meningism
	Paralytic spinal	Flaccid paralysis in the limbs
	Paralytic bulbar	Often seen in infants with facial weakness, dysphagia and hoarseness
	Paralytic spinal and bulbar	Often seen in adults with short-lived bulbar symptoms
	Encephalitis	Rare presentation with confusion and coma and has a high mortality

Infantile hemiplegia is seen in cases of cerebral palsy – an umbrella term describing a non-progressive brain lesion acquired in the perinatal period that can have motor, sensory and cognitive effects. In reviewing adults who have suffered with infantile hemiplegia the affected lower limb(s) will be grossly growth stunted and exhibit pyramidal weakness rather than LMN signs.

ALS/MND: there would be both LMN and UMN signs with fasciculations and the neurological findings would tend to be bilateral.

Lumbosacral myelopathy: compressive myelopathy in the lumbosacral region from either degenerative spine disease or extramedullary tumours can cause a unilateral lower limb weakness but this would produce LMN signs at the site of the lesion and UMN signs below the lesion. Antero-lateral lesions can behave like a hemisection of the cord and produce Brown–Séquard syndrome, describing ipsilateral pyramidal weakness, loss of light touch, proprioception and vibration sense, and contralateral loss of pain and temperature sensation.

HIV-related myelopathy: this would usually present bilaterally and with UMN weakness, and may be associated with dementia.

Multiple sclerosis could present with unilateral limbs weakness but this would present with a UMN pattern and there are almost always brain lesions with cranial nerve signs in the presence of spinal cord disease.

Peripheral neuropathy tends to present symmetrically and be length dependent, with more advanced distal than proximal signs together with sensory neuropathy.

Acute flaccid paralysis: in the acute stages of polio presenting with flaccid paralysis important differentials would include:

- **Infection**: Japanese encephalitis, non-polio enterovirus, varicella-zoster virus, tetanus infection, botulism, diphtheria, Lyme disease, paralytic rabies
- **Spinal disease**: acute transverse myelitis, spinal shock and spinal cord infarction, epidural abscess
- **Neuropathy**: Guillain–Barré syndrome
- **Toxins**: lead poisoning, curare poisoning
- **Iatrogenic**: vaccine-associated paralytic poliomyelitis, acute traumatic sciatic neuritis after gluteal injection.

Clinical judgement and maintaining patient welfare

Investigations
Virology: isolation of polio virus from stool, upper respiratory or CSF specimens. PCR analysis can be used to determine if infection is with wild-type or vaccine-related virus strain.

Lumbar puncture: CSF analysis will show increased protein and lymphocytosis. Investigations for acute flaccid paralysis will include analysis for oligoclonal bands seen with MS or autoantibodies associated with Guillain–Barré syndrome.

Neuroimaging: MRI of the spinal cord and brain will show inflammation of the spinal cord and help rule out demyelination.

EMG: can show characteristic findings in paralytic polio or PPS.

Management
There is no cure for polio and in the acute stages management is supportive with regular neurological monitoring and preparation for intubation in severe cases.

Ongoing care for paralytic polio or symptoms of PPS requires a multidisciplinary approach including orthopaedic input for joint surgery.

SCENARIO 30. INVOLUNTARY MOVEMENTS AND HUNTINGTON'S DISEASE

There are several ways of categorising involuntary movements (Table 3.9). Often several types of involuntary movement can be present in one patient.

Identifying physical signs

The case below describes the physical features of Huntington's disease.

General observation

The patient may appear **fidgety**. There are **continuous involuntary movements at rest** that affect different body parts in a **random** order, which can appear **'dance like'.** The patient may try to mask the chorea by **incorporating the jerks into purposeful movements**. There are occasional more striking, involuntary limb movements **(hemiballismus)**. The **chorea is exacerbated by activity**, such as asking the patient to pick something up off the table. **Motor impersistence** can be seen when shaking the patient's hand – the grip strength alternates ('milkmaid's grip'), and there is non-sustained attempted tongue protrusion or eye closure.

Cranial nerve examination

This may be normal or there could be impaired smooth pursuit when examining eye movements.

Table 3.9 Types of involuntary movement

Movement type	Clinical features
Hypokinesia or bradykinesia	Insufficient movement
Hyperkinesia or dyskinesia	Too much movement
Jerky movements	
Myoclonus	Sudden, brief, non-rhythmic shock-like movements
Chorea	Continuous, random and distributed, non-rhythmic movements which can be 'dance like'. May show motor impersistence with inability to sustain an action
Ballismus	Proximal, large amplitude, choreatic movements
Tics	Stereotyped movements associated with urge
Non-jerky movements	
Dystonia	Sustained abnormal postures with muscle contraction
Athetosis	Distal mobile dystonias; can be writhing
Tremor	Rhythmic alternating movement with changes in amplitude but fixed frequency

Disturbed saccadic movements may cause the patient to turn the head when asked to follow a moving finger with the eyes, or to blink repeatedly, thereby breaking fixation. The patient may have **slurred dysarthria**.

Upper and lower limb examination

Tone may be reduced. Power is usually preserved and **deep tendon reflexes may be reduced or exaggerated**. The plantar response is usually downward. There are **no sensory changes**. There may be a **broad-based ataxic gait**, made more unsteady with involuntary movements. There may be additional **bradykinesia** with impaired initiation of voluntary movement and **postural instability**.

Additional

Request to **test cognition** and take a **drug history**.

Differential diagnosis of chorea

- Vascular:
  - Cerebrovascular disease
  - Chronic subdural haematoma
- Inherited:
  - Huntington's disease
  - Wilson's disease
  - Spinocerebellar ataxias
- Infectious:
  - HIV
  - Subacute sclerosing panencephalitis
  - Lyme disease
  - Creutzfeldt–Jakob disease
- Endocrine:
  - Chorea gravidarum
  - Thyrotoxicosis
  - Hypoparathyroidism
- Autoimmune:
  - Sydenham's chorea
  - Systemic lupus erythematosus
  - Paraneoplastic syndromes
- Drugs:
  - Dopamine antagonists
  - Levodopa
  - Lamotrigine
  - Methadone
  - Lithium
  - Combined oral contraceptive pill.

Huntington's disease

Huntington's disease is an autosomal dominant neurodegenerative disease caused by expansion of a CAG trinucleotide repeat sequence within the gene that encodes the huntingtin protein. The abnormal huntingtin protein cross-links and is resistant to degradation. It is not known how this accumulation of abnormal huntingtin protein leads to Huntington's disease but it is thought to interfere with normal cellular function including mitochondrial metabolism. Neuronal loss is seen within the striatal areas of the putamen and caudate nucleus, in addition to changes within the cerebral cortex, globus pallidus, subthalamic nucleus and cerebellum.

Clinical onset is usually between the ages of 30 and 50 years, but shows anticipation within families. Clinical features include chorea, ataxia, dystonia, personality changes, cognitive impairment and psychiatric symptoms. Death usually occurs within 15 years of disease onset.

Clinical judgement and maintaining patient welfare

Investigations

Genetic testing: CAG repeat testing can provide a definitive diagnosis and has predictive potential for future offspring.

MRI: may show striatal atrophy.

Management

There are no disease-modifying treatments but depressive symptoms can be treated, and to some extent the movement and behavioural disorders can be helped.

Depression is treated along standard lines:

- Behavioural symptoms can be treated with antipsychotics such as olanzapine or mood stabilisers.
- Chorea can be treated with tetrabenazine.

- As disease progresses, bradykinesia and rigidity overtake chorea symptoms and dopamine agonists can be used.

The treating team should advise patients on relevant issues as necessary, such as work, driving, long-term care, family planning and counselling, preimplantation genetic testing and advanced directives.

STATION 4

The Communication and Ethics Examination

COMMUNICATION SKILLS AND ETHICS STATION

Many candidates feel that they are already skilled in communication and do not prepare adequately for this station. Communication in this context is more than an exchange of information. A common mistake is to forget that you are being assessed not only on imparting information in a clear and empathetic manner but also on listening and adapting to the information that you are given by the patient or relative as the interaction progresses.

A key principle is that complex ideas or concepts must be addressed only once understanding of more basic or straightforward information has been established. The ideal candidate should guide and 'build' the interaction towards the main goal of the consultation.

Doing this naturally yet speedily is a difficult skill that requires practice. An overly formulaic approach can be hackneyed and irritating for both examiner and patient. For example, although it is essential to establish at the beginning of any consultation what your participant already knows and understands, robotically invoking the infamous 'ICE' acronym by asking 'What are your ideas, concerns and expectations?' risks immediately extinguishing any rapport with your participant.

In difficult scenarios, some decision may be required of the patient or relative which may be difficult for them to come to terms with, eg asking a taxi driver to stop driving and inform the DVLA of his recent suspected epileptic fit. This requires not only building understanding but also shepherding the patient towards a sensible course of action. Done properly, this demands highly advanced communication skills, avoiding confrontation and allowing individuals to reach a difficult or emotionally challenging conclusion themselves by building a 'proximal scaffold'. (Educational psychologist Lev Vygotsky's scaffolding theory describes a supportive framework

of incremental concepts that helps a person build his or her own permanent system of understanding. It avoids didactic delivery of facts or concepts that can be readily recited by a learner but not necessarily believed or understood.)

For example:

Doctor: *'One really important thing we should talk about is the dangers of losing consciousness suddenly and unexpectedly like this again in the future, which has probably been playing on your mind. Things like swimming alone, for example, should be avoided, for obvious reasons. Riding a bike would be very risky to yourself and to pedestrians. There has been a case where a patient who had a seizure while cycling knocked over and seriously injured a small child, and as you can imagine this was devastating for him.'*

Pause

Patient: *'I suppose this means I shouldn't drive then, doctor.'*

This chapter covers all the types of scenarios that a candidate may be expected to deal with and suggests a 'build' for each one. This covers the 'Clinical communication skills' and 'Managing patients' concerns' elements of the marking scheme.

However, you are also expected to have some knowledge of both medical ethics and medicolegal issues pertaining to everyday clinical practice. In addition, candidates are asked to explain common procedures and obtain consent for specific situations. This is assessed in the 'Clinical judgement' and 'Maintaining patient welfare' elements of the marking scheme. This requires some essential knowledge which is covered in each relevant scenario.

Communication skills and ethics: common scenarios

Ethics is traditionally taught at medical school within a framework of four principles: *autonomy* (the right to self-determination), *beneficence* (promote the wellbeing of others), *non-maleficence* (do no harm) and *justice* (the fair distribution of resources). Although this may be a useful checklist if asked to consider the ethical considerations of a specific case, it is otherwise of limited use for success in this station.

The following categories provide a more useful means of tailoring the way in which you build the discussion according to the type of scenarios that commonly arise.

End-of-life decisions and breaking bad news

These account for around a third of all cases and just under half of these involve a discussion with a relative rather than the patient. The cases vary from telling a family member that a relative has died suddenly, to giving a patient the results of a diagnostic test with major implications for their future.

Approach
Almost invariably, these scenarios begin with breaking bad news. This is usually not the only task at hand; often a difficult choice must also be explained and a decision sought. A common error is to do these three things in the wrong order.

Common scenarios

- Brain-stem death and organ donation
- Do not attempt resuscitation (DNAR) decisions
- An unexpected death and request for a postmortem examination
- Clinical deterioration and enactment of advanced directives

Negotiating a plan

It is not unusual for a patient or relative to have objections to some or all of a treatment plan, or request an alternative treatment that he or she wishes to pursue. Negotiating an agreed action

plan within the boundaries of a patient's best interests is a common PACES scenario and can be one of the most challenging. Alternatively, scenarios may involve taking consent for a proposed procedure. Candidates should know how these procedures are performed and the risks associated with them. Often these cases involve an ambivalent or nervous patient.

Approach
Classic negotiation skills, as taught in business schools (eg anchoring an aggressive starting position beyond your actual requirements), are counterproductive here. You are working within tight ethical and legal boundaries centred around the best interests of your patient, with little room for manoeuvre. As in all cases, start by establishing what the patient understands already and identify the root source of their concern or disagreement. It is often a simple misunderstanding that is readily resolved. Failing to convince a relative or patient of a plan of action is not equivalent to failing the station.

Common scenarios

- Relative disagrees with management plan
- Patient disagrees with management plan
- Consent for an investigation or treatment

Errors and complaints

These scenarios encompass failings and shortcomings – real, perceived or potential – in the care provided to a patient. They often involve talking to a relative rather than the patient.

Approach
In some scenarios there has been a clear professional failure; in other cases you will have limited information about an alleged shortcoming or mistake. No matter how emotionally charged the scenario becomes, remain calm and avoid the three Cs at all costs:

- **C**onfrontation ('You're being a little unreasonable')

- Collusion ('I know, you're right, the nurses are awful on this ward')
- Confabulation ('We are normally very good at this procedure at this hospital').

As with all other scenarios, begin from the patient/relative's understanding of events. Prioritise the concerns and deal with the easiest first. Make sure that the consultation ends with a plan for addressing both the immediate clinical shortcoming and further investigation of how it came about and how it can be improved.

Common scenarios

- Dealing with issues of potential neglect or abuse by a colleague or team
- Discussing a mistake made by the medical team with a patient or relative
- Explaining why an expensive treatment may not be available through NHS funding

Complex explanations

In these scenarios, candidates have to convey complex or multiple concepts about a condition to a patient or relative.

Approach

Many candidates mistakenly confuse this scenario with an assessment of their knowledge of a given condition and proceed to tell the individual everything they know about it. This is not the task at hand and a barrage of superfluous or confusing information is a sure way to fail. As in all scenarios, information must be conveyed incrementally, building on a person's current understanding until this is sufficient to make informed choices about his or her care.

Common scenarios

- Explanation of a diagnosis with multiple treatment options
- Diagnoses with uncertain/unpredictable outcomes
- Diagnoses with complex implications for the patient and others

Confidentiality and third parties

It is often the case in the communication skills station that the main subject of the discussion is not in the room. Obtaining crucial information from a relative or friend without divulging confidential details about the patient can be difficult. In some scenarios, information emerges in which a third unknown party is at risk. In others, a wider responsibility to the general public may conflict with a duty of confidentiality to the patient.

Approach

It is crucial in discussions with relatives to identify what they are already aware of (and can therefore be discussed cautiously within limits) and what they are not (wherein discussion would break confidentiality). Risking confidentiality to protect a third party is a major threat to the patient–doctor relationship. It is best to first explain any risk to others and seek cooperation from the patient in order to mitigate risk to others while preserving confidentiality. It is unusual in PACES to encounter a person who wishes to protect his or her confidentiality at all costs once you have explained the potential risks to others.

Common scenarios

- Contact tracing a third party who may have been exposed to a sexually transmitted infection
- Informing the DVLA of impaired fitness to drive
- General approach to the communication skills station for PACES

Part 1: 5 minutes outside the room to read the provided instructions

Work out what type of category this scenario falls into (**end-of-life decisions, negotiating a plan, errors and complaints, complex explanations, confidentiality and third parties**). Read the instructions very carefully and start to design your 'build' of the key information that needs to be conveyed. Establish the hierarchy of the information that you wish to convey, deciding which information or news cannot be absorbed or understood until a foundation of more basic information has been established. Invariably the foundation of any discussion is what the patient knows and understands already; *this must be the first thing that you clarify in any interaction.*

A classic example is approaching the issue of organ transplantation with a relative of a patient who has just been diagnosed with brain-stem death. In this scenario, approaching the issue of organ transplantation is futile unless the concept of brain-stem death has been adequately conveyed. A less dramatic example is obtaining consent for a procedure. It is impossible to understand or weigh the risks and benefits until these and the basic principles of the procedure have been explained.

Part 2: The interview – 15 minutes (including 1 minute to gather one's thoughts at the end)

Introduce yourself and explain your role.

Build the discussion
Establish the expectations and knowledge of the patient with open questions. Establish why this patient has presented to you at this particular time, eg 'We've not met before but I understand you have come today to talk about your kidney problems. What do you know already about what is going on?'.

Key principles

- Allow pauses for patients to digest information
- It is far better for the patient to have secured one or two key facts rather than a huge jumbled blur of information

Under certain circumstances it is reasonable not to cover all the possible information from the instructions, or even not to reach the 'goal' of the consultation towards which you were building, eg discussing resuscitation status in a patient who is clearly in shock after being told that the cancer has returned may need to be delayed.

Before finishing
- Summarise the consultation
- Try to give the patient choices rather than instructions
- Ask if the patient wants anything repeated or has any questions
- Ask if there are any important issues that have not been covered
- Make a shared management plan for the future
- Arrange another appointment if necessary.

Gathering thoughts – 1 minute
Order the information in your mind and anticipate the likely discussion points with the examiners.

Part 3: 5 minutes of discussion with examiners
The following issues are likely to be discussed:

- How you think it went: good areas and bad areas?
- Things that could be done differently
- What you think the patient has understood
- How you would approach follow-up consultations
- Which areas were not covered
- Have the needs of the patient been met?
- Legal and ethical issues surrounding the case
- Further management and follow-up arrangements.

Communication skills and ethics scenarios

1. Breaking bad news and organ donation

2. Breaking bad news and DNAR decisions

3. Breaking bad news and requesting a postmortem examination

4. Breaking bad news and advance directives

5. Consent for a procedure

6. Relative disagrees with management plan

7. Patient disagrees with management plan

8. A medical error

9. Request for a treatment not available through the NHS

10. Neglect or abuse by a colleague

11. Diagnosis with multiple treatment options

12. Diagnosis with uncertain/ unpredictable outcomes

13. Diagnosis with implications beyond the patient

14. Informing the DVLA of impaired fitness to drive

15. Risking confidentiality for public/third party protection

END-OF-LIFE SCENARIOS

SCENARIO 1. BREAKING BAD NEWS AND ORGAN DONATION

'You have been looking after a 28-year old man on ICU since he was knocked off his bicycle 1 week ago. He has been on a life support machine since admission. You have agreed with the father the need to do brain-stem tests and he has made an appointment with you to discuss the results. The tests have confirmed that his son is brain-stem dead.

'Please inform the father of the results and discuss organ donation with him. The son did carry a donor card (which is 11 years old), but no advanced directive, and he is not on the national register of organ donors.'

Clinical judgement and maintaining patient welfare

The Human Tissue Act 2004 and code of practice

If those close to the deceased person object to the donation, for whatever purpose, when the deceased person has explicitly consented, the healthcare professional should seek to discuss the matter sensitively with them. They should be encouraged to accept the deceased person's wishes and it should be made clear that they do not have the legal right to veto or overrule those wishes. The emphasis in these difficult situations

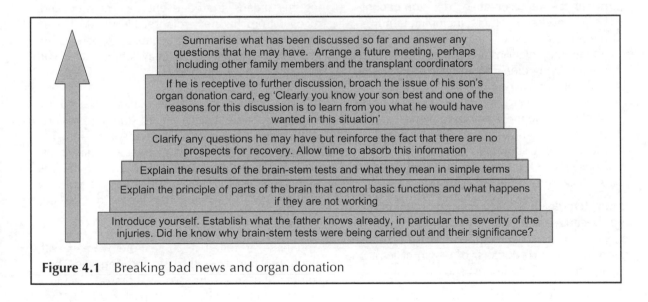

Figure 4.1   Breaking bad news and organ donation

should be placed on having an open and sensitive discussion with those close to the deceased where the process is explained fully to them. Healthcare professionals should also consider the impact of going ahead with a procedure in light of strong opposition from the family, despite the legal basis for doing so.

Somewhat conflictingly, the final sentence suggests that it is valid for physicians to ignore the deceased's wishes if they fear that it will be detrimental to a family in opposition, despite the fact that the family have no legal right to veto. In reality, therefore, although the legal requirement of relative's consent was removed by the 2004 act, few organ harvests go ahead when relatives strongly oppose it.

- If the deceased's wishes are unknown, the family or a person previously nominated by the deceased (a nominated representative) must give consent for organ donation. The nominated representative's decision cannot be overridden by others, including family members or next of kin.
- 'Qualifying relationships' for next of kin have the following hierarchy for giving or refusing consent: spouse/partner > parent or child > brother or sister > grandparent or grandchild > niece or nephew > step-father or stepmother > half-brother or half-sister > friend of long standing.
- Consent can be withdrawn up until the point of incision to retrieve the organs.

Brain-stem death is a key concept in organ donation because most organs for transplantation are harvested in this context. Assessment should be performed by two doctors, of whom at least one is a consultant. Criteria are as follows:

- Irreversible brain damage of known aetiology in the absence of depressant drugs, hypothermia, reversible endocrine/circulatory/metabolic/endocrine disturbance, muscle relaxants and cervical cord injury
- Fixed pupils unresponsive to light
- Absent corneal reflex

- Absent oculovestibular reflexes – no eye movements following the slow injection of at least 50 mL ice-cold water into each ear in turn (the caloric test)
- Absent response to supraorbital pressure
- Absent cough reflex to bronchial stimulation or gagging response to pharyngeal stimulation
- No respiratory effort in response to disconnection of the ventilator for long enough to ensure elevation of the arterial partial pressure of CO_2 to at least 6.0 kPa (6.5 kPa in patients with chronic CO_2 retention).

Variations

'You are about to discharge a 28-year-old man with primary progressive multiple sclerosis. He was recently admitted with a chest infection after a major relapse. He would like to discuss donating his organs in the event that he does not recover from his next relapse. He would like to make these wishes clear because his parents are Jehovah's witnesses and may object to organ donation on religious grounds.'

'A 54-year-old man with liver metastases from a resected pancreatic carcinoid tumour has recently been assessed for liver transplantation. The transplant committee have decided that transplantation would be unlikely to extend his lifespan more than 2 years and therefore will not add him to the waiting list. Please discuss this with him.'

'You have admitted a 29-year-old woman with alcohol-related liver disease and end-stage liver failure. She has had two withdrawal seizures, having drunk heavily for the past 2 weeks, then stopped abruptly 2 days ago. Her notes indicate that she is on a liver transplant waiting list at another hospital. The transplant team will need to be informed of this admission and there is a strong chance that she will be de-listed as a consequence. Please discuss this with her.'

SCENARIO 2. BREAKING BAD NEWS AND DNAR DECISIONS

'An 80-year-old man, previously alert and independent, has been brought in with a massive haemoptysis. He has been resuscitated and stabilised, and bronchoscopy has revealed a probable bronchial carcinoma, but histology is awaited. Ultrasonography shows multiple liver metastases but an enhanced CT head scan is normal. He remains acutely confused but his wife is understandably anxious and wishes to know what is going on. Your consultant has decided that he should not be for resuscitation in the event of a cardiac arrest and she would like you to discuss this with his wife. She has as yet been given very little information.'

Clinical judgement and maintaining patient welfare

DNAR decisions are frequently made summarily without proper consultation with the patient or relatives. Reasons for a DNAR order can be divided into two broad categories:

1. Resuscitation would be unsuccessful
2. If successful, the burdens of prolonging life would outweigh the benefits.

The former is a purely clinical decision, the latter only partially so. The expected level of recovery, awareness and likelihood of unmanageable pain if CPR is successful are all matters for clinical judgement. However, every patient and relative will weigh these factors against their subjective perception of the benefits of prolonged life, so their wishes and beliefs are of paramount importance.

* On the face of it, a DNAR order for 'an octogenarian with metastatic lung cancer and massive haemoptysis' may seem a straightforward decision. However, the most likely cause of a cardiorespiratory arrest in this case would be further bleeding, which should be reversible. The presence of incurable metastatic cancer does not mean that CPR itself will be futile. Furthermore, his confusion should resolve and his quality of

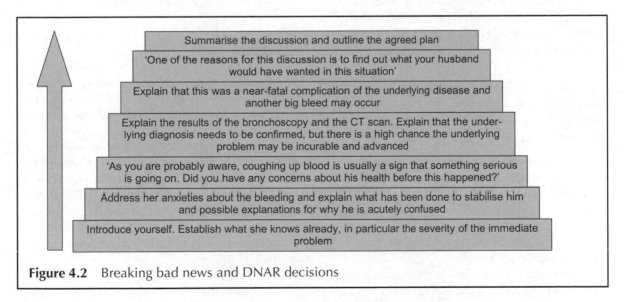

Figure 4.2   Breaking bad news and DNAR decisions

life before admission was good. The bleed or its treatment may or may not result in pain, although the progression of his cancer certainly could. But will this be *unmanageable* pain? There is no coherent argument for age as a valid independent factor in a DNAR decision.

- Clearly, the patient's (or relative's) wishes need to be explored rather than being simply 'informed' of the DNAR decision. This is often uncomfortable or distressing for both doctor and patient and thus commonly avoided (or, as in this case, delegated). The consultation may end with the wife expressing strong opposition to a DNAR order, in which case you should arrange a further discussion between her and the consultant. Remember, the overall clinical responsibility for decisions about DNAR orders rests with the most senior clinician in charge of the patient's care. Although you may fear disappointing them (or the examiners) for inadequately 'making the case', remember that, where the burdens and benefits of prolonged life must be weighed, understanding of the wishes and beliefs of the patient and/or relative is essential. Also, most consultants would rather be aware of patient/relative's wishes or beliefs that conflict with their initial judgement.

Other key points from the British Medical Association (BMA), Resuscitation Council and Royal College of Nursing (RCN) joint statement on DNAR orders (2007) are as follows:

- Decisions about CPR must be made on the basis of an *individual* assessment of each patient's case.
- Advance care planning, including making decisions about CPR, is an important part of good clinical care for those at risk of cardiorespiratory arrest.
- It is not necessary to initiate discussion about CPR with a patient if there is no reason to believe that the patient is likely to suffer a cardiorespiratory arrest.

- Where no explicit decision has been made in advance there should be an initial presumption in favour of CPR.
- If CPR would not re-start the heart and breathing, it should not be attempted. Neither patients, nor those close to them, can demand treatment that is clinically inappropriate. However, a second opinion should be offered.
- Where the expected benefit of attempted CPR may be outweighed by the burdens, the patient's informed views are of paramount importance. If the patient lacks capacity, those close to the patient should be involved in discussions to explore the patient's wishes, feelings, beliefs and values.
- A DNAR decision does not override clinical judgement in the unlikely event of a reversible cause of the patient's respiratory or cardiac arrest that does not match the circumstances envisaged.
- If a patient with capacity refuses CPR, or a patient lacking capacity has a valid and applicable advance decision refusing CPR, this should be respected.
- DNAR decisions apply only to CPR and not to any other aspects of treatment.

Variations

'A 56-year-old man with motor neuron disease has been admitted with type 2 respiratory failure. He is having intermittent non-invasive positive pressure ventilation. The consultant from the ICU has assessed him and believes that he would not benefit from intubation and ventilation should he deteriorate because successful weaning from a ventilator would be highly likely to fail. He has therefore suggested that the patient be made 'not for resuscitation', but has not discussed this with the patient. Please discuss resuscitation status with the patient.'

'A 96-year-old man has been admitted to A&E with a Glasgow Coma Score of 6/15. He was intubated by the anaesthetist on arrival and is now being mechanically ventilated. He is known to live alone with a helper who visits once a week to do cleaning and washing for him. The cause of his sudden decline is not yet known – a CT of the head has been arranged. Notes from his previous admission 2 months ago with a UTI include a DNAR form signed by the patient and consultant. His daughter would like nothing further to be done for him. Please discuss this with her.'

SCENARIO 3. BREAKING BAD NEWS AND REQUESTING A POSTMORTEM EXAMINATION

'The on-call team informs you that a 63-year-old man under your team's care died during the night. He was admitted 48 hours earlier with pneumonia and appeared to be stable. Unfortunately he deteriorated suddenly overnight and had an asystolic arrest. Attempted resuscitation was unsuccessful. The cause of death remains uncertain, although progressive pneumonia or pulmonary embolus is suspected. The daughter has been in close contact with her father during his admission, but was not contactable last night. She has arrived on the ward and has been seated in a private relatives room. She is unaware that her father has died.

'Please explain to her what has happened and discuss the possibility of a postmortem examination.'

Note that, in PACES, you are rarely required to break news of a death and then just manage the emotions that follow. You are usually also re-quired to impart a further piece of information (eg a drug error may be responsible for their relative's death), seek further information (eg was the patient at risk of neglect/abuse?) or make a request (eg organ donation or postmortem examination).

In real life, responses to sudden loss vary greatly. In PACES, the actor will typically have been instructed to cycle rapidly through disbelief/denial, anger/blame, then despair, and finally recover some degree of composure such that you have an opportunity to fulfil the additional aim of your task.

Disbelief/denial is usually managed by gently reinforcing or repeating the sequence of events. The anger/blame phase must be managed cautiously and sympathetically because it can be exacerbated by an evasive or defensive response, leaving you stuck and unable to complete the task at hand.

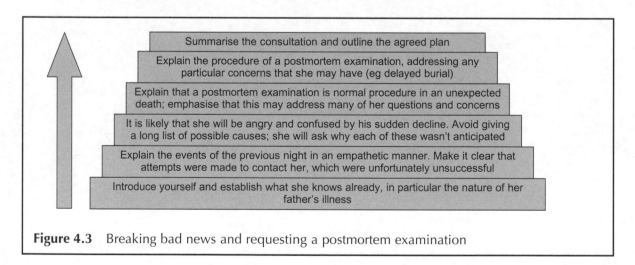

Figure 4.3   Breaking bad news and requesting a postmortem examination

Clinical judgement and maintaining patient welfare

Postmortem examinations or postmortems (PMs) can be requested by the hospital or the coroner.

Coroner requested PM

This usually follows referral to the coroner for the following reasons:

- If the death was sudden and unexpected.
- If the death was violent or unnatural, or if it occurred under suspicious circumstances.
- If the death was a result of an accident.
- If the death occurred during medical treatment or in hospital.
- If the doctor treating the deceased person had not seen him or her within 14 days before death.

If a coroner requests a PM then the consent of relatives is not required, nor can they countermand the coroner's instruction.

Hospital requested PM

Where establishing the cause of death may be useful to address relatives' concerns, for training or research purposes, or to determine a diagnosis that may have implications for the relatives (eg heritable conditions), the hospital may request a PM. In this situation the written consent of the relative is required.

PM is usually carried out within 3 days. The pathologist will usually accommodate requests, for religious reasons, to carry out a PM within 24 h.

Variations

'A 60-year-old man under your team's care deteriorated suddenly during coronary catheterisation for suspected LAD stenosis and could not be resuscitated. The cause of death is unclear. His daughter has told the nursing staff that she would like a full enquiry and wants a postmortem examination performed at a different hospital. Please discuss this with her.'

'An 84-year-old woman with known dementia was admitted under your team's care 14 days ago with confusion and multiple broken ribs. She developed pneumonia as an inpatient, which proved fatal despite antibiotics and non-invasive ventilation. Her son has requested the body be released for burial within 24 hours for religious reasons. Please discuss the need to inform the coroner of her death and the likelihood that a postmortem examination may be requested.'

'You are looking after a 74-year-old man who was admitted last night with a GI bleed. Subsequent endoscopy, which stopped the bleeding initially, has shown that this was due to a known underlying gastric carcinoma and a CT scan this morning has demonstrated widespread disease including brain metastases. He is a widower who has repeatedly stated that he does not want any intervention. His old notes have been obtained and include an advance directive that clearly stipulates that he does not want any intervention should he deteriorate, other than symptom control. He has not allocated lasting power of attorney to anyone. After the endoscopy he is confused and disoriented. Over the course of today, his haemoglobin has dropped 4 g/dL. His younger brother has arrived and would like to know the management plan.

'Please discuss this further with him.'

Clinical judgement and maintaining patient welfare

Situations where consent is not possible

Unconscious patients are unable to give the necessary consent required for treatment. Under these circumstances doctors can give emergency treatment if it is in the best interests of the patient, the 'doctrine of necessity'. The 2005 Mental Capacity Act made several key changes to the older Act:

- Advance directives became legally enforceable. However, patients can opt in or out only of specific future treatment opinions and cannot stipulate specific wants.
- It is a criminal offence to take advantage of someone with impaired capacity.
- The process for allocating management of financial affairs changed.
- There is a new code of practice for assessment and documentation of capacity which applies to all health professionals (see below).

There are five key principles of the Mental Capacity Act 2005:

1. Individuals have the right to make their own decisions and must be assumed to have capacity to do so unless it is proved otherwise.
2. Individuals must be supported to make their own decisions – people must be given all appropriate help before anyone concludes that they cannot make their own decisions.

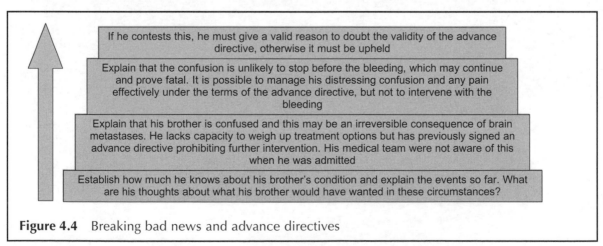

Figure 4.4   Breaking bad news and advance directives

3. Individuals must retain the right to make what might be seen as eccentric or unwise decisions.
4. Anything done for or on behalf of people without capacity must be in their best interests.
5. Anything done for or on behalf of people without capacity should be the least restrictive of their basic rights and freedoms.

Advanced directives are made prospectively in order to convey one's wishes on specific matters in case one is unable to give subsequent consent due to incapacity for whatever reason. They are recognised in law and must be respected as long as completed by a competent, witnessed adult. Patients should seek the help of a medical practitioner when completing an advance directive. Review of advance directives is recommended periodically.

Assessing capacity

Capacity is assessed in the context of a particular decision at a particular time. It is not a generic assessment of decision-making ability. There are two stages.

1. Diagnostic test
If it is suspected that there is impairment of mental function a diagnostic test with objective criteria must be applied to demonstrate this and the result documented (eg Mini-Mental State Examination or MMSE).

2. Functional test
- Can the individual **understand** the information relevant to the decision once information has been presented in a fashion relevant to the circumstances?

- Can the individual **retain** this information for long enough to make the decision? (Note: it is not necessary to retain the information until the proposed procedure takes place.)
- Can the individual **use and weigh the information** to arrive at a choice (which requires an understanding of the consequences)?
- Can the individual **communicate** the decision?

If the individual is unable to fulfil one of these criteria then he or she is deemed to lack capacity to make a decision.

Variations

'A 74-year-old woman has been admitted from her nursing home following general deterioration and not eating. She has advanced Alzheimer's disease. Her 44-year-old son has seen other patients at the nursing home fed through a percutaneous gastrostomy and would like this to be inserted as soon as possible because she is 'wasting away'. The medical notes include a letter written by the patient 5 years ago to her elderly care consultant indicating that she should not be fed artificially under any circumstances should she be unable to eat normally. Please discuss this with her son.'

'A 32-year-old man with cystic fibrosis has worsening lung function after his second lung transplantation 2 years ago. Chronic rejection has been difficult to control and he has been told by the consultant that he may require a third transplantation. He has discussed this with his wife and decided not to undergo transplantation again. He has some requests about his care in the future and wants to make sure that these are not ignored. Please discuss this with him.'

NEGOTIATING A PLAN

SCENARIO 5. CONSENT FOR A PROCEDURE

'A 21-year-old man has undergone extensive small bowel resection for Crohn's disease. He continues to lose weight despite overnight naso-gastric feeding and now requires supplemental parental nutrition. This will be administered through a tunnelled central venous (CV) subcla-vian line. Please consent him for the insertion procedure.'

Clinical judgement and maintaining patient welfare

Administering treatment to a patient of sound mind who has refused it is battery in law, whether or not physical injury occurs. Consent must be voluntary, informed and given by some-one who has capacity to make the decision. There are legal precedents in which each of these key aspects of consent have been contested.

- **Voluntary:** the decision must be made alone without coercion by staff, family or friends

- **Informed:** the patient must be informed of a procedure's benefits, risks and **alternatives**
- **Capacity:** see above.

The Bolam case (*Bolam v Friern Hospital Man-agement Committee* (1957) QBD) infers that doc-tors need not inform patients of risks if it is not common or accepted medical practice to do so. This was applied in the Sidaway case (*Sidaway v Bethlem Royal Hospital Governors and others* (1985) AC 871) in which a woman undergoing surgery for nerve root impingement suffered da-mage to the spinal cord and was rendered para-plegic. She was warned of the risk to the nerve root (approximately 2%) but not the spinal cord (<1%). The judge confirmed the duty of the doctor to provide adequate information, but ac-cepted that there is a limit to the range of information that can be given. A patient will never be 'fully' informed of the risks of nerve root release to the same degree as an experienced senior neurosurgeon, for example. This case re-sulted in the common assumption that risks <1%

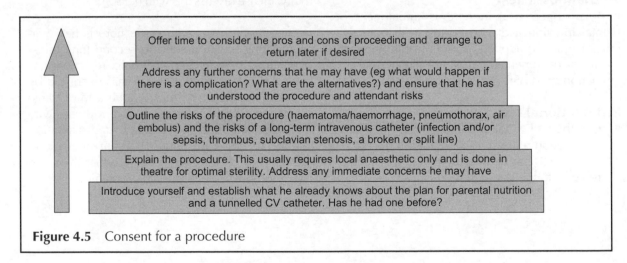

Figure 4.5   Consent for a procedure

need not be mentioned during the consent process. However, this has never been tested in case law. Quoted risk rates are subject to geographical variation and vulnerable to statistical scrutiny. Should, for example, the upper range of the confidence interval of the mean risk rate be lower than 1%?

The notion that a common or accepted medical practice should be an adequate defence (the Bolam test) was rejected in the more recent Bolitho case (*Bolitho v City and Hackney Health Authority* (1997) 3 WLR 1151). Here it was determined that a doctor must also be able to provide evidence of the good sense behind a decision, inferring that logical decisions and accepted practice are not always convergent.

In taking consent, for example, it may be prudent to warn of risks that are very small and not commonly mentioned, but may have dramatic consequences for the patient, eg warning a professional singer of the risk of recurrent laryngeal nerve injury with a tunnelled line insertion may be wise, despite the risk being well below 1%.

Rarely, in PACES, the proposed procedure will be unsuitable for the patient. More commonly, however, there is no such 'trick' in the scenario and the candidate is being tested simply on his or her ability to explain a complex concept in a concise and clear fashion. A classic error is to mention only the risks of the procedure (often with some precisely recalled statistics) and forget to mention the benefits or alternatives – all three are integral to making an 'informed' decision.

Variations

'This 45-year-old man, who is a hypertensive smoker, has had a recent exercise tolerance test which was positive (he does not know the result). He has had his blood pressure controlled and been advised to stop smoking. He will need coronary angiography. He has mentioned before that he was keen to avoid any invasive procedures after his sister died during a coronary bypass operation. Please discuss the result of the exercise test with him and the need for coronary angiography.'

'Ms Jones is a 55-year-old woman who was admitted with obstructive jaundice, and ultrasound scan and MRCP suggest that gallstones may be the cause although imaging also showed a mass in the head of the pancreas. She has been booked for an ERCP on tomorrow's list. There are no contraindications. Please discuss the ERCP procedure with her.'

SCENARIO 6. RELATIVE DISAGREES WITH MANAGEMENT PLAN

'An 84-year-old man has been admitted having been found confused at home. He lives alone in a warden-controlled flat. On admission 2 weeks ago he had an MMSE score of 1/10 but after treatment of his urinary tract infection this improved to 8/10. The medical and nursing staff think that he is safe to go home and he has been assessed by the occupational therapist and physiotherapist with a successful home visit. The patient wishes to return home, but his daughter is extremely concerned about him and 'refuses' to let him home. The daughter has made an appointment to see you to discuss her father, who has been deemed to have full capacity and given verbal consent for you to discuss any aspect of his case with her.'

Note: avoid confrontation at all costs – the

daughter has no legal right to veto her father's discharge, but it is clearly in his best interests to have an appropriate plan that she supports. The high readmission rate of patients after this kind of inpatient episode is testimony to how frequently the timing of discharge is misjudged.

Clinical judgement and maintaining patient welfare

Next of kin and lasting/enduring power of attorney

Next of kin (or 'nearest relative') can deputise another relative for this role or be reassigned by the patient. Next of kin do not have any legal rights or responsibilities for a patient except under the 2005 Mental Capacity Act, and these

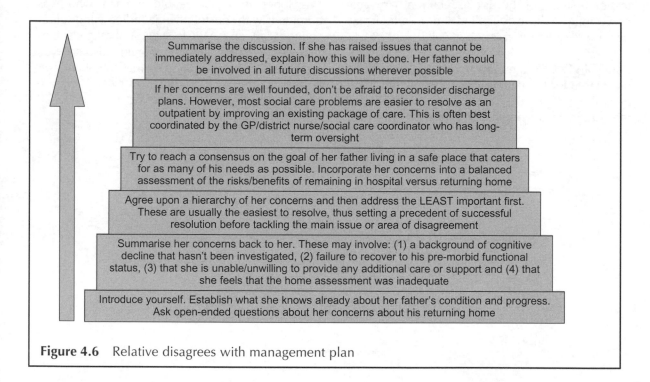

Figure 4.6   Relative disagrees with management plan

mostly relate to the right to be consulted and informed of detention of a patient under the 1983 Mental Health Act.

If mental capacity is impaired or fluctuating – as in this case – legal responsibility for the patient's wellbeing remains with the clinical care team (inpatient and outpatient).

If the nearest relative has applied for and been given lasting power of attorney by the Office of the Public Guardian, the situation is different. A relative with a lasting power of attorney can accept or refuse treatment on a patient's behalf and make decisions about his or her long-term care. This does not, of course, extend to changing the options offered by healthcare teams.

Variations

'You have admitted a 44-year-old woman with a known inoperable frontal lobe glioma. She has a probable chest infection but is refusing all therapy including cannulation for intravenous antibiotics. She has been assessed by the liaison psychiatrist and neurologist who have both deemed that she has full capacity. Her husband is concerned that she has been behaving increasingly strangely recently and thinks her judgement is being directly affected by the tumour. Please discuss this with him.'

'You have seen an 80-year-old man in A&E on behalf of the on-call medical team. He has a UTI with dysuria and increased frequency but no other symptoms. The consultant on-call has seen him and thinks the UTI can be managed at home on oral antibiotics. The patient is slow on his feet but independently mobile and otherwise well. He lives with his daughter who reports that he has had two episodes of urinary incontinence and she is finding it difficult to manage this. She would like him to remain in hospital for treatment. Please discuss this with her.'

'You are the junior doctor on the acute medical ward. Mr Philips is a 29-year-old patient with a history of intravenous drug use. He has been treated successfully for cellulitis of his left leg. Investigations (ultrasound scan) revealed no underlying DVT or other pathology, and he is ready for discharge. However, he now describes ongoing chronic leg pain for 2 years, which has worsened and will be relieved only by the oxycodone that his GP has previously prescribed for exacerbations. There is no record in his hospital notes of previous oxycodone use. He takes regular methadone and denies ongoing heroin use. He refuses to leave the ward until this has been included in his discharge medications. Please discuss his analgesia with him.'

Clinical judgement and maintaining patient welfare

Preconceived notions of illness, disease, pain and disability vary greatly between individuals. These are readily further distorted by the fear, discomfort and anxiety of being unwell. Indeed, most doctors can recount instances of lapses in their clinical judgement when they or a loved one becomes sick. Agreeing a plan of action that marries the 'ideas, concerns and expectations' of a patient with an evidence-based, objective appraisal of clinical need is one of the great challenges of medicine. (It is as yet unclear how this complex challenge fits into the current reductionist view of healthcare as a marketplace, with patient as empowered customer and doctors as competing providers.)

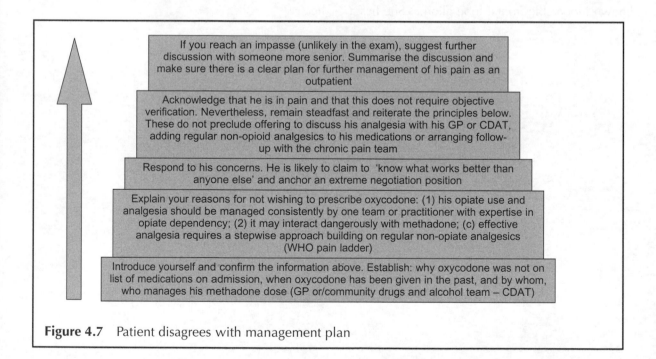

If you reach an impasse (unlikely in the exam), suggest further discussion with someone more senior. Summarise the discussion and make sure there is a clear plan for further management of his pain as an outpatient

Acknowledge that he is in pain and that this does not require objective verification. Nevertheless, remain steadfast and reiterate the principles below. These do not preclude offering to discuss his analgesia with his GP or CDAT, adding regular non-opioid analgesics to his medications or arranging follow-up with the chronic pain team

Respond to his concerns. He is likely to claim to 'know what works better than anyone else' and anchor an extreme negotiation position

Explain your reasons for not wishing to prescribe oxycodone: (1) his opiate use and analgesia should be managed consistently by one team or practitioner with expertise in opiate dependency; (2) it may interact dangerously with methadone; (c) effective analgesia requires a stepwise approach building on regular non-opiate analgesics (WHO pain ladder)

Introduce yourself and confirm the information above. Establish: why oxycodone was not on list of medications on admission, when oxycodone has been given in the past, and by whom, who manages his methadone dose (GP or/community drugs and alcohol team – CDAT)

Figure 4.7   Patient disagrees with management plan

This scenario is not a test of negotiation skills, in which classically both sides begin by anchoring their positions and then make concessions until they meet somewhere in the middle. Examiners expect you to remain steadfast to a course of action that is in the patient's best interests and make no concessions that may risk harm, even in the face of angry insistence. You may attempt to address any underlying misconceptions or strongly held beliefs that have resulted in the patient's unhappiness with the proposed plan of action, but this – as in life – will not necessarily change their position (and is not a requirement to pass).

Variations

'A 45-year-old woman with worsening asthma has attended a respiratory clinic. She was started on oral steroids by her GP 2 days ago. She is nervous about weight gain and would like to stop these. She has also heard that aloe vera can dramatically improve asthma but is expensive and would like to know if it is available on prescription. Please discuss this with her.'

'A 19-year-old man with severe ulcerative colitis has been on intravenous steroids and anti-TNF-α monoclonal antibody therapy for 8 days as an inpatient under your team. His colitis has failed to improve and the gastroenterology consultant and surgeon have agreed that he requires a colectomy. He may require a defunctioning ileostomy for some months before reanastomosis and ileoanal pouch formation can be attempted. However, he would like to avoid surgery and try other anti-TNF-α agents that he has been told are superior. Please discuss this with him.'

ERRORS AND COMPLAINTS

SCENARIO 8. A MEDICAL ERROR

'As a junior doctor in the acute medicine team, you discover that one of your patients with pyelonephritis was given too much gentamicin for pyelonephritis over the weekend by the on-call team, despite documented levels being too high. She has since developed impaired renal function, but is unlikely to need dialysis.

'Please discuss the situation with the patient.'

Clinical judgement and maintaining patient welfare

Negligence
Three separate issues are involved in demonstrating negligence in the UK:

1. A duty of care between the doctor and patient must be established.
2. A breach of this duty of care must be demonstrated (the treatment was not in accordance with a reasonable body of medical opinion).

3. This breach of duty of care caused harm.

Any claim of negligence should be brought within 6 years of the action occurring, unless under exceptional circumstances (eg the complainant was unaware of the breach of duty until >6 years after the event).

In the UK, financial reward for a successful claim is aimed at compensating the individual or family rather than punishing the guilty parties. The Woolf reforms (2000) made the process of a claim quicker and easier. Most cases should be settled out of court, and a claim should be acknowledged within 21 days.

Clinical governance
A discussion about aspects of clinical governance is not uncommon in this station of PACES.

Clinical governance is a framework through which NHS organisations are accountable for continuous improvement of the quality of service. It is a systematic approach to quality assurance

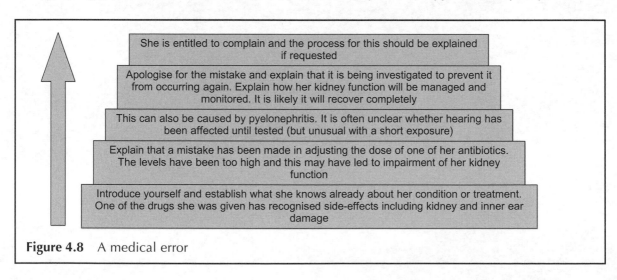

She is entitled to complain and the process for this should be explained if requested

Apologise for the mistake and explain that it is being investigated to prevent it from occurring again. Explain how her kidney function will be managed and monitored. It is likely it will recover completely

This can also be caused by pyelonephritis. It is often unclear whether hearing has been affected until tested (but unusual with a short exposure)

Explain that a mistake has been made in adjusting the dose of one of her antibiotics. The levels have been too high and this may have led to impairment of her kidney function

Introduce yourself and establish what she knows already about her condition or treatment. One of the drugs she was given has recognised side-effects including kidney and inner ear damage

Figure 4.8   A medical error

and must work at a local level. Clinical governance is upheld by the statutory duty of healthcare
trusts to monitor the quality of care provided.
Much of this framework was established after the
Bristol Royal Infirmary enquiry into paediatric
cardiac surgery (www.bristol-inquiry.org.uk). The
more recent Mid-Staffordshire NHS Foundation
Trust Public Inquiry (www.midstaffspublicinquiry.
com) has identified some significant weaknesses
in this framework.

Mistakes and errors are usually multidimensional
and often identify several shortfalls in the system
of healthcare delivery. The 'pillars' of clinical
governance should address these proactively:

- Clinical audit
- Clinical effectiveness
- Communication
- Research
- Audit
- CPED (continuing professional education and
  development)
- Risk management.

Complaints

From 1 September 2006, changes to the NHS
complaints regulation came into force that are
designed to make the complaints procedure
clearer.

Two bodies can be approached for help:

1. The Independent Complaints Advocacy
   Service (ICAS)
2. The Patients' Advice Liaison Service (PALS)

Individuals can complain if they feel that the NHS
adversely affected their life or care. Someone can
complain on another person's behalf with his or
her consent. This should take place within 6
months of the event. The first stage is to complain
locally, which should be done by writing to the
complaint manager of the specific institution.
Patients should receive a response within 25
working days. If patients are unhappy with the
result of this, they can ask for an independent
review from the Healthcare Commission.

Variations

'A 55-year-old man on the ward has developed a
rash after being given one dose of oral amoxicillin despite being penicillin allergic. He has no
other symptoms. The same thing happened a year
ago when he was treated for a gastric ulcer and
he was assured that processes would be changed
to stop it from happening again. On this occasion, it seems that he was prescribed amoxicillin
when it was meant for another patient on the
ward with a similar name. Please explain this to
him and address his concerns.'

'A 74-year-old man has developed *C. difficile*
diarrhoea after a course of intravenous antibiotics
for a lower respiratory tract infection. He has
been moved to a side room. He noticed that one
of the junior doctors in your team failed to wash
his hands or wear gloves before examining him
on one occasion before he developed the diarrhoea. He believes that this is the source of the
infection and would like to make a complaint.
Please discuss this with him.'

'A 55-year-old woman with advanced renal cancer has come to an oncology clinic. She would like to find out more about a new drug that she has read about which can improve life expectancy by 2 months. The drug is licensed and widely used in the USA and Europe, but was turned down by the National Institute of Health and Care Excellence (NICE) and is not available within your trust. She would like to know why she hasn't been told about it, and how and when she can start treatment. Please discuss this with her.'

Clinical judgement and maintaining patient welfare

The quality-adjusted life-year (QALY) threshold of NICE is currently considered to be around £30 000. If a treatment costs more than £30 000 per annum per QALY gained it is usually rejected. It is inadvisable to mention this exact figure in such a consultation because it evokes either the accusation that 'the NHS has put a price on my life' or the assumption that £30 000 must be found to fund further treatment. The existence of such a threshold, and whether it should be revised upward or downward, is the source of much debate.

Examiners often ask how therapeutic or preventive efficacy is measured and you should be familiar with the following terms:

- The **absolute risk** describes the percentage difference in risk of an event or outcome in a treatment (or exposed) group compared with a control group and takes into account overall risk of an event, eg if people undergoing treatment have a risk of lung cancer of 2% compared with 3% in an untreated group, the absolute risk reduction is 1%.

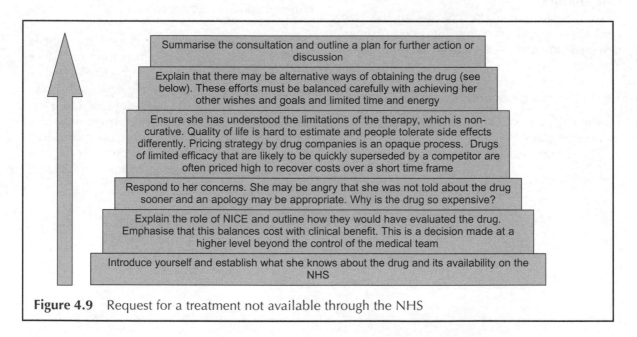

Figure 4.9   Request for a treatment not available through the NHS

- The **relative risk** is a comparison of risk between groups without reference to overall risk, eg if people undergoing treatment A have a risk of lung cancer of 2% compared with 3% in an untreated group, the relative risk reduction is 33%.
- The **number needed to treat (NNT)** is the inverse of the *absolute* risk reduction, eg if the absolute risk reduction is 1%, 100 people will need to be treated for one to benefit.

Options for non-NHS-funded therapies

1. Clinical Commissioning Group funding on a single-case basis: patients have the right to appeal any rejected application.
2. Patient-funded treatment: following the Richards Report (2008), additional drugs can be funded by a patient but have to be administered in a private clinic. This will not forfeit monitoring or further care, which can continue under the NHS.
3. Participate in clinical trials: as these are often blinded and controlled, there is no guarantee that the new treatment will be received.
4. Apply to discretionary disease-specific funds, eg the current UK government Cancer Drugs Fund.
5. Exploit the 'patient choice' system: since April 2009, a patient has the legal right to choose any hospital offering a suitable treatment that meets NHS standards and costs. As some trusts will offer treatments that others have deemed too expensive, this is a means of getting access to treatment that is locally unavailable. Travel costs can be applied for through the Healthcare Travel Cost Scheme.

The notion that one should 'fight' a terminal illness by exploring all avenues of therapies has become deeply ingrained in modern society. This is not without its drawbacks. The refusal to acknowledge the imminence of death may mean delaying important tasks or conversations until it is too late. Patients may opt for further rounds of uncomfortable therapy because they feel a sense of obligation to their loved ones to hold out for as long as possible. They may fear that turning down the option of potentially life-extending therapy seems weak, defeatist or even selfish.

Such decisions are often finely balanced and therefore exquisitely sensitive to the way in which doctors portray the available options. In particular, the notion of 'never giving up' is powerfully supported by a parallel principle upheld by many doctors that 'one should never take away hope' from a patient.

There are marked differences across the healthcare professions in how one approaches this issue. Medical oncologists, for example, may be more inclined to encourage patients to seek palliative chemotherapy than a palliative care nurse.

The guiding principle is to attempt to describe further options in the most objective fashion possible and help patients reach a decision that is compatible with their own values, beliefs and wishes (as long as they fall within legal boundaries). This often requires suspending one's own professional and personal prejudices and biases, which must first be identified if they are to be effectively countered.

Variations

'A 54-year-old man with metastatic bladder cancer would like to discuss a new treatment for his type of tumour that he has read about. He is aware that this new therapy has been turned down by NICE but would like to fund the therapy himself. He has been told by a friend that this means that he will have to switch to entirely private care and is not sure that he can afford this on top of the drug costs. Please discuss this with him.'

'A 54-year-old man with pemphigus vulgaris has steroid-dependent disease despite azathioprine. His consultant applied to the local primary care trust for funding of rituximab therapy but this was recently rejected. The patient has attended the

clinic because he has just discovered that rituximab is readily available through a tertiary centre
dermatologist in a different region and would like
to be referred there. Please discuss this with him.'

SCENARIO 10. NEGLECT OR ABUSE BY A COLLEAGUE

'A 50-year-old woman would like to discuss the care of her 86-year-old mother, who has advanced dementia. Her mother was admitted for treatment of a UTI 2 weeks ago and has remained bed-bound since admission. Her daughter is very concerned that her mother has developed a sacral pressure sore and thinks that this is because she is not receiving adequate attention from the nursing staff. She normally looks after her mother in her own home and is both her main carer and her next of kin.

'The nursing notes make first mention of a pressure sore 2 days ago and an assessment by the tissue viability nurse has been requested (pending). There is no mention of the pressure sore in the medical notes.

'Please discuss this with her.'

Clinical judgement and maintaining patient welfare

With the exception of wilful neglect of a child by a parent, English law rarely criminalises the failure of individuals to act in situations where their actions would prevent harm. However, doctors and nurses can be charged with wilful neglect of a mentally incapacitated patient under current mental health legislation. Some are campaigning for this to include all types of patient, as is the case in French law.

This scenario involves a patent with impaired capacity and there may be grounds under the 2007 Mental Health Act for criminal charges of wilful neglect to be brought against medical staff. The stakes are thus high and, although transparency is paramount, acceptance of responsibility

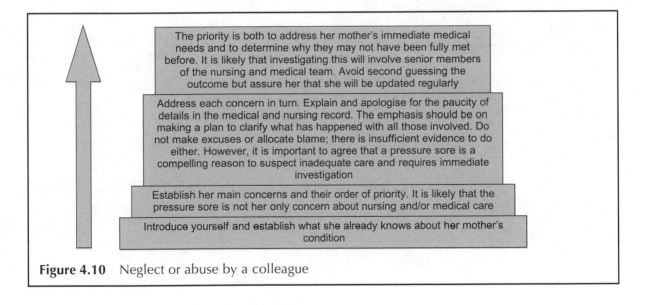

The priority is both to address her mother's immediate medical needs and to determine why they may not have been fully met before. It is likely that investigating this will involve senior members of the nursing and medical team. Avoid second guessing the outcome but assure her that she will be updated regularly

Address each concern in turn. Explain and apologise for the paucity of details in the medical and nursing record. The emphasis should be on making a plan to clarify what has happened with all those involved. Do not make excuses or allocate blame; there is insufficient evidence to do either. However, it is important to agree that a pressure sore is a compelling reason to suspect inadequate care and requires immediate investigation

Establish her main concerns and their order of priority. It is likely that the pressure sore is not her only concern about nursing and/or medical care

Introduce yourself and establish what she already knows about her mother's condition

Figure 4.10   Neglect or abuse by a colleague

and culpability 'on behalf of the medical team' before a thorough investigation risks wide-ranging consequences in the long term.

Variations

'Overnight one of the patients under your team's care was prescribed fluids by the on-call house officer. This was given through an existing cannula while the patient was asleep. The cannula had "tissued" resulting in a very swollen arm the next morning. The patient, a 54-year-old man recovering from gastroenteritis, is angry that the fluids were started while he was asleep without his consent. Please address his concerns.'

'A 78-year-old patient has alleged that one of the nursing staff was rude and abrupt towards her after she wet the bed. She was recovering from a coronary angiography and says that she called for a bedpan several times but no one came. Her daughter is upset by this and would like to make a complaint. Please discuss this with her.'

COMPLEX EXPLANATIONS

SCENARIO 11. DIAGNOSIS WITH MULTIPLE TREATMENT OPTIONS

'You are the junior doctor in the endocrinology clinic and the biochemical results on the next patient, a 32-year-old woman, confirm the clinical suspicion that she has Graves' disease. These show a grossly elevated free T_4 and suppressed TSH with strongly positive anti-thyroid antibodies. She has moderate exophthalmoses and is a smoker.

'Please discuss with her the subsequent management of her condition.'

Clinical judgement and maintaining patient welfare

Some cases in the communication skills station will require knowledge of a condition and its treatment. However, you are not being assessed on your depth of knowledge, rather which key pieces of information you choose to convey to your patient and how you do this.

A good approach is to build an explanation around what she already knows about thyroid disease (many patients will have a relative or friend with this common condition). It is important to emphasise that the condition is readily treatable. If the patient wants to know more, outline the three modalities of treatment for hyperthyroidism in Graves' disease (surgery, radioiodine therapy and medical therapy), and their risks and benefits. The goal of this scenario is not to establish which modality is most suited to the patient – this requires information that is not yet at hand.

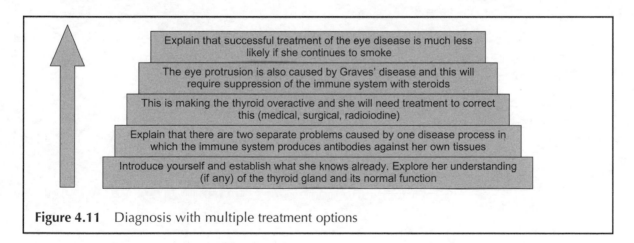

Figure 4.11   Diagnosis with multiple treatment options

Variations

'Your next patient in the rheumatology clinic is a 33-year-old woman with probable rheumatoid arthritis, principally affecting the small joints of her hand. At her last clinic appointment she was started on steroids to which she responded well. Please outline the concept of long-term immuno-suppression with steroid-sparing agents and their major risks and benefits.'

'A 44 year old with end-stage renal failure will soon require dialysis. He had a brief period of haemodialysis through a temporary vascular catheter 1 year ago after an episode of sepsis. Please outline the main features of peritoneal haemodialysis and explore his suitability and preferences.'

SCENARIO 12: DIAGNOSIS WITH UNCERTAIN/UNPREDICTABLE OUTCOMES

'A 33-year-old woman has a consultation with you to discuss the results of her recent MRI, which you had organised at her previous neurology appointment. She has a 3-year-old daughter but is actively trying for a second child. For the last 3 months she has noticed several episodes of visual disturbance and intermittent weakness of her legs. Her MRI is consistent with the diagnosis of multiple sclerosis.

'Please discuss this result with her.'

Clinical judgement and maintaining patient welfare

Scenarios where a diagnosis must be given and explained are frequent in PACES. Do not fall into the trap of trying to use your interaction with the patient to demonstrate your extensive knowledge of the condition at hand to the examiners. 'Clin-

ical judgement' in this context is more concerned with what information you choose to leave out, such that the patient walks away with a clear understanding and plan. With any condition, try to ensure that the following are conveyed clearly and simply:

• Level of diagnostic certainty and whether other tests are needed
• How current symptoms and/or functional impairment might be managed
• Treatments and their limitations or risks
• What they can expect (in broad terms) in the short, medium and long term.

Although all of these should be covered, in the limited time available it is best to focus on the factors that are causing most concern.

Things to avoid:

• Predicting survival time/duration of remission/response to treatment

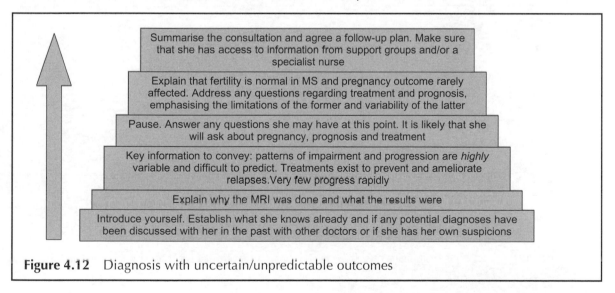

Figure 4.12   Diagnosis with uncertain/unpredictable outcomes

- Giving worst- or best-case outcomes (only the former will be remembered)
- Overloading the patient with information
- Ignoring seemingly trivial specific concerns (eg will treatment make my hair fall out, doctor?).

Variations

'A 34-year-old woman with alopecia, a butterfly rash and bilateral arthritis in her hands attends her first rheumatology clinic appointment. Blood tests requested by her referring GP show positive ANA, high ESR and a positive anti-dsDNA anti-body. Her renal function is normal and there are no neurological signs or symptoms. Please explain the likely diagnosis of systemic lupus erythematosus and outline the treatment and prognosis.'

'A 54-year-old woman has just had a coronary angiography and stent insertion for a 50% left anterior descending artery occlusion. There was a 20% right coronary artery stem stenosis seen, which was not treated. She has known hypercholesterolaemia and is a smoker. Please discuss the likelihood of needing further treatment and address any concerns that she may have.'

SCENARIO 13: DIAGNOSIS WITH IMPLICATIONS BEYOND THE PATIENT

'You are a junior doctor in the neurology clinic. The next patient is a 42-year-old woman who presented previously with chorea and forgetfulness. Her father died in his early 50s from an undiagnosed neurological condition. The locum consultant who saw her previously suspected Huntington's disease and arranged a CT of the head. This has showed changes in the caudate nuclei characteristic of the disease. She has two daughters aged 4 and 7, and three younger brothers who are fit and well. Explain the results of the scan and discuss genetic testing.'

Clinical judgement and maintaining patient welfare

You have been asked to discuss genetic testing, not take consent for the test itself. This scenario is about genetic testing for confirmation of the diagnosis and not the pros and cons of testing for other family members. The latter is a highly complex issue and is subject not only to her own genetic status but also to the individual choices of those at risk. An open-ended discussion in the consultation is perfectly acceptable – it is likely

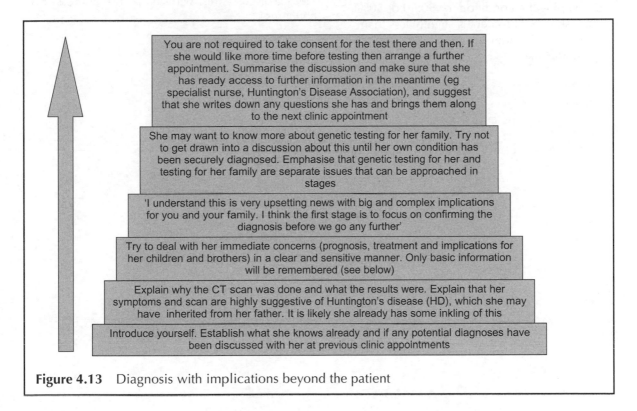

Figure 4.13   Diagnosis with implications beyond the patient

that she will eventually opt for testing and it is crucial that she does not feel rushed into confirming such burdensome foreknowledge of her family's future. The diagnosis is a devastating one – attempting to address all the complex implications in one sitting is likely to result in dealing with none of them adequately.

Basic information about Huntington's disease that you may be required to discuss:

- There is no cure.
- Treatment is supportive and there are medications to manage symptoms.
- It is progressive (usually >15–20 years).
- If she carries the genetic fault, then each of her children have a one in two risk of developing the condition (or 50:50 or 50%).
- The risk to her brothers is slightly less than 50% given that they are now adults and asymptomatic.

Variations

'A 54-year-old woman with two teenage daughters has recently had successful treatment for early stage breast cancer found at mammography screening. She has two sisters with the disease and your consultant has suggested that she should undergo testing for *BRCA1* and *BRCA2* mutations. Please discuss this with her.'

'A 31-year-old man has attended A&E asking for help. He is not registered with a local GP. His father has recently returned from Pakistan where he was diagnosed with tuberculosis and commenced on medications. He is concerned that his 4-year-old son might be at risk of infection. Please discuss this with him and address his concerns.'

CONFIDENTIALITY

SCENARIO 14. INFORMING THE DVLA OF IMPAIRED FITNESS TO DRIVE

'A 48-year-old taxi driver who has type 2 diabetes is attending your diabetic clinic. He has had multiple laser photocoagulations for pre-proliferative retinopathy and now has a fixed field defect that does not fulfil DVLA requirements for driving. He says that he cannot afford to give up driving because he is the only income earner in the family and has three small children.

'Please discuss this with him.'

Clinical judgement and maintaining patient welfare

It is his legal obligation to inform the DVLA. If he does not do so, you will have to break confidentiality and do so.

DVLA medical requirements are more stringent for group 2 entitlement drivers (buses, large lorries) than group 1 drivers (cars and motorcycles). Group 2 standards encompass taxi drivers,

although the responsibility for enforcing this lies with the local authority and not the DVLA. However, a visual field defect that fails DVLA criteria will preclude driving at both group 1 and group 2 levels.

Common sense largely dictates which conditions should require informing the DVLA. DVLA medical criteria of fitness to drive are complex and both group and condition specific. You are not expected to know them off by heart, or second guess what the DVLA assessment might be.

Variations

'A 21-year-old fashion model was recently admitted with her second suspected epileptic seizure. This was controlled with IV lorazepam. Regular phenytoin – which she has previously refused – has been commenced. She has been told on a previous admission by a consultant neurologist to stop driving. It emerges during her

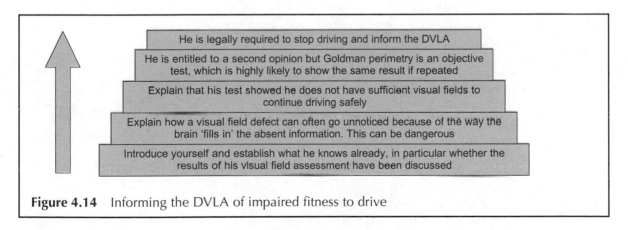

He is legally required to stop driving and inform the DVLA

He is entitled to a second opinion but Goldman perimetry is an objective test, which is highly likely to show the same result if repeated

Explain that his test showed he does not have sufficient visual fields to continue driving safely

Explain how a visual field defect can often go unnoticed because of the way the brain 'fills in' the absent information. This can be dangerous

Introduce yourself and establish what he knows already, in particular whether the results of his visual field assessment have been discussed

Figure 4.14   Informing the DVLA of impaired fitness to drive

inpatient stay that she was driving at the time of the second seizure. Please discuss this with her.'

'A 33-year-old investment banker has just been admitted with a suspected non-ST elevation myocardial infarction. He has a documented past history of cocaine use. The NSTEMI occurred while driving and he discloses that an accident ensued involving another car but he drove on without stopping. Another patient had been admitted just an hour previously with severe trauma following a road traffic accident in which the other party failed to stop. The police have asked to be informed of any other admissions of people on the same day who may have been involved in an RTA. Please discuss this with the patient.'

(Note that the Road Traffic Act 1988 obliges anyone, including healthcare professionals, to provide the police, on request, with any information that might identify a driver who is alleged to have committed a traffic offence.)

SCENARIO 15 RISKING CONFIDENTIALITY FOR PUBLIC/THIRD PARTY PROTECTION

'You are about to discharge a 34-year-old woman who was admitted with mild jaundice 3 days ago. She has been diagnosed with acute hepatitis B virus (HBV) infection and her liver function tests are now resolving. A follow-up appointment has been arranged in 6 months to determine whether she has cleared the infection or requires treatment. It is likely that she acquired HBV after sex with a colleague 5 weeks ago. She is married and has two young children. Please discuss barrier contraception and the need to test her husband for HBV infection.'

Clinical judgement and maintaining patient welfare

Index patients presenting with a sexually transmitted infection should be given the choice of informing partners themselves (patient referral), or allowing notification by a health adviser. Occasionally conditional referral is agreed wherein partners are contacted if they have not attended by an agreed time.

This is straightforward only if the index patient is cooperative. In scenarios where confidentiality will be jeopardised – even by anonymous contact tracing – the index patient may be resistant to giving details of sexual contacts.

The Venereal Disease Regulations 1974 state that information about anybody diagnosed with a sexually transmitted infection shall not be disclosed except:

(a) For the purpose of communicating that information to a medical practitioner, or to a person employed under the direction of a medical practitioner in connection with the treatment of persons suffering from such disease or the prevention of the spread thereof, and

(b) For the purpose of such treatment and prevention.

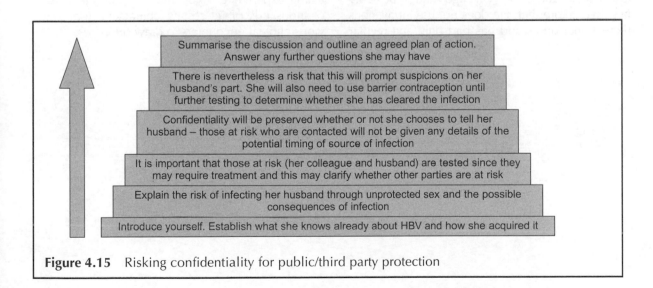

Figure 4.15   Risking confidentiality for public/third party protection

There is no legal precedent for forcing index patients to disclose details of sexual contacts if they are reluctant to do so. However, this does not mean that likely contacts (such as spouses) cannot be researched and contacted by sexual health workers, even without the index patient's consent and if doing so may jeopardise their confidentiality. This is a consultant decision and is usually taken after legal advice.

There have now been several convictions in the UK for grievous bodily harm in cases where known HIV-positive individuals have recklessly infected a sexual partner through unprotected sex. Civil cases involving a range of STIs from genital herpes to HIV, facilitated by a growing personal injury lawyer industry, are increasingly common. An index patient reluctant to give details for contact tracing may be legally culpable for any harm that comes to those individuals as a result of inadequate preventive measures or treatment.

Variations

'A 33-year-old man with HIV on HAART has recently been diagnosed with hepatitis C. The test was negative 1 year ago and repeatedly negative before that. He does not use intravenous recreational drugs and has had only one regular male sexual partner for the last 4 years. Please outline further investigations and treatment and discuss getting his partner tested.'

'A 44-year-old restaurateur and chef has been admitted with bloody diarrhoea and diagnosed with campylobacter gastroenteritis. Your consultant has asked you to inform Public Health England of his case. Please discuss this with the patient.'

Using this chapter

Throughout this chapter we have provided techniques and approaches that you can apply successfully to any scenario, rather than exhaustive coverage of everything that you might encounter.

It is essential now to practise communication skills scenarios with a revision partner. We have given key examples in each category of how you might 'build' a discussion towards a goal, followed by examples of common variations on the same theme, which you can use to form the basis of your practice. It is remarkable how easy it is to play the role of patient or relative without any acting experience – you have a back catalogue of thousands of interesting characters from previous clinical encounters to draw upon.

STATION 5

Integrated Clinical Assessment

STRUCTURE OF THE ICA

The older Station 5 (until 2009) involved a series of three short cases based around examination of the eyes, an endocrine disorder or rheumatological condition. Like the other examination stations, this involved a ritualised examination followed by presentation of findings to the examiners. There are still 'echoes' of this old format in many textbooks and courses; skin, locomotor and endocrine scenarios have been shoe-horned into an 'integrated clinical assessment' (ICA) format. This slightly misrepresents the content of the exam, which is highly varied and demands far more than an ability to elicit clinical signs. Indeed, this is the only station of the PACES exam that assesses candidates in all categories of the marking scheme.

Station 5 is organised as follows:

- Two 10-minute cases known as **'brief clinical consultations'**.
- The candidate has 8 minutes with the patient to take a focused history, carry out a relevant examination, reach a diagnosis or identify a clinical problem and then communicate this **to the patient.**
- The remaining 2-minute discussion with the examiners will not begin until these 8 minutes have elapsed.
- The examiner will ask the candidate to state the positive physical findings, their concluding diagnosis and differential diagnoses (if appropriate) based on their assessment.

CONTENT AND MARKING OF THE ICA

The cases found in Station 5 typically involve a presenting complaint that guides you to the relevant system for a targeted examination. Alternatively, there may be obvious clinical signs (eg thyroid eye disease) and a rather vague history.

The seven areas in which candidates are scored are summarised below, with candidates being scored on a three-point scale: satisfactory, borderline or unsatisfactory.

Clinical communication skills

- Eliciting a history relevant to the complaint
- Explaining information to the patient in a focused, fluent and professional manner

Physical examination

Performing an examination in a correct, appropriate, practised and professional manner

Clinical judgement

Selecting a sensible and appropriate investigation and treatment plan

Managing patient's concerns

- Detecting, acknowledging and attempting to address patient's concerns
- Listening
- Demonstrating empathy

Identifying physical signs

- Identifying the correct physical signs
- Not finding signs that are not present

Differential diagnosis

Constructing a sensible differential diagnosis, including the correct diagnosis

Maintaining patient welfare

Treating the patient respectfully and sensitively, ensuring comfort, safety and dignity

A formal marksheet is shown on page can be found on the MRCPUK website.

INFORMATION GIVEN TO CANDIDATES, PATIENTS AND EXAMINERS

Before each Station 5 examination, each candidate, patient and examiner will be given some information.

Below is a worked example of the information given to each person based on guidance on the MRCP website (www.mrcpuk.org).

Information to candidate

You will be asked to see two patients at this station. The clinical information about one of these patients is given in the box below. You should have a second sheet giving you information about the other patient.

- You have 10 minutes with each patient. The examiners will alert you when 6 minutes have elapsed and will stop you after 8 minutes.
- In the remaining 2 minutes, one examiner will ask you to report abnormal physical signs (if any), your diagnosis or differential diagnosis, and your plan for management (if not already clear from your discussion with the patient).

Your role: You are the medical doctor on call

Patient name: Mrs Beverley Gordon – age 39 years

This lady was admitted to the orthopaedic ward for a carpal tunnel release operation.

She mentioned to the orthopaedic doctors that she has swelling in her neck and they have asked for the opinion of a physician. You were asked by your consultant to see the patient and to assess the suspected swelling in her neck.

Your task is to assess the patient's problems and address any questions or concerns raised by the patient.

- You should assess the problem by means of a relevant clinical history and a relevant physical examination. You do not need to complete the history before carrying out appropriate examination.
- You should respond to any questions the patient may have, advise the patient of your probable diagnosis (or differential diagnoses) and your plan for investigation and treatment where appropriate.
- You have 8 minutes to complete the task.

Accompanying notes are given to each patient and may take the following format.

Information for patients

The doctors sitting the examination have been asked to assess your problem. They will have 8 minutes to ask you about the problem and any other relevant issues. They will also examine you. They should explain to you what they think is wrong and what action should be taken and answer any questions you have, for example about the diagnosis, tests that may be needed, or treatment. One of the examiners will ask them to describe any abnormal examination findings and give their diagnosis.

Your history is described below.

You are: Mrs Beverley Gordon – age 39 years

Your problem: A swelling in your neck

You are in the orthopaedic ward and you mentioned to the admitting doctor that your neck seemed swollen. One of the medical doctors has been asked to see you about this.

You have been suffering from pain in your right forearm and a numb or tingly feeling in your right hand – affecting your third, fourth and fifth fingers. The aching in your arm is worse at night and you have found it more and more difficult to get comfortable. The problem has been present for several years and was worse when you were pregnant with your daughter, 3 years ago, but improved for a time after that.

A trapped nerve in the wrist has been diagnosed. You are having a short admission to have the nerve released.

You mentioned that you thought your neck was swollen when the admitting doctor was examining you. You have not mentioned this to a doctor before, but your sister has been commenting on it for a few years. Your sister is 36 and has an underactive thyroid.

You do not have any of the symptoms your sister had when her thyroid was underactive.

Indeed you feel well. Your weight is stable. Your skin and hair are normal. You do not seem to feel the heat or the cold any more than anyone else. Your bowel works normally. You do not have any problem with swallowing.

You should ask why your neck seems swollen and whether there is something wrong with your thyroid gland. You should ask if any tests are required and, if so, what these tests will be.

Finally, for the same worked example, the examiners have the following information, which would typically list the findings the candidate would be expected to observe or elicit.

Information for examiners

Patient: Mrs Beverley Gordon – age 39 years

Examiners should discuss and agree the criteria for pass and for fail in the competencies being assessed.

As a general guide, candidates would be expected to:

- Note the history of neck swelling and the family history of thyroid disease
- Enquire about symptoms of disturbed thyroid function
- Examine the neck and identify the smooth and symmetrical thyroid enlargement. Note absence of bruit
- Examine for signs of overactive and underactive thyroid gland and confirm clinical euthyroid state
- Confirm to the patient that her thyroid gland does seem enlarged but reassure her that the gland seems to be working normally judging from clinical examination. Advise on appropriate further investigations.

The lead examiner should:

(a) Advise the candidate after 6 minutes have elapsed that 'You have two minutes remaining with your patient'
(b) Ask the candidate to describe any abnormal physical findings that have been identified
(c) Ask the candidate to give the preferred diagnosis and any differential diagnosis that is being considered
(d) Ensure any remaining areas of uncertainty, eg regarding the plan for investigation or management of the problem, are addressed in any time that remains.

THE APPROACH TO STATION 5

It is very easy to fall into the familiar modes of the history-taking station or the examination stations, then find, with a minute remaining, that you have either almost wordlessly examined your patient without garnering any information about their symptoms or that you have taken a thorough history but examined nothing. You may choose to attempt to divide each consultation between history and examination, but we strongly recommend taking a history and examination in parallel, just as you would during a busy on-call or clinic.

It is also crucial to remember that the examiners are not looking for the ritualised, detailed and complete examination of systems as in other stations, or for a full history. They are testing your ability to perform a targeted examination and elicit the most salient symptoms. This is not solely for the purpose of forming a differential diagnosis – don't forget that you have been specifically asked to address the patient's principal concerns and must therefore explain to them what you think the underlying problem is and how you are going to investigate and manage it.

Each of the Station 5 cases in this chapter is based around a flow chart that gives a worked example of how you might perform an 'integrated clinical assessment' (ICA) for a given presenting condition.

All cases can be divided into a new condition or an exacerbation of an existing chronic illness. These require slightly different emphasis in the history taking and examination, and this is reflected in each flow chart.

An important feature of this approach is the 'callback', wherein towards the end of the consultation candidates re-state the presenting complaint of the patient and any other specific concerns they raised during the consultation. This is an easy way of demonstrating to the examiners that you have registered and understood the patient's main concern (which is not necessarily the main clinical priority). It also gives the patient an opportunity to mention other salient points which the candidate missed. If you have built a good rapport with the patients/actor, they may help you out at this stage by volunteering important information.

The consulation should end with you describing:

- How you will address the patient's main concern (eg analgesia)
- What you think the diagnosis may be
- What investigations and initial treatments are necessary.

This is an oppurtunity to demonstrate to the examiner that you have come to a reasonable differential diagnosis and formed a safe and efficient investigation and management plan.

EXAMINATION TECHNIQUES FOR STATION 5

Station 5 often requires examination routines not encountered elsewhere in PACES, for example examination of a goitre. These are described below.

Examination of the hands

It is important to ensure the patient is comfortable and to rest the hands on a pillow. Expose the hands and forearms up to and including the elbows. A large proportion of the patients may have painful and tender joints and it is imperative therefore to ask about this before palpating the joints, which should be done after careful inspection.

A rheumatological examination typically involves inspection, palpation, neurological assessment, functional assessement and examination for extra-articular signs. However, you may not have time to do all of these completely.

1. Inspection

The bulk of the available information will be gathered by inspection rather than palpation or active movement.

- Peripheral accessories, eg walking stick
- Peripheral arthropathies, eg knees, ankles
- Systemic sclerosis – tight, shiny, stretched skin with beaked nose +/– telangectasia
- Cushingoid appearance – steroid treatment
- Horner's syndrome – T1 lesion (see page. .....)
- Ears for evidence of psoriasis, or gouty tophi in helix of ear.

Then make an assessment of:

- **Nails** – pitting, onycholysis, clubbing, nail fold infarcts, Beau's lines
- **Skin** – tight shiny skin over dorsum of hand or fingers (scleroderma); tissue paper thin +/– purpura (steroid therapy); surgical scars (joint replacement); tar staining
- **Muscles**
  - bilateral wasting of the small muscles with dorsal guttering (rheumatoid arthritis, syringomyelia, motor neurone disease)
  - unilateral wasting of the small muscles of the hand (C8/T1 root lesion, eg cervical rib, Pancoast tumour)
  - unilateral wasting involving thenar eminence (median nerve, eg carpal tunnel syndrome)
  - unilateral wasting sparing thenar eminence (ulnar nerve, eg elbow trauma)
- **Joints** (in order to describe the location of the abnormality accurately, candidates should know the names of the bones and joints)
- **Distribution** of any abnormalities – symmetrical (eg rheumatoid arthritis) or asymmetrical (eg seronegative arthritides); proximal or distal joints
- **Specific deformities** eg 'swan neck', 'Boutonniere', Z-shaped thumb, subluxation, ulnar deviation, Heberden's nodes, gouty tophi
- **Inflammation** – calor, rubor, dolor, tumor and loss of function
  - NB rubor is replaced with shininess of the skin in those with dark skin

Once the hands have been inspected, an assessment of the elbows is essential, as this can reveal

psoriatic plaques or rheumatoid nodules (indicating sero-positive rheumatoid arthritis).

The whole examination can be achieved by three
movements – assessment of the dorsum of the
hand, then plantar aspect, followed by crossing
the arms over and exposing the extensors surface
of the elbows.

2. Palpation (with caution)

This must only be assessed with extreme caution
on the examination and only where there is an
absolute requirement to do so in the time given,
such as if there is a specific complaint by the
patient (ie painful joints) or inspection has
demonstrated a specific abnormality.

- Palm – Dupuytren's contracture
- Elbow nodules
- Joints – palpate any swelling to determine
  whether it is soft and boggy (rheumatoid
  arthritis) or hard and bony (Heberden's nodes
  or gouty tophi)
- Skin – tightness or calcinosis in finger pulps
  (scleroderma/CREST).

This does not mean that you need to examine every
joint in the hands, but merely the joints involved, eg
MCP joints.

3. Functional assessment of the hands

You will be expected to perform this assessment
if the patient reports reduced function.

- First, you can ask the patient to make a fist,
  followed by the prayer sign, followed by the
  reverse prayer sign.
- Finally, you could ask the patient to do up a
  button on a shirt or hold a pen.

These manoeuvres have been validated against
more complex assessments of function and provide
a quick means of assessing the likelihood of impaired function in daily activities.

Neurological assessment – if relevant to the presenting complaint (eg symptoms of carpal tunnel
syndrome), one should proceed to perform a

neurological assessment focusing particularly on
the median and ulnar nerve. Single nerve lesions
are occasionally encountered in this station.

4. Extra-articular signs

Having screened for symptoms suggestive of systemic manifestions of joint disease, examination
should then focus on the **affected system**.

Examination of the axial spine

A patient may present with stiffness of the axial
spine and restricted movements (eg as in ankylosing spondylitis and other spondylarthropathies).

Inspection is crucial again. For example, the
'question mark posture' (loss of lumbar lordosis,
fixed kyphoscoliosis of the thoracic spine with
extensive of the cervical spine) of ankylosing
spondylitis can be a 'spot diagnosis'. The characteristic posture is usually immediately evident
**unless the patient is lying down with the head
supported by pillows.**

The following examination routine should stage
disease and detect associated signs:

1. Establish restricted spinal movement

Two quick tests can be perfomed:

Lumbar spine: modified Shober's index:
With the patient standing upright, place two
marks 10 cm apart on the lumbar spine in the
midline. The lower mark is at the level of the
posterior superior iliac spines. The patient then
flexes forward (ask them to touch their toes) and
at maximal flexion the distance is re-measured.
In normal subjects there is an expansion of at
least 5 cm between the two marks. Lower values
indicate decreased mobility of the lumbar spine.

Thoracic spine: Occiput-to-wall distance:
The subject stands with their back against a wall
(both heels and buttocks must be touching the
wall) with a horizontal gaze. In normal subjects

the occiput will touch the wall. Any wall-to-occiput gap is a measure of restriction of the thoracic and cervical spines.

2. Examine for sacroiliitis/enthesitis

Examine (carefully) for tenderness over the sacroiliac joints. Palpate for evidence of other enthesitides over the heels, costochondral joints and iliac crest.

Tell the examiner you would like to perform the FABERE (flexion, abduction, external rotation and extension) test. The patient places one ankle on the opposite knee and allows the ipsilateral knee to fall outwards (external rotation at the hip) to form a figure '4'. If this causes pain over the sacroiliac joint, sacroiliitis should be suspected.

3. Exclude extra-articular manifestations from head to toe:

If a spondylarthropathy is suspected (eg ankylosing spondylitis), a focused history should include questions related to the extra-articular manifestations associated with these conditions.

*   **Eyes**: acute uveitis
*   **Mouth**: mucosal inflammation manifesting as oral ulceration is common
*   **Chest**: apical fibrobullous disease (1%)
*   **Cardiac**: aortic root dilatation and associated aortic valve incompetence
*   **Abdomen**: 15–20% will develop symptomatic Crohn's disease (stoma present?). Look for evidence of amyloidosis (hepatomegaly, evidence of renal failure or replacement therapy)
*   **Nervous system**: paraesthesia, signs of cord compression
*   **Feet**: Achilles tendonitis and plantar fasciitis

Examination of thyroid status

The assessment of the thyroid status of a patient is a fundamental clinical skill that should not present difficulties provided that the following scheme is followed. For obvious reasons, patients with severe hyper- or hypothyroidism are unlikely to appear, but over/under-replacement of thyroxine is quite a common scenario.

General observation
*   Hypothyroidism
    *   Pale dry skin
    *   'Peaches and cream' complexion
    *   Dry hair
        *   Note: Loss of the outer one-third of the eyebrows is unreliable and non-specific
*   Hyperthyroidism
    *   Anxious, fidgety patient
    *   Staring eyes (lid retraction)
    *   Sweating

Hands
Shake their hands

*   Warm and sweaty or cool and dry?
*   Fine tremor – hands outstretched with a piece of paper resting on fingers
*   Pulse
    *   Rate
    *   Rhythm (AF often occurs in thyrotoxicosis)
    *   Volume (typically large volume and collapsing in hyperthyroidism)
*   Thyroid acropachy – a rare feature of Graves' disease
*   Tar staining – Graves' ophthalmopathy is worse in smokers

Neuromuscular manifestations
*   Reflexes: Slow relaxing in hypothyroidism; brisk in thyrotoxicosis
*   Proximal myopathy: Thyrotoxicosis – ask the patient to stand from a chair unaided

Dermatological manifestations of thyroid disease
*   Graves' dermopathy

Sheet-like myxoedema – coarse diffuse skin with non-pitting oedema
Nodular localised – violaceous infiltrative waxy area on the shin, resembling erythema nodosum
Horny – papilliform irregular firm red dermopathy on shin/upper foot

Examination of the thyroid gland

Follow the sequence of inspection, palpation and percussion. If you find a goitre, it would be prudent to comment on the thyroid status, combining reported symptoms and a formal examination of thyroid status as above. You must also comment on the most likely aetiology.

Inspection
Ask the patient to swallow a sip of water and look for upward movement of the thyroid gland. NB a thyroglossal cyst will move upwards both on swallowing and protrusion of the tongue, and can be trans-illuminated.

Is there any evidence from the history or examination that the thyroid is compressing any of the following:

- Trachea
  - monophonic syncope (rare), but the history may suggestmsome dyspnoea, particularly on lying flat
- Recurrent laryngeal nerve
  - hoarseness
- Oesophagus
  - dysphagia, very rarely odynophagia
- Venous return from the head
  - superior vena cava obstruction (very rare)

Look carefully for a scar – previous hemi/total thyroidectomy

Palpation
Stand behind the patient and gently palpate the gland, located two finger widths below the thyroid cartilage, with one hand on each side and the neck gently flexed.

- If a goitre is present, comment on its:
  - Size
  - Consistency
    - soft
    - firm
    - hard

Note: Soft – 'like lips', firm – 'like the tip of the nose' and hard 'like the forehead' is a good aide memoir to remember (but not repeat in the exam) when thinking about how to measure the consistency of the goitre.
- Diffuse or nodular
  - If nodular – multinodular or a single nodule
- Tender – suggests thyroiditis
- Lymphadenopathy
- Tethered – this suggests cancer.

Percussion
Percuss gently for retro-sternal extension.

Auscultate
Bruit – classically occurs in Graves' thyrotoxicosis.

Examination of thyroid eye disease

This may not be necessary in the exam unless the patient is complaining of eye symptoms or if on inspection the patient has obvious thyroid eye disease.

Note that lid lag and lid retraction are signs of hyperthyroidism rather than Graves' disease, although the two may clearly co-exist.

Lid retraction
Indicated by visible sclera above the superior limbus of the cornea

This results from sympathetic stimulation of levator palpabrae superioris of **any** aetiology, eg thyrotoxicosis, anxiety, β-agonists.

Lid lag
Ask the patient to follow the slow downward movement of your finger at a distance of about 50 cm. The upper lid lags behind the descending eyeball.

Look for clinical features of Graves's affecting the eyes

Exophthalmos
Sclera visible below the inferior limbus of the cornea with the patient sitting at the same level as you and looking straight ahead.

This sign only occurs in Graves' disease (cv), the term is synonymous with proptosis; it can be unilateral, although a retro-orbital tumour should always be excluded.

Other features of Graves'
● Periorbital oedema
● Chemosis
● Conjunctival injection
● Opthalmoplegia

If Graves' ophthalmopathy is present on inspection it is necessary to perform a more detailed examination and take further history.
● Are the eyes painful in any way? Are they gritty or dry? Also ask if any part of the subsequent exam causes pain or discomfort.
● Is eyelid closure adequate?
  ● With exophthalmos there is a greater volume of eye to be covered with each blink, the frequency of blinking is reduced and the time of each blink is increased.
● Ask patient to follow your finger (and to say if they experience diplopia) as you test all directions of gaze.
  ● Limitation of upward gaze is the most common abnormality in Graves' ophthalmopathy.
  ● However, the combination of enlarged ocular muscles +/− subsequent fibrosis may lead to complex ophthalmoplegia that is not explained by either single nerve or muscle disease.
● Ptosis – a very rare occurrence in either Graves' disease or hyperthyroidism. Its presence should raise the possibility of co-existent myasthenia gravis.
● Acuity (see page 405) – full assessment (with ophthalmoscopy) rather than gross assessment

of acuity may be unnecessary, unless there is a high suspicion this has been compromised.
● Since the most important concern of Graves' ophthalmopathy is a threat to the sight, it is critical to assess vision in the following fashion.
  ● Acuity using a Jaeger chart or Snellen chart (+ pinhole)
  ● Colour vision – either using Ishihara plates or a red pin to look for desaturation
  ● Fields – compression of the nerve head at the orbital apex can cause constriction of the fields
  ● Ophthalmoscopy
  ● Is there papilloedema or consecutive optic atrophy?
  ● If closure is poor or you have concerns about the cornea you may want an ophthalmologist to perform slit lamp examination to look for corneal scars or ulcers – you should state this to the examiner. One can get a reasonable view with a direct ophthalmoscope, but not good enough to preclude a proper examination.

Examination of a skin lesion/rash

The dermatology cases in the Station 5 ICA require a special mention. Classically, the history associated with the condition may not be long or detailed, and most of the differentiating information is gleaned from examination. Furthermore, the presentation of the examination is essential too. Remember that many dermatological conditions reflect underlying medical conditions that should not be overlooked.

It is important to ensure you are fluent with the common terminology:

Macule	Circumscribed area of erythematous change without elevation
Papule	Solid raised lesion < 1 cm in size
Nodule	Solid raised lesion ≥ 1 cm in size

Plaque	Circumscribed elevated confluence of papules ⩾ 1 cm in size
Pustule	Circumscribed area containing pus
Vesicle	Circumscribed fluid-filled area < 1 cm in size
Bulla	Circumscribed fluid-filled area ⩾ 1 cm in size

When examining the patient, you need to expose the patient as much as the situation will allow (which the examiner should guide) and inspect the patient as a whole, considering:

- Is there a rash and what is its distribution?
- Is there any hair growth or loss?
- Are there any features of systemic disease?

And more specifically:

- If there is a rash – is it red or not?
- Is the rash macular, papular, in patches or plaques?
- Are there scales or evidence of excoriation?
- Are there fluid-filled lesions?
- Are these vesicles, pustules or blisters?
- Are there signs of systemic disease giving clues as to the aetiology of the skin lesion, eg a colostomy bag suggesting ulcerative colitis?

On presenting your findings, use the correct terminology and be succinct. If there is a suggestion from the history that the dermatological condition is associated with an underlying condition (eg erythema nodosum and inflammatory bowel disease), then an examination of the relevant system may be necessary.

For example:

'There is a vesicular rash bilaterally on the extensor aspects of the elbow, with associated evidence of excoriation, on a background of a patient with symptoms consistent with coeliac disease, suggesting that this is dermatitis herpetiformis.'

This gives a clear and precise description of the rash, its location, associated excoriation and links it to the most likely underlying aetiological cause.

Examination of the eyes

As with the dermatology ICA cases, the history associated with an ophthalmological condition may be brief, but the examination is crucial. Taking a history and examining simultaneously can be easily achieved. Be cautious, however, since red flag symptoms must not be missed (such as in papilloedema or diabetic retinopathy), as some conditions reflect very serious underlying medical conditions or even malignancy.

This does not mean, however, that all aspects of the eye examination must be completed in the examination. For example:

In a patient with a **painful red eye** you may consider examining:

- Visual acuity – may be reduced
- Fundoscopy – may show anterior uveitis or corneal scarring
- Pupil – may be irregular, small, or unreactive

However, you might expect visual fields and eye movements to be normal and tell the examiner you would include the examination of these as part of your further investigations.

In a patient with a history of **progressive deterioration in vision** you may consider examining:

- Visual acuity
- Fundoscopy – retinitis pigmentosa, diabetic retinopathy
- Eye movements
- Visual fields – peripheral loss first

It is important to **tailor** your examination according to the presenting complaint.

However, it is still important to know how to examine the eye in a systematic way. Fundoscopy is a core skill for a practising clinician and MRCP candidate, but one with which many have considerable difficulty.

General appearance of the eye

Look carefully for symmetry of the eyelids, pupils and general eye movements. In particular, check for signs such as ptosis, lid retraction or irregular pupils.

Look for clues suggesting decreased visual acuity, eg white stick, adjacent Braille books, or for evidence of other systemic diseases such as diabetes, eg glucose testing sticks, diabetic drinks, foot ulcers or evidence of co-existent dialysis.

Visual acuity

Assess acuity with the patient wearing their normal glasses.

Ask the patient if they can see from each eye, and then assess individually by use of a Snellen chart. Visual acuity is defined as $V = d/D$ where $d =$ distance at which numbers are read and $D =$ distance at which they should be read.

Pupillary reflexes

Each eye should be tested in turn for direct and consensual pupilary reflexes with a pen torch while the patient faces forward with eyes focused directly ahead.

Visual fields

Visual fields should be assessed by confrontation with you sitting approximately 1 metre from the patient and with your eyes at the same level. When assessing the patient's right eye, ask them to cover up their left eye, and after covering your right eye, slowly bring an object in from the periphery in a plane equal between you and the patient.

What should the object be? A moving finger is commonly used and may be fine for a screening test if examining the cranial nerves. The top of a pen, placed in the quadrants in turn, is better, but do not bring it inwards too quickly, as the patient must have the time to say when they first see it.

A red pin can be used for assessing central colour vision that is located around the macula.

Where it is first visible gives a good indication of peripheral vision.

Eye movements (see p 225)

Fundoscopy

This should be performed in a dark room – if it is not dark ask to turn the lights off.

A mydriatic (dilating the pupil) such as tropicamide may have been used. It is essential that you examine the patient's right eye with your right eye and their left eye with your left eye. The latter is a routine many candidates have difficulty with, but failure to do this, for whatever reason, is frowned upon.

Find the red reflex, keep it in view and get in close!

Although the temptation and tendency is to go straight to the retina, you should get into the routine of gradually racking down through the lens strengths, examining first the front of the eye and gradually, by reducing the strength of the lens, moving to the retina, which is usually observed with a zero or a slightly negative lens, depending on whether or not the patient is myopic.

The disc and each quadrant of the retina should be identified and studied in turn.

Disc – note its shape, colour (pale in optic atrophy), margins and if there is papilloedema.

Retinal blood vessels – examine the vessels, noting their diameter (arteries are narrower than veins) and the point at which they cross. Is there A–V nipping?

Look for arterial emboli (arteries become much thinner or thread like) or venous thrombosis (veins become engorged with surrounding haemorrhages).

Each retinal quadrant should be examined for the presence of:

- Haemorrhages
  - dot, blot or flame shaped
- Microaneurysms
- Pigmentation
  - Exudates, distinguish between:
    - hard – white/yellow and shiny with well-defined edges
    - soft ('cotton wool spots')
- The presence of new vessels should be identified and any previous photocoagulation scars.

The macula – It should be specifically examined as the surrounding area is, as the name suggests, the site of diabetic maculopathy.

Examine the peripheries of the retina, looking particularly for evidence of retinitis pigmentosa.

Considering the cases you might be asked to see; look around the bedside for clues.

FINAL THOUGHTS

Remember that Station 5 is very different from the other stations. You are somewhat liberated from the regimented examination routines of the other stations. However, you need to gather a great deal of information and communicate a plan to the patient in a very short space of time. It is perhaps the most accurate and global reflection of how you will perform as a registrar in clinic or on-call. This should not be intimidating – if in doubt just resort to what you would normally do in exactly that scenario at work!

Integrated Clinical Assessment

1. Acromegaly
2. Addison's disease
3. Ankylosing spondylitis
4. Anterior uveitis
5. Asthma
6. Atrial fibrillation
7. Coeliac disease
8. Congestive cardiac failure
9. Cranial nerve III palsy
10. Crohn's disease/bloody diarrhoea
11. Cushing's disease
12. Dermatomyositis
13. Diabetic retinopathy
14. Eczema
15. Erythema nodosum
16. Gout
17. Graves' disease
18. Henoch–Schönlein purpura
19. Hereditary haemorrhagic telangiectasia
20. Herpes zoster
21. Horner syndrome
22. Hypothyroidism
23. Impetigo
24. Marfan syndrome
25. Osteogenesis imperfecta
26. Paget's disease
27. Papilloedema
28. Pemphigus
29. Pleural effusion
30. Psoriasis
31. Psoriatic arthropathy
32. Pyoderma gangrenosum
33. Retinitis pigmentosa
34. Rheumatoid arthritis
35. Scleroderma
36. Systemic lupus erythematosus
37. Tremor
38. Turner syndrome
39. Vitiligo

SCENARIO 1: ACROMEGALY

<table>
<tr><td rowspan="4">1–2 minutes</td><td colspan="2" align="center">Introduce yourself</td></tr>
<tr><td colspan="2">Confirm the information you've been given and patient details: this 36-year-old man has presented with headaches. Please assess him.</td></tr>
<tr><td colspan="2">'What is the main problem from your point of view?' 'For the last 3 months I have been having headaches, and I am worried about my vision as I have recently crashed my car into a parked car when driving along the road. A friend has commented that my appearance has changed.'</td></tr>
</table>

<table>
<tr>
<td rowspan="8" valign="top">5 minutes</td>
<td valign="top">

New condition

Focused history of the presenting complaint and relevant systems enquiry. This should include screening for endocrine disturbance (any aspect of the hypothalamic–pituitary axis can be disrupted) and for localising neurology (eg diplopia, visual field defect, carpal tunnel syndrome)

Identify alarm symptoms: sudden headache, diplopia, ptosis (may imply pituitary apoplexy). Polyuria/polydipsia may imply either diabetes insipidus or diabetes mellitus

Pre-existing conditions: hypertension, diabetes, colonic polyps, sleep apnoea

Social/occupational/family circumstances: especially if driving professionally (eg taxi driver, group 1 driver)

Drug history – antihypertensives, oral hypoglycaemics
DRUG ALLERGIES

Other medical conditions: any co-morbidity that might preclude hypophysectomy (eg bleeding diathesis)?

</td>
<td valign="top">

Begin a **targeted** examination of relevant area/system and continue while taking the history

General appearance (see Figure 5.1)

- Prominent supraorbital ridges, nose and lips
- Pronounced jawline (prognathism)
- Macroglossia and increased interdental separation
- Enlarged sweaty hands with thickened skin

In addition

- Examine visual fields for bitemporal hemianopia. There may be optic atrophy if the adenoma extends into the parasellar region
- Assess for cranial nerves palsies, especially nerves III, IV and VI (if raised intracranial pressure)
- Examine for carpal tunnel syndrome/scars from previous decompression
- Myopathy (especially proximal) and arthropathy is common, but no synovitis will be found
- Examine for associated endocrine features, including goitre, gynaecomastia and/or hirsutism
- Perform a cardiac and abdominal examination if has symptoms, looking for associated cardiomegaly and hepatomegaly
- Measure blood pressure, assess for glycosuria (may reflect associated impaired glucose tolerance/diabetes mellitus)

Any old photographs of the patient available?

</td>
</tr>
</table>

<table>
<tr><td colspan="2">CALLBACK: 'You said at the beginning that the main problem was headaches, change in vision and appearance. Is there anything else troubling you that we haven't covered?</td></tr>
</table>

<table>
<tr><td rowspan="4" valign="top">1–2 minutes</td><td colspan="2" align="center">RESPOND TO PATIENT'S CONCERNS (1–2 min)</td></tr>
<tr><td>1.</td><td>I think that your headaches, change in vision and appearance are due to a condition resulting from acromegaly, which is caused by a benign growth in the pituitary gland that produces too much growth hormone</td></tr>
<tr><td>2.</td><td>For your headaches, I can give you some painkillers as a temporary measure. However, it is very important to establish the diagnosis by doing some urgent investigations. As your vision is impaired, I am afraid that you will have to stop driving immediately because of the risk to yourself and other road users</td></tr>
<tr><td>3.</td><td>I am going to organise some urgent blood tests (glucose tolerance tests, IGF-1, other pituitary hormones). We will need to arrange an urgent MRI of your pituitary gland and ask the eye specialists to see you to assess to what extent this growth has affected your vision</td></tr>
<tr><td colspan="2" align="center">Thank the patient</td></tr>
</table>

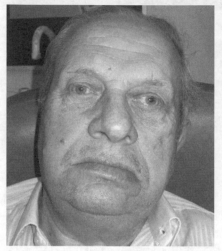

Acromegalic facies

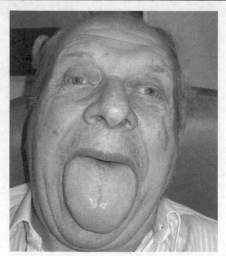

Large tongue

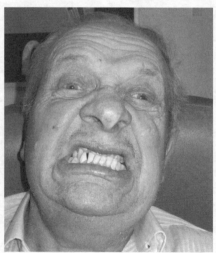

Increased interdental spacing

Figure 5.1 Acromegaly

Differential diagnosis	Clinical communication skills and managing patient concerns	Physical examination and identifying physical signs	Clinical judgement and maintaining patient welfare
Craniopharyngioma A relatively rare tumour, consisting of both solid and liquid components, which arises in Rathke's pouch	Symptoms of raised intracranial pressure (headache, nausea and vomiting), visual field defects and endocrine deficiencies (eg pubertal delay from gonadotrophin deficiency)	Visual defects In contrast to other pituitary adenomas; this starts by causing a bitemporal inferior quadrantanopia, because the suprasellar lesion initially compresses the optic chiasma from above. Over time, this may progress to bitemporal hemianopia	Diagnosed by characteristic appearances on pituitary imaging Transcranial frontal surgery is the major modality of treatment, either with or without radiotherapy A large proportion of patients will require hormone replacement
Pituitary adenoma These may be either hormone secreting or non-secreting	Symptoms of mass effects, visual field defects and endocrine disorders	*Mass effects* May first present with headache, nausea and vomiting Visual defects: initially bitemporal superior quadrantanopia, as outlined above *Endocrine disorders* In hormone-secreting adenomas, clinical features reflect the particular hormone being secreted excessively (eg Cushing's disease from a corticotroph adenoma) As tumours expand, they may disrupt other hormone axes and cause symptoms and signs of hormone deficiency	Tumours are often diagnosed on pituitary imaging, with MRI being the preferred modality Assessment of pituitary function to assess for hormone hypersecretion and/or any associated hormone deficiencies Visual field testing should be performed at the start of treatment and thereafter to assess efficacy of treatment Transsphenoidal surgery, either with or without radiotherapy. Careful ongoing pituitary function assessment will be needed to assess if long-term hormone replacement is indicated
Pseudoacromegaly Excessive insulin secretion and associated insulin resistance	Symptoms very similar to true acromegaly as described below. No visual field defects	Clinical phenotype similar to acromegaly without visual field defects Disturbance of other hormone axes rare	Investigation focuses on exclusion of growth hormone-secreting adenoma

Clinical judgement and maintaining patient welfare

Acromegaly is a clinical syndrome resulting from the hypersecretion of growth hormone (GH). Most cases are caused by GH-secreting adenomas situated in the anterior pituitary. Approximately three-quarters of these are macroadenomas (ie >10 mm diameter) at the time of diagnosis. These adenomas account for approximately a third of all hormonally secreting pituitary adenomas. Rare causes of acromegaly include growth hormone-releasing hormone (GHRH) secretion from hypothalamic tumours, or ectopic GHRH or GH secretion (eg from neuroendocrine tumours).

Adenomas tend to grow very slowly; it is estimated that there is an average delay of more than 10 years between initial symptoms and diagnosis. The most consistent early symptoms (and those most likely to form the stem of a Station 5 question on the condition) include headaches and visual disturbance. Other relatively early features are those of endocrine disturbance, particular gonadotrophin deficiency, ie oligo-/amenorrhoea in women, or erectile dysfunction, loss of libido and testicular atrophy in men. As the condition progresses, a large number of organ systems may be affected, and a number of physical signs may develop, as described in the differential diagnosis table. There may also be signs of treatment of the condition (eg scars around the nose reflecting previous transsphenoidal surgery).

Acromegaly incurs a significantly increased mortality rate (estimated as at least twice as high) as the healthy population, with those with the highest GH levels at the greatest risk of premature death. This is mostly attributable to increased cardiovascular disease.

Investigations

1. Establish the presence of GH excess
- Random GH plasma levels in themselves are not diagnostic, because these fluctuate greatly between individuals and at different times of the day. However, serum insulin-like growth factor 1 (IGF-1) levels are elevated in almost all patients with acromegaly.
- The most effective means of diagnosing GH excess is with an oral glucose tolerance test; although GH levels suppress to very low levels after a glucose load in healthy individuals, GH levels will fail to suppress or paradoxically rise in patients with acromegaly.

2. Establish the aetiology (Table 5.1)
- Pituitary imaging should be performed; MRI is the most sensitive modality.
- Establish whether a pituitary adenoma is functional.

3. Look for complications
- Visual perimetry: to establish visual fields.
- ECG, echocardiogram and chest radiograph: if cardiomyopathy is suspected.

Table 5.1 Differentiation between anterior and posterior pituitary causes

Anterior pituitary	Posterior pituitary
Corticotroph: 9 am cortisol. If <500 nmol/L, perform a dynamic test, ie insulin or glucose tolerance test Thyrotroph: T_4, T_3 and TSH Gonadotroph: LH, FSH, testosterone and SHBG or estradiol Lactotroph: prolactin	ADH secretion – plasma and urinary sodium and osmolality. A water deprivation test may also be required

- Oral glucose tolerance test: used to make the diagnosis, but also to establish the presence of associated impaired glucose tolerance/ diabetes mellitus.
- Nerve conduction studies: if an associated carpal tunnel syndrome is suspected.
- Sleep studies: if obstructive sleep apnoea is suspected.
- Colonoscopy: surveillance for polyps and colorectal malignancies, a recognised complication of acromegaly.
- Bone profile and parathyroid hormone: the combination of acromegaly and hyperparathyroidism raises the possibility of multiple endocrine neoplasia type 1 (MEN-1) syndrome; there should be a low threshold to investigate for a possible pancreatic tumour.

Treatment

Surgical
- Transsphenoidal hypophysectomy is successful in up to 90% of patients with microadenomas and 50% of those with macroadenomas in the hands of the most experienced neurosurgeons.
- Long-term deficiency in one or more of the pituitary hormones will develop in approximately 70% of patients.

Radiotherapy
- Pituitary external irradiation is indicated for patients unfit for or not cured by surgery. It results in a 50% decline in GH levels by 2 years, but with a continuing exponential decline thereafter.
- There is a significant risk of late hypopituitarism, with other complications including cranial neuropathies and visual field impairment.

Medical
- Somatostatin analogues (eg octreotide or lancreotide) are administered subcutaneously. They reduce serum GH in 90% of patients, and to a level of GH that will prevent adenoma growth in approximately 50% of patients. Side effects are nausea and gallstones (approximately 50% by 5 years).
- Dopamine agonists (eg bromocriptine, cabergoline) are effective in only 10% of patients.
- Pegvisomant is a GH receptor antagonist, administered subcutaneously daily, which normalises serum IGF-1 in >90% of patients, helping to reduce many of the clinical features. However, it does not reduce GH secretion or constrain tumour growth, so it is currently reserved for patients with ongoing disease despite surgery, radiotherapy and other medical therapies.

Maintaining patient welfare

It is important in managing acromegalic patients to think not only about the immediate treatment for the condition, but also about the means of minimising long-term complications. Candidates can show that they are aware of these by suggesting colonoscopic screening for colonic malignancy (this is currently recommended every 3 years), and minimising the patient's risk of cardiovascular disease by optimising their blood pressure, lipid profile and smoking cessation advice.

SCENARIO 2 ADDISON'S DISEASE

Introduce yourself

Confirm the information you've been given and patient details: this 50-year-old woman presents with symptoms of fatigue and light-headedness on standing. Please assess her.

'What is the main problem from your point of view?' 'Over the past few weeks, I have felt tired all the time, as well as feeling light-headed on standing up or when I get out of bed in the morning.'

New condition

Focused history of the presenting complaint and relevant systems enquiry. Exclude common causes of fatigue (eg anaemia (blood loss?), hypothyroidism, diabetes mellitus, sleep apnoea, postviral syndrome) and hypotension (eg fluid loss (diarrhoea, diuresis), autonomic neuropathy (eg diabetes mellitus)) before considering failure of the hypothalamic–pituitary–adrenal axis

Identify alarm symptoms: collapse, loss of consciousness, symptoms suggestive of neoplasia (eg malaise, unintentional weight loss, constitutional upset)

Pre-existing conditions/risk factors: other autoimmune diseases (eg vitiligo), tuberculosis, HIV, current steroid use, previous pituitary surgery

Social/occupational/family circumstances: smoking, examples of prolonged illness/infection after physiological stress, exposure to TB

Drug history: exclude current or recent steroid use. **DRUG ALLERGIES**

Other medical conditions: as above, including inflammatory diseases that require long-term steroid use (eg asthma). Has the steroid dose been reduced recently?

Begin a **targeted** examination of relevant area/system and continue while taking the history

General appearance: thin, pale, although may be cushingoid if recently on long-term steroids

Skin: pigmentation of skin creases, mouth and any scars; also, assess for hypopigmented skin (if vitiligo present)

Abdomen: for scars of possible previous adrenalectomy

Chest: if history is suggestive of TB

Blood pressure: request assessment of blood pressure lying and standing

CALLBACK: 'You said at the beginning that the main problem was feeling light-headed and fatigued. Is there anything else troubling you that we haven't covered?

RESPOND TO PATIENT'S CONCERNS (1–2 min)

1. I think that your symptoms may be caused by your body not producing enough natural steroids from your adrenal glands – a condition called Addison's disease
2. It is very important that we make a diagnosis so that we can start effective treatment, the mainstay of which is replacing those steroids
3. If we assume that it is Addison's disease and start treatment, this will interfere with the diagnostic test. As such, I think we need to admit you to hospital for further tests, as well as investigations to exclude other possible causes for your symptoms (such as anaemia or diabetes)

Thank the patient

1–2 minutes

5 minutes

1–2 minutes

Differential diagnosis	Clinical communication skills and managing patient concerns	Physical examination and identifying physical signs	Clinical judgement and maintaining patient welfare
Nelson's syndrome The growth of a corticotrophic pituitary adenoma due to loss of hormonal negative feedback to the pituitary after a bilateral adrenalectomy performed for Cushing's disease	Symptoms of intracranial mass and disturbance of other hormone axes Symptoms of hypoadrenalism: postural hypotension, lethargy, collapse	Pigmentation – after bilateral adrenalectomy in the context of Cushing's disease, huge amounts of pro-opiomelanocortin (POMC) are produced by the adenoma. This is broken down to ACTH and a number of other products, including melanocyte-stimulating hormone (MSH). Both ACTH and MSH can bind the melanocortin receptor, resulting in pigmentation Mass effects: growth of a pituitary adenoma may result in neurological deficits (cranial neuropathies, visual impairment)	*Investigations* ACTH levels are greatly elevated Neuroimaging will demonstrate a pituitary adenoma *Treatment* Dexamethasone, to suppress tumour secretion of ACTH Radiotherapy of the pituitary Neurosurgery, typically transsphenoidal resection
Secondary adrenal failure Low ACTH resulting in understimulation of adrenal glucocorticoid production	Symptoms of pituitary disease or their causes, eg intracranial tumours (or complications related to their treatment) Vascular lesions (eg pituitary apoplexy) Infiltrative disease: infective (eg TB), inflammatory (eg sarcoidosis) or malignant (ie metastases) Symptoms of hypoadrenalism: postural hypotension, lethargy, collapse	Postural hypotension and loss of secondary sexual hair are common. No pigmentation will occur, as little ACTH is produced There may also be features related to other hormone deficiencies Intracranial mass effects – see above	*Investigations* Blood tests; plasma sodium and potassium are relatively well preserved, because this condition is associated with glucocorticoid but not mineralocorticoid deficiency. Baseline ACTH will tend to be very low (in contrast to Addison's disease), but cannot in itself make the diagnosis. A useful dynamic test is insulin-induced hypoglycaemia; the cortisol response will be blunted in those with secondary adrenal failure. Full pituitary function will also need to be assessed MRI or CT of the pituitary will help establish the cause of hypopituitarism Visual field perimetry *Treatment* Treatment of the underlying cause, including neurosurgery and/or radiotherapy for pituitary tumours
Tertiary adrenal failure	A history of long-term steroid use that has been abruptly stopped	Patients will have certain typical features of Addison's disease (eg postural hypotension), but lack certain others (ie no pigmentation)	Usually first suspected from history alone Investigations as per Addison's disease (see Clinical judgement section) Treatment involves restoring provision of exogenous steroids and tapering dose

Clinical judgement and maintaining patient welfare

Addison's disease is defined as primary failure of function of the cortex of the adrenal gland, with clinical features all related to the associated lack of production of glucocorticoid and mineralocorticoid.

Candidates should be aware that the case may not be a 'pure' case of Addison's disease; there will often be clues in the history or examination for the presence of other autoimmune diseases, or possibly for features of a polyglandular autoimmune syndrome.

The causes of the condition are

- **Autoimmune**: the most common cause in the developed world.
- **Infections**: TB is the most common cause worldwide. Other infectious causes include disseminated fungal infections (eg histoplasmosis) and HIV (either directly, or related to opportunistic infections associated with the virus, eg CMV, *Mycobacterium avium-intracellulare*).
- **Metastatic disease**: lung, breast, melanoma and intra-abdominal malignancies.
- **Haemorrhage/infarction**: Waterhouse–Friderichsen syndrome (as found in meningococcal septicaemia), but also associated with anticoagulants, thrombophilic and haemorrhagic diseases, and trauma.
- **Infiltrative metabolic diseases**: including amyloidosis and haemochromatosis.
- **Drugs**: reduce cortisol production (eg ketoconazole and metyrapone, as used in the treatment of Cushing syndrome), or drugs that increase cortisol catabolism (eg rifampicin and phenytoin).
- **Congenital**: eg congenital adrenal hyperplasia, adrenoleukodystrophy.

Investigations

- Haematology: eosinophilia, neutropenia, lymphocytosis and normochromic normocytic anaemia are characteristic.
- Biochemistry: hyponatraemia and hyperkalaemia (reflects mineralocorticoid deficiency) and hypoglycaemia (reflects glucocorticoid deficiency).
- Immunology: >80% of those with autoimmune Addison's disease will have autoantibodies detectable in the serum. These are most commonly autoantibodies focused against the enzyme 21-hydroxylase, but may be one of several other autoantibodies instead (eg anti-17-hydroxylase). It is appropriate to screen for autoantibodies found in other associated conditions (eg thyroid autoantibodies).
- Endocrinology: 9 am ACTH will be inappropriately raised in Addison's disease. A very low ACTH level in the context of other relevant clinical features may imply secondary adrenal failure.
- Short Synacthen test (SST): the patient's plasma cortisol level is measured before, and 30 and 60 min after, injection of Synacthen, an ACTH analogue. If the cortisol level increases to >550 nmol/L, then Addison's disease may be excluded. Note that, although a 9 am cortisol may be useful (with a level >500 nmol/L making adrenal failure very unlikely), it is not as sensitive a test as the SST.

Imaging
- Chest radiograph: to assess if evidence of malignancy or TB.
- CT adrenal glands: this is useful in cases of suspected infiltrative or haemorrhagic disease.

Management
If a patient first presents with the condition in adrenal crisis, he or she will need rapid resuscita-

tion with fluids and hydrocortisone to restore haemodynamic stability.

Once resuscitated (or if first diagnosed in a more stable state), the patient will require steroid replacement of both glucocorticoid (with hydrocortisone or prednisolone) and mineralocorticoid (ie fludrocortisone 0.025–0.15 mg, adjusted depending on the degree of postural hypotension).

Clinically obvious pigmentation tends to suggest inadequate replacement. However, even with adequate replacement, ACTH levels may still be modestly elevated.

Maintaining patient welfare
If the scenario involves explaining a possible new case of Addison's disease, candidates should offer a MedicAlert book/bracelet, explain the importance of close attention to steroid replacement and outline what to do when unwell (eg doubling hydrocortisone dose during illness).

SCENARIO 3: ANKYLOSING SPONDYLITIS

1–2 minutes

Introduce yourself

Confirm the information you've been given: this 33-year-old man has been experiencing worsening lower back pain and stiffness over the past 2 years. Please assess him.

'What is the main problem from your point of view?' 'I've been getting severe lower back pain which is worse at night and in the mornings. It's really difficult to get going in the morning and my back feels very stiff. I've tried yoga which has helped a bit, but now both hips and my right knee also seem to be affected.'

5 minutes

New Condition

Focused history of the presenting complaint and relevant systems enquiry. Obtain further details about the pain/stiffness of the back, and the degree of joint involvement. Screen for features of possible enthesitis (eg heel pain of Achilles tendonitis). Ask about a relevant family history

Screen for extra-articular manifestations, eg breathing difficulties, palpitations, visual impairment, change in bowel habit, mouth ulceration

Alarm symptoms: loss of sensation/weakness in lower limbs, sphincter disturbance, to exclude back pain reflecting a spinal syndrome

Existing treatments: eg NSAIDs, and common side effects (nausea, GI bleeding). **DRUG ALLERGIES**

Degree of physical impairment/immobility: are there any occupational/social consequences to the current level of immobility/pain?

Pre-existing associated conditions: eg inflammatory bowel disease

Begin a **targeted** examination of relevant area/system and continue while taking the history
Back pain/restricted movement

- **Establish restricted spinal movement/kyphosis**
  General appearance – look for the 'question mark' posture of AS (neck hyperextension accompanied by severe kyphosis, with loss of the cervical and lumbar lordosis)
  Specialised tests, eg Flesche's test, modified Schober's test and chest expansion (see main text)
- **Examine for sacroiliitis/enthesitis**
  FABERE (flexion, abduction, external rotation and extension) test for sacroiliitis
  For signs of enthesitis, focus on the posterior and inferior surfaces of the calcaneum (Achilles tendon and plantar fascia insertions, respectively)

Joint pain

- **Examine for peripheral large-joint arthritis and enthesitis**
  Examine for extra-articular features (the 'As') supporting the diagnosis of AS
- **A**nterior uveitis – affects approximately a third of patients
- **A**ortic regurgitation and **a**trioventricular conduction defects
- **A**pical pulmonary fibrosis
- **A**chilles tendonitis
- **A**tlantoaxial subluxation
- **A**myloid and IgA nephropathy causing renal disease

Urine dipstick (proteinuria/haematuria?): abdomen: 15–20% will develop symptomatic Crohn's disease (stoma present?). Evidence of amyloidosis (hepatomegaly, evidence of renal failure or replacement therapy)

CALLBACK: 'You said at the beginning that the main problem was pain and stiffness, especially in your back but also in some large joints. Is there anything else troubling you that we haven't covered?'

1–2 minutes

RESPOND TO PATIENT'S CONCERNS (1–2 min)

1. Lower back pain is common and often a specific cause cannot be found. In some instances it is caused by your own immune system attacking the spine and other joints, a condition called ankylosing spondylitis. This may be the case here
2. We need to address the immediate issue of your pain and I think anti-inflammatories, painkillers and physiotherapy are the best way to address this while we investigate further
3. We will need to do some further tests (blood tests for inflammatory markers, radiograph ± MRI of spine) to work out if this is AS. If so, in addition to the anti-inflammatories and physiotherapy, we will need to consider medications that help to 'dampen down' the immune system

Thank the patient

Differential diagnosis	Clinical communication skills and managing patient concerns	Physical examination and identifying physical signs	Clinical judgement and maintaining patient welfare
Reactive arthritis (formerly Reiter's syndrome)	Typically a mono- or oligoarthritis occurring between days to weeks after an infection. May be associated with a number of other systemic symptoms, including those of conjunctivitis and urethritis. Preceding symptoms of associated infections (diarrhoea, urethritis). History of new sexual contacts/STI risks	Clinical features include Arthritis: usually an acute asymmetrical oligoarthritis involving the lower limbs May include sacroiliitis Enthesitis: including Achilles tendonitis and plantar fasciitis Eyes: conjunctivitis, although may also include anterior uveitis Genital: urethritis and *circinate balanitis* (painless ulceration of the glans penis) Skin: *keratoderma blenorrhagica* (red, painless raised pustules on the hands and feet) and erythema nodosum Hands and nails: dactylitis and nail pitting	*Investigations* Blood tests: raised inflammatory markers Rheumatoid factor negative Microbiology: urethral swabs, urinalysis and stool culture may detect a precipitating diarrhoeal infection/STI, eg *Campylobacter, Shigella, Salmonella* and *Yersinia* spp. and *Chlamydia trachomatis* Imaging: sacroiliitis may be seen even on plain radiographs *Management* Antibiotics if evidence of ongoing precipitating infection Analgesia and anti-inflammatories. NSAIDs may be used initially, but intra-articular steroid injections may also help arthritis. DMARDs and anti-TNF-α therapy may also be appropriate in severe cases Physio- and occupational therapy
Back pain secondary to infection	Symptoms of TB (night sweats, fevers, weight loss, cough) Symptoms of brucellosis ('Malta fever': anaemia, diaphoresis, orchitis, back pain) Symptoms/history of other focal infection (eg line sepsis) from which metastatic infectious spread has lead to discitis	An extremely variable clinical spectrum, ranging from dull back pain through to paraparesis with or without an associated sepsis syndrome	Investigations These will vary depending upon the nature of the suspected infection **Management** This will include • Minimisation of any precipitating source of sepsis (eg removal of infected central venous catheter) • Antimicrobial therapy • Neurosurgical/orthopaedic intervention where there is vertebral/spinal instability or abscess

(continued)

Differential diagnosis	Clinical communication skills and managing patient concerns	Physical examination and identifying physical signs	Clinical judgement and maintaining patient welfare
Mechanical back pain	History of trauma or recent heavy lifting/unusual activity Be mindful of back pain after minimal exertion/movement suggestive of pathological vertebral fracture (malignancy, osteoporosis) History of steroid use	Clinical examination should focus on excluding focal neurology or evidence of disc impingement on the spinal cord	*Investigations* MRI of the spine if evidence of nerve impingement (urgent if cord compression suspected, less urgent for radicular impingement) Exclusion of osteoporosis (bone densitometry) in vertebral compression fractures *Management* • Bone protection (bisphosphonates) • Surgery • Analgesia
Psoriatic arthritis	See Psoriatic arthropathy (Scenario 31)		
Enteropathic arthritis	see Psoriatic arthropathy (Scenario 31)		
Rheumatoid arthritis	See Rheumatoid arthritis (Scenario 34)		
Osteoarthritis	See Gout differential diagnosis table (Scenario 16)		

Clinical judgement and maintaining patient welfare

Ankylosing spondylitis (AS) is a chronic inflammatory disease of the spine and sacroiliac joints of unclear aetiology. It is more common in men, and tends to first present before age 30 years. It belongs to the group of *seronegative spondyloarthropathies*, so called because, in contrast to other rheumatological diseases (eg rheumatoid arthritis, SLE, etc), there is no easily measurable diagnostic serum antibody. The seronegative spondyloarthropathies, in addition to AS, are

- Psoriatic arthropathy
- Reactive arthritis
- Enteropathic arthritis: as found in association with inflammatory bowel disease.

The seronegative spondyloarthropathies have a number of common features

- No detectable serum markers of rheumatological disease
- Arthritis affecting the axial skeleton (spinal joints, including the sacroiliac region) and/or peripheral arthritis (usually manifesting as large joint mono- or asymmetrical oligoarthritis)
- Extra-articular manifestations, eg skin changes in psoriatic disease, and eye and genital features in reactive arthritis
- Disease at the site of tendon insertion (*enthesitis*) and whole digit disease (*dactylitis*).

Investigations
As part of the examination there are a number of specialised tests that are useful in assessing patients with suspected AS

- Flesche's test: although healthy people can touch the wall with the occiput, patients with AS cannot as a result of their spinal deformity.
- Reduced chest expansion: this may reflect both spinal deformity and intercostal tendon enthesitis. It is best measured at the fourth intercostal space.

- Modified Schober's test: find the level of the posterior iliac spines at the level of the 'dimples of Venus', and mark 10 cm above and 5 cm below this point. When healthy adults bend forward, these marks will be at least 5 cm further apart; however, they will not extend this far in patients with AS.

The seronegative spondyloarthropathies are diagnosed clinically. However, a number of investigations may help towards making the diagnosis

- Blood tests: inflammatory markers are raised in active disease and are useful for monitoring the efficacy of treatment. HLA-B27 is found in most patients with AS, but is also found in up to 6% of the healthy population.
- Imaging: plain radiographs alone may be suggestive of sacroiliitis, although MRI is more sensitive.

Management
This will require a multidisciplinary approach, with input from both primary and secondary care

- Physical therapies
  - Exercise, physiotherapy and occupational therapy may reduce pain and stiffness and allow sufferers to adapt to any physical disability.
- Pharmacological
  - Analgesia/anti-inflammatories: NSAIDs are a useful first-line therapy
  - Glucocorticoids: either pulsed corticosteroids or intra-articular steroid injection
  - DMARDs: sulfasalazine is the only DMARD with established efficacy in AS
  - Anti-TNF-α therapy: this is now licensed and approved by NICE for use when AS sacroiliitis has not responded to at least two first-line therapies.
- Surgical
  - Total hip replacement and spinal surgery may be indicated.

Managing patient welfare
- In a young patient with progressive lower back pain, the candidate should screen for neurological symptoms and assess the peripheral neurological system if appropriate to exclude a spinal syndrome.
- Patients may develop considerable disability that may impact on themselves and their family. Referral to support groups (eg NASS) may be helpful.

Resources
National Ankylosing Spondylitis Society (NASS): www.nass.co.uk.

SCENARIO 4: ANTERIOR UVEITIS

1–2 minutes

Introduce yourself

Confirm the information you've been given and patient details: this 32-year-old man has presented with blurred vision, photophobia and painful red right eye. Please assess him.

'What is the main problem from your point of view?' 'I have a painful right eye, with blurred vision and sensitivity to light. Recently, I have also had problems with joint pain.'

5 minutes

New condition

Focused history of the presenting complaint and relevant systems enquiry

Differentiate from other causes of a painful red eye – purulent discharge, gritty pain (conjunctivitis, corneal ulcer); nausea, vomiting, headache, severe visual loss (acute closed-angle glaucoma); recurrent episodes (episcleritis); trauma; etc

Photophobia or blurred vision (involvement of the muscle of the iris)

Identify alarm symptoms: systemic upset and photophobia (meningitis); severely painful red eye (glaucoma); breathlessness/dry cough (sarcoid); bloody diarrhoea (IBD); arthritis (seronegative arthritis, connective tissue disorder); genital ulcers (syphilis)

Social/occupational/family circumstances: sexual history; family history of IBD/seronegative arthritis

Drug history: anti-inflammatory medications, antibiotics, previous need for eye drops. **DRUG ALLERGIES**

Other medical conditions: known arthritis, IBD, sarcoidosis

Begin a **targeted** examination of relevant area/system and continue while taking the history

General appearance: conjunctival pallor, oral ulcers (may both imply IBD)

Examination of the eye

General: 'circumlimbal injection' (erythema around the cornea, dilated blood vessels)

Fundoscopy: anterior chamber inspection may show cloudy fluid ('*flare*'), white clumps of inflammatory cells (*keratitic precipitates*), and possibly *hypopyon* (protein-rich fluid/pus in lower chamber of eye)

Visual acuity: acutely, may be decreased

Fields: typically normal

Pupils: often small, non-reacting, irregular pupil

Movement: typically normal

Additional examination

Joints: if seronegative arthritis/connective tissue disorder suspected, looking for deformity/synovitis

Abdominal: if IBD suspected (also tell examiner you would do a rectal examination)

Respiratory: if sarcoidosis suspected

CALLBACK: 'You said at the beginning that the main problem was a painful right eye, blurred vision, and sensitivity to light. You also have had some joint pain. Is there anything else troubling you that we haven't covered?'

1–2 minutes

RESPOND TO PATIENT'S CONCERNS (1–2 min)

1. I think that your symptoms are caused by acute anterior uveitis. This is where the front of your eye is inflamed. Usually no cause is found, but it can be associated with other inflammatory conditions
2. I will refer you immediately to an eye specialist (ophthalmologist) for a more detailed slit-lamp examination of your eye. It is important that you stay in hospital for now, as I want to exclude other conditions that need urgent treatment such as glaucoma and an ulcer on your cornea
3. If it is acute anterior uveitis, then steroids eye drops will normally successfully treat this. It would be important to investigate your joint pain with blood tests and radiographs to exclude an associated inflammatory form of arthritis that requires urgent treatment

Thank the patient

Differential diagnosis	Clinical communication skills and managing patient concerns	Physical examination and identifying physical signs	Clinical judgement and maintaining patient welfare
Conjunctivitis	Patients describe a gritty, itchy, eye, often sticky in the morning Given the possibility of *Chlamydia sp.* as a cause, a sexual history may be appropriate	Presents as an acute red eye. There may be associated lid swelling, conjunctival injection, papillae or follicles. Patients may also develop discharge from the eye (purulent in bacterial disease, but usually watery in other causes) Severe cases may progress to corneal inflammation (*keratitis*) and *corneal ulceration*	*Investigations* Eye swabs to identify underlying infection Corneal ulceration diagnosed with slit-lamp examination *Management* Topical aciclovir for herpes conjunctivitis, topical antibiotics (eg chloramphenicol) for bacterial disease
Scleritis	A red eye with pain on eye movement Patients may give a history of associated autoimmune diseases, including rheumatoid arthritis, SLE and vasculitides, eg Wegener's granulomatosis	The sclera is often injected and thickened, although may become thin and transparent in acute severe necrotising scleritis Make a careful assessment of visual acuity	*Investigations* Slit-lamp examination Autoantibody/vasculitis screen *Management* NSAIDs for mild cases, systemic steroids (or other immunosuppressives) for severe cases Rapid diagnosis and treatment is key because **a quarter of patients may develop significant visual loss**
Episcleritis	An aching red eye, less painful than scleritis Only rarely associated with systemic diseases	Injected sclerae Much lower risk of visual loss than scleritis	*Investigations* Diagnosed via slit-lamp examination *Management* Normally resolves with topical NSAIDs or steroids, with only minimal risk of prolonged visual impairment

(continued)

Differential diagnosis	Clinical communication skills and managing patient concerns	Physical examination and identifying physical signs	Clinical judgement and maintaining patient welfare
Acute angle-closure glaucoma	The condition typically presents with an acutely painful eye and associated nausea and vomiting. Common triggers include tricyclic antidepressants and H_2-receptor antagonists. Patients will often complain of a significant loss of vision and the presence of haloes	Examination of the eye reveals a red eye with a minimally reactive, mid-dilated pupil and a cloudy, oedematous cornea that lacks a red reflex	*Investigations* The diagnosis is made clinically. Tonometry (eye pressure) and gonioscopy (examines the trabecular meshwork for outflow obstruction) *Management* Medical treatments include β blockers, pilocarpine and acetazolamide. Surgical therapies (eg laser iridotomy) improve flow of aqueous humour into the anterior chamber
Subconjunctival haemorrhage	A history of a painless, red eye, usually of sudden onset	Presents as bright red blood seen under the conjunctiva. May occur spontaneously or in response to trauma	*Investigations* Diagnosed clinically *Management* Usually resolves spontaneously
Trauma			

Clinical judgement and maintaining patient welfare

Anterior uveitis (also known as iritis) is a relatively common form of inflammatory eye disease that may occur either acutely or chronically. Many cases of anterior uveitis are idiopathic. However, the reason that it is a common examination topic is that the condition has a number of associations with systemic diseases (Table 5.2).

In addition, there are a number of conditions ('masquerade syndromes') that have very similar clinical findings to anterior uveitis, but are not caused through a primary inflammatory process. One example is B-cell lymphoma of the eye/central nervous system; this may first be suspected if a condition previously diagnosed as anterior uveitis fails to settle with steroid therapy.

Table 5.2 Associations of anterior uveitis

Category of disease	Examples
Rheumatological	Seronegative spondyloarthropathies Juvenile idiopathic arthritis Behçet's disease
Respiratory	Sarcoidosis
Gastroenterological	Inflammatory bowel disease
Infections	Tuberculosis Syphilis Herpes simplex Herpes zoster Lyme disease Leptospirosis

Investigations
- **Blood tests**: inflammatory markers may be raised in autoimmune and infective causes. Serum calcium and ACE may be elevated in sarcoidosis. Serological assays (combined with appropriate cultures) may help diagnose infective causes.
- **Imaging**: a chest radiograph will be useful in suspected sarcoidosis or tuberculosis. Joint imaging (by plain radiograph, MRI or other modality) can help in the diagnosis of associated seronegative spondyloarthropathies.
- **Endoscopy**: lower GI imaging, endoscopy and biopsy are appropriate in investigating suspected inflammatory bowel disease.

Management
The mainstay of treatment for anterior uveitis is immediate treatment with steroid eye drops or ointment, every 2 hours initially to ensure a rapid response. A topical mydriatic such as cyclopentolate may also be used to minimise the risk of adhesions forming between the iris and lens. Systemic corticosteroids and immunosuppressants may be indicated in the most severe cases. In most cases, vision returns to normal.

Maintaining patient welfare
- Patients in MRCP (PACES) with apparent anterior uveitis will almost always have an underlying systemic medical disorder. A plan to systematically exclude associated conditions should be made during the assessment.
- It is important to give patients practical advice about activities that they should limit while their vision is impaired, including adaptations that they may need to make at work or home, and at least temporary cessation of driving.

SCENARIO 5. ASTHMA

Introduce yourself

Confirm the information you've been given and patient details: this 20-year-old woman with asthma has presented with increasing dyspnoea and wheeze over the last few days. Please assess her.

'What is the main problem from your point of view?' 'Over the last 2 days I have been getting more wheezy and short of breath. I am not able to walk up the stairs at work without feeling wheezy and my inhalers do not seem to be making any difference.'

(1–2 minutes)

Exacerbation of a chronic illness

Existing treatment/surveillance. Confirm current diagnosis, duration of disease, frequency of flares and responsiveness to previous therapy

How well/poorly has disease been controlled? Intensive care/high dependency admissions, best peak flow rate and recent readings, steroid use, compliance with medications

Brief account of this flare/exacerbation, focusing on severity (increased nocturnal cough, response to salbutamol inhaler), duration and whether obvious precipitant (ie dust, dander, cold, exercise)

Alarm symptoms: unable to talk in full sentences, previous intubation

Social/occupational/family circumstances: smoking, pets, living/work environment. Family history of atopy. What do the symptoms stop the patient from doing?

Drug history: current and previous failed medications. Inhaler technique and compliance. Previous or current steroid use. **DRUG ALLERGIES**

Other medical conditions: eczema, hay fever, nasal polyps, previous skin testing

Begin a **targeted** examination of relevant area/system and continue while taking the history

Establish

- **Key diagnostic signs**
  - Examine respiratory system, looking for lung expansion (if unilateral reduction, consider pneumothorax), prolonged expiratory phase, expiratory wheeze, and/or bronchial breathing
- **Disease severity** (although significant exacerbations unlikely to be found in MRCP (PACES))
  - Not able to talk in full sentences, tachypnoea, tachycardia, reduced peak expiratory flow measurement, oxygen saturations
  - Ask to check inhaler technique
- **Signs of therapy**
  - eg cushingoid features

(5 minutes)

CALLBACK: 'You said at the beginning that the main problem was being wheezy and short of breath. Is there anything else troubling you that we haven't covered?'

RESPOND TO PATIENT'S CONCERNS (1–2 min)

1. I think the cause of your shortness of breath and wheeziness is a flare of your asthma
2. We need to get your symptoms and your breathing under control quickly with a combination of different medications, including inhalers/nebulisers and steroids
3. We need to perform tests (including peak flow spirometry) now and after increasing your treatment to check that it is working. A key element of your treatment will be using inhalers regularly rather than just when you feel wheezy
4. I think that the cause of this flare of your asthma is ... (eg exercise, exposure to allergenic trigger, respiratory tract infection); we will need to get this under control (eg with antibiotics)

Thank the patient

(1–2 minutes)

Differential diagnosis	Clinical communication skills and managing patient concerns	Physical examination and identifying physical signs	Clinical judgement and maintaining patient welfare
Chronic obstructive pulmonary disease (COPD)	A chronic progressive inflammatory airways disease characterised by airway obstruction with minimal or no reversibility. COPD was previously described as either chronic bronchitis or emphysema • Emphysema – a condition diagnosed pathologically, defined by enlargement of airway spaces distal to the terminal bronchioles and destruction of their walls. • Chronic bronchitis – a condition diagnosed clinically by the presence of a productive cough on most days for at least three months during two consecutive years. The vast majority of cases are attributable to smoking, although other risk factors are also well-recognised (eg coal dust).	Clinical features include • On inspection – use of accessory muscles of respiration and pursed lip breathing. In advanced disease, chronic hypoxia may result in polycythaemia (look for plethoric facies) and/ or cor pulmonale (suggested clinically by raised venous pressure and peripheral oedema). • On palpation – hyperexpanded lungs. • On percussion – hyper-resonance. • On auscultation – prolonged expiratory phase with polyphonic expiratory wheeze.	**Investigations** • Pulmonary function tests: Will demonstrate an obstructive deficit, ie $FEV_1 < 80\%$ predicted, with $FEV_1 / FVC < 70\%$ predicted. • Chest radiograph: Hyperexpansion. The radiograph also helps exclude other mimicking conditions, and identifying pneumonic precipitants for exacerbations. **Management** • General measures: Smoking cessation, vaccination against influenza/ *Pneumococcus*. Pulmonary rehabilitation is also of benefit. • Pharmacological: A combination of inhaled β2 agonists (short and/ or long acting), inhaled anti-cholinergics (i.e. tiotropium) and inhaled corticosteroid. Oral corticosteroid and/ or nebulisers useful in exacerbations. • Oxygen therapy: Long-term oxygen therapy for COPD is indicated in non-smoking patients with resting $PaO_2 < 7.3$ kPa, or those with resting PaO_2 of $7.3 – 8$ kPa in the context of polycythaemia or cor pulmonale. • Surgical: A limited role in COPD, but may include bullectomy, lung volume reduction surgery, or transplantation.
Congestive cardiac failure	See Cardiac Failure ICA (Scenario 8).		

(continued)

Differential diagnosis	Clinical communication skills and managing patient concerns	Physical examination and identifying physical signs	Clinical judgement and maintaining patient welfare
Churg–Strauss syndrome	This is a form of small vessel vasculitis characterised by a triad of features • An asthma/rhinitis-like illness. • Eosinophilia and eosinophilic infiltration into tissues. • Vasculitic illness involving multiple organs.	Clinicians should consider particularly Churg–Strauss syndrome in the following circumstances • If a patient thought to have asthma suddenly develops rapidly progressive respiratory disease that does not respond promptly to conventional asthma therapy. • If a patient thought to have asthma develops multi-system disease consistent with vasculitis, eg mononeuritis, conjunctivitis, nephritic syndrome, arthritis, purpuric skin lesions, etc.	**Investigations** • Blood tests: Marked eosinophilia, raised inflammatory markers. Approximately one-half of patients will be positive for pANCA. • Histology: eg of affected skin lesions; the definitive means of confirming the diagnosis. **Management** • Steroids, cyclophosphamide and/or plasmapheresis.
Allergic broncho-pulmonary aspergillosis (ABPA)	A condition occurring through a hypersensitivity reaction to *Aspergillus fumigatus*. Over time, chronic inflammation of the lungs results in mucus plugging and a bronchiectasis-like condition.	Clinical features include • Wheeze and dyspnoea that may mimic asthma. • Recurrent cough with large volumes of sputum.	**Investigations** • Laboratory tests: Marked eosinophilia and raised plasma IgE. *Aspergillus* often detectable in sputum, and skin tests against it are usually positive. • Chest radiograph: Consolidation or bronchiectatic-type changes. **Management** • Symptomatic treatment of wheeze with inhalers. • Oral corticosteroids for exacerbations. • Some evidence for the use of long-term anti-fungals, eg itraconazole.

SCENARIO 6. ATRIAL FIBRILLATION

1–2 minutes

Introduce yourself

Confirm the information you've been given and patient details: this 68-year-old woman has presented with palpitations and chest pain intermittently for the last month. Please assess her.

'What is the main problem from your point of view?' 'I get episodes where I feel that my heart is racing. The heart beat doesn't feel regular when this happens. I also get chest pain, and sometimes feel short of breath too. I am worried about having a heart attack.'

5 minutes

New condition

Focused history of the presenting complaint and relevant systems enquiry. Identify exact nature of 'palpitations', including how fast the heart beat is perceived, whether regular or irregular, the nature of onset and termination of symptoms (ie abrupt or gradual onset; whether an obvious associated trigger, such as caffeine), and how frequently attacks occur

Explore whether pain sounds ischaemic in nature, and strength of association with palpitations with exertion and dyspnoea. Screen for causes of AF (eg symptoms of thyrotoxicosis). Exclude anxiety-related phenomena (eg perioral/fingertip paraesthesia)

Identify alarm symptoms: crescendo angina, presyncope, focal neurological signs that may suggest stroke

Pre-existing conditions: cardiorespiratory disease, previous stroke, hyperthyroidism, hypertension

Drug history: ask about thyroid hormone replacement (and when last TFTs check if so), medications associated with arrhythmia (eg salbutamol) and other cardiac medication (eg antihypertensives, lipid-lowering medications). Screen for contraindications to anticoagulation where AF is suspected. **DRUG ALLERGIES**

Social history: ask about impact of symptoms on daily activities, and use of alcohol and recreational drugs (including amphetamines and cocaine)

Begin a **targeted** examination of relevant area/system and continue while taking the history

General appearance: features of thyrotoxic eye disease, short of breath

Pulse: irregularly irregular in AF

Hands: tar staining, splinter haemorrhages, tremor, sweaty palms, palmar erythema

Face and neck: malar flush, carotid bruits, goitre

Cardiac: examine for features of mitral stenosis (undisplaced tapping apex beat, mid-diastolic murmur, opening snap, etc), mitral regurgitation (displaced apex, pansystolic murmur, radiating to axilla) and/or peripheral signs of cardiac failure (raised venous pressure, peripheral and sacral oedema, etc)

Chest: bibasal crepitations and pleural effusions of cardiac failure

Neurology: focal neurological deficit from previous stroke

To finish: ask for blood pressure

CALLBACK: 'You said at the beginning that the main problem was palpitations, chest pain and breathlessness. Is there anything else troubling you that we haven't covered?'

1–2 minutes

RESPOND TO PATIENT'S CONCERNS (1–2 min)

1. I think the cause of your palpitations is an (occasional) irregular heart beat, called (paroxysmal) atrial fibrillation (AF), which is usually easily managed. We can either get the heart back into a normal rhythm, or try to stop it from beating too fast. The cause is often not found but we need to look for underlying problems and treat these. The fact that you get pain and shortness of breath suggests that there may be a problem with the blood supply to the heart itself through the coronary arteries
2. Initially, we will need to investigate you by also performing an ECG, ultrasound of your heart (echocardiogram) and a 24-hour measurement of your heart rhythm. We may also need to perform other tests (eg stress echocardiogram, coronary angiogram) to check the blood supply to the heart
3. If the ECG confirms AF, we can start treatment right away

Thank the patient

Differential diagnosis	Clinical communication skills and managing patient concerns	Physical examination and identifying physical signs	Clinical judgement and maintaining patient welfare
Extrasystole	Atrial extrasystole Ventricular extrasystole	Typically perceived as a 'missed beat, pause, then an extra-strong beat' May generate an irregularly irregular pulse that restores to sinus rhythm on exercise	Diagnosed clinically or on ECG Usually (certainly in the absence of other cardiac disease) benign, with no further intervention needed
Supraventricular tachyarrhythmia (SVT)	Atrial flutter	Similar to AF, atrial flutter may be diagnosed incidentally, or present with palpitations, dyspnoea, chest pain and/or features of cardiac failure	Diagnosed through the presence of flutter waves on ECG Management broadly similar to that of AF
	Atrioventricular re-entry tachycardia (AVRT) and atrioventricular nodal re-entry tachycardia (AVNRT) – arrhythmias occurring because of accessory conducting pathways	Patients with AVNRT may describe the sensation of palpitation in the neck, reflecting cannon 'a' waves as a result of atrioventricular dissociation Patients may describe polyuria at the time of the tachycardia, reflecting atrial stretch and release of atrial natriuretic peptide Patients may have noted that the Valsalva manoeuvre terminates the arrhythmia	Diagnosed on ECG, as a regular narrow complex tachycardia. There may be features of Wolff–Parkinson–White syndrome, ie delta waves After initial stabilisation (with adenosine, β blocker, amiodarone, etc), may be managed pharmacologically or with catheter ablation of the accessory pathway
Ventricular tachyarrhythmia	Ventricular tachycardia (VT)	Typically presents as presyncope/syncope with severe haemodynamic compromise, including cardiac arrest Often occurs in the context of severe cardiac disease, with features found on clinical assessment being those of the underlying aetiology	Diagnosed on ECG, as a broad complex regular tachycardia Should be treated as a life-threatening emergency, with DC cardioversion and amiodarone administration if haemodynamically compromised. Survivors of a VT cardiac arrest should have an implantable cardioverter defibrillator (ICD) inserted

(continued)

Differential diagnosis	Clinical communication skills and managing patient concerns	Physical examination and identifying physical signs	Clinical judgement and maintaining patient welfare
Bradyarrhythmia	Sinoatrial node disease – includes sinus bradycardia, vasovagal attacks and carotid sinus hypersensitivity Atrioventricular block – all forms of heart block	Presyncope or syncope is the common presenting feature There may be no abnormal physical signs in even high-level heart block apart from a slow pulse	ECG will make the diagnosis of heart block. Ambulatory ECG monitoring or loop recorder insertion may be merited in cases of suspected infrequent bradyarrhythmia Once stabilised (with atropine and/or other medications), patients with high-level heart block will require permanent pacemaker insertion
Non-cardiac	Metabolic disease, eg thyrotoxicosis, hypoglycaemia	Thyrotoxicosis may generate sinus tachycardia, atrial fibrillation/flutter or SVT. See Scenario 17. Graves' disease	See Scenario 17. Graves' disease
	Anaemia	May be diagnosed clinically, eg pallor of the conjunctivae	Confirmed through detection of a low haemoglobin level, with investigations dependent on the clinical scenario and the mean cell volume
	Drugs and toxins: including alcohol, caffeine, thyroid hormone, β agonists and stimulants (eg amphetamines)		Often sinus tachycardia is the only abnormality found. However, medications may also be associated with life-threatening cardiotoxicity (eg tricyclic antidepressant overdose resulting in long QT segments and polymorphic VT). As such, telemetry should be undertaken wherever drug-related cardiotoxicity is suspected
	Psychiatric disease: anxiety disorders, panic attacks, etc		

Clinical judgement and maintaining patient welfare

Atrial fibrillation (AF) is the most common persistent arrhythmia encountered in clinical practice, affecting more than a sixth of those aged >80 years. AF represents chaotic electrical activity within the atrial muscle, with atria contracting up to 600 times/min; the AV node reacts to this only intermittently, resulting in irregular ventricular contractions. Many cases of AF have no obvious precipitating cause (so-called 'lone AF'), but the condition also has a number of well-recognised triggers, including

- Cardiac precipitants: ischaemic, hypertensive and valvular heart disease (particularly valvular disease of the mitral valve), cardiomyopathy and infective endocarditis.
- Non-cardiac precipitants: hypermetabolic states (eg thyrotoxicosis, phaeochromocytoma), drugs and toxins (eg alcohol, amphetamines), or any acute illness resulting in physiological stress (particularly respiratory conditions, including pneumonia, exacerbations of COPD, etc).

Clinical features

An irregularly irregular pulse is found in AF. This may also be found in patients with frequent ventricular ectopic beats; note that ectopics usually reduce or stop entirely with exercise, but not AF.

Investigations

- **ECG**
  - Irregular QRS complexes and the absence of the P waves on ECG define the condition. Where paroxysmal AF is suspected, ambulatory ECG monitoring is useful for confirming the diagnosis and/or differentiating from other arrhythmias.
- **Chest radiograph**
  - Useful for establishing if there is evidence of cardiac failure where AF is suspected to be secondary to established cardiac disease
  - Also helps in assessing for a respiratory precipitant to AF, eg consolidation.
- **Blood tests**
  - Biochemistry: abnormalities in electrolytes may exacerbate AF
  - Endocrine: thyroid function tests should be checked in all cases. Hypoglycaemia may manifest clinically as palpitations, and glucose should be checked in cases of diagnostic doubt. Assays for serum and urinary catecholamines and their derivatives should be performed where phaeochromocytoma is suspected.
- **Echocardiogram**
  - This will help establish if there is underlying structural cardiac disease that may be contributing to AF, eg mitral regurgitation. It is also important as part of the assessment for whether anticoagulation is appropriate (see below).
- **Other tests**
  - Ischaemia investigations: stress echocardiogram, myocardial perfusion scan and/or coronary angiogram
  - Implantable loop recorders
  - Electrophysiological study (EPS): where arrhythmia is suspected but has not been captured, an EPS may be used to trigger it. If an arrhythmia is identified, then a catheter ablation may be performed.

Management

- *General measures*
  - Treat any precipitating cause (eg anti-thyroid medications if thyrotoxicosis, correction of electrolytes).
  - Patients with AF with an accelerated ventricular rate should be managed according to national resuscitation guidelines. The ventricular rate may be slowed pharmacologically (eg metoprolol, verapamil, digoxin and amiodarone), although immediate DC cardioversion

may be required if there are features of cardiovascular instability.

- *Antiarrhythmic therapy* – rhythm vs rate control strategies
  - There is ongoing debate about whether the aim of antiarrhythmic therapy in AF should be to restore the patient to sinus rhythm, or only to control the ventricular rate. Extensive research shows no difference in either long-term morbidity or mortality between patients managed by either strategy. However, given that AF is associated with an increased risk of stroke (see below), sinus rhythm is preferable to AF wherever possible.
  - Current guidelines (NICE and the European Society of Cardiology) recommend that the following group of patients be treated with a rhythm control strategy
    - New-onset AF
    - Patients with symptoms attributable to AF (including features of heart failure)
    - Patients with AF secondary to a clear precipitant, eg pneumonia.
  - Rhythm control is most successfully achieved with DC cardioversion. This should be taken only after several weeks of anticoagulation because of the risk of thromboembolisation and stroke. Given that AF will recur in up to half of cardioverted patients, patients should also be treated pharmacologically to try to minimise the chance of cardioversion back into AF. β blockers are the mainstay of therapy, with amiodarone and sotalol used as second-line therapies.
  - Rate control may be achieved with β blockers, non-dihydropyridine calcium channel antagonists (eg verapamil), digoxin and amiodarone. β blockers and calcium channel antagonists should not be used together because of the risk of high-level heart block.

- *Anticoagulation*
  - Patients with permanent AF have a risk of stroke as high as 10% per year, principally reflecting systemic thromboembolisation from the heart. A number of trials have concluded that this risk may be reduced significantly (by >50%) through the use of warfarin, with studies consistently finding that warfarin (or novel oral anticoagulants (NOACs)) is far superior in this role compared with anti-platelet therapy.
  - However, these same studies have also identified that certain patient cohorts with AF (ie patients aged <65 years, lone AF, etc) gain much less benefit in this regard from anticoagulation than others. As anticoagulation is of course associated with significant potential complications (principally bleeding), risk stratification should be taken for patients with AF to gauge whether anticoagulation is appropriate. A number of different means of risk stratification are used, but that most widely used in current practice is the **CHA$_2$DS$_2$-VASC** score (see box opposite).
  - Patients with a score of at least 2 will gain significant benefit from anticoagulation.
- **Other therapies for AF**
  - *Electrophysiological*: specialised cardiac electrophysiology centres may attempt to terminate AF through radiofrequency ablation within the left atrium/pulmonary veins, or – in very difficult cases – ablation of the AV node and permanent pacemaker insertion.
  - *Surgical*: a number of techniques have been tried, including the Maze procedure, ie surgical myocardial ablation in an attempt to optimise electrical conduction between fibrillating atria and adjacent ventricles.

CHA$_2$DS$_2$-VASC score	
Risk factor	**Score**
Congestive cardiac failure/reduced left ventricular function	1
Hypertension	1
Age ⩾75 years	2
Diabetes mellitus	1
Stroke/TIA/previous thromboembolic disease	2
Vascular disease (including myocardial infarction, peripheral vascular disease)	1
Age 65–74 years	1
Sex category (female)	1

Maintaining patient welfare

Careful counselling must be undertaken before starting anticoagulation for AF, with the advantages balanced against possible disadvantages (eg risk of bleeding after falls and injury).

SCENARIO 7. COELIAC DISEASE

Introduce yourself

Confirm the information you've been given and patient details: this 29-year-old man has presented to out-patients with a history of diarrhoea, abdominal pain, weight loss and an itchy blistering skin rash on both of his elbows. Please assess him.

'What is the main problem from your point of view?' 'For the last 3 months, I have had diarrhoea and abdominal pain, I've lost 2 stone in weight, and I've now developed a rash on my elbows.'

New condition

Focused history of the presenting complaint and relevant systems enquiry: differentiate infective causes (acute onset, bloody diarrhoea, anorexia, fever, recent travel) from inflammatory (slower onset, preserved or increased appetite). Assess for relationship between symptoms and consumption of gluten-containing foods. What were the results of previous investigations (eg stool microscopy by GP) or self-imposed dietary exclusions?

Identify alarm symptoms: B symptoms, bloody diarrhoea, jaundice, weight loss

Pre-existing conditions/risk factors: nearly all autoimmune conditions are associated with coeliac disease

Social/occupational/family circumstances: impact on daily activities, family history of coeliac disease, etc

Drug history: ask about new medications that may cause a pruritic rash. Have antihistamines been tried? **DRUG ALLERGIES**

Other medical conditions: any other autoimmune condition? Seronegative arthritis/iritis/erythema nodosum suggest IBD rather than coeliac disease

Begin a **targeted** examination of relevant area/system and continue while taking the history

General: make a global assessment of nutritional status; looks well nourished or cachectic?

Face: pale, angular stomatitis, glossitis

Hands: koilonychia in severe cases

Eyes: look for jaundice, pale conjunctiva, iritis (IBD)

Skin: pruritic vesicular rash on elbows may represent dermatitis herpetiformis (may also be on trunk, knees, or buttocks)

Abdomen: soft, non-tender in coeliac disease (in contrast to IBD – abdomen may be tender with a mass)

Extras: consider examining other systems if evidence of other autoimmune disorders, eg hand arthritis of small joints consistent with rheumatoid arthritis

CALLBACK: 'You said at the beginning that the main problem was diarrhoea, weight loss and a rash. Is there anything else troubling you that we haven't covered?'

RESPOND TO PATIENT'S CONCERNS (1–2 min)

1. I think your symptoms suggest inflammation in the gut. From your story and the associated itchy rash, I think that this is likely to be caused by an overreaction to gluten – a condition called coeliac disease. However, we need to exclude other inflammatory conditions of the gut that require different treatments
2. Coeliac disease usually responds very well to exclusion of gluten from the diet. As gluten is found in anything containing wheat (eg bread and pasta), this is not easy
3. It's therefore essential that we first confirm the diagnosis with a biopsy of the small bowel and some blood tests. The biopsy is done by endoscopy of the upper gut which is a quick and safe procedure

Thank the patient

1–2 minutes

5 minutes

1–2 minutes

Differential diagnosis	Clinical communication skills and managing patient concerns	Physical examination and identifying physical signs	Clinical judgement and maintaining patient welfare
Crohn's disease	See Scenario 10. Crohn's disease flowchart		
Small bowel bacterial overgrowth	A condition with many different risk factors Functional small bowel disease: diabetes mellitus, systemic sclerosis Structural abnormalities: secondary to surgery, strictures related to Crohn's disease, etc Other causes: immunodeficiency, cirrhosis, etc	Abdominal pain, diarrhoea and weight loss that occurs in association with any of the known risk factors for the condition	*Investigations* Glucose hydrogen breath test: a positive test detects hydrogen released by bacteria metabolising glucose Jejunal aspirate and culture: the 'gold standard' for diagnosis *Management* Treatment of the underlying precipitant Dietary changes Rotating courses of antibiotics
Chronic pancreatitis	Progressive failure of pancreatic endocrine and exocrine function Particularly associated with chronic alcohol excess	Typical features include: Severe epigastric pain, radiating to the back Steatorrhoea (once 90% of pancreatic exocrine function lost) Diabetes (related to loss of pancreatic endocrine function)	*Investigations* Imaging: pancreatic calcification may be seen on plain radiographs; ultrasonography, CT and MRI give more detail MRCP: to visualise biliary/pancreatic ducts. ERCP and endoscopic ultrasonography may also be of use Pancreatic function tests: now rarely used *Management* Alcohol cessation and dietary modification Pancreatic enzyme supplementation Analgesia
Giardiasis	Caused by the protozoan *Giardia lamblia*. Typically an imported infection, although may be contracted in UK with faeco-oral transmission	Ongoing diarrhoea, altered bowel habit and bloating/belching after an episode of acute diarrhoea	*Investigations* Stool sample: cysts/trophozoites identified on microscopy *Management* Tinidazole or metronidazole

(continued)

Differential diagnosis	Clinical communication skills and managing patient concerns	Physical examination and identifying physical signs	Clinical judgement and maintaining patient welfare
Tropical sprue	A chronic diarrhoeal disease of presumed infective aetiology found in residents of the tropics	Chronic diarrhoea/steatorrhoea and weight loss May be features of vitamin and haematinic deficiency, eg glossitis	*Investigations* Jejunal biopsy: shows partial villous atrophy and round cell infiltration of the lamina propria *Management* Prolonged course (>3 months) of tetracycline and folic acid
Lactose intolerance	Common in many regions of the world; caused by lactase deficiency May be a primary or a secondary disorder (eg post-gastroenteritis)	Diarrhoea associated with milk ingestion	Diagnosed either clinically or through breath testing Treated through avoidance of lactose-containing foods
Eosinophilic enteritis	A rare but increasingly recognised condition. Some overlap with Churg–Strauss syndrome	Chronic diarrhoea and weight loss	Should be considered in those with chronic diarrhoea and raised eosinophil counts after exclusion of parasite infection Dietary modification and steroids may be useful treatments

Clinical judgement and maintaining patient welfare

Coeliac disease (also called gluten-sensitive enteropathy) is a condition characterised by increased immunological responsiveness to dietary gluten associated with malabsorption. The exact aetiology is unknown but probably involves both environmental and genetic factors; a number of twin and family studies have identified a number of predisposing genetic loci. Pathologically, the disease is associated with T-cell activation causing patchy damage to the small intestinal mucosa.

Clinical features
Common presenting clinical features in adults include chronic diarrhoea with steatorrhoea, abdominal pain and bloating.

Clinical examination may be normal or reveal features of vitamin, mineral and haematinic deficiency, eg angular stomatitis, glossitis or koilonychia.

Coeliac disease has a strong association with *dermatitis herpetiformis*; as such, coeliac disease should be high on the differential in any case of diarrhoea and rash found in MRCP (PACES). Dermatitis herpetiformis presents as a pruritic vesiculopapular rash, found symmetrically on extensor surfaces, particularly the elbows.

Investigations
- **Blood tests**: may demonstrate anaemia (caused through haematinic deficiency). May also demonstrate low albumin, calcium, vitamin D and micronutrient levels as a result of malabsorption.
- **Serological tests**: there are a number of associated antibodies, including IgG and IgA gliadin, IgA reticulin, IgA anti-endomysial and tissue transglutaminase antibodies (TTGs). Immunoglobulins should be measured simultaneously to check total IgA levels (selective IgA deficiency – found in 5% of the population – may give a false-negative TTG

result). Antibodies should be assayed while the patient is on a gluten-containing diet.
- **Upper GI endoscopy**: histology remains the gold standard for diagnosis. At least four duodenal biopsies should be taken because the disease is patchy in nature. The classic histological finding is of *partial villous atrophy*.
- **Barium follow-through**: may demonstrate loss of fine feathery mucosal pattern, although this is performed infrequently now.
- **Skin biopsy**: in cases where dermatitis herpetiformis is suspected but there is diagnostic doubt, a skin biopsy may be performed. Immunofluorescence will show granular IgA deposition at the dermoepidermal junction.

Management
- Diet: strictly gluten free (exclude wheat, rye, oats and barley). Repeat biopsy may be undertaken after 6 months to assess response to dietary changes, when villous regeneration should be seen.
- Patients should be given dietetic support if having compliance issues (especially young women/girls, who may use gluten to effect weight control).
- Any nutritional deficiencies should be corrected (ie folate, iron and calcium supplementation) and patients should have a baseline DXA scan to look for osteopenia/ osteoporosis.
- Immunosuppressants may be required in those not responding to dietary modification, including prednisolone and azathioprine.

Dermatitis herpetiformis will also usually improve with instigation of the above management steps, although dapsone may be of use.

Coeliac disease is associated with other conditions with an autoimmune element (including diabetes mellitus, thyroid disease, primary biliary cirrhosis and rheumatoid arthritis), and these should be screened for if appropriate.

It is important to exclude complications if there is no improvement despite a gluten-free diet. Common causes of recurrent symptoms include

- **Non-compliance** with a gluten-free diet.
- Associated autoimmune disease, eg associated thyrotoxicosis.
- **Refractory disease**: some patients do not respond to a gluten-free diet; immunosuppression may be necessary.
- **GI malignancy**: coeliac disease is associated with an increased risk of GI T-cell lymphoma, squamous cell carcinoma of the oesophagus and small intestinal adenocarcinoma.
- **Collagenous sprue**: a thick band of collagen forms beneath the basement membrane of the mucosal epithelium impeding absorption. Parenteral nutrition is often required.

Maintaining patient welfare

Symptoms such as diarrhoea can have a huge impact on work, relationships and dependants. Patients may be embarrassed by their symptoms and therefore conceal many of them even from close family and friends. Lifestyle may be affected by inability to go into open spaces or public transport because of fear of 'accidents' and incontinence.

- Candidates would be expected to offer patients practical advice including which foods they should avoid and where they might obtain dietary advice. They would also be expected to consider referral to a dietician if appropriate. Certain patients with the condition in the UK qualify for prescriptions for gluten-free food from their general practitioner. Candidates could also suggest that the patient contacts the support group Coeliac UK.
- Patients may have their own concerns about symptoms such as fear of cancer or other serious underlying pathologies.

Resources

Coeliac UK: www.coeliac.org.uk

SCENARIO 8. CONGESTIVE CARDIAC FAILURE

Introduce yourself

Confirm the information you've been given and patient details: this 66-year-old man with known heart failure has noticed that he is increasingly short of breath, has more swollen ankles and is having difficulty sleeping. Please assess him.

'What is the main problem from your point of view?' 'I am feeling short of breath most of the time, even at rest, and my shoes no longer fit. I am not sleeping at night, so I am tired throughout the day.'

1–2 minutes

5 minutes

Exacerbation of a chronic illness

Existing treatment/surveillance: medical therapy (diuretics, ACE inhibitors, β blockers, etc), interventions (ICD, CRT, bypass surgery, etc)

How well/poorly has disease been controlled? Usual exercise tolerance. Assess risk factors for heart failure and their level of control, eg risk factors for ischaemic heart disease, hypertension, valvular heart disease, arrhythmias

Brief account of this exacerbation: identify progression with increasing severity from swollen ankles → reduced exercise tolerance → orthopnoea → PND → chest pain. What changes may have exacerbated symptoms recently (eg diuretics stopped)?

Social/occupational/family circumstances: smoking history, impact of symptoms on activities of daily living (see NYHA score in Clinical judgement section)

Drug history: identify recent changes that may have exacerbated symptoms. **DRUG ALLERGIES**

Other medical conditions: particularly risk factors for ischaemic heart disease (ie hypertension, hypercholesterolaemia, family history, smoking, diabetes, previous cardiovascular events)

Begin a **targeted** examination of relevant area/system and continue while taking the history

General appearance: dyspnoea at rest, cyanosis

Hands: may be peripherally cyanosed and cool

Pulse: character will depend on the cause of heart failure, eg slow rising in aortic stenosis, pulsus alternans in severe cardiac failure

Neck: raised JVP (may be systolic 'v' waves in tricuspid regurgitation)

Praecordium and chest: features may include displaced apex beat, murmur(s) (eg pansystolic murmur of functional mitral regurgitation), third ± fourth heart sounds, bibasal inspiratory crackles, pleural effusion(s)

Ankle/sacral oedema: pitting oedema

Extra features: if evidence of tricuspid regurgitation, may identify pulsatile hepatomegaly on abdominal examination

Finally: ask for blood pressure (hypertension is a risk factor for heart failure)

CALLBACK: 'You said at the beginning that the main problem was shortness of breath and swollen ankles. Is there anything else troubling you that we haven't covered?'

1–2 minutes

RESPOND TO PATIENT'S CONCERNS (1–2 min)

1. I think the cause of your shortness of breath and swollen ankles is congestive heart failure; your heart muscle is not pumping as effectively as it should, so fluid collects on the lungs and peripheries
2. We can start treatment right away – we need to increase your water tablets (diuretics), as well as alter some of your other medications (ACE inhibitors, β blockers) to help your heart work more effectively
3. I would like to do a number of investigations to assess the function of your heart (ECG, echocardiogram) and blood tests (FBC, U+Es, LFTs, BNP, etc) to ensure that no other factors are causing your symptoms

Thank the patient

Differential diagnosis	Clinical communication skills and managing patient concerns	Physical examination and identifying physical signs	Clinical judgement and maintaining patient welfare
COPD	See differential diagnosis table of Scenario 5. Asthma	Long-standing COPD may be complicated by pulmonary hypertension/cor pulmonale over time. Characteristic features include: Inspection: raised venous pressure, with systolic 'v' waves. Palpation: parasternal heave and thrill. Auscultation: loud P2; pansystolic murmur at lower left sternal edge heard loudest during inspiration (representing tricuspid regurgitation); early diastolic murmur heard loudest at upper left sternal edge on inspiration (representing pulmonary regurgitation; 'Graham–Steell' murmur)	See differential diagnosis table of Scenario 5. Asthma for management of COPD Management of cor pulmonale is as for cardiac failure in general
Chronic thromboembolic disease	Patients with recurrent venous thromboembolism may present with progressive dyspnoea, chest pain and leg swelling which may initially be suspected to represent cardiac failure	As the disease progresses, the patient may develop features of right-sided heart failure, including the features of pulmonary hypertension outlined above	Diagnosis of venous thromboembolic disease is via conventional means (ie CT pulmonary angiogram to assess pulmonary vasculature) Treatment is with anticoagulation
Pulmonary fibrosis			

Clinical judgement and maintaining patient welfare

Cardiac failure is a condition defined by the inability of the heart to generate a cardiac output appropriate to the patient's physiological needs. The usual reason for the inadequate cardiac output is heart muscle impairment (*low-output cardiac failure*). However, in less common cases (so-called *high-output cardiac failure*), the condition occurs because of high systemic metabolic demand that the heart cannot match (eg thyrotoxicosis, beri-beri). Heart failure is a common condition (affecting up to 10% of those aged >65 years in western countries) and increasingly prevalent, reflecting an ageing population in general, but also improvements in treatment of heart disease which mean that patients survive for longer periods. There is a wide variety of causes of heart failure, but the most common include coronary/ischaemic disease, hypertension, cardiomyopathies and valvular heart disease.

Clinical features
A useful measure of the degree of disease progression is to ascertain a patient's usual level of exercise tolerance/function, and what it is like at present. One simple way of establishing this is with the New York Heart Association (NYHA) breathlessness classification, ie

- NYHA class I: no symptoms on ordinary levels of activity
- NYHA class II: slight breathlessness on ordinary activity
- NYHA class III: symptoms on minimal exertion, eg walking around the house
- NYHA class IV: breathlessness present even at rest.

As described in the flowchart, clinical findings will depend on the underlying aetiology of cardiac failure, and whether the disease is predominantly affecting the left ventricle, the right ventricle or both.

Investigations
- **Blood tests**
  - Anaemia, deranged electrolytes and abnormal thyroid function may all exacerbate cardiac failure.
  - B-type natriuretic peptide (BNP) is a protein released from the ventricles in cardiac failure. It is a relatively non-specific but highly sensitive marker for the condition, helping to differentiate dyspnoea secondary to cardiac failure from that attributable to other causes.
- **ECG**
  - This may show evidence of the cause of cardiac failure (eg ischaemic changes), or some of the sequelae (eg left ventricular hypertrophy).
- **Chest radiograph**
  - Classic changes seen in heart failure include diversion of blood to the upper lobes of the lungs, perihilar oedema, cardiomegaly, pleural effusions and Kerley B lines (representing interstitial oedema).
- **Echocardiogram**
  - The key test for diagnosing heart failure, helping to define an aetiology to heart failure (eg valvular disease) and the degree of impairment of ventricular function.
  - Further functional imaging may also be contributory, eg dopamine stress echocardiogram, cardiac MR.

Management
- **General measures**
  - No added salt diet and restricted fluid intake.
  - Adjust modifiable risk factors, ie smoking, hypertension, diabetes.
  - Stop medications promoting fluid retention where possible (eg NSAIDs, steroids, calcium channel blockers, etc).
  - Weight reduction and rehabilitation/exercise programmes.
  - Seasonal influenza immunisation.

- **Pharmacological treatments**
    - Diuretics: predominantly loop diuretics (eg furosemide), but also some role for thiazide diuretics (eg metolazone). They are of symptomatic but not prognostic benefit.
    - ACE inhibitors/angiotension receptor blockers: these have been shown to cause ventricular remodelling where there is impaired function. These are of both symptomatic and prognostic benefit.
    - β blockers: β$_1$-adrenoceptor-selective blockers (eg metoprolol) have prognostic benefit in NYHA II–IV cardiac failure. They may be contraindicated for a number of reasons (eg asthma or severe COPD).
    - Spironolactone: this is of prognostic benefit in NYHA III–IV cardiac failure. Its use may be limited by side effects, eg hyperkalaemia.
    - Digoxin: useful if symptoms are still uncontrolled after above therapy (even if in sinus rhythm), through its role as a mild positive inotrope, but of no prognostic benefit.
    - Hydralazine/long-acting nitrates: of symptomatic and prognostic benefit in black people, or people intolerant of ACE inhibitors.
    - Ivabradine: a funny current antagonist with a growing role in cardiac failure management.
- **Interventional/surgical**
    - Implantable cardioverter defibrillator

(ICD): of prognostic benefit for patients with NYHA II–III cardiac failure and left ventricular ejection fraction <35%.
- Cardiac resynchronisation therapy (CRT): a dual-chamber pacemaker with an additional left ventricular lead. It has prognostic benefit for patients with NYHA II–III cardiac failure, left ventricular ejection fraction <35% and QRS interval >120 ms.
- Surgical: CABG or valvular surgery is of benefit if indicated. In severe cases, cardiac transplantation may be considered; technological improvements mean that cardiac devices (eg left ventricular assist device) are increasingly used as an adjunct while patients are waiting for transplants to become available.

Maintaining patient welfare

- Candidates should demonstrate an appreciation of the many non-pharmacological components to management. A community heart failure team (often led by specialist nursing staff) can educate patients about their condition and facilitate community exercise/rehabilitation programmes.
- Cardiac failure may be severely debilitating and has a relatively poor prognosis in those with a high NYHA grade/poor ventricular function. Palliative care has an important role in certain patients.

SCENARIO 9. CRANIAL NERVE III PALSY

Introduce yourself

Confirm the information you've been given and patient details: this 46-year-old woman presents with diplopia. Please assess her.

'What is the main problem from your point of view?' 'I have double vision, and my husband says my right eye is pointing outward.'

New condition

Focused history of the presenting complaint and relevant systems enquiry. Differentiate between causes of diplopia, eg all directions, but especially when the affected eye gazes medially and superiorly (CN III palsy), vertical diplopia (CN IV palsy), on lateral gaze to affected side (CN VI palsy) and diplopia not following a particular direction (internuclear ophthalmoplegia)

Identify alarm symptoms: painful onset ('surgical' causes, eg berry aneurysm of the posterior communicating artery, brainstem tumour); peripheral sensorimotor symptoms (consider mononeuritis multiplex, eg diabetes mellitus); history of confusion or meningitic symptoms (eg meningoencephalitis)

Social/occupational/family circumstances: smoking history, occupational history (eg group 1, taxi driver)

Drug history: insulin or oral hypoglycaemics, antihypertensives. **DRUG ALLERGIES**

Other medical conditions: diabetes, hypertension, vasculitis, etc

Begin a **targeted** examination of relevant area/system and continue while taking the history

General appearance: in CN III palsy, affected eye has ptosis, and is fixed in a down and out position in primary gaze, from which it will not move. Also look for other clues to aetiology, eg BM testing marks on fingertips in patients with diabetes

Examination of the eye

Visual acuity: typically normal, but may be decreased if macular damage (eg diabetes)

Pupils: fixed and dilated pupil in complete CN III palsy ('surgical' causes, eg tumour, aneurysms); spared pupil in partial CN III palsy ('medical' causes, eg diabetes)

Movement: if CN IV palsy, affected eye will fail to adduct and look down (the eye will intort); if CN VI palsy, affected eye will fail to abduct. Use the *cover test* – cover each eye in turn at the point of maximum diplopia – it will be the outer image that will disappear when the involved eye is covered

Fundoscopy: may find, for example, papilloedema if intracranial tumour, haemorrhages and exudates if diabetic retinopathy, etc

Additional examinations

Tell the examiner that you would like to test urine for glycosuria and check blood pressure (to exclude hypertension)

Suggest cranial and peripheral nervous examinations if the assessment suggests other focal neurology

CALLBACK: 'You said at the beginning that the main problem was double vision and your eye pointing outward. Is there anything else troubling you that we haven't covered?'

RESPOND TO PATIENT'S CONCERNS (1–2 min)

1. I think the double vision and your eye pointing outwards may be caused by one of the nerves that controls the muscles in the eye not working properly, called a third nerve palsy. This can be caused by a number of things, including diabetes and high blood pressure

2. To help you with your double vision we can put a patch temporarily over your eye/glasses. You will need to stop driving for the time being

3. However, we need to investigate you further to find the cause of this before we can treat you fully. I will initially do some blood tests (eg fasting glucose, lipids, vasculitis/autoantibody screen) and you may require some imaging tests before a final treatment plan can be made

Thank the patient

(left margin) 1–2 minutes   5 minutes   1–2 minutes

Differential diagnosis	Clinical communication skills and managing patient concerns	Physical examination and identifying physical signs	Clinical judgement and maintaining patient welfare
Horner's syndrome	Unilateral ptosis may also be found in Horner's syndrome; see Scenario 21.		Diagnosed clinically Investigations and management dictated by the presumed underlying cause
Trochlear (cranial nerve IV) palsy	Causes include: Traumatic, after head injury: the most common cause Mononeuritis multiplex Space-occupying lesions: of the brain stem and cavernous sinus (see Table 5.3) Congenital Idiopathic	This palsy means failure of superior oblique, which moves the eye in and down. Clinical features include • The affected eye is higher than the other, especially on attempted lateral gaze • The affected eye will depress from vertical gaze when abducted but not when adducted • The head is often tilted to the opposite side of the affected eye in an attempt to minimise diplopia	
Abducens (cranial nerve VI) palsy	Causes include: Mononeuritis multiplex Space-occupying lesions: of the pons and the cavernous sinus (see Table 5.3) Subacute chronic meningitis Idiopathic	The affected eye looks inwards at primary gaze, and fails to abduct – reflecting loss of the abductor lateral rectus Given the close positioning between the nucleus/fibres of the abducens nerve and that of other cranial nerves (ie facial nerve) and the pyramidal tract within the pons, examine the cranial nerves and the peripheral nervous system fully to assess their involvement	
Internuclear ophthalmoplegia (INO)	(See Station 3)		

Clinical judgement and maintaining patient welfare

Ophthalmoplegia is a common case in MRCP (PACES), both as part of the neurological examination in Station 3 (Scenario 22. Ophthalmoplegia) and as part of Station 5. This discussion focuses on the approach for isolated oculomotor nerve palsy, with the above differential diagnosis table providing more information on other ophthalmoplegia syndromes.

Clinical features
As described in the flowchart, clinical features of oculomotor nerve palsy include

- *Ptosis of the affected eye*: this reflects involvement of the axons of the oculomotor nerve that supply the levator palpebrae superioris muscle. As fibres from the oculomotor nerve on one side of the brain stem supply both the ipsilateral *and* the contralateral levator palpebrae superioris, there may also be a degree of ptosis of the contralateral eye.
- *Affected eye looking down and out*: the eye looks laterally because of the palsy of medial rectus. The eye looks down because the superior oblique (a depressor supplied by the trochlear nerve) is intact, but there is palsy of the elevators supplied by the oculomotor nerve (ie superior rectus and inferior oblique).
- *Dilated pupil, unresponsive to light and accommodation*: pupil dilatation implies involvement of the parasympathetic fibres from the Edinger–Westphal nucleus which supply the sphincter pupillae muscles of the iris. These fibres lie on the outside of the oculomotor nerve. They are most commonly

affected by compressive lesions, such as tumour and haemorrhage ('surgical' causes). Cases where the pupil is not involved are more suggestive of an intrinisic neuropathic process, such as mononeuritis multiplex ('medical' causes).

Investigations
This depends on the differential diagnosis being considered within the particular scenario. Causes of oculomotor nerve palsy include those in Table 5.3.

Investigations that may be considered include

- Blood tests: including testing for diabetes mellitus, autoantibodies, serological markers of relevant infections and tumour markers
- Lumbar puncture: where a meningitic disease is suspected
- Neuroimaging: imaging of the circle of Willis, brain stem, cavernous sinus or superior orbital fissure is indicated where space-occupying lesions are suspected.

Maintaining patient welfare
Candidates should demonstrate an appreciation of how unpleasant and distressing diplopia may be for the patient. They should suggest practical steps that may be taken to help symptoms while further investigations are undertaken (eg eye patching). It is also expected that candidates will have an appreciation of some of the broader implications that diplopia or other forms of visual impairment may have on patients, eg the need to inform the DVLA, the possible indication for disability benefit and occupational therapy input in order to maintain day-to-day activities.

Table 5.3 Causes of oculomotor nerve palsy

Differential	Examples
Mononeuritis multiplex	Metabolic causes (eg diabetes mellitus) Infectious disease (Lyme disease, leprosy, syphilis, etc) Autoimmune conditions (eg SLE, rheumatoid arthritis, vasculitis) Malignancy (eg lymphoma, paraneoplastic) Other conditions (eg hypertension)
Space-occupying lesions	Posterior communicating artery aneurysms Cavernous sinus disease, eg vascular disease (carotid artery aneurysms, thrombosis, etc), tumour, inflammation (eg from infective sinusitis or autoimmune involvement from vasculitis) Brain-stem disease, eg malignancy, haemorrhage, infarct, demyelinating lesions Superior orbital fissure disease, eg trauma, tumour infiltration
Subacute/chronic meningitis	Malignant: lymphoma, carcinoma, paraneoplastic Infectious, eg mycobacterial, fungal
Idiopathic	A diagnosis of exclusion

SCENARIO 10. CROHN'S DISEASE/BLOODY DIARRHOEA

1–2 minutes

Introduce yourself

Confirm the information you've been given and patient details: this man has attended the accident and emergency department because of bloody diarrhoea and abdominal pain. Please assess him.

'What is the main problem from your point of view?' EITHER 'I think my Crohn's – which I've had for 30 years – is flaring up. I have blood in my stool and I'm going up to five times at night. It's been going on for about 3 weeks.' **OR** 'I've had bloody diarrhoea and stomach ache for the last 3 weeks. I've also lost a lot of weight – I'm only 25, surely this can't be cancer?'

5 minutes

Exacerbation of a chronic illness   OR   New condition

Brief account of this exacerbation: number of stools per day, blood/mucus, systemic symptoms, screening questions for extraintestinal manifestations. Any obvious source of possible GI infection/relevant travel history?

Existing treatment/surveillance, eg biologics such as infliximab, blood tests if on thiopurines/methotrexate, prior surgery? Other possible cause of immunosuppression (eg HIV+, chemotherapy)? How many flares per year? Receiving surveillance colonoscopies?

Extent of previous disease (eg small bowel, large bowel, perianal or combinations of the above)

Focused history of the presenting complaint and relevant systems enquiry: Passage of blood/mucus, perianal symptoms, abdominal pain, weight loss, obstructive symptoms. Joint, eye or skin changes, mouth ulcers

Identify alarm symptoms: extreme weight loss, obstructive symptoms, systemic symptoms (fevers, rigors, etc). Immunosuppressed? Travel history or other obvious source of infection?

Investigations/treatments so far: blood tests, imaging (including MRI/CT, contrast studies, radiographs), endoscopy

Predictors of severity: continued smoking, young age of onset, extensive disease, perianal disease

Begin a **targeted** examination of relevant area/system and continue while taking the history

General appearance: pale, cachectic, cushingoid features (moon face, striae, supraclavicular fat pad, etc)

Abdomen: laparotomy scars, sites of previous ileostomy/colostomy, abdominal masses and tenderness

Mouth: aphthous ulcers, angular stomatitis

Briefly examine key areas of **other systems** that may be relevant

Hands: clubbing, koilonychia

Skin: erythema nodosum, pyoderma gangrenosum, scratch marks (pruritis)

Rheumatological: sacroiliac tenderness, kyphosis, scars from surgery for previous osteomalacia-related fractures

Eyes: looking for anterior uveitis, episcleritis and jaundice

Finally: explain that would normally perform rectal examination

Social/occupational/family circumstances: other family members with Crohn's disease/ulcerative colitis, difficulties with toilet access at work/social environment, incontinence concerns, stoma care. Smoker (as exacerbates Crohn's disease)?

Drug history: including steroids, aminosalicylates, thiopurines (ie azathioprine/6-MP), methotrexate, biologics (infliximab, adalimumab, etc). Drug side effects and **DRUG ALLERGIES**

Other medical conditions: seronegative spondyloarthropathies, primary sclerosing cholangitis (and possible cholangiocarcinoma), anterior uveitis, erythema nodosum, pyoderma gangrenosum, renal calculi, colorectal malignancy

1–2 minutes

CALLBACK: 'You said at the beginning that the main problem was bloody diarrhoea and weight loss. Is there anything else troubling you that we haven't covered?'

RESPOND TO PATIENT'S CONCERNS (1–2 min)

1. There are a number of conditions that cause bloody diarrhoea, and cancer is a very unlikely cause in someone of your age. It is more likely that you have an exacerbation of your Crohn's disease (inflammation of the bowel) caused by an overactive immune system
2. IBD is usually readily managed with medications. Surgery to remove the affected bowel is only occasionally needed. Once we've excluded an infectious cause (of your exacerbation) we can start treatment right away
3. We will need to look at the bowel directly by endoscopy and take biopsies as well as taking stool samples and performing some blood tests

Thank the patient

Differential diagnosis	Clinical communication skills and managing patient concerns	Physical examination and identifying physical signs	Clinical judgement and maintaining patient welfare
Infectious	*Infectious colitis*: pain, diarrhoea (sometimes bloody) and fever. Causes include • Dysenteric bacteria, eg *Shigella*, *Yersinia*, spp. • Pseudomembranous colitis – *Clostridium difficile* • CMV colitis, eg HIV-positive, transplant recipients	Abdominal findings are a spectrum from normal to guarding suggestive of peritonitis	*Investigations* Stool culture: to identify precipitating bacterial or viral causes Abdominal radiograph: large bowel dilatation and wall thickening consistent with toxic megacolon in severe cases Sigmoidoscopy: will allow direct visualisation and biopsy of affected tissue to aid diagnosis. However, this should be used with caution in acute severe colitis because of the risk of perforation *Management* Antimicrobial/antiviral therapy: including oral metronidazole for *C. difficile*, ganciclovir for severe CMV colitis, etc Surgery: colectomy is indicated for toxic megacolon with a high risk of perforation
	Abdominal TB: accounts for approximately 2% of all manifestations of the disease. It particularly affects the ileum	Typically presents with constitutional symptoms (fever, night sweats, etc), abdominal pain and a change of bowel habit Clinical features include abdominal tenderness and masses, particularly in the right iliac fossa There may be clinical findings consistent with TB in other organ systems too, including lymphadenopathy and apical fibrotic lung disease	*Investigations* Immunological studies: a Mantoux test and interferon-γ release assay may be helpful in diagnosing TB Ascitic tap: this will be exudative with high levels of adenosine deaminase. *Mycobacterium tuberculosis* may be cultured from the fluid but often this is hard to detect in ascites, even by PCR Imaging: inflammatory changes (including abscesses) may be seen, particularly in the ileum. CT is the usual imaging modality Endoscopy: to obtain tissue for mycobacterial culture *Management* Combination anti-TB chemotherapy. All patients with a new diagnosis of TB should have their HIV status ascertained

(continued)

Differential diagnosis	Clinical communication skills and managing patient concerns	Physical examination and identifying physical signs	Clinical judgement and maintaining patient welfare
Inflammatory	*Ulcerative colitis* – although Crohn's disease may affect the entire GI tract, disease in UC is confined to the rectum, colon and ileum ('backwash ileitis'). Disease in UC is continuous, in contrast to the skip lesions found in Crohn's disease	See flowchart	See flowchart for investigations; Crohn's disease and UC have very distinctive histological changes, helping to differentiate the two conditions Immunosuppressive therapy and surgery are the mainstays of treatment; see flowchart
	Coeliac disease	See Scenario 9. Coeliac disease	
	Behçet's disease: this is a rare vasculitic disease of unclear aetiology, found particularly in the so-called 'silk route' which extends from eastern Europe through to the Far East	Eye and neurological disease: including anterior uveitis, aseptic meningitis, sagittal sinus thrombosis and cranial neuropathies Skin disease: ulcers (perioral, genital), and pathergy (ie sterile pustular lesions that develop at sites of pressure on the skin) Rheumatological: usually an oligoarthritis GI disease: may present with GI symptoms that closely mimic IBD, reflecting gut vasculitic changes	Diagnosed clinically, with investigations helping to exclude mimicking conditions Oral or intravenous immunosuppressants (steroids, azathioprine, ciclosporin, etc) are the mainstay of treatment of active disease
	Radiation colitis/proctitis: inflammation of the lower GI tract as a result of previous radiotherapy for cancer treatment (eg prostatic, gynaecological)	There will be a variable degree of abdominal tenderness dependent on the degree of disease. Strictures and fistulae may be challenging to differentiate from IBD on clinical grounds alone Look for scars and/or radiotherapy burns from previous cancer treatment	*Investigations* The diagnosis is usually first suspected clinically, with the changes seen on endoscopy and biopsy used as confirmation *Management* Pharmacological therapies include corticosteroids and antibiotics, with endoscopic treatments (including argon plasma coagulation to treat haemorrhagic lesions, dilatation and stenting of strictures, etc) also of efficacy Surgical adhesiolysis and/or resection of affected areas may also be indicated in severe cases

(continued)

Differential diagnosis	Clinical communication skills and managing patient concerns	Physical examination and identifying physical signs	Clinical judgement and maintaining patient welfare
Inflammatory	*Microscopic colitis:* a condition most often found in middle-aged/elderly women. The aetiology is unclear, but there is an association with NSAIDs and autoimmune diseases (eg coeliac disease, thyroid disease)	Typically presents with symptoms including persistent diarrhoea, abdominal pain and unintentional weight loss Often no abnormal physical findings	*Investigations* Colonoscopy: often diagnosed through the finding of abnormal histology from colonic biopsies, even though the mucosa may have appeared normal. Typical histology changes are of increased intraepithelial lymphocytes, and/or a subepithelial strip of collagen ('collagenous' colitis) *Treatment* A number of pharmacological agents have confirmed efficacy, including budesonide and mesalazine
Malignant	*Intestinal malignancies:* colonic malignancies may present with rectal bleeding, whereas small bowel tumours (eg GI lymphoma) typically cause pain, obstructive symptoms and/or diarrhoea	May mimic IBD by presenting with abdominal pain, altered bowel habit and constitutional upset (ie B symptoms such as fever and night sweats)	*Investigations* CT and endoscopy *Management* Dependent on the underlying tumour, but likely to involve surgery and/or chemotherapy
Ischaemic	*Ischaemic colitis:* a condition associated with vascular compromise of the colon, with high morbidity and mortality Most often occurs due to a drop in perfusion pressure of the colon combined with microvascular disease rather than an embolism Commonly affects the splenic flexure; a 'watershed area' between the regions of the colon supplied by the superior and inferior mesenteric arteries. The rectum has a dual supply from the iliac artery and is usually spared	The typical clinical picture is with abdominal pain out of proportion to examination findings. There may also be rectal bleeding as colonic infarction occurs	*Investigations* Blood tests: elevated plasma lactate, as a result of diminished oxygenated blood supply to the colon Endoscopic appearances are often characteristic (dusky, purple, ulcerated mucosa) and biopsies are useful to exclude other causes Imaging: CT (ideally with angiography) is the most useful modality to confirm the diagnosis *Management* This will depend upon the severity of the disease – 50% require surgery for acute (perforation) or chronic (strictures) complications

Clinical judgement and maintaining patient welfare

The IBDs of Crohn's disease and ulcerative colitis (UC) are chronic inflammatory diseases that are associated with a high level of morbidity. The aetiology is complex, including a genetic component (twin/familial studies demonstrate significant concordance within families), as well as a number of environmental factors (eg epidemiological studies have identified a relationship with certain intestinal infections).

Clinical features

Where a Station 5 scenario in MRCP (PACES) concerns Crohn's disease, there are two main focuses that the assessment may take

1. A new diagnosis of the condition – with candidates expected to identify possible differential diagnoses
2. A flare of known Crohn's disease – with candidates required to assess for factors causing the exacerbation.

The typical presenting features of Crohn's disease include diarrhoea (which may be bloody), abdominal pain, weight loss and constitutional upset (lethargy, fever, etc). The first presentation of the condition is often at the extremes of age, ie usually either in patients aged between 16 and 30 years, or in those older than 70 years. There are a number of differential diagnoses to consider but most involve intestinal infection. The history should therefore assess for possible sources of gastrointestinal infection including travel history, immunosuppression and risk factors for TB. As outlined in the flowchart, Crohn's disease has many associated extraintestinal manifestations.

Investigations
- **Blood tests**
  - Haematological investigations often show anaemia. This may be microcytic (reflecting iron malabsorption), macrocytic (reflecting vitamin B_{12} and/or folate malabsorption) or normocytic (reflecting chronic disease and/or mixed haematinic

malabsorption). White blood cell count, platelet count and ESR are often raised in active disease.
  - Biochemical investigations will demonstrate raised CRP and low albumin levels.
- **Microbiology and virology**
  - Stool analysis (for microscopy, culture and sensitivity, *C. difficile* toxin, ova, cysts and parasites, and CMV) is indicated to exclude intestinal infection.
  - Assays may be required to exclude intestinal tuberculosis (eg Mantoux test, interferon-γ release assay, tissue biopsy).
- **Imaging**
  - Contrast studies: small bowel follow-through has been the conventional means for trying to identify small bowel stricturing and fistulating disease.
  - MRI of the small bowel is increasingly used for making the diagnosis of enteric Crohn's disease and complications thereof (Crohn's disease may affect the entire GI tract, whereas UC involves only tissue distal to the ileum). MRI of the pelvis is useful to assess perianal disease, including deep abscesses and fistulae.
- **Endoscopy**
  - Sigmoidoscopy/colonoscopy will show the degree of mucosal inflammation and ulceration, and allow biopsies to be obtained to confirm the diagnosis. The classic histological findings in Crohn's disease are of patchy areas of transmural inflammation with granulomas. Note that changes consistent with Crohn's disease may be identified histologically even if the mucosa appears grossly normal endoscopically.
  - Regular lower GI endoscopy is also indicated in those who have had IBD for >10 years as surveillance for colonic malignancy (although rates of this are much higher in those with UC than in those with Crohn's disease).
  - Gastroscopy (with enteroscopy) and capsule endoscopy are useful for assessing

upper GI and enteric Crohn's disease, and for treatment (eg dilatation of strictures).

Management

Management of Crohn's disease is complex, with high interpatient variability in response to treatment. It requires a multidisciplinary team approach.

- **General measures**
  - Patient education: includes advice about ways of minimising disease flares, eg stopping smoking. Many centres have IBD nurse specialists.
  - Dietician input: low-fibre diets may be of benefit where there is stricturing disease, whereas elemental diets may contribute towards remission in enteric disease.
- **Pharmacological**
  - A large number of different pharmacological agents are available, including those shown in Table 5.4.

Table 5.4 Pharmacological agents in Crohn's disease

Agent	Uses	Side effects
Antibiotics	Particularly metronidazole and ciprofloxacin. These are effective where infection is thought to be either a precipitant or a complication of a Crohn's disease flare, and are of particular benefit in perianal disease	Fluoroquinolone antibiotics increase the rate of *C. difficile* infection, which is already much more common in patients with IBD
5-Aminosalicylate acids (5-ASAs)	5-ASAs (such as mesalazine) slightly reduce the risk of Crohn's disease relapse after surgery but are generally of limited efficacy in Crohn's disease	5-ASAs may rarely cause tubulointerstitial nephritis. As such, patients should have their renal function checked prior to starting 5-ASAs, and at regular intervals afterwards
Corticosteroids	These may be administered intravenously (ie hydrocortisone, used in severe flares), rectally or orally (either as tablets such as prednisolone, or as topical steroids such as budesonide, used in mild-to-moderate flares) to induce remission	Corticosteroids appear to induce remission but do not reduce the rate of relapse of Crohn's disease With frequent use, patients may become steroid dependent. In addition, steroid side effects may develop with long-term use

(continued)

Table 5.4 (*continued*)

Agent	Uses	Side effects
Azathioprine	Has been demonstrated both to induce remission and to help reduce relapse rates. However, it may require up to 10 weeks before benefits are seen If efficacious, azathioprine will allow weaning off any long-term steroids	Patients will require assay of TPMT level before starting (this is the enzyme that metabolises the active component of azathioprine, 6-mercaptopurine (6-MP)) Side effects include • Myelosuppression • Pancreatitis • Hepatotoxicity As such, patients will require regular monitoring of their blood counts and liver function tests
Methotrexate	Often introduced in those failing to respond to azathioprine. When efficacious, will allow weaning off steroids	Side effects include • Myelosuppression • Hepatotoxicity • Teratogenicity (partly explained through folate depletion)
Anti-TNF-α treatments	Including infliximab and adalimumab These agents have been shown to induce remission in severe disease refractory to other therapies.	Expensive therapies that are contraindicated in a significant number of patients, with the following conditions • Pregnant/lactating • Sepsis – including possible latent TB • Malignancy • Demyelinating disease

- **Surgery**
  - Indicated for obstructing or fistulating disease refractory to medical therapy
  - Multiple small bowel resections may result in short gut syndrome.

Maintaining patient welfare

Patients first presenting with Crohn's disease are often young people who are studying or trying to establish themselves in jobs or relationships. The condition may cause a heavy psychological burden for patients for a number of reasons, such as social embarrassment from frequent diarrhoea, the effect on sexual function that pelvic/perianal disease may cause, or the need to visit medical staff frequently for monitoring by patients taking immunomodulatory agents. As such, patients should be assessed sensitively and holistically. They may benefit from input from a support group, such as Crohn's and Colitis UK (details below).

Resources

Crohn's and Colitis UK:
  www.crohnsandcolitis.org.uk

SCENARIO 11. CUSHING'S DISEASE

1–2 minutes

Introduce yourself

Confirm the information you've been given and patient details: this 29-year-old man has presented with weight gain, difficulty climbing the stairs and worsening acne. Please assess him.

'What is the main problem from your point of view?' 'I have gained weight rapidly on my face and stomach, and now have acne. I am also feeling weak in the legs and struggling to climb the stairs at work.'

5 minutes

New condition

Focused history of the presenting complaint and relevant systems enquiry: exclude common causes of weight gain (diabetes, hypothyroidism, medications, eg psychotropic agents) and/or proximal myopathy (thyroid disease, myositis, statins). Focused psychiatric history if relevant (as mood change/depression may be the first symptom)

Identify alarm symptoms: visual field loss (pituitary adenoma), cough (ectopic ACTH from lung carcinoma), severe headache (malignant hypertension)

Pre-existing conditions/risk factors: including diabetes or hypertension

Social/occupational/family circumstances: interests (such as body building; could there be steroid abuse?), depression, alcohol excess. Do the symptoms affect the patient's daily routine?

Drug history – excluding previous or current corticosteroids. **DRUG ALLERGIES**

Other medical conditions, eg depression, chronic inflammatory conditions requiring long-term steroid use

Begin a **targeted** examination of relevant area/system and continue while taking the history

General appearance (see Figure 5.2): hirsute, increased bruising, thin skin, scars from surgery for previous fractures (as Cushing's disease is associated with osteoporosis)

Face: moon-like face, plethoric, acne, hirsute

Mouth: oral candidiasis

Back: acne, supraclavicular and interscapular fat pads, kyphoscoliosis

Abdomen and chest: truncal obesity, striae

Lower limbs: proximal myopathy

Important extras

- Check visual fields
- Ask to measure blood pressure
- Test for glycosuria

1–2 minutes

CALLBACK: 'You said at the beginning that the main problem was weight gain, acne and difficulty climbing stairs. Is there anything else troubling you that we haven't covered?'

RESPOND TO PATIENT'S CONCERNS (1–2 min)

1. I think your symptoms may be because of an overproduction of steroids by your body, which is called Cushing syndrome. The best way of treating your symptoms is through treating the underlying cause of your condition, which we will investigate
2. To confirm the diagnosis, I need to collect all your urine for 24 hours (24-hour urinary free cortisol) and perform a test called an overnight dexamethasone suppression test. I also need to perform a chest radiograph

Thank the patient

Differential diagnosis	Clinical communication skills and managing patient concerns	Physical examination and identifying physical signs	Clinical judgement and maintaining patient welfare
Pseudo-Cushing syndrome A disorder of cortisol excess that may mimic Cushing syndrome clinically and biochemically	It is particularly associated with alcohol excess, depression and obesity	Patients may have many of the typical features of Cushing syndrome, but do not generally develop proximal myopathy or any of the associated skin changes	*Investigations* These are as for Cushing syndrome Results from the low-dose dexamethasone test can help to distinguish between Cushing syndrome and pseudo-Cushing syndrome; the test is generally positive in the former but not the latter (see Clinical judgement section) *Management* Treatment is through reversing the precipitating condition
Polycystic ovarian syndrome (PCOS) A condition of unclear aetiology characterised by multiple ovarian cysts, hypersecretion of androgens by the ovaries and reduced insulin sensitivity	Oligo-/amenorrhoea: the condition is often first diagnosed during investigation for subfertility	Clinical symptoms and signs include: Features of excessive androgen secretion – including hirsutism, acne and male pattern balding Impaired glucose tolerance and weight gain – presumed secondary to excessive insulin secretion Acanthosis nigricans	*Investigations* Blood tests: include LH:FSH >2:1, elevated testosterone and also elevated prolactin in certain cases. An oral glucose tolerance test will help identify impaired glucose tolerance Pelvic ultrasonography: the typical findings for a woman on transvaginal ultrasonography are multiple follicles within the ovaries ('string-of-pearls' appearance) *Management* Weight loss: this has been demonstrated to reduce many of the clinical features Oral contraceptive pill: has been demonstrated to reduce the effects of androgen secretion Metformin: appears to be of particular benefit to obese patients in helping to improve fertility. Other diabetic medications are also undergoing investigation for efficacy Clomifene: may be prescribed to aid fertility

Clinical judgement and maintaining patient welfare

Cushing syndrome is a disorder resulting from prolonged excess corticosteroid. There are a number of different causes, often classified into either ACTH-dependent or ACTH-independent causes (Table 5.5).

Clinical features

The initial clinical features may be non-specific. It may be only after the development of a constellation of typical clinical features (eg weight gain, poorly controlled hypertension, erectile dysfunction in men or oligomenorrhoea in women) that the condition is first expected.

The exact pattern of clinical features found may help point to the underlying aetiology, eg patients with ectopic ACTH production often develop extremely high ACTH plasma concentrations, with prominent muscle wasting, pigmentation, severe hyperglycaemia and features consistent with hyperaldosteronism (ie hypokalaemia, metabolic alkalosis).

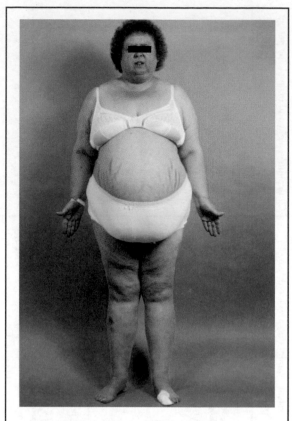

Figure 5.2 Cushing syndrome

Table 5.5 ACTH-dependent and -independent causes of Cushing syndrome

ACTH-dependent causes	ACTH-independent causes
Cushing's disease: a disease characterised by an ACTH-secreting pituitary adenoma **Ectopic ACTH production**: typically caused by malignancies, especially small cell lung cancer and carcinoid tumours **Ectopic CRH production**: very rare, but associated with malignancies including prostatic carcinoma	**Iatrogenic**: prolonged exogenous steroids **Adrenal adenoma/carcinoma** **Adrenal nodular hyperplasia** **Primary pigmented nodular adrenal disease (PPNAD)**: may occur sporadically, or in association with other disorders, eg Carney's syndrome

Investigations

A diagnosis of Cushing syndrome requires a systematic approach

1. **Initial screen**: measurement of random cortisol levels is of no help, because these are highly variable between individuals and at different times of the day.
    *   **24-hour urinary free cortisol**: usually recommended to be performed at least three times.
    *   **Overnight dexamethasone suppression test**: dexamethasone is given at midnight, with cortisol levels measured before administration and again in the early morning (ie 8 am). The dexamethasone normally causes negative feedback and suppresses ACTH and cortisol release, but this inhibition will not occur in Cushing syndrome.

2. **Confirmation of the diagnosis**: this involves a test that is more highly specific and sensitive than the screening assays
    *   **Midnight cortisol**: cortisol levels change during the day as part of the circadian rhythm, with the nadir at midnight. However, the midnight level will be significantly elevated in Cushing syndrome.
    *   **Low-dose dexamethasone suppression test**: dexamethasone is given every 6 hours for 2 days. As in the overnight test, cortisol suppression will occur in normal individuals but will not occur in those with Cushing syndrome. This test tends to be positive in Cushing syndrome but not in pseudo-Cushing syndrome states (see differential diagnosis table on previous page), helping to distinguish the two conditions.

3. **Establishing the aetiology**
    *   *Suspected ACTH-dependent Cushing's syndrome*: a number of specialised tests are indicated
        *   **High-dose dexamethasone suppression test**: large doses of dexamethasone are given orally every 6 hours for 2 days. In Cushing's disease, there is suppression of cortisol because the pituitary still retains some control of feedback. However, in ectopic disease, no cortisol suppression will occur.
    *   **CRH test**: after administration of CRH, there will be a marked increase in cortisol levels in Cushing's disease (because the pituitary adenoma is sensitive to CRH). However, there will be no increase in cortisol production in ectopic disease, because ACTH-secreting tumours usually have no receptors for CRH.
    *   **Inferior petrosal sinus sampling**: ACTH levels are measured from the peripheral blood and the inferior petrosal sinuses on both sides (using radiological guidance). Levels are measured before and after administration of CRH. An increase in ACTH in the inferior petrosal sinus greater than in the periphery, in response to CRH stimulation, indicates a pituitary adenoma. If the ACTH increase is more marked in one inferior petrosal sinus than the other, then this helps to localise on which side of the pituitary the adenoma is sited.
    *   **Imaging**: imaging of the pituitary (ideally with MR) will help to identify pituitary adenomas; however, up to 10% of the population may have evidence of non-functioning pituitary adenomas on pituitary imaging, which can make interpretation difficult. Imaging of the neck, chest and abdomen (by plain radiographs, CT or MR) will help to identify tumours producing ACTH ectopically.
    *   *Suspected ACTH-independent Cushing syndrome:* This may be suspected through the finding of very elevated cortisol levels with a highly suppressed ACTH level. Further investigations would include imaging by CT or MR of the adrenal glands to assess for adenoma or carcinoma.

Treatment

This depends on the underlying aetiology. In the case of iatrogenic Cushing syndrome, this may involve reducing the dose of exogenous steroids or converting to a steroid-sparing medication if possible. In other cases, medications can initially be used to try to reduce corticosteroid production (ie metyrapone and ketaconazole) before definitive management. Further treatments include

- Adrenal tumour or ectopic ACTH-producing tumour: surgical resection with or without radiotherapy
- Cushing's disease: ideally treated with transsphenoidal hypophysectomy, with or without radiotherapy. Before this procedure became widely available, many patients were treated with bilateral adrenalectomy. Regardless of the form of surgery, patients need close follow-up and assessment of their hormone axes, with hormone replacement as necessary.

Management also involves treating complications of the condition (eg controlling hypertension, preventing osteoporosis).

Maintaining patient welfare

- The examiner will not be impressed if the candidate demonstrates all the signs of Cushing syndrome thoroughly, but does not take the time to listen to the patient properly and explain that, for example, his or her recent depression may be caused by the disease and may well respond to treatment of the condition.
- Other practical ways that patients can be helped include physiotherapy or occupational therapy (eg if they have developed kyphoscoliosis), or to engage patients with a support group (see below).

Resources

The Pituitary Foundation: www.pituitary.org.uk

SCENARIO 12 DERMATOMYOSITIS

Introduce yourself

Confirm the information you've been given and patient details: this 45-year-old man is finding it difficult to climb stairs and has noticed a rash around his eyes. Please assess him.

'What is the main problem from your point of view?' 'I have noticed that I have pain in my muscles, I'm struggling to climb the stairs and I've had a rash around my eyes for the past few months.'

5 minutes

New condition

Focused history of the presenting complaint and relevant systems enquiry: differentiate common causes of muscle weakness (endocrine causes are usually painless, whereas tenderness implies inflammation and myositis). Aim to differentiate proximal myopathy (eg difficulty in standing up from sitting) from distal myopathy (eg difficulty with fine movements, such as using keys). Screen for symptoms of underlying malignancy

Alarm symptoms: features of malignancy (strong association with lung, gastrointestinal, ovarian, breast), and ask about dyspnoea (may reflect interstitial lung disease or respiratory muscle weakness, etc). Dysphagia may occur secondary to myositis of oesophageal muscles

Social/occupational/family circumstances: smoking history, effect on daily activities

Drug history: statins, hydroxyurea, chloroquine (proximal myopathy). **DRUG ALLERGIES**

Begin a **targeted** examination of relevant area/ system and continue while taking the history

General appearance: cachexia may be present

Eye: lilac-coloured 'heliotrope rash' around eyes, often associated with mild oedema

Nails: erythema around the nailbed, irregular or distorted cuticles, Raynaud's phenomenon

Hands: violaceous, scaly, papular rash on knuckles (elbows or knees also), so-called Gottron's papules

Chest: photosensitive rash on chest and neck ('V' shaped) and shoulders ('shawl sign'); bibasal inspiratory crackles may be present due to associated interstitial lung disease

Locomotor: proximal muscle weakness and *tenderness*, weakness of neck flexors, intact or absent deep tendon reflexes

Additional examination

- If history suggests occult malignancy, examine the relevant system

CALLBACK: 'You said at the beginning that the main problem was difficulty climbing the stairs, pain in your muscles and a rash around your eyes. Is there anything else troubling you that we haven't covered?

RESPOND TO PATIENT'S CONCERNS (1–2 min)

1. I think the cause of your symptoms and your rash is a condition called dermatomyositis, which can result in weakness and pain in your muscles and cause this type of rash
2. We can address the pain and soreness immediately with anti-inflammatory medications. However, I will need to confirm you have this condition and then start you on specific medication (ie oral steroids) to treat the underlying cause
3. We will need to perform blood tests (eg CK, FBC, ESR, ANA), perform specific tests on the electrical conduction in your muscles (eg EMG), and then think about performing a muscle biopsy. Assuming that we confirm the diagnosis, we may also need to investigate for other associated problems that we know can precipitate this disease

Thank the patient

Differential diagnosis	Clinical communication skills and managing patient concerns	Physical examination and identifying physical signs	Clinical judgement and maintaining patient welfare
Proximal myopathy			
Polymyalgia rheumatica (PMR) A rheumatological condition affecting middle-aged and elderly people of unclear aetiology	Progressive pain and stiffness in the proximal limbs	May be associated with the clinical features of giant cell arteritis (GCA), a condition closely associated with PMR Muscles usually non-tender	*Investigations* Essentially a clinical diagnosis, but investigations will help to exclude mimicking conditions Blood tests: raised CRP and ESR (>40 mm/h), normocytic anaemia, raised ALP. Usually negative autoantibodies MR of girdle muscles: may demonstrate patterns of tenosynovial inflammation characteristic of the condition *Management* Symptoms normally rapidly respond to high-dose corticosteroids. Patients may be weaned off steroids based on clinical response
Muscular dystrophies Progressive muscular dysfunction of heterogenetic origin	The pattern of myopathy and rate of progression of disease is dependent upon the exact condition (eg Duchenne versus Becker muscular dystrophy). Typically diagnosed in childhood/adolescence so rare in PACES	Cardiac abnormalities including hypertrophy, arrhythmias Compensatory calf muscle hypertrophy	Often first suspected clinically, with genetic analysis used to confirm the diagnosis Management is generally supportive, with genetic counselling also indicated where appropriate
Thyrotoxicosis	See flowchart of Scenario 17. Graves' disease		
Cushing syndrome	See flowchart of Scenario 11. Cushing's disease		
Osteomalacia	See differential diagnosis table for Scenario 25. Osteogenesis imperfecta		

(continued)

Differential diagnosis	Clinical communication skills and managing patient concerns	Physical examination and identifying physical signs	Clinical judgement and maintaining patient welfare
Drugs and toxins	There are a number of associated drugs that may cause proximal myopathy, as described in the main text (eg steroids) A number of toxins may also cause a similar picture, in particular alcohol		
Paraneoplastic syndrome	A history suggestive of underlying malignancies, eg small cell lung cancer	The particular pattern of neuromuscular deficit is variable between patients • Cerebellar ataxia and degeneration (lung, ovary or breast, Hu/Ro/Yi antibodies) • Lambert–Eaton myasthenic syndrome (small cell lung cancer, anti-calcium channel antibodies) • Stiff person syndrome (breast, lung, thymoma, amphiphysin antibodies) • Encephalomyelitis (small cell lung cancer, Hu antibodies) • Myasthenia gravis (thymoma, ACh-receptor antibodies, anti-skeletal muscle antibodies)	Investigate underlying malignancy (syndrome may precede emergent tumour by many months/years) Antibody tests as opposite Nerve conduction studies and EMG
Myasthenia gravis	See differential diagnosis table of Scenario 21. Horner's syndrome and Station 3 Neurological Scenario 9	May present with a syndrome that may mimic the proximal myopathy of dermatomyositis. However, the fatigability that is characteristic of myasthenia gravis is not found in dermatomyositis	

(continued)

Differential diagnosis	Clinical communication skills and managing patient concerns	Physical examination and identifying physical signs	Clinical judgement and maintaining patient welfare
Skin changes			
Atopic eczema	See Scenario 14. Eczema flowchart	Atopic eczema may involve the face including the eyelids, and may mimic a heliotrope rash	
Psoriasis	See Scenario 30. Psoriasis flowchart	Both seborrhoeic dermatitis and contact dermatitis may involve the face and mimic a heliotrope rash The scaly nature of Gottron's papules may also be confused with psoriatic plaques	
SLE and DLE	See Scenario 36. SLE flowchart and differential diagnosis table for Scenario 30. Psoriasis	The skin changes of SLE are characteristically photosensitive in nature, as in dermatomyositis	
Rosacea A chronic inflammatory facial dermatosis	Facial flushing is often reported	Characteristic features include inflammatory facial skin lesions (often initially macular and later papulopustular) and multiple telangiectasia In advanced cases, *rhinophyma* (ie enlargement of the nose as a result of hyperplasia of the sebaceous glands and connective tissue within it) may occur	The diagnosis is made clinically Treatment initially consists of topical antibiotics (often metronidazole), topical benzoyl peroxide or salicylic acid. In cases that fail to respond, systemic antibiotics (eg tetracycline) may also be tried. Oral isotretinoin and light therapy are reserved for the most severe cases

Clinical judgement and maintaining patient welfare

Dermatomyositis is a rare disease in the category of idiopathic inflammatory myopathies. Although, as the name implies, these disorders have an unclear pathogenesis, they are believed to be autoimmune in nature.

Clinical features

The typical presentation is with the combination of proximal myopathy and characteristic skin changes (as outlined in the flowchart), often associated with underlying malignancy. Patients diagnosed with the condition should undergo a respiratory examination because a minority of patients will also develop interstitial lung disease; other patients may develop diaphragmatic/inter-costal muscle weakness as part of the underlying myopathic process. The drug history will need to be established carefully; particular medications can result in a proximal myopathy (eg steroids), skin changes similar to dermatomyositis (eg hy-droxyurea) or both (eg statins).

Investigations

- **Blood tests**
  - Biochemistry: CK will often be significantly raised, and will fall in response to therapy.
  - Immunology: ANAs will be positive in most patients. Anti-Jo 1 is positive in a subgroup of patients with the so-called

'anti-synthetase syndrome', characterised by fever, acute myositis, symmetrical polyarthritis, fever, Raynaud's phenomenon and interstitial lung disease. Other antibodies (including anti-Ro, -La, -Sm or RNP) suggest myositis occurring in the context of another autoimmune disease, eg SLE.

- **Radiology**
  - High-resolution CT chest will help confirm the presence of interstitial lung disease where suspected.
  - Cross-sectional imaging with ultrasonography, CT or MR may be relevant when an underlying malignancy is suspected.
  - MR may also be useful to identify a site of marked myositis that is suitable for biopsy (quadriceps is usually the favoured site).
- **Electromyogram** (EMG)
  - Typical changes include spontaneous fibrillation.
- **Tissue biopsy**
  - Muscle biopsy is the most definitive means of confirming the diagnosis but not always necessary in the presence of a raised CK, rash and muscle tenderness.
  - Biopsy of skin lesions may also be of use.

Management

- **General measures**
  - Avoiding excessive sunlight exposure/use of suncreams will minimise skin changes.
  - Physiotherapy may aid mobility and minimise contractures where myositis is present.
- **Pharmacological**
  - High-dose oral corticosteroids should be instigated. Patients can be weaned off them based on clinical progress and the CK. Topical steroids (and/or hydroxychloroquine) may be used for skin disease.
  - Other immunosuppressants that may be used as 'steroid-sparing' agents include methotrexate and azathioprine. Intravenous immunoglobulin may be

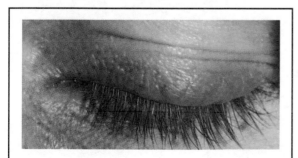

Figure 5.3 Heliotrope rash

considered in cases that are particularly severe or refractory to other treatments.

Maintaining patient welfare

- The association between this condition and malignancy is so strong that most clinicians will thoroughly investigate patients aged >40 years for an underlying cancer, even in the absence of obvious focal symptoms. The rationale for these investigations will need to be explained honestly but sensitively to the patient.
- The diagnosis is very rare so few patients diagnosed with the condition will have heard of it previously. Patients should be offered details of a support group if they feel that this would be of help, such as the Myositis Support Group in the UK.

Resources

Myositis Support Group: www.myositis.org.uk

SCENARIO 13. DIABETIC RETINOPATHY

Introduce yourself

Confirm the information you've been given and patient details: this 66-year-old woman has been referred with a deterioration in her vision. Please assess her.

'What is the main problem from your point of view?' 'I have been having regular check-ups with my doctor for my diabetes but my eye sight has got worse in the last few weeks and I am now struggling to read the newspaper.'

Exacerbation of a chronic illness

Existing treatment/surveillance: diet controlled/oral hypoglycaemics/insulin. When was the last ophthalmological examination?

How well/poorly has disease been controlled? HbA1c and frequency of hyper-/hypoglycaemia. Other diabetic complications (nephropathy, neuropathy, etc)?

Brief account of this exacerbation: sudden or gradual deterioration in vision? Floaters, flashes or the perception of a 'curtain' over vision suggests retinal detachment or tear

Social/occupational/family circumstances: is the patient still driving? Smoking history, compliance with medications, family history of cardiovascular disease

Drug history: current and previous medications for diabetic care. Medications for other risk factors (eg antihypertensives, lipid-lowering drugs). **DRUG ALLERGIES**

Other medical conditions: hypertension, hypercholesterolaemia, smoking history, cardiovascular events (eg MI, CVA)

Begin a **targeted** examination of relevant area/system and continue while taking the history

Examination of the eye

Visual acuity: a drop to <6/12 suggests maculopathy

Fields and movement: there may be a central scotoma if maculopathy. Movement often reduced if partial CN III and/or VI lesions as part of diabetic mononeuritis multiplex

Fundoscopy: look in anterior eye for cataracts. Examine the fundus thoroughly, and assess whether there are features consistent with *background retinopathy, pre-proliferative retinopathy, proliferative retinopathy, maculopathy* or *advanced diabetic eye disease* (see Clinical judgement section). Examine carefully for treated retinopathy, ie photocoagulation scars (See Figure in Neuro Examination)

Finally

- Ask to test urine for glycosuria, or for BM if available
- Check postural blood pressure (a postural drop implies autonomic neuropathy, which is associated with more severe retinopathy)

CALLBACK: 'You said at the beginning that the main problem was your eyesight. Is there anything else troubling you that we haven't covered?'

RESPOND TO PATIENT'S CONCERNS (1–2 min)

1. I think the reason your eyesight has deteriorated is because your diabetes has affected the blood vessels in the back part of your eye, called the macula, which is very important for vision
2. To help with your symptoms, we need you to see a specialist ophthalmologist urgently, who will need to take a more detailed look at your eyes. I will help to get your blood glucose under closer control, because this is very important. It's essential that you stop driving until we know how severely your eyesight has been impaired
3. The ophthalmologist will most likely need to perform laser treatment (photocoagulation) on the blood vessels at the back of your eye so that your eyesight does not get any worse. This is painless and usually very successful

Thank the patient

1–2 minutes

5 minutes

1–2 minutes

Differential diagnosis	Clinical communication skills and managing patient concerns	Physical examination and identifying physical signs	Clinical judgement and maintaining patient welfare
Hypertensive retinopathy	Visual impairment may be minimal	The Keith–Wagener–Barker classification of hypertensive retinopathy is as follows: Grade I: arteriolar narrowing, appearing as 'silver wiring' or tortuous vessels Grade II: arteriovenous 'nipping' Grade III: cotton-wool spots, hard exudates, flame-shaped haemorrhages Grade IV: papilloedema Note that the papilloedema found in grade IV hypertensive retinopathy is distinguishable from that of other causes in a number of ways, including the associated arteriolar changes, and the presence of haemorrhages and exudates far beyond the disc	Diagnosed clinically Management is focused on appropriate treatment of hypertension
Retinal vein occlusion	Acute painless loss of vision. The reduction in visual acuity may range from mild to very profound There are a number of conditions associated with retinal vein occlusion, including diabetes mellitus, hypertension and thrombophilias, although cases may also be idiopathic	Characteristic fundoscopic changes include: Tortuous, dilated retinal veins Retinal haemorrhages Cotton-wool spots The degree of fundoscopic change depends on whether it is a central or branch retinal vein that is involved. Where central retinal veins are involved, there is often a swollen optic disc, macular oedema and a very marked reduction in visual acuity	Diagnosis is clinical Treatment is of any precipitating condition. Laser treatment may also be used to attempt to reduce macular oedema, and to minimise the neovascularisation within the ischaemic retina

Clinical judgement and maintaining patient welfare

Diabetic eye disease is globally one of the most common causes of visual impairment and the most frequently occurring 'ophthalmology case' in Station 5. It is estimated that 25% of all patients with diabetes are affected by retinopathy. The risk of the condition is related to the length of time that the patient has had diabetes, with approximately 100% of those with type 1 diabetes and 60% of those with type 2 diabetes developing the condition by 20 years after diagnosis. Risk factors associated with diabetic retinopathy include poor glycaemic control, hypertension, smoking, dyslipidaemia, other microvascular complications (particularly nephropathy) and pregnancy.

The most commonly used classification for diabetic retinopathy is summarised in the Table 5.6.

As well as retinal disease, patients with diabetes are at increased risk of a number of other eye conditions, including the following

- Cataracts.
- Lens disease: those with newly diagnosed diabetes who have just started therapy may experience rapid changes in blood glucose with associated osmotic effects on the lens. This manifests clinically as acute changes in visual acuity. Acuity normally settles once the patient has stabilised on therapy.
- Impaired eye movements: reflecting diabetic neuropathy affecting cranial nerves III, IV and VI.
- Eye infections: patients with diabetes have an increased propensity to soft-tissue infections, meaning that patients are more prone to conjunctivitis, periorbital cellulitis, etc.

Management

Screening
All patients aged >12 years with diabetes should undergo annual retinal photography (more frequently during pregnancy). Although the risk of significant retinopathy is very low in patients with type 1 diabetes until at least 5 years after diagnosis, screening also serves a role in teaching patients about minimising risk factors for retinopathy, and may reveal other eye disease.

Prevention
There is now good evidence that optimal management of risk factors for diabetic retinopathy can prevent/slow down the progression of the condition, ie

- *Glycaemic control:* the DCCT study of patients with type 1 diabetes demonstrated that tight glycaemic control was associated with a relative risk reduction of developing retinopathy by 6.5 years of 76% compared with standard glycaemic control.
- *Hypertensive control:* the UKPDS trial of patients with type 2 diabetes demonstrated that tight control of blood pressure was associated with a reduction in retinopathy by approximately a third compared with standard blood pressure control. There is some evidence that ACE inhibitors/ angiotension receptor blockers may be more effective than other antihypertensives, but trials are ongoing.

Ophthalmological
All patients with pre-proliferative or proliferative retinopathy, or maculopathy regardless of the degree of retinopathy, should be referred for urgent ophthalmological assessment for ocular laser therapy. There is very good evidence for laser photocoagulation significantly reducing the rate of serious visual loss in advanced retinopathy and maculopathy; however, there are also possible complications, including scotoma formation and retinal vein thrombosis. Photocoagulation produces characteristic scars that should be obvious. Modalities of laser therapy include

- Panretinal photocoagulation: this is used in severe pre-proliferative and proliferative retinopathy to obliterate the ischaemic portions of the retina to minimise the possibility of neovascularisation.

Table 5.6 Classification of diabetic retinopathy

Classification	Clinical features
Background	Typical features include: Microaneurysms, ie dilatations of capillaries Dot haemorrhages: occur as microaneurysms break down Blot haemorrhages: larger than dot haemorrhages, reflecting haemorrhage into deeper retinal layers Hard exudates: yellow-coloured lesions composed of protein and lipid that has leaked from retinal capillaries
Pre-proliferative	Includes all the features of background retinopathy, but with a number of additional features representing retinal microvascular ischaemia: Large haemorrhages and hard exudates: across increasingly large areas of the retina as the disease progresses 'Cotton-wool spots': similar to hard exudates, but larger and with poorly defined borders. These represent nerve fibre layer infarction due to retinal arteriolar occlusion Venous abnormalities: including venous looping and beading
Proliferative	Includes all the features of severe pre-proliferative retinopathy, but in addition *neovascularisation*, ie bundles of new vessels developing in response to microvascular ischaemia. These may occur either from disc vessels ('intraretinal microvascular abnormalities' (IRMAs)), or from vessels elsewhere in the retina
Maculopathy	Maculopathy is the most feared complication of diabetic eye disease, because it presents the greatest threat to vision. It may occur at any stage of retinopathy, and should be particularly suspected if the visual acuity of a diabetic patient falls to ≤6/12 Maculopathy may be diagnosed by fundoscopy alone, but may require slit-lamp examination or fluorescein angiography to accurately make the diagnosis Significant macular oedema is defined as: Retinal thickening within 500 µm of the macula. Retinal thickening/oedema is suggested by the presence of a greyish discoloration of the retina Hard exudates within 500 µm of the macula. These often have a circinate pattern ('macular star') At least one area of retinal thickening of at least one disc diameter (1500 µm) located within one disc diameter of the macula
Advanced diabetic eye disease	This term is used to describe patients with all the features of advanced proliferative retinopathy and maculopathy, but with additional features too: Vitreous haemorrhage: the new vessels formed in proliferative retinopathy are thin, fragile, and prone to haemorrhage Retinal detachment: new vessels are associated with fibrotic tissue that may attach to the retina. Over time, these may cause retinal detachment through traction Iris rubeosis: this is new vessel formation at the iris, and may result in a severe glaucoma

- Focal laser photocoagulation/macular grid therapy: this is used in maculopathy to reduce ongoing leak and to maximise resorption of macular oedema.

Other ophthalmological procedures may also be appropriate, eg vitrectomy for severe vitreous haemorrhage.

Future treatments
There are ongoing trials for a number of other potential therapies for diabetic retinopathy, including the use of intravitreal VEGF-inhibiting monoclonal antibodies (eg bevacizumab) and intravitreal corticosteroids (eg triamcinolone).

Maintaining patient welfare
- Many patients will be understandably petrified about the risk of going blind. It is important to make a sympathetic and realistic assessment of their chances of severe visual loss based on their history and clinical findings, and to outline the full range of lifestyle, medical and ophthalmological changes that may be appropriate to minimise progression.
- Where patients already have severe visual impairment related to diabetic retinopathy, it is important to take a holistic view of what services may help, including disability benefits, occupational therapy and psychological support. Drivers with diabetes will have to discuss their diagnosis with the DVLA and may have to stop driving, because of either visual impairment or other diabetic complications (eg hypoglycaemia unawareness).

SCENARIO 14 ECZEMA

Introduce yourself

Confirm the information you've been given and patient details: this 18-year-old hairdresser has presented with worsening erythema and pruritus in the web spaces and back of his hands. Please assess him.

'What is the main problem from your point of view?' 'I've had eczema since childhood but never this badly. The back of my hands have been really itchy and sore, and it is affecting my work now – my clients have noticed and say it's unsanitary.'

Exacerbation of a chronic illness

Existing treatment/surveillance: current treatment, compliance, and when it stopped working. Usual areas affected compared with now. Previous skin-prick/patch testing and results

How well/poorly has disease been controlled? Topical therapy only vs systemic therapy/ phototherapy

Brief account of this flare/exacerbation: duration, severity, coverage, response to therapy escalation, new precipitants (eg new cosmetics)

Social/occupational/family circumstances: occupational precipitants; family history of atopy

Drug history: if on maintenance emollients, topical steroids or treatment for other inflammatory conditions. **DRUG ALLERGIES**

Other medical conditions: asthma, hayfever, etc

Begin a **targeted** examination of relevant area/ system and continue while taking the history

Examination of the skin

Location: principally flexural regions of elbows, wrists, hands, fingers, ankles, toes and feet; may also affect the face

Description: this will depend upon the acuity of the eczema

- *Acute*: initially a pruritic macular rash with associated oedema, before development of a vesicopapular rash. Vesicles break down and release exudate
- *Chronic*: dry, erythematous skin, with excoriation. May become scaled, lichenified, and hyper- or hypopigmented. Fissures may develop over time

Additional examination features

- Superimposed infection
- If erythema is severe in hands, assess for functional impairment

CALLBACK: 'You said at the beginning that the main problem was redness and itching of the web spaces and back of the hands which was affecting your work. Is there anything else troubling you that we haven't covered?'

RESPOND TO PATIENT'S CONCERNS (1–2 min)

1. I think this is worsening of your atopic eczema, which may have been exacerbated by your work and exposure to solvents or other chemicals
2. For your itching I can prescribe you some medication (ie antihistamines). As you work as a hairdresser, there may be a way of adapting your work so that you are not exposed to potential irritants/precipitants, such as wearing protective gloves
3. We do not need to do any further investigations, but we should start treatment with a mild topical steroid cream and emollients to keep the skin from getting dry

Thank the patient

1–2 minutes

5 minutes

1–2 minutes

Differential diagnosis	Clinical communication skills and managing patient concerns	Physical examination and identifying physical signs	Clinical judgement and maintaining patient welfare
Lichen planus	Patients may report pruritus, or emergence of lesions at the sites of previous skin trauma (Koebner's phenomenon)	Clinical features include: Small, shiny, pruritic, flat-topped, polygonal, purplish papules with an overlying network of fine white lines (*Wickham's striae*) Affects the flexor aspect of the wrists, the forearms, shins, trunk and lower back, usually in a symmetrical distribution Other features include: Buccal mucosa: may also demonstrate Wickham's striae Nails: longitudinal areas of thinning Scalp: may develop scarring alopecia	Diagnosis is usually clinical Mild cases usually require no treatment, although topical steroids and oral antihistamines are the mainstay for more symptomatic cases In cases of severe/widespread disease, oral prednisolone is indicated (eg 20–30 mg/day for 4–6 weeks). Hypertrophic plaques may require intralesional steroid injection
Psoriasis	See Scenario 30. Psoriasis flowchart		
Rosacea	See Scenario 12. Dermatomyositis differential diagnosis table		

Clinical judgement and maintaining patient welfare

Eczema is a common inflammatory disorder that affects people of all ages, and may affect the skin of any area of the body. One difficulty in describing eczema is the lack of a consistent classification, but Table 5.7 summarises the main forms commonly found in practice.

Table 5.7 Main forms of eczema seen

Categories	Details
Atopic eczema	The most common form, occurring through the same mechanism as (and associated with) other atopic conditions Often intensely pruritic, and tends to be focused on flexural areas
Contact dermatitis	Caused through continued exposure of the skin to either an irritant (eg solvents) or an allergen (eg nickel) Particularly found over the hands and face, although the exact distribution will depend on the underlying precipitating agent
Seborrhoeic dermatitis	A form of chronic eczema of the scalp and face particularly characterised by greasy, scaly skin Associated with certain fungal skin infections, especially *Pityrosporum ovale*
Xerotic/asteatotic eczema	Characterised by dry, fissured, pruritic, scaly skin, with a clinical appearance sometimes described as 'crazy paving' Associated with dehydration and dry weather
Pompholyx	Associated with a pruritic vesicular rash on the finger and palms (and also possibly the soles) Particularly occurs in young adults, with onset usually in warm weather
Discoid/nummular eczema	Typified by dry, round or oval eczematous lesions, usually found symmetrically on the lower legs Most often found in elderly male patients
Venous/gravitational eczema	Chronic venous insufficiency predisposes to this dry, scaly form of eczema that affects the lower legs, especially the medial malleolus Appears to predispose to venous ulcers
Neurodermatitis (lichen simplex chronicus)	This is pigmented lichenified eczema that occurs in response to frequent habitual scratching or rubbing Usually occurs as a single lesion, most often located on the leg, neck or perineum

One major complication of eczema is infection; this may be with either bacteria (often staphylococci or streptococci) or viruses (eg eczema herpeticum, where herpes simplex infection occurs in skin chronically inflamed from atopic eczema).

Investigations

The diagnosis is usually made clinically. Where superadded infection is suspected, swabs are useful for directing antimicrobial/antiviral therapy. To identify precipitants, a number of immunological tests may be used. Patch testing detects type IV hypersensitivity reactions (and will therefore help to identify triggers to contact dermatitis), whereas skin-prick testing detects type I hypersensitivity reactions (thus aiding the detection of relevant allergens in atopic eczema). Patients with atopic eczema will often have elevated plasma IgE titres during exacerbations.

Management

- General measures
  - Keep skin moist, eg where the hands are affected wash only in warm water and use emollients as soap substitutes regularly throughout the day.
  - Avoid known allergens/irritants where possible. Where this is not possible (eg exposure as part of a job), wearing gloves may be necessary.
- Pharmacological
  - Topical therapies
    - Topical steroids: effective in most forms of the condition. As a result of possible side effects (eg skin atrophy), patients should use the least potent steroid for the shortest time possible to control the inflammation.
    - Topical tacrolimus: particularly of use in areas where steroids are not suitable, such as the face.
    - Coal tar: a number of different uses, including as a shampoo (either with or without salicylic acid) to treat seborrhoeic dermatitis, or incorporated into a bandage and applied overnight to help particularly lichenified eczema.
    - Potassium permanganate: incorporated into dressings as a means of treating pompholyx.
  - Systemic therapies
    - Immunosuppressants: a variety of potent oral immunosuppressants – including azathioprine and ciclosporin – may be tried in severe atopic eczema.
    - Antihistamines: for pruritus.
    - Antibiotics/antivirals: for superinfection.
- Phototherapy
  - UVB and PUVA may both be considered in severe atopic eczema.

Maintaining patient welfare

Patients may find having eczema particularly challenging for a number of reasons. These include the strain that it might place on them carrying on their current job, the discomfort that they experience from chronic pruritus, the psychological difficulty from having a condition affecting the skin of the face, or the possible side effects that they may have to deal with from the treatments available. Candidates should therefore assess patients with the condition sensitively and gauge carefully what is of most concern to them at present. Management plans should offer practical support, and should, if relevant, enquire as to whether patients feel that they may benefit from support groups (such as the UK National Eczema Society, details below).

In light of these challenges, where the scenario calls for candidates to assess patients with chronic eczema in whom the condition has suddenly worsened, they should think broadly about what the trigger may be. Common causes include poor compliance with emollients/steroids, or changes to their job and lifestyle that have brought them into contact with new precipitants.

Resources

National Eczema Society: www.eczema.org

SCENARIO 15. ERYTHEMA NODOSUM

1–2 minutes

Introduce yourself

Confirm the information you've been given and patient details: this 29-year-old Asian woman presents with painful nodules on her shins. Please assess her.

'What is the main problem from your point of view?' 'I have developed painful red lumps on both of my shins for the last few days.'

5 minutes

New condition

Focused history of the presenting complaint and relevant systems enquiry: establish symptoms suggestive of underlying causes, eg diarrhoea, abdominal pain and weight loss may imply underlying IBD; fever and constitutional upset may imply infection (eg streptococci, *Yersinia* sp., etc.) or inflammation (eg sarcoidosis, Behçet's disease)

Identify alarm symptoms: eg dyspnoea and respiratory failure may imply sarcoidosis, TB, group A β-haemolytic streptococci or *Mycoplasma pneumoniae*

Pre-existing conditions/risk factors: IBD, sarcoidosis, Behçet's disease, pregnancy, exposure to TB, foreign travel. Sexual history may be appropriate, given association with *Chlamydia* sp. and syphilis

Social/occupational/family circumstances: recent foreign travel, close contacts with TB/other associated infections

Drug history: in particular, the oral contraceptive pill, penicillin and sulfonamides. **DRUG ALLERGIES**

Other medical conditions: previous infectious diseases, history of IBD or sarcoidosis, pregnancy

Begin a **targeted** examination of relevant area/system and continue while taking the history

Examination of the skin

Location: particularly shins, bilaterally in pre-tibial distribution (but occasionally thighs)

Description: tender, nodular lesions, usually 2–6 cm in diameter. Initially erythematous, becoming more red–purple in colour as begin to resolve

Additional examination

- **Respiratory**: if suggestion of TB, sarcoidosis
- **Abdomen**: if suggestion of IBD, or gastrointestinal symptoms
- **Joints**: if arthralgia is mentioned
- Suggest a **pregnancy test**

1–2 minutes

CALLBACK: 'You said at the beginning that the main problem was painful lesions on your shins. Is there anything else troubling you that we haven't covered?'

RESPOND TO PATIENT'S CONCERNS (1–2 min)

1. I think your painful shins are caused by a condition called erythema nodosum. This usually goes away by itself, but can indicate a problem elsewhere
2. To help with the pain, I can give you some painkillers (eg paracetamol, NSAIDs). Cold compresses can also help with the symptoms of this condition. However, we need identify the underlying cause
3. The best way to do this is by performing blood tests, a throat swab and a chest radiograph in the first instance. We will ask a dermatologist to look at your legs, and he or she may decide that a biopsy is necessary to confirm the diagnosis

Thank the patient

Differential diagnosis	Clinical communication skills and managing patient concerns	Physical examination and identifying physical signs	Clinical judgement and maintaining patient welfare
Cutaneous vasculitis A term that describes various different forms of dermatoses that occur through autoimmune mechanisms	Some forms of cutaneous vasculitis have an association with TB and a number of autoimmune/vasculitic diseases, although most cases are idiopathic	The major form of cutaneous vasculitis that may be confused with erythema nodosum (EN) is **nodular vasculitis (erythema induratum)**, another form of panniculitis. Nodular vasculitis is characterised by painful subcutaneous erythematous nodules, often of the lower legs. Unlike EN, lesions may involve the posterior aspects of the legs, and have a propensity to ulcerate	Often diagnosed clinically, with biopsy used to confirm diagnosis where doubt exists. Treatment is of the underlying disorder. In addition, dapsone and immunosuppression (eg prednisolone) may help to accelerate recovery of the condition
Subcutaneous skin infections	Enquire about risk factors of skin infections, including diabetes mellitus, immunosuppression, etc	The formation of pustules is useful to differentiate from EN	Microbiological assays from skin usually cultures typical pathogenic skin organisms, especially streptococci and staphylococci
Thrombophlebitis	Enquire about underlying malignancy, associated with thrombophlebitis migrans. Trauma, surgery or infection may trigger superficial vein thrombosis	Thrombophlebitis of the superficial veins of the breast or anterior chest wall is known as Mondor's disease. In the axilla it is known as axillary web syndrome	Clots can extend to deep veins and embolise, causing pulmonary thrombosis. Doppler ultrasonography to exclude DVT is therefore useful. NSAIDs are the mainstay of treatment, although some guidelines advocate anticoagulation to prevent deep vein extension

Clinical judgement and maintaining patient welfare

Erythema nodosum is a condition characterised by the appearance of red (or purple), painful, subcutaneous nodules, usually bilaterally in a pre-tibial location. It is more common in women than men and is most likely to occur in people in their 20s and 30s. At least half of patients will present with other symptoms including fever and arthralgia.

The exact pathogenesis of this delayed hypersensitivity reaction is unclear. There are a considerable number of known precipitants; honing in on these in the history and examination is key to success in a Station 5 in which EN appears.

The known associated conditions/precipitants for EN include those shown in Table 5.8.

Table 5.8 Conditions or precipitants associated with erythema nodosum

Category	Specific examples	
Idiopathic	Up to three-quarters of cases may have no precipitant identified	
Infectious diseases	Bacterial	Group A β-haemolytic streptococci – worldwide, the cause most commonly associated with EN *Yersinia* sp. *Salmonella* sp. *Campylobacter* sp. *Shigella* sp. *Chlamydia* sp. *Mycoplasma pneumoniae* Syphilis
	Mycobacterial	Tuberculosis Leprosy
	Viral	HIV
	Fungal	Coccidioidomycosis Histoplasmosis
Multisystemic non-infectious diseases	Inflammatory bowel disease Sarcoidosis Behçet's disease	
Malignancy	Some evidence of association, particularly with lymphoma	
Drugs	Including: Oral contraceptive pill Antibiotics (penicillin, sulfonamides, isotretinoin, etc)	
Other causes	Pregnancy	

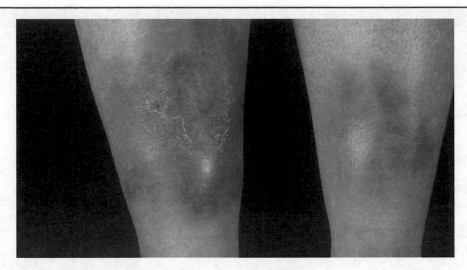

Figure 5.4 Erythema nodosum

Investigation and management

EN is usually diagnosed clinically. Where there is diagnostic doubt, a wedge biopsy may be performed from an affected area. The histological features will be of a panniculitis, with inflammation and thickening of the septa of the subcutaneous fat.

Initial investigations for a precipitant will depend on the clinical scenario, but a basic screen would include

- **Blood tests**: FBC, CRP, ESR
- **Microbiology**: anti-streptolysin O titre, cultures of throat swabs, stool and blood
- **Chest radiograph**: to look for evidence of TB, sarcoidosis or lymphoma.

Other investigations that may be relevant include

- Where TB is suspected: Mantoux test, interferon-γ release assay, mycobacterial sputum cultures, bronchoscopy, etc
- Where sarcoidosis is suspected: serum ACE, CT of the chest, bronchoscopy, etc

- Where IBD is suspected: endoscopy and biopsy, intestinal imaging (plain films, ultrasonography, CT or MR), etc.

Lesions of EN typically resolve within 8 weeks, and usually the only treatment required is that of any underlying condition. However, if lesions are particularly painful then NSAIDs may be useful (unless the patient has Crohn's disease, in which case a flare may be precipitated by NSAIDs). Corticosteroids may also be used sometimes, although the evidence for their benefit is sparse.

Maintaining patient welfare

- A sexual history may be appropriate, which should be approached sensitively with reassurances about confidentiality.
- Where patients have EN that has been precipitated by group A β-haemolytic streptococci, there is little evidence that antibiotics will help improve the condition. Patients will require a careful explanation that EN occurs as an immunological phenomenon rather than due to the infection directly.

SCENARIO 16. GOUT

Introduce yourself

Confirm the information you've been given: this 58-year-old man has severe pain in his right foot. Please assess him.

'What is the main problem from your point of view?' 'I have severe pain in my right big toe. I've also noticed painful swellings on my elbows and left ear.'

New condition

Focused history of the presenting complaint and relevant systems enquiry: differentiate between septic arthritis (spiking fever with rigors, symptoms of infective foci elsewhere, immunosuppression, etc) and inflammatory crystal arthropathy (low-grade fever, risk factors (see below), typical joint involvement (ie first metatarsophalangeal joint in gout))

Identifying alarm symptoms: night sweats or fevers, B symptoms or features suggestive of a haematological malignancy

Pre-existing conditions/risk factors: obesity, current cancers with or without chemotherapy, chronic kidney disease, alcohol excess, recent changes in medications

Social/occupational/family circumstances: pain affecting work, tophi affecting cosmetic appearance, history of alcohol excess

Drugs: diuretics, previous colchicine, NSAIDs, renal replacement therapy. **DRUG ALLERGIES**

Pre-existing conditions: haematological malignancies, chronic kidney disease, hypertension, chronic inflammatory disorders, obesity and/or insulin resistance syndromes

Begin a **targeted** examination of relevant area/system and continue while taking the history

General appearance: in pain, walking tentatively, obese, BM testing finger pricks

Look at the painful region for

- Erythema, warmth, swelling
- Limitation of movement
- Extreme tenderness of affected joints (beware!)

Particularly observe the first metatarsophalangeal joint (podagra; involved in 90% of gout cases), inflamed Heberden's or Bouchard's nodes, and bursitis of the olecranon or patella bursae

Also look for evidence of chronic tophaceous gout

- Hard, **painless**, nodular, calcified swellings
- Look at the pinnae of ears, hands and feet, ulnar surface of forearm (resembling rheumatoid arthritis) and Achilles tendons

Also look for/consider the following

- Signs of chronic kidney disease/renal replacement therapy
- Lymphadenopathy, hepatosplenomegaly, conjunctival pallor, petechiae (could there be an underlying haematological malignancy?)
- Complete the assessment by asking for blood pressure and blood glucose/urine dipstick for glycosuria

CALLBACK: 'You said at the beginning that the main problem was painful right foot and swelling around the left ear and your elbows. Is there anything else troubling you that we haven't covered?'

RESPOND TO PATIENT'S CONCERNS (1–2 min)

1. I think the pain in your right foot is caused by gout and this accounts for the swellings on the ear and elbows. They are called tophi. This may have been exacerbated by your pre-existing kidney problem
2. First, we need to help with the pain by giving you some strong painkillers and anti-inflammatories
3. To confirm the diagnosis we should draw some fluid from the painful joint. This is crucial to make sure that there is no infection, which could destroy the joint quickly. In the long term, you will need medication to prevent further episodes of gout (eg allopurinol)

Thank the patient

1–2 minutes

5 minutes

1–2 minutes

Differential diagnosis	Clinical communication skills and managing patient concerns	Physical examination and identifying physical signs	Clinical judgement and maintaining patient welfare
Septic arthritis	History of systemic upset (eg fever, rigors) may be present More common in patients who are elderly, have diabetes or alcohol problems, and those with pre-existing joint disease (eg rheumatoid arthritis, previous joint surgery) Sexual history is also important to exclude gonococcal arthritis	Hot, tender joint with surrounding erythema Systemic inflammatory response (tachycardia, hypotension, high temperature, sweating) May also be tenosynovitis and pustular skin lesions in gonococcal infection	*Investigations* Blood tests: FBC (raised WBC), CRP, ESR, blood cultures Joint aspiration: urgent Gram staining and culture (for staphylococci, streptococci, *Pseudomonas* sp., gonococci or TB). Synovial fluid is usually turbid with a high neutrophil count Joint imaging: to exclude other causes of monoarthritis. MRI may be needed to exclude osteomyelitis *Management* Needs emergency intervention Intravenous antibiotics: start *before* diagnosis is made (typically empirical flucloxacillin + fusidic acid + gentamicin) Orthopaedic referral for arthroscopic joint washouts
Pseudogout A form of arthropathy associated with calcium pyrophosphate crystals	There are a number of well-recognised risk factors/associated conditions, including: Haemochromatosis Hyperparathyroidism Hypothyroidism Osteoarthritis Low phosphate and magnesium levels Chronic kidney disease	Classically presents as monoarthritis or oligoarthritis. Over 50% of cases affect the knee, with the wrist and hip also commonly affected **Not** associated with tophi May also rarely present as a chronic oligo-/polyarthritis that may be confused with osteoarthritis or rheumatoid arthritis	*Investigations* Blood tests: raised inflammatory markers Joint radiograph: shows *chondrocalcinosis*, representing crystal deposition within joint cartilage Joint aspiration: rhomboidal, weakly positive, birefringent calcium pyrophosphate crystal deposits on polarised light microscopy *Management* Typically self-limiting Analgesia/anti-inflammatories: NSAIDs or colchicine Glucocorticoids: oral or intra-articular steroids may be used once sepsis has been excluded Joint aspiration: may ease the pain

(continued)

Differential diagnosis	Clinical communication skills and managing patient concerns	Physical examination and identifying physical signs	Clinical judgement and maintaining patient welfare
Osteoarthritis	Typically presents with chronic progressive joint pain usually involving several joints; made worse by movement and relieved by rest However, may rarely present with acute single joint pain and swelling that is difficult to distinguish from other causes of monoarthritis	Hands: bony swellings at the distal interphalangeal joint (*Heberden's nodes*) and proximal interphalangeal joints (*Bouchard's nodes*), and a 'squared' appearance to the first metacarpophalangeal joint Large joints: often affected asymmetrically. There may be marked deformities (eg varus deformity of the knee). Crepitus and sometimes 'locking' often on examination of affected joints. The gait may be antalgic, and *Trendelenburg's test* may be positive if the hip is affected (ie standing on one leg, the pelvis drops onto the non-weight-bearing leg, implying weakness of the hip stabilisers on the weight-bearing side)	*Investigations* Joint radiograph: loss of joint space, marginal osteophytosis, subchondral sclerosis and subchondral cysts Joint aspiration: clear fluid, no crystals and a low WBC count *Management* Analgesia: including intra-articular steroids Physiotherapy and occupational therapy Joint replacement in severe disease
Rheumatoid arthritis	See Scenario 34. Rheumatoid arthritis flowchart		
Seronegative arthropathy	See Scenario 3. Ankylosing spondylitis flowchart, Scenario 31. Psoriatic arthropathy and Scenario 10. Crohn's disease		

Clinical judgement and maintaining patient welfare

Gout is caused through the deposition of mono-sodium urate (MSU) crystals in joints, bone and/or soft tissues. The greater the serum uric acid concentration the higher the possibility of MSU crystal formation, and therefore the greater the risk of gout occurring. Uric acid is produced through the catabolism of purines in the liver by the enzyme xanthine oxidase. As such, risk factors for gout include conditions associated with increased uric acid production, and those associated with reduced uric acid excretion (Table 5.9).

Attacks of gout may occur without an obvious trigger, but typical precipitants include dehydration, starvation, exercise, changes in diet (particularly alcohol excess) and changes in medications.

Investigations
- **Blood tests**
  - Raised inflammatory markers may be found. These are useful for monitoring the condition during treatment, but not specific in making the diagnosis.
  - Where an infectious cause of acute monoarthritis is being considered, blood cultures should be sent, along with any relevant serology (eg borrelia serology, if appropriate).
  - Serum urate level is **not** useful in diagnosing acute gout – levels may be normal at the time of an acute gout attack, or conversely may be raised in those who do not have gout.
- **Synovial fluid aspiration and analysis**
  - In gout, polarised light microscopy of synovial fluid will show *negatively birefringent needle-shaped MSU crystals*. Microscopy will show high neutrophil counts in both crystal arthropathy and septic arthritis.
  - Synovial fluid Gram stain has only approximately 60% sensitivity for detecting septic arthritis. Synovial fluid culture has a higher sensitivity (about 80%) but this is negligible if antibiotics have already been given, and much lower in gonococcal infections.
- **Radiographs**
  - Chronic tophaceous gout is sometimes indistinguishable from rheumatoid arthritis. In gout, erosions are usually

Table 5.9 Risk factors for gout

Risk factor	Examples
Increased uric acid production	High purine diet: particularly meat, seafood and beer Lymphoproliferative and myeloproliferative disorders: reflecting high cell turnover Chronic inflammatory disorders (eg psoriasis): again, reflecting high cell turnover Obesity: associated with increased new purine production Drugs: particularly the use of chemotherapy in haematological malignancy ('tumour lysis syndrome')
Reduced uric acid excretion	States associated with raised organic acids: dehydration and starvation, ketoacidosis, lactate acidosis Chronic kidney disease Hypertension Drugs: including aspirin, ACE inhibitors, diuretics and immunosuppressants (eg ciclosporin)

'punched out' with sclerotic margins; they are often distant from the joint and sometimes outside the joint capsule. In contrast, rheumatoid erosions are always within the joint capsule and near the joint margin. Furthermore, joints affected by gout do not develop narrowed joint space or periarticular osteopenia.

Management

Most attacks of acute gout are self-limiting, but the following may be used

- Treatment of any precipitant, eg treatment of ketoacidosis.
- Analgesia/anti-inflammatories: NSAIDs are a useful first-line therapy but are not appropriate for all (eg chronic kidney disease). An effective alternative is colchicine, although its use may be limited by diarrhoea.
- Corticosteroids: intra-articular steroids may be used where sepsis has been excluded.

Measures used to prevent further gout attacks/in treatment of chronic tophaceous gout include

- Reduction in risk factors, eg dietary changes, review of medications.
- Allopurinol: this is a xanthine oxidase inhibitor that is used in people with recurrent gout. Low-dose colchicine or an NSAID should be prescribed in a prophylactic manner before its initiation to prevent an attack of acute gout. Treatment is normally life-long. Where allopurinol is contraindicated or not tolerated, other uricosuric medications may be tried (eg probenecid).

Maintaining patient welfare

- Emphasise to patients (and therefore examiners) the urgency of excluding septic arthritis.
- Explain appropriate changes to the patient's diet or medications that may be needed to minimise further attacks of crystal arthropathy
- Demonstrate an appreciation of the pain and disability that may result from chronic tophaceous gout and how this may impact on the patient's life. Appropriate help includes referral to physiotherapy and occupational therapy, advice on any disability benefit and discussion about support groups (eg Arthritis Care, UK Gout Society, etc).

Resources

UK Gout Society: www.ukgoutsociety.org

SCENARIO 17. GRAVES' DISEASE

Introduce yourself

Confirm the information you've been given and patient details: this 41-year-old woman has presented with intermittent palpitations and feeling anxious and sweating excessively for the last month. Please assess her.

'What is the main problem from your point of view?' 'I feel that my heart is racing while doing my housework and even in bed at night. I am feeling anxious and sweating most of the time, and am finding it difficult to concentrate properly'.

1–2 minutes

5 minutes

New condition

Focused history of the presenting complaint and relevant systems enquiry: differentiate symptoms of hyperthyroidism (palpitations, sweating/heat intolerance, tremor, oligomenorrhoea, weight loss, diarrhoea, etc) from other causes (eg anxiety states (ask about psychiatric history), or phaeochromocytoma (intermittent symptoms))

Identify alarm symptoms: intrinsic cardiac disease gives increased propensity to arrhythmias (mitral valve disease, IHD, etc). Also assess with regard to eye symptoms (eg diplopia; suggestive of Graves' disease)

Pre-existing conditions: other autoimmune disorders, previous thyroid disease

Social/occupational/family circumstances and impact of disease: impact on work and family life. Smoking history (especially if eye signs suggestive of Graves' disease)

Drug history: β blocker (will mask tachycardia). Ask about medications that affect the thyroid axis (eg amiodarone). Ask about pregnancy risk (as will influence treatment options for hyperthyroidism). **DRUG ALLERGIES**

Other medical conditions: other autoimmune disorders

Begin a **targeted** examination of relevant area/system and continue while taking the history

Thyroid status: tachycardia (± irregular), tremor, lid lag, lid retraction, hyperkinesia, sweaty palms

Neck: goitre – diffuse or nodular mass that moves with swallowing. Evidence of retrosternal extension? Is it possible to auscultate a bruit?

Eyes: characteristic features of Graves' ophthalmopathy include exophthalmos (risks corneal ulceration), proptosis, ophthalmoplegia (usually most marked on upward gaze), conjunctival oedema (*chemosis*), periorbital oedema

Fundoscopy: severe Graves' disease may result in optic nerve compression and optic atrophy

Extras: proximal muscle weakness. *Thyroid acropachy* is a complication of Graves' disease characterised by digits that appeared clubbed, but is actually caused through excessive new periosteal bone. *Pretibial myxoedema* may also be found in a small number of patients with Graves' disease, ie bilateral, asymmetrical, pink–brown, shiny plaques found in the pre-tibial area, with surrounding oedema

CALLBACK: 'You said at the beginning that the main problem was palpitations, anxiety and excessive sweating. Is there anything else troubling you that we haven't covered?'

RESPOND TO PATIENT'S CONCERNS (1–2 min)

1–2 minutes

1. I think the cause of your palpitations is an overactive thyroid gland. This is also making you feel anxious and causing you to feel excessively sweaty. We will perform an urgent blood test (thyroid function test) to confirm the diagnosis, and an ECG to ascertain the cause of the palpitations. Assuming that the blood test confirms my suspicions, we can give you medication (β blocker) that will control some of the symptoms right away
2. I am concerned that your thyroid problem is because of a condition called Graves' disease which may also affect your eyes. I will therefore also need to refer you to an eye specialist
3. There are three main ways to treat an overactive thyroid: medications, surgery and radioiodine; we will need to talk again once we have the test results to establish which is most appropriate for you

Thank the patient

Differential diagnosis	Clinical communication skills and managing patient concerns	Physical examination and identifying physical signs	Clinical judgement and maintaining patient welfare
Sick euthyroid disease	Any systemic disease causing physiological stress may result in derangement of thyroid hormone status, with T_3/T_4 and TSH either increased or decreased	No distinguishing clinical features	As a result of sick euthyroid disease, TFTs are difficult to interpret at times of physiological stress, eg during sepsis Where deranged TFTs have been found but the suspicion is of sick euthyroid disease, tests should be repeated several weeks after resolution of the current illness
Phaeochromocytoma Very rare catecholamine-secreting tumours. They arise from sympathetic paraganglia cells, and are usually based in the adrenal medulla	Clinical features are classically transient in nature. These include: General: sweating, subjective fever, heat intolerance Cardiological: palpitations, dizziness, chest pain, dyspnoea Neurological: anxiety, tremor, headache, visual obscurations Gastrointestinal: altered bowel habit, nausea, abdominal pain Most cases are idiopathic, although approximately 25% occur as part of a genetic cancer syndrome, eg von Hippel–Lindau syndrome Phaeochromocytomas are rare and anxiety disorders very common. The symptoms are very similar. Severe or labile hypertension is the most useful clinical differentiator	Phaeochromocytomas should be considered in cases of severe hypertension that is refractory to treatment, especially if occurring in the context of any typical symptoms	*Investigations* These include 24-hour urinary free catecholamines: usually performed at least three times to increase sensitivity Plasma catecholamines/metanephrines: where available, these have a slightly higher sensitivity than urinary catecholamines and similar specificity CT and MRI of the abdomen: to directly visualise the tumour [123I]MIBG scintigraphy: a nuclear medicine scan that allows tumour localisation, because the isotope is taken up by the tumour. PET is also increasingly recognised as valuable in diagnosis *Management* Ideally surgical where feasible Before surgery, patients will need treatment with both α-adrenergic blockade (ie phenoxybenzamine) and β-adrenergic blockade; α blockade is administered first to minimise a hypertensive/metabolic crisis from unopposed α-adrenergic stimulation Genetic counselling/screening is appropriate where there are grounds to suspect a familial syndrome
Anxiety disorders	Patients with anxiety disorder may complain of palpitations, tremor, light-headedness and mood changes which may be confused with thyrotoxicosis or phaeochromocytoma		There should be a low threshold for checking TFTs in any patients presenting with anxiety

Clinical judgement and maintaining patient welfare

Thyrotoxicosis is the clinical syndrome resulting from excessive secretion of thyroid hormones. Most cases result from primary pathology of the thyroid gland. Very rarely, the syndrome may occur as a result of hypothalamic–pituitary disease or other endocrine conditions. The differential diagnosis for thyrotoxicosis is shown Table 5.10.

Graves' disease is one of the most common causes of thyrotoxicosis, and hence one of the most frequently occurring 'thyroid cases' appearing in MRCP (PACES). It is an autoimmune condition, most often occurring in young and middle-aged women, caused by the production of autoantibodies that target and activate the TSH receptor.

This results in the enlargement of thyroid follicles and excessive hormone production. As described in the flowchart, there are certain clinical features in the assessment of a patient with thyrotoxicosis that are specific for a diagnosis of Graves' disease, including

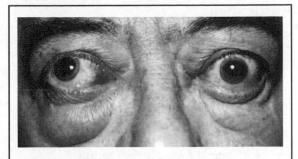

Figure 5.5 Exophthalmos

Table 5.10 Differential diagnosis for thyrotoxicosis

Category	Causes	Specific examples
Primary hyperthyroidism	Immune and inflammatory	Graves' disease. Subacute (de Quervain's) thyroiditis: a normally self-limiting form of thyroid inflammation, associated with viruses including Coxsackie virus Postpartum thyroiditis Infective thyroiditis Hyperthyroid phase as part of Hashimoto's disease ('hashitoxicosis')
	Nodular	Toxic multinodular goitre Toxic adenoma
	Drugs	Excessive thyroid hormone replacement, excessive iodine Amiodarone Lithium
	Ectopic sources of thyroid hormone	Struma ovarii (ie ovarian teratoma containing thyroid tissue) Metastatic follicular thyroid carcinoma
Secondary hyperthyroidism	Hypothalamic–pituitary disease	TSH-secreting pituitary adenoma The hCG-secreting trophoblastic tumours

- Graves' ophthalmopathy
- Thyroid acropachy
- Pre-tibial myxoedema.

Note that, although goitre is often found in Graves' disease, it is not specific for the condition.

Investigations

- **Blood tests**: these include
    - Thyroid function tests: thyrotoxicosis is defined by an increase in plasma free T_3 and T_4 levels. TSH levels are suppressed in primary hyperthyroidism and are increased only in the very rare syndrome of TSHoma. The presence of normal T_4/T_3 with reduced TSH is defined as *subclinical hyperthyroidism.* The interpretation of TFTs is summarised in Table 5.11.
    - Anti-thyroid antibodies: anti-thyroid peroxidase antibodies may be detected in a proportion of patients with an autoimmune aetiology to their thyrotoxicosis. TSH receptor-stimulating antibodies may be detected in the serum of those with Graves' disease.
    - Full blood count: there may be an associated normocytic anaemia secondary to impaired erythropoiesis.
    - Biochemistry: corrected calcium levels may also be increased. Inflammatory markers may be raised in de Quervain's thyroiditis.
- **Radioisotope uptake scan**: ^{99m}Tc or more rarely ^{123}I
    - This is most useful in helping to diagnose toxic adenoma, in which the scan will show a well-defined area of high uptake and suppressed activity elsewhere.
    - Findings in other conditions will include
        - Graves' disease: globally increased uptake.
        - Thyroiditis: globally low uptake.
        - Toxic multinodular goitre: several different areas of increased uptake.
- Ultrasonography
    - Typically quite a limited role, but may be useful in skilled hands for assessing dominant nodules/dominance within

Table 5.11 Interpretation of thyroid function tests

	Free T_4	Free or total T_3	TSH
Primary hyperthyroidism	Usually ↑ or →	Usually ↑ or →	Always undetectable
Primary hypothyroidism	Usually ↓ or →	↓ or →	Always ↑
Pituitary disease	Usually↓ or →	Usually ↓ or →	Usually ↓ or low →
TSHoma	Usually ↑ or →	Usually ↑ or →	Detectable or modestly ↑
Sick euthyroid	↓ or ↑ or →	↓ or ↑ or →	↓ or ↑ or →
Amiodarone	Usually ↑	Usually ↓	Usually modestly ↑
Thyroid hormone resistance	→	→	Elevated

nodules when neoplasia is a possibility and fine-needle aspiration is being considered.

Management

- β-Adrenergic blockers (eg propranolol)
  - These provide symptomatic relief until euthyroid. Often large doses are required.
- Anti-thyroid medications (eg carbimazole or propylthiouracil)
  - These are the first-line medical treatments. They can be administered either by titrating the dose by biochemical response or through use of a 'block-and-replace' regimen (ie high-dose carbimazole to completely suppress thyroid hormone activity, then supplemental thyroxine). In Graves' disease, such medications are given for at least 1 year before an attempt at withdrawal occurs; approximately half of patients will relapse.
  - Patients should be warned of side effects (ie rash – approximately 1 in 200; agranulocytosis – approximately 1 in 2000; patients should be told to seek an urgent FBC if they develop a sore throat or other infection).
- ^{131}I-labelled radioiodine
  - This is useful for long-term treatment, although 50% of the patients will become hypothyroid.
  - Radioiodine therapy is contraindicated in pregnancy and lactation. In addition, there is some evidence that it may worsen ophthalmopathy, especially in smokers (although this risk may be reduced by the administration of steroids).
- Surgery: total or subtotal thyroidectomy depending on local practice
  - Risks include haemorrhage, damage to the recurrent laryngeal nerve palsy, and hypothyroidism and hypocalcaemia through the removal of thyroid and parathyroid tissue, respectively.
- Some additional points about treatment

- In the context of a 'thyroid storm', iodide may be administered after anti-thyroid medications have been given to minimise further thyroid hormone release. There is also evidence that dexamethasone may be useful in this context by preventing the conversion of T_4 to T_3, thus also reducing thyroid hormone effects.
- Thyroid eye disease is an emergency. Treatments for exophthalmos (see Figure 5.5) include lubricating eye drops, eye patching, prism glasses and consideration of lateral tarsorraphy. Where the full features of Graves' ophthalmopathy are present, patients should be given corticosteroids (to reduce oedema), and be considered for urgent radiotherapy and/or decompressive surgery of the orbit.
- Management of thyroid disease in pregnancy is difficult; the fetus is at risk of either hyperthyroidism (passage of thyroid-stimulating antibodies across the placenta) or hypothyroidism (due to transfer of anti-thyroid drugs). Propylthiouracil is preferred to carbimazole because it crosses the placenta and saturates in breast tissue to a lesser degree. Monitoring of fetal heart rate is the best measure of disease activity.

Maintaining patient welfare

- Although the diagnosis of thyroid storm may be made relatively easily, it is not unusual for the diagnosis of thyrotoxicosis to be initially missed. Clinicians should have a low threshold for checking thyroid function tests if any symptoms that may be associated with the syndrome are present.
- All patients on anti-thyroid medication should be counselled carefully about the risk of agranulocytosis. Female patients should be advised to inform medical services if they become pregnant, because they will require very close monitoring of their thyroid function and possible changes in their treatment regimen.

SCENARIO 18. HENOCH–SCHÖNLEIN PURPURA

1–2 minutes

Introduce yourself

Confirm the information you've been given and patient details: this 20-year-old woman has a non-blanching rash on the back of her legs, aching joints and abdominal pain. Please assess her.

'What is the main problem from your point of view?' 'I have discomfort in my stomach, and my joints are also aching. I have also developed a purple rash on the back of my legs.'

5 minutes

New condition

Focused history of the presenting complaint and relevant systems enquiry: recent fever and coryzal illness (streptococcal upper respiratory tract infection is the most common precipitant)

Differentiate from other causes of arthralgia and abdominal colic/pain (ie IBD, Behçet's disease, reactive arthritis, autoimmune hepatitis, etc)

Differentiate from other causes of purpuric rash, including infection (meningococcal, streptococcal, etc), vasculitis (eg cryoglobulinaemia), connective tissue diseases (SLE, polyarthritis nodosa, etc) and drug reaction (recent penicillin, sulfonamides and/or NSAIDs)

Identify alarm symptoms: macroscopic haematuria and peripheral swelling (raises possibility of glomerulonephritis/nephrotic syndrome)

Social/occupational/family circumstances: effect on employment during illness

Drug history: including ACE inhibitors, penicillin, sulfonamides, thiazide diuretics. **DRUG ALLERGIES**

Other medical conditions: connective tissue diseases, vasculitis, etc.

Begin a **targeted** examination of relevant area/system and continue while taking the history

Examination of the skin

Location: extensor surfaces of lower limbs and buttocks (only occasionally on hands and face)

Description: non-blanching *palpable* purpuric rash

Additional examinations

Abdominal examination: GI haemorrhage is a common complication (33%); may be attributable to intussusception. If haemorrhage is present, tell examiner that you would perform a rectal examination

Joint(s) examination: HSP may be complicated by a non-deforming arthritis, typically found in hands, elbows, knees and ankles

Assess for oedema: as nephrotic syndrome is a possible complication

Ask to perform blood pressure and urine dipstick (for microscopic haematuria – either nephritic or nephrotic syndrome may occur as complications)

CALLBACK: 'You said at the beginning that the main problems were aching joints, abdominal pain and a purple rash on the back of your legs. Is there anything else troubling you that we haven't covered?

1–2 minutes

RESPOND TO PATIENT'S CONCERNS (1–2 min)

1. I think the cause of your symptoms and your rash is a condition called Henoch–Schönlein purpura. It is caused by inflammation of your small blood vessels, called a vasculitis
2. For your painful joints and abdomen, I will give you some painkillers (eg paracetamol, not NSAIDs). I will need to confirm that you have this condition before I can decide if you need any further treatment. In particular, we need to ensure that your kidneys have not been affected
3. To investigate this condition, we will need to perform blood tests (eg FBC, U+Es, CRP, ESR, complement) and take a sample of your urine (eg urine dipstick and microscopy). If things are still unclear after that, we may need to perform a biopsy of your skin and even kidneys to confirm the diagnosis (eg for IgA or C3 immunofluorescence)

Thank the patient

Differential diagnosis		Clinical communication skills and managing patient concerns	Physical examination and identifying physical signs	Clinical judgement and maintaining patient welfare
Non-palpable				
Primary cutaneous disorders	These include: Trauma Solar purpura	Ask about a history of purpura following trauma or light exposure	Purpuric lesions represent extravasation of red blood cells from capillaries into the skin, and are by definition non-blanching under pressure	*Investigations* These will depend on the differential diagnosis, but may include:
Systemic disorders	Disorders of the platelet and/ or coagulation system, including: Thrombocytopenia: of any cause Abnormal platelet function, eg chronic kidney disease, chronic liver disease Haemophilic disorders: both inherited (eg haemophilia A and B) and acquired (eg disseminated intravascular coagulation) Anti-platelet/anti-thrombotic therapy: or reaction to it	Patients may volunteer previous haematological investigations or a family history of excessive bleeding The history should include a drug history about use of aspirin, clopidogrel, warfarin or other anti-platelets/anticoagulation	Palpable purpura represents an inflammatory infiltrate within the vessel wall (with red blood cells forming part of this infiltrate), whereas conditions with non-palpable purpura tend to be non-inflammatory in nature Palpable purpura may be accompanied by other features of vasculitic disease, eg splinter haemorrhages, vasculitic ulcers (see Scenario 15. Erythema nodosum differential diagnosis table)	Haematology: FBC (to assess platelet number), clotting profile (to assess the function of the coagulation system), and blood film (to assess for platelet clumping) are the minimal investigations required Biochemistry: renal function and urine dipstick should be obtained where a multisystem disorder (eg vasculitis) is suspected Immunology: an autoimmune screen is necessary whenever vasculitis/autoimmune disease is suspected *Management* Dependent on the underlying diagnosis
	Disorders associated with vascular fragility: Increased vascular pressure, eg chronic venous disease Disorders with primary vascular fragility/dermal weakness, eg steroid purpura, Ehlers–Danlos syndrome, HHT, amyloidosis, scurvy, etc			
	Disorders associated with embolisation: Fat emboli Cholesterol emboli	Fat emboli may be suggested by purpura occurring post-bony trauma Cholesterol emboli may be considered if the patient has had recent vascular intervention, eg angioplasty		

(continued)

Differential diagnosis		Clinical communication skills and managing patient concerns	Physical examination and identifying physical signs	Clinical judgement and maintaining patient welfare
Palpable				
Vasculitic/ autoimmune disorders	Small vessel vasculitides, including: Cryoglobulinaemia type 2 or 3 ANCA-positive disorders, ie granulomatosis with polyangiitis (Wegener's granulomatosis), Churg–Strauss syndrome, microscopic polyangiitis	Symptoms would vary depending on the underlying disorder		
	Autoimmune diseases, including: SLE Rheumatoid arthritis Sjögren's syndrome Behçet's disease Polyarteritis nodosa Cryoglobulinaemia type 1			
Infections	This includes: Bacterial infections: meningococci, gonococci, group A β-haemolytic streptococci, *Staphylococcus aureus*, bacterial endocarditis Viral infections: hepatitis B and C Rickettsia: Rocky Mountain spotted fever			
Drugs	This includes: Penicillins Sulfonamides Thiazide diuretics	May be established from the drug history		

Clinical judgement and maintaining patient welfare

Assessing a patient with purpura is a relatively common Station 5 case in MRCP (PACES), with Henoch–Schönlein purpura (HSP) an important differential to consider. This is a condition that may be found in patients of all ages, but predominantly occurs among children. In most cases, no precipitant is found; however, epidemiological studies have identified a number of potential precipitants, including infections (particularly streptococcal upper respiratory tract infections) and medications (such as ACE inhibitors and antibiotics such as vancomycin). Pathologically, HSP is a small vessel vasculitis that is characterised by deposition of immune complexes containing IgA in affected organs. Most cases resolve without any long-term adverse sequelae, although a small percentage of patients will develop ongoing dysfunction in affected organs (eg chronic kidney disease occurs in approximately 1% of patients).

Clinical features

As outlined in the flowchart, HSP is characterised by four major clinical features: (1) palpable purpura, (2) arthritis, (3) gastrointestinal disease (often haemorrhage) and (4) renal disease (ranging from asymptomatic right up to nephritic or nephrotic syndrome). Very rarely, the vasculitic process may also involve other organ systems, eg patients may develop haemoptysis as a manifestation of lung involvement.

Investigations

The diagnosis is usually made clinically. However, investigations are useful for excluding differential diagnoses, and for helping to establish the severity of the condition where the diagnosis has been confirmed. These include

- Laboratory investigations
  - Haematological investigations reveal a normal or raised platelet count and a normal coagulation profile (in contrast with other conditions associated with purpura).
  - Biochemical investigations will

demonstrate raised inflammatory markers, and a variable level of renal dysfunction. IgA levels are elevated in approximately half of patients. A urine dipstick (for haematuria) and urinary protein:creatinine ratio will help to establish the degree of glomerular blood and protein loss.
- Imaging
  - Abdominal imaging and/or endoscopy is merited when patients have severe abdominal pain/GI haemorrhage.
- Biopsy
  - Skin biopsy: not performed routinely, but where there is diagnostic uncertainty about the cause of purpura. Under immunofluorescence, IgA and complement C3 deposition are seen in HSP.
  - Renal biopsy: performed only rarely. In HSP, this will demonstrate histological changes identical to those seen in IgA nephropathy, including mesangial IgA deposition and crescenteric changes.

Management

Most cases resolve spontaneously. Only a small percentage of affected patients will have a recurrence of disease or permanent organ dysfunction. Analgesics are usually the only measure required during the active phase of disease (although NSAIDs should be avoided, given their potential adverse effects on renal function). The only indication for immunosuppressive therapy is severe renal involvement (eg pulsed methylprednisolone when there is extensive renal disease on biopsy).

Maintaining patient welfare

Although only a minority of patients will develop progressive renal disease, it is important that these patients are not missed. Patients with renal involvement will need frequent investigations and close monitoring, because patients can develop advanced CKD and even end-stage kidney disease with only a minimum of symptoms. It will need to be explained why follow-up is crucial, and why unpleasant, invasive procedures such as renal biopsy may be important, even though they may be asymptomatic.

SCENARIO 19: HEREDITARY HAEMORRHAGIC TELANGIECTASIA

1–2 minutes

Introduce yourself

Confirm the information you've been given and patient details: this 20-year-old woman has been referred to outpatients for investigation of tiredness and vascular lesions on mucosal membranes. Please assess her.

'What is the main problem from your point of view?' 'It started with red spots in my mouth and lips and nosebleeds, and now I feel tired all the time.'

5 minutes

New condition

Focused history of the presenting complaint and relevant systems enquiry: exclude other causes of tiredness (symptoms of thyroid disease, depression, sleep apnoea, etc) from anaemia. Differentiate causes of anaemia (epistaxis, GI bleeding (50% of patients), menstrual loss, etc)

Differentiate different causes of telangiectasia, eg systemic sclerosis (typical facial features, Raynaud's phenomenon, etc), spider naevi (history of or risk factors for chronic liver disease)

Identify alarm symptoms: signs of severe anaemia (eg breathlessness, angina, presyncope), severe bleeding (melaena, haematemesis, haemoptysis) and/or neurological features (eg sensorimotor symptoms or visual impairment, which may imply cerebral or spinal AVMs)

Social/occupational/family circumstances: family history of Osler–Weber–Rendu syndrome (hereditary haemorrhagic telangiectasia (HHT))

What is the patient's fatigue preventing her from doing?

Drug history: iron supplementation. **DRUG ALLERGIES**

Other medical conditions: previous GI or gynaecological investigations for bleeding

Begin a **targeted** examination of relevant area/system and continue while taking the history

Signs of anaemia/iron deficiency

Pallor (especially conjunctivae), koilonychia, tachycardia, low blood pressure, flow murmur

Features of HHT

- Telangiectasia of the face, lips, tongue, oral cavity and nasal mucosa
- Telangiectasias blanch on pressure

Additional examinations

- **Neurological examination**: of a focused region if there are localising neurological symptoms
- **Abdominal examination:** if there is a history of GI bleeding, tell examiner that you would perform a per rectum examination
- **Respiratory examination**: if there is a history of haemoptysis; pulmonary AVMs may cause bruits
- **Fundoscopy (if appropriate)**: risk of retinal haemorrhage

CALLBACK: 'You said at the beginning that the main problem was nosebleeds, red spots in your mouth and tiredness. Is there anything else troubling you that we haven't covered?'

1–2 minutes

RESPOND TO PATIENT'S CONCERNS (1–2 min)

1. I think your symptoms are caused by a condition called Osler–Weber–Rendu syndrome (hereditary haemorrhagic telangiectasia), where blood vessels called telangiectasias bleed without warning. As this happens over time, it can make you anaemic and so you feel tired
2. The diagnosis is based on finding telengiectasias throughout the body. The treatment involves treating the anaemia with iron replacement and trying to stop the blood vessels from bleeding
3. I will need to check your blood to see how anaemic you are, and check that your clotting system is working and that your platelet levels are satisfactory. I will need to refer you for endoscopy (OGD/colonoscopy) and imaging (CT angiogram) to ensure that there are no abnormal blood vessels elsewhere in the body
4. This is an inherited condition, and it may also be of benefit for you to see a geneticist, especially if you are thinking of having children

Thank the patient

Differential diagnosis	Clinical communication skills and managing patient concerns	Physical examination and identifying physical signs	Clinical judgement and maintaining patient welfare
Essential telangiectasia			This diagnosis may be made only after exclusion of secondary causes (see below)
Ataxia–telangiectasia This is an autosomal recessive disorder associated with telangiectasia along with a range of neurological features	This should be suspected if there is a history of telangiectasia in association with neurological deficit, particularly if there is also a suggestive family history	Clinical features include: Telangiectasia: particularly around the face, neck and conjunctivae Neurological disease: principally a progressive cerebellar syndrome Recurrent infections: particularly recurrent respiratory, with increased propensity to bronchiectasis and interstitial lung disease Increased rate of malignancy: particularly haematological malignancies	*Investigations* The condition may be first suspected clinically or because of a family history, with genetic testing for mutations in the *ATM* gene helpful for confirming the diagnosis. *Management* There is no specific treatment, with management consisting of symptom control for affected organs Genetic counselling is warranted
Capillary malformation – AVM syndromes A range of conditions associated with vascular malformations of capillaries in the skin along with postcapillary venules	There may be a history of migraine or visual impairment	These vascular malformations classically lead to 'port wine stains' which may occur anywhere in the body (although the face is most often affected). They usually continue to grow as the child grows Other features depend on the underlying disorder, eg in Sturge–Weber syndrome, there is classically a triad of facial 'port wine stain', leptomeningeal angiomatosis (resulting in variable levels of neurodisability) and eye disease (including visual field defects, glaucoma, etc)	*Investigations* Such conditions are normally first suspected on clinical grounds. Genetic studies useful in confirming the diagnosis Axial imaging is required to establish the degree of AVM disease *Management* Treatment is generally supportive

(continued)

Differential diagnosis	Clinical communication skills and managing patient concerns	Physical examination and identifying physical signs	Clinical judgement and maintaining patient welfare
Carcinoid syndrome Note that carcinoid tumours are neuroendocrine tumours, most often found in the GI tract, which may secrete hormones derived from the amino acid tryptophan; the *carcinoid syndrome* is the term used to describe the range of symptoms and signs generated in response to the different hormones that these tumours produce, eg serotonin	Patients may present with any of a number of symptoms related to serotonin excess, including facial flushing, bronchospasm, diarrhoea and palpitations	Other clinical features may include Telangiectasia Heart failure: particularly right sided due to tricuspid valve dysfunction	*Investigations* The initial screening tests are the detection of increased levels of urinary 5-HIAA (the end-product of serotonin metabolism), and/or the detection of raised plasma serotonin/chromogranins Imaging is then used to localise the tumour, including CT, MRI, PET and/or octreotide scanning (ie a nuclear medicine scan employing octreotide, an analogue of somatostatin) *Management* Localised tumours may be surgically resected, whereas metastatic disease is treated with chemotherapy, interferon or somatostatin analogues
Spider naevi Abnormalities of the vasculature consisting of a central arteriole with multiple smaller surrounding vessels	They are found in chronic liver disease and pregnancy	These are found on the chest, upper limbs and face	These are diagnosed clinically No treatment is required
Systemic sclerosis scleroderma	See Scenario 35. Scleroderma		
Rosacea	See Scenario 12. Dermatomyositis differential diagnosis table		

Clinical judgement and maintaining patient welfare

Hereditary haemorrhagic telangiectasia (HHT; also known as Osler–Weber–Rendu syndrome) is a disorder with autosomal dominant inheritance that is characterised by widespread telangiectasia with a propensity to chronic haemorrhage. In addition, the condition is also associated with arteriovenous malformations (AVMs) which may occur in any of a number of different organ systems.

Clinical features

These are as outlined in the flowchart. Recurrent epistaxis is the most frequently occurring feature, affecting >90% of patients. GI bleeding is the next most common occurrence, with up to half of all patients affected. Patients can develop severe iron-deficiency anaemia even in the absence of overt bleeding.

The degree of AVM formation is variable between patients, and responsible for much of the morbidity and mortality associated with the condition. Within the central nervous system, cerebral AVMs may lead to subarachnoid haemorrhage, whereas those in the spine may result in paraparesis. Pulmonary AVMs may cause left-to-right shunting of blood, which increases the risk of ischaemic stroke (via paradoxical embolism), brain abscess/mycotic AVMs or – in the most severe cases – severe cardiorespiratory failure, with haemoptysis, cyanosis and clubbed digits. Up to a third of patients may be affected by hepatic AVMs, with those with the most severe disease at risk of developing cirrhosis and portal hypertension. There may also be shunting from the portal circulation directly into the inferior vena cava, putting the patient at risk of right-sided heart failure.

Investigations

The diagnosis of HHT is based on the use of the Curaçao criteria (see Resources)

- Epistaxis: spontaneous and recurrent

- Telangiectases: multiple, at characteristic sites – lips, oral cavity, fingers, nose
- Visceral lesions: GI telangiectasia, pulmonary, hepatic, cerebral or spinal AVMs
- Family history: a first-degree relative with HHT according to these criteria.

At least three criteria indicate a 'definite' diagnosis of HHT, two a 'suspected' diagnosis, with 0 or 1 criterion making the diagnosis 'unlikely'.

There are at least five different genes involved in the condition, and over 600 different confirmed mutations. The genes involved code for the Endoglin, ALK-1 and Smad4 proteins among others; these proteins are all involved in modulating cell signalling by TGF-β. Mutational analysis is increasingly being used clinically to help confirm the diagnosis of HHT, and is particularly useful in patients with two of the Curaçao criteria, and/or as part of prenatal diagnosis.

Once the diagnosis has been made, there should be a low threshold for screening for AVMs in common sites. This will include use of imaging modalities such as CT or MR angiography (for liver, lung and CNS AVMs), as well as the use of endoscopy for GI lesions. AVMs and telangiectasias can enlarge with age, and patients will therefore require close follow-up.

Management

Treatment of chronic anaemia may involve oral or intravenous iron supplementation or even blood transfusions. There may also be a role for a number of other medical therapies to reduce bleeding, including oestrogen therapy, aminocaproic acid, tranexamic acid and anti-VEGF treatments such as bevacizumab.

Recurrent epistaxis merits ENT input, when cauterisation or laser treatment may be appropriate. Gastrointestinal lesions may be treated endoscopically, often with argon plasma coagulation. AVMs may be embolised by interventional radiologists, but may also require surgical treatment in the most severe cases.

Maintaining patient welfare

- The fact that the condition is autosomal dominant means that patients may benefit from the input of a genetics service, particularly if at the stage of family planning.
- HHT is a relatively rare condition, and patients newly diagnosed with the condition are extremely unlikely to have much prior knowledge of it (unless a strong family history is present). As such, patients may benefit from input from a support group, such as the UK Telangiectasia Self Help Group (see weblink below).

Resources

Telangiectasia Self Help Group: www.telangiectasia.co.uk

Faughnan ME, Palda VA, Garcia-Tsao G, et al. International guidelines for the diagnosis and management of hereditary haemorrhagic telangiectasia. *J Med Genet* 2011;48:73–87.

SCENARIO 20. HERPES ZOSTER

1–2 minutes

Introduce yourself

Confirm the information you've been given and patient details: this 55-year-old man has presented to outpatients with a painful rash on the trunk. Please assess him.

'What is the main problem from your point of view?' 'It started with severe pain across my body and then this rash developed a few days later.'

5 minutes

New condition

Focused history of the presenting complaint and relevant systems enquiry: elicit typical history of prodrome (ie pain and paraesthesiae, followed by dermatomal vesicular eruption)

Identify alarm symptoms: visual disturbance (corneal ulcers/scarring), motor weakness (CN VII palsy), shortness of breath (varicella pneumonia), confusion (encephalitis)

Pre-existing conditions/risk factors: haematological malignancy (especially Hodgkin's disease), immunosuppressed state (eg HIV positive, chemotherapy, transplant recipients)

Social/occupational/family circumstances: exposure to pregnant women, immunosuppressed people or those who have not had chickenpox

Drug history: chemotherapy, immunosuppression. **DRUG ALLERGIES**

Other medical conditions: previous history of chickenpox

Begin a **targeted** examination of relevant area/ system and continue while taking the history

Examination of the skin (Figure 5.6)

Location: trunk (50%) in a dermatomal distribution. In elderly people, involvement of the ophthalmic division of the trigeminal nerve is relatively common

Description: grouped, clear, fluid-filled vesicles surrounded by erythema, becoming pustular and crusting

Additional examinations

- **Cranial nerve examination**: if cranial nerve palsy or meningoencephalitis is suspected
- **Peripheral nerves**: if an associated motor palsy is suspected
- **Eye**: corneal ulcer/scars (especially in shingles affecting the ophthalmic division of the trigeminal nerve)
- **Respiratory**: if there is a suggestion of dissemination to the lungs

CALLBACK: 'You said at the beginning that the main problem was a painful rash across your chest. Is there anything else troubling you that we haven't covered?'

1–2 minutes

RESPOND TO PATIENT'S CONCERNS (1–2 min)

1. I think your rash is a condition called shingles, which is caused by a virus called herpes zoster
2. I will prescribe you painkillers, and you will also need to rest and recover. Calamine lotion will help dry the rash. As the rash has only just started (presented within 48 hours of vesicle eruption), I will prescribe you an antiviral tablet called aciclovir which should help the rash resolve quicker
3. The diagnosis is obvious clinically, although we will take a viral swab for culture. The virus is shed in the fluid from the vesicles, so you should especially avoid people who have not had chickenpox, pregnant women and those who have a weakened immune system until the rash dries out

Thank the patient

Differential diagnosis	Clinical communication skills and managing patient concerns	Physical examination and identifying physical signs	Clinical judgement and maintaining patient welfare		
Herpes simplex infection A highly contagious viral infection, often acute and self-limiting but sometimes chronic in nature	In similarity to herpes zoster infection, HSV infection is associated with a localised area of pain and sensory disturbance before the appearance of a vesicular rash The history will require candidates to ask if patients have been in contact with others with a similar rash; this will include a sexual history	Infection is characterised by a vesicular rash that may be confused with herpes zoster Classically, HSV type 1 infection is associated with facial/mouth lesions, whereas HSV-2 infection is associated with genital lesions, although practically this distinction is not so clear-cut. Initial HSV-1 infection is often first subclinical at a very young age, whereas HSV-2 infection is usually first encountered at the age of sexual maturity Crusts will form at the site of lesions in <48 hours, and the rash tends to resolve completely within a week. Rarely, HSV infection may occur in a dermatomal distribution. In all cases, recurrence is common Complications vary greatly in severity between relatively mild (eg bacterial superinfection/impegitinisation of affected regions) and life threatening (eg herpes encephalitis)	*Investigations* The diagnosis is often made clinically, but may be confirmed through swabbing of lesions and viral culture *Management* Topical aciclovir has been shown to reduce the length of attacks when applied early to facial herpetic lesions. Oral antivirals are indicated for severe attacks of facial herpetic infection or genital disease, with intravenous aciclovir reserved for very severe cases (eg immunosuppressed patients, suspected herpes encephalitis) Given the potentially sexually transmitted nature of the infection, contact tracing may be appropriate		
Dermatitis herpetiformis	See Scenario 7. Coeliac disease flowchart				
Acute dermatitis	Particularly contact dermatitis; see Scenario 14. Eczema flowchart				

Clinical judgement and maintaining patient welfare

After infection with varicella-zoster virus (VZV), the virus will remain dormant in the dorsal root ganglion of sensory nerves within the spinal cord. In response to particular triggers, the virus can reactivate, begin replicating and migrate along the length of the nerve. As this occurs, the typical features of shingles begin to develop.

Clinical features

These are as described in the flowchart. Candidates will be expected to show an appreciation for complications, including

- Corneal ulcerations: these may endanger vision unless rapidly diagnosed and treated. Other ophthalmic complications are also recognised, including acute retinal necrosis.
- Ramsay Hunt syndrome: this should be suspected in patients with the constellation of facial nerve palsy, otalgia and vesicular lesions seen on otoscopy. Alterations in taste perception and hearing, and spontaneous lacrimation may all also be found.
- Postherpetic neuralgia: ongoing dermatomal pain and sensory disturbance may occur in up to a third of patients. In many cases this

resolves within weeks to months, although it may last much longer in certain patients.
- Motor neuron involvement: although VZV almost exclusively affects sensory nerves, it may translocate into the anterior horn of the spinal cord and cause a motor neuropathy. VZV may also cause more extensive spinal cord disease, resulting in transverse myelitis.
- Encephalitis: a form of sterile meningitis is also recognised. Other neurological complications include Guillain–Barré syndrome and stroke-like syndromes.
- Skin disease: haemorrhagic vesicles and gangrenous/necrotic skin disease may occur in severe cases, with immunosuppressed patients particularly at risk.
- Varicella pneumonitis: may initially present with non-specific respiratory symptoms, but may be rapidly progressive with a high mortality unless suspected early.

Investigations and management

The diagnosis is usually made clinically, although swabbing of lesions and viral culture are used to confirm the diagnosis.

In mild cases of shingles, the mainstay of treatment is analgesia and the use of drying agents

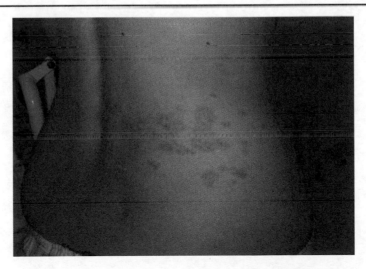

Figure 5.6 Herpes zoster

such as calamine lotion. If patients present within 48 hours of eruption of the vesicular rash, oral aciclovir will reduce viral shedding, length of time until resolution and the risk of postherpetic neuralgia. There is evidence that the early administration of oral prednisolone may also reduce the incidence of postherpetic neuralgia. Antibiotics – either topical or systemic – are indicated where impetiginisation occurs. In severe disease (particularly pneumonitis or encephalitis, or where immunosuppressed patients are affected), intravenous aciclovir is appropriate.

Maintaining patient welfare

- Patients with shingles need to be informed that they should avoid those who have never had chickenpox, who are pregnant or who are immunocompromised until resolution of the condition.
- Candidates should think broadly about what may have precipitated the attack of shingles. In patients with particularly severe attacks with no obvious precipitant, it would be important to check a patient's FBC, immunoglobulin counts and complement levels, as well as HIV status.
- Candidates should appreciate how postherpetic neuralgia may severely affect patients. As well as suggesting the use of neuropathic analgesic agents (amitriptyline, pregabalin, etc), candidates should consider whether physiotherapy, occupational therapy or pain clinic review is appropriate.

SCENARIO 21. HORNER SYNDROME

Introduce yourself

Confirm the information you've been given and patient details: this 58-year-old man presents with a unilateral drooping of his eyelid. Please assess him.

'What is the main problem from your point of view?' 'Over the last few weeks I have noticed my left eyelid is drooping. I've also developed a chest infection that I can't seem to shift.'

New condition

Focused history of the presenting complaint and relevant systems enquiry: screen for symptoms associated with disease along the sympathetic chain to anatomically localise potential lesions (including headache, speech change, visual changes, sensorimotor deficit, etc). Any suggestion of fatigability? Recent trauma (levator palpebrae disinsertion)?

Identify alarm symptoms: particularly for features of possible apical lung cancer (cough, dyspnoea, haemoptysis, constitutional upset, etc)

Pre-existing conditions/risk factors: smoking, recent central line insertion, neck/chest surgery

Social/occupational/family circumstances: impact on job if driving, smoking history, occupational risk of lung malignancy

Drug history: confirming other conditions implied by medication list. Use of eye drops? **DRUG ALLERGIES**

Other medical conditions: MS, trauma to base of neck, carotid artery dissection, carotid endarterectomy, aortic dissection, thyroid disease, syphilis (Argyll Robertson pupil)

Begin a **targeted** examination of relevant area/system and continue while taking the history

Horner syndrome: isolated ptosis, miosis, pseudo-enophthalmos, possible anhidrosis

Cranial nerve III palsy: associated ophthalmoplegia

Pupillary syndromes: small, unequal pupils with no light reflex/preserved accommodation (Argyll Robertson pupil); unilateral dilated pupil with slow reflexes (Holmes–Adie syndrome)

Briefly examine key areas of other systems that may be relevant

Neck: scars, masses (eg lymphadenopathy, tumours), carotid aneurysm

Chest: signs of an apical mass (eg Pancoast's tumour), scars, cervical rib

Hands/limbs: clubbing, tar-staining, wasting of the small muscles (ie supplied by T1) in the hand; may be consistent with Pancoast's lesion. Dissociated sensory impairment may be suggestive of syringomyelia. Fatigability may imply myasthenia gravis. Reduced/absent tendon reflexes may imply Holmes Adie syndrome

Cranial nerves: examine for bulbar palsy and cranial neuropathies that may imply brain-stem disease (eg multiple sclerosis)

CALLBACK: 'You said at the beginning that the main problem was your eye drooping and a cough. Is there anything else troubling you that we haven't covered?'

RESPOND TO PATIENT'S CONCERNS (1–2 min)

1. I think your eyelid drooping and cough may be related and be a condition called Horner syndrome
2. There is no specific treatment for this condition until the cause of it is known. This is usually benign
3. We need to perform a number of investigations, including in the first instance a chest radiograph and blood tests. Depending on these results, further investigations may be necessary, including a scan of the brain and neck

Thank the patient

Differential diagnosis	Clinical communication skills and managing patient concerns	Physical examination and identifying physical signs	Clinical judgement and maintaining patient welfare
Oculomotor (CN III) palsy		Unilateral ptosis may also be found in oculomotor nerve palsy; see Scenario 9. Cranial nerve III palsy flowchart and Station 3, Scenario 22. Ophthalmoplegia	
Myasthenia gravis (MG) An autoimmune condition associated with autoantibodies that target the nicotinic acetylcholine receptor, resulting in impaired neuromuscular transmission. See Station 3, Scenario 9.	The major clinical feature is progressive muscle weakness with fatigability. The patient may present with limb or facial weakness, or even diplopia from extraocular muscle involvement Note that MG is found in association with other autoimmune conditions, and may be precipitated by certain medications (β blockers, quinine, penicillamine, procainamide, opiates, etc)	Typical muscle groups involved include: Extraocular muscles: examination usually reveals bilateral ptosis, although may be unilateral; particularly marked on prolonged upgaze Bulbar: dysarthria, dysphagia Facial: giving 'myasthenic snarl' on smiling Limbs: particularly proximal weakness/ fatigability, with preserved reflexes and no muscle wasting Neck Torso The condition is also associated with enlargement of the thymus	*Investigations* Blood tests: anti-ACh receptor antibodies detected in most patients Tensilon test: administration of edrophonium results in improvement in muscular weakness Neurophysiology: progressively decreased muscle response to repetitive nerve stimulation Thymus imaging: association between MG and thymus malignancy *Management* Acetylcholinesterase inhibitors (eg pyridostigmine) and immunosuppression (typically prednisolone) are the mainstay of treatment IV immunoglobulin, plasmapheresis and/ or thymectomy may be considered in severe disease
Levator palpebrae disinsertion	Trauma may result in disinsertion of the aponeurosis of the levator palpebrae superioris muscle	Patients will have a unilateral ptosis, but will have no miosis or other features of Horner's syndrome	Diagnosed clinically May be treated with surgical reinsertion
Anterior uveitis	See Scenario 4. Anterior uveitis flowchart	May give a unilateral miosis, but will not be accompanied by any of the other features of Horner's syndrome. In addition, tends to present with an acutely red, painful eye	

(continued)

Differential diagnosis	Clinical communication skills and managing patient concerns	Physical examination and identifying physical signs	Clinical judgement and maintaining patient welfare
Drugs	Recent use of pilocarpine eye drops will give unilateral miosis	None of the other features of Horner's syndrome will be present	
Argyll Robertson pupil A cause for a small pupil, believed to result from a midbrain lesion	The best-established cause is neurosyphilis, with other causes including diabetes mellitus, and various causes of midbrain lesion (including tumours and vascular lesions)	Typical clinical features include: Unequal pupils, but both tending to be small Very delayed or minimal reaction to light, but maintained accommodation reflex However, **not** associated with ptosis, allowing differentiation from Horner's syndrome	Diagnosed clinically Investigations are those for precipitating disorders, eg VDRL for suspected syphilis
Holmes–Adie (myotonic) pupil A cause for unequal pupil size associated with damage to parasympathetic fibres		Typical clinical features include: Usually a unilaterally dilated pupil, but may be a unilateral miotic pupil (especially if long-standing) Associated with a slow/absent reflex to both light and accommodation May be associated with reduced/absent tendon reflexes and evidence of autonomic neuropathy (eg postural hypotension) (so-called Holmes–Adie syndrome) However, **not** associated with ptosis, allowing differentiation from Horner's syndrome	Diagnosed clinically

Clinical judgement and maintaining patient welfare

Horner's syndrome is a condition resulting from interruption of the sympathetic innervation of the eye. The sympathetic supply of the eye com-mences in the hypothalamus and ends within the orbit, and consists of a pathway of three neurons with two intervening synapses; lesions may occur anywhere along this course. Table 5.12 describes the anatomy of the three nerves, and pathologies that may cause lesions.

Table 5.12 Anatomy of three nerves causing lesions

Category of neuron	Anatomy	Examples of possible lesions
First neuron	Arises in the hypothalamus, and descends through the dorsolateral brain stem into the cervical cord Synapses at the T1 root ganglion either in the intermediomedial or in the intermediolateral cell column of the spinal cord	Hypothalamic, brain-stem or cervical cord space-occupying/structural lesions, including Haemorrhage Tumour Demyelination Oedema (eg secondary to ischaemic stroke or meningitis) Syringomyelia Trauma
Second neuron	Ascends from the T1 root ganglion across the lung apex before forming the cervical 'sympathetic chain' Eventually synapses in the superior cervical ganglion, found at the level of the bifurcation of the common carotid artery	Neck and chest pathologies that may impinge the T1 root ganglion, including Tumours: Pancoast's tumours, thyroid malignancies, etc Aortic aneurysms Cervical rib Lymphadenopathy Lower brachial plexus lesions (eg secondary to birth trauma) Trauma (eg thyroid or cardiothoracic surgery, central venous line insertion)
Third neuron	Straight after the superior cervical ganglion, the nerve gives off branches responsible for control of sweating and vascular tone within the face which join the external carotid artery The main nerve fibres continue along the path of the internal carotid artery and cavernous sinus before entering the orbit and innervating the pupil via the long ciliary nerves	Principally carotid artery disease, either Structural (eg dissection, fistula to cavernous sinus), or Functional (eg spasm secondary to migraine)

Certain other conditions can affect more than one neuron in the pathway, eg severe varicella-zoster.

Clinical features

The classic clinical features of Horner's syndrome are of unilateral partial ptosis (see Figure 5.7), miosis, pseudo-enophthlamos and (in certain cases) anhidrosis. One way of differentiating the site of the lesion in Horner's syndrome is by evaluating whether anhidrosis is present. Specifically, lesions that affect the first- and second-order neurons in the sympathetic pathway will cause anhidrosis (because the lesion occurs proximal to nerve branches responsible for sweating), whereas lesions in the third-order neuron in the pathway occur distal to those branches, so anhidrosis is not found.

In addition, there is a congenital form of Horner's syndrome featuring heterochromia of the irides, which is not found in other causes of the syndrome.

Investigation and management

This will depend on the clinical scenario. However, a basic work-up would include

- **Blood tests**
  - For example, thyroid function tests/ antibodies if there was suggestion of a thyroid mass, acetylcholine receptor antibodies in suspected myasthenia gravis, etc.
- **Imaging**
  - Chest radiograph: may demonstrate Pancoast's tumour, cervical rib or other relevant pathologies.
  - CT of the chest and neck: if there is the

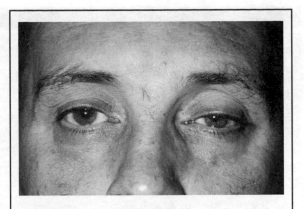

Figure 5.7 Horner's syndrome

suggestion of primary lung, aortic or thyroid pathology.
- MR brain/brain stem and neck: if there is the suspicion of a structural neurological lesion to explain a Horner's syndrome, eg brain-stem tumour.

Treatment will depend on the underlying aetiology.

Maintaining patient welfare

Patients may find it very distressing to have a condition that affects their vision and facial appearance, which may be irreversible. If Horner's syndrome occurs secondary to a generalised neurological condition (eg brain-stem MS) imminent neurodisability may require considerable physical, psychological and social support. The diagnosis must be explained carefully, with a sensitive but realistic overview of treatment options and prognosis.

SCENARIO 22. HYPOTHYROIDISM

1–2 minutes

Introduce yourself

Confirm the information you've been given and patient details: this 45-year-old woman has presented with lethargy and weight gain. Please assess her.

'What is the main problem from your point of view?' 'I am feeling increasingly tired, and have gained weight without any change in my diet or the amount of exercise I have done. I also feel cold the whole time.'

5 minutes

New condition

Focused history of the presenting complaint and relevant systems enquiry

Neurological: fatigue, low mood/depression, cognitive impairment, psychotic symptoms, hearing difficulties, change in voice

Gastrointestinal: unintentional weight gain, constipation

Metabolic: cold intolerance, menorrhagia

Other: generalised myalgia, neck lump (although goitre only found in particular cases of hypothyroidism, eg Hashimoto's thyroiditis)

Pre-existing conditions/risk factors: previous history of hyperthyroidism, previous radioiodine treatment and/or goitre surgery, and history of autoimmune disease

Social/occupational/family circumstances: impact on work, family history of thyroid disease

Drug history: also consider past treatments. Ask about drugs that may affect thyroid status, eg amiodarone, lithium. **DRUG ALLERGIES**

Other medical conditions: may be misdiagnosed as depression.

Begin a **targeted** examination of relevant area/system and continue while taking the history

General appearance: increased BMI, dry skin with erythema ab igne, nail changes (onycholysis, longitudinal ridging, etc)

Face: periorbital swelling, xanthelasma, thin and brittle hair

Neck: goitre; look for thyroidectomy scar

Cardiac: bradycardia, features of cardiac failure

Neurology: cerebellar syndrome, carpal tunnel syndrome, proximal muscle weakness, slow relaxing tendon reflexes, peripheral neuropathy (also consider coexisting explanations for any neuropathy, eg pernicious anaemia).

Finally: ask for blood pressure (often raised; may be postural drop in coexisting Addison's disease) and urine dipstick for glycosuria (association with diabetes mellitus)

1–2 minutes

CALLBACK: 'You said at the beginning that the main problems were tiredness, weight gain and feeling cold. Is there anything else troubling you that we haven't covered?'

RESPOND TO PATIENT'S CONCERNS (1–2 min)

1. I think the cause of your tiredness and weight gain is an underactive thyroid gland which is not producing enough of the hormone thyroxine
2. The best way to treat your symptoms is by replacing the thyroxine that is not being produced
3. Before starting treatment, we need to confirm the diagnosis by performing thyroid function tests as well as other blood tests (full blood count, autoantibodies) to exclude other possible causes of your symptoms

Thank the patient

Differential diagnosis	Clinical communication skills and managing patient concerns	Physical examination and identifying physical signs	Clinical judgement and maintaining patient welfare
Addison's disease	See Scenario 2. Addison's disease flowchart		
Sick euthyroid disease	See Scenario 17. Graves' disease flowchart		
Depression	The low mood that may be a feature of hypothyroidism can be confused with depression Other physical conditions with a probable psychological component (eg fibromyalgia, chronic fatigue syndrome, etc) may also present with symptoms overlapping with hypothyroidism		There should be a low threshold for checking TFTs before the diagnosis of depressive illness if there are any accompanying features of the condition

Clinical judgement and maintaining patient welfare

Hypothyroidism is a syndrome with multiorgan effects that result from a deficiency of thyroid hormones (thyroxine (T_4) and triiodothyronine (T_3)). There are a large number of different causes, as described in Table 5.13.

Investigations
- **Blood tests**: these include
  - Thyroid function tests: hypothyroidism is defined by a reduction in free plasma thyroxine levels. Thyroid-stimulating hormone (TSH) levels will be increased in primary hypothyroidism and reduced in secondary hypothyroidism. The presence

Table 5.13 Causes of hypothyroidism

Category	Causes	Specific examples
Primary hypothyroidism	Prior treatment for hyperthyroidism/thyroid masses	Previous radioiodine therapy Previous thyroid surgery Excess use of anti-thyroid medications (eg carbimazole)
	Iodine deficiency	Often from dietary deficiency – the most common cause of the condition worldwide
	Autoimmune disease	*Hashimoto's thyroiditis:* an autoimmune condition, particularly found in middle-aged and elderly women, associated with plasma cell and lymphocyte infiltration of the thyroid gland *Primary atrophic thyroiditis:* an autoimmune condition, particularly found in women, associated with diffuse lymphocytic infiltration of the thyroid gland
	Other causes	Congenital thyroid aplasia Infiltrative disease, eg malignancy, sarcoidosis, amyloidosis Other forms of thyroiditis, eg subacute, postpartum; such conditions are associated more with thyrotoxicosis, but also often cause transient hypothyroidism Drugs, eg amiodarone, lithium
Secondary hypothyroidism	Hypothyroidism secondary to hypothalamic and/or pituitary disease	Any cause of hypothalamic–pituitary disease, including Tumours Vascular lesions Infiltrative diseases (eg amyloidosis, sarcoidosis)

of normal T_4/T_3 with raised TSH is defined as *subclinical hypothyroidism.*

- Anti-thyroid antibodies: anti-thyroglobulin and anti-thyroid peroxidase (anti-TPO) antibodies are detectable in plasma in most patients with Hashimoto's thyroiditis or primary atrophic thyroiditis.
- The 9 am cortisol: this should be the very minimum assessment of adrenal status in cases of hypothyroidism. Addison's disease can cause the biochemical picture of hypothyroidism or exist as an additional autoimmune disease, either in isolation or as part of a polyglandular autoimmune syndrome.
- Full blood count: most typically macrocytic anaemia.
- Biochemistry: total cholesterol and triglycerides are often increased. Creatine kinase is also often raised.

- **Thyroid imaging**
  - An ultrasound scan may be useful to confirm the presence of a suspected goitre. It is also useful where infiltrative disease of the gland (eg malignancy) is suspected. However, thyroid imaging need not be done routinely.

Management

Any reversible cause should be treated, eg adjustment of drug regimen where the condition is attributable to medications. The mainstay of treatment is the replacement of thyroid hormone, usually with levothyroxine. Once started, a repeat clinical assessment and set of TFTs should occur at 6–8 weeks, and changes to dosing made as appropriate. Some complexities in treating hypothyroidism include

- In the case of suspected myxoedematous coma, patients will require very close monitoring with aggressive treatment of hypoglycaemia, hypothermia, electrolyte disturbances and any precipitating event (eg sepsis). Where there is a delay in obtaining results of TFTs and/or cortisol levels, intravenous hydrocortisone should be administered (adrenal insufficiency should always be corrected before correcting thyroid hormone deficiency). Thyroid hormone replacement may be via nasogastric tube or intravenously where required.
- Elderly patients are particularly sensitive to the effects of thyroid hormones, and should start with lower doses, eg levothyroxine 25 µg/day as a starting dose, rather than the typical 50 µg/day used in younger patients.
- Some specialists will use liothyronine alongside levothyroxine, at least initially, because there is some evidence that this more naturally mimics the physiological pattern of thyroid hormone release.
- There is still ongoing disagreement about which patients with subclinical hypothyroidism should receive treatment, but most specialists will treat patients with TSH levels >10 mU/L. Other risk factors for progression from subclinical to clinical disease include previous treatment for hyperthyroidism, and the presence of thyroid autoantibodies within serum.
- Pregnant patients with hypothyroidism may experience large increases in their thyroid hormone needs as the pregnancy progresses. TFTs should be checked at least once during every trimester.

Maintaining patient welfare

Patients may find it difficult to appreciate that the wide number of symptoms that they are experiencing may all stem from hypothyroidism. They should be counselled on the importance of compliance with thyroid hormone replacement.

SCENARIO 23. IMPETIGO

1–2 minutes

Introduce yourself

Confirm the information you've been given and patient details: this 16-year-old girl has presented to out-patients with a pustular rash on her face. Please assess her.

'What is the main problem from your point of view?' 'It started with a rash on my face which is now yellow and crusted.'

5 minutes

New condition

Focused history of the presenting complaint and relevant systems enquiry: differentiate from other blistering rashes (eg herpes simplex, acne, dermatophyte infections) and establish if primary or secondary to pre-existing conditions (eczema, psoriasis, scabies, or even herpes simplex infections)

Pre-existing conditions/risk factors: prior diagnosis of chronic skin disease; plus risk factors for soft-tissue infection in general, including diabetes mellitus, immunocompromise, etc

Social/occupational/family circumstances: exclude history of contagion from other family members. There is an increased risk of spread in those living in poor sanitary conditions

Drug history: treatments for other skin conditions. **DRUG ALLERGIES**

Other medical conditions: skin conditions as above

Begin a **targeted** examination of relevant area/system and continue while taking the history

Examination of the skin

Location

- Typically face or extremities, although severe infections can be widespread

Description

- Typically starts with a papular rash, and progresses to vesicles with surrounding erythema. Vesicles become pustular and rupture, leaving thick, 'golden-yellow', crusted exudates
- There are also recognised bullous forms of the disease, where bullae of 1–2 cm diameter may develop
- There is also a rare severe form of the condition called *ecthyma*, characterised by painful, pus-filled vesicopustular lesions that extend into the dermis. They may exude thick grey–yellow pus and cause local lymphadenopathy as they break down, leaving ulcers that produce scars as they heal

Additional examination

- Tell the examiner that you want to perform a urine dipstick and blood pressure measurement (glomerulonephritis is a complication of a *Streptococcus pyogenes* infection)

1–2 minutes

CALLBACK: 'You said at the beginning that the main problem was a yellow crusted rash on your face. Is there anything else troubling you that we haven't covered?'

RESPOND TO PATIENT'S CONCERNS (1–2 min)

1. I think your rash is an infection called impetigo which is caused by a bacterial infection of the skin
2. To treat this we need to remove the crusts with saline and apply a topical antibiotic (eg fusidic acid). If this does not settle the rash, then you will need oral antibiotics
3. The diagnosis is made on its appearance clinically, although we will also take a swab for culture. It is very important to have good hand hygiene to avoid this spreading to other people because this infection is contagious

Thank the patient

Differential diagnosis	Clinical communication skills and managing patient concerns	Physical examination and identifying physical signs	Clinical judgement and maintaining patient welfare
Herpes simplex infection	See Scenario 20. Herpes zoster differential diagnosis table		
Herpes zoster	See Scenario 20. Herpes zoster flowchart; vesicles may initially be confused between the two conditions		
Acne vulgaris/rosacea	See Scenario 12. Dermatomyositis differential diagnosis table.	This often includes a papulopustular rash as part of the disease syndrome	
Folliculitis Bacterial infection of hair follicles	Most associated with *Staphylococcus aureus* infections Risk factors include obesity and diabetes mellitus	Typically will present with a cluster of pustules and surrounding erythema found around an area densely populated by hair follicles In men, this may develop in the beard area (*sycosis barbae*), becoming particularly noticeable after shaving In severe cases, there may be the development of a *carbuncle* (an abscess deep to an area of hair follicles) or *furuncles* (boils – pustular, erythematous masses prone to rupture)	*Investigations* Diagnosed clinically, with swabs from affected sites aiding choice of antimicrobials *Management* Management involves minimising any precipitating factors (eg optimising diabetic control), and topical and oral antibiotics Carbuncles will require surgical drainage
Hidradenitis suppurativa A chronic suppurative disease that may progress to sinus and fistula formation	This typically first presents in patients in their 20s to 30s, with risk factors including diabetes, smoking and obesity	The condition starts with painful, pruritic erythematous nodules, typically in the axillae and groin Over time, lesions progress to large pustular nodules, and may heal with scar formation	*Investigations* Diagnosed clinically, with swabs from affected sites helping with the choice of antimicrobials CT or MR is indicated where sinus formation or fistulae are suspected *Management* Antibiotics are useful for treating infective pustules, with some patients with chronic disease requiring cyclical courses of antibiotics Surgical treatment of sinuses/fistulae is required in severe cases

(continued)

Differential diagnosis	Clinical communication skills and managing patient concerns	Physical examination and identifying physical signs	Clinical judgement and maintaining patient welfare
Dermatophyte infection Fungal infection of the skin		Tinea corporis (ie superficial fungal infection of the skin) typically gives plaques with overlying scale and surrounding erythema. However, lesions may also develop vesicles which may pustulate, especially on areas densely covered with hair	*Investigations* Usually diagnosed clinically, although skin scrapings and mycological culture may be useful Viewing the lesions under Wood's lamp may also be useful in cases of diagnostic doubt *Management* Most cases respond to general measures (eg keeping the site dry) and topical treatments, eg clotrimazole In more severe cases, systemic antifungal treatment (eg terbinafine) may be appropriate
Perioral dermatitis Eczematous involvement in the perioral region		This will usually start as a maculopapular rash in the perioral region. From here, may progress to vesicular lesions which may pustulate	Treatment is that of eczema in general (see Scenario 14. Eczema flowchart).

Clinical judgement and maintaining patient welfare

Impetigo is a form of bacterial skin infection that is particularly found in young children. It may occur either in previously normal skin or in skin with existing disease (eg eczema, psoriasis). The most common offending organism is *Staphylococcus aureus,* with β-haemolytic streptococci being the other class of bacteria commonly associated with the condition. The condition is contagious, spread by close contact and/or poor sanitary conditions (eg children at nursery school). Other risk factors for the condition include those for soft-tissue infection in general, eg diabetes mellitus.

Investigation and management
The condition is diagnosed clinically, with typical features as described in the flowchart. A swab from the affected site may be useful in guiding antimicrobial therapy.

General measures in management include reducing the risk of transmission (normally by improving hygiene, eg hand washing) and through saline washes of affected areas to remove crusts. Treatment is with topical antibiotics with cover for *Staphylococcus aureus* and β-haemolytic streptococci, eg fusidic acid. In the case of lesions not responding to topical antibiotics and/or severe cases, oral antibiotics (eg flucloxacillin, clindamycin) may be used.

Maintaining patient welfare
The contagious nature of the condition should be explained, including practical steps (particularly improved hand washing) to minimise transmission.

SCENARIO 24. MARFAN SYNDROME

Introduce yourself

1–2 minutes

Confirm the information you've been given: this 28-year-old man has had a spontaneous pneumothorax on the left side on two occasions in the past year. He has had mild asthma since he was a teenager. Please assess him.

'What is the main problem from your point of view?' 'I'm fine at the moment but when the lung collapsed the second time it was really alarming. I was very short of breath. I thought I was having a severe asthma attack which is strange because I've barely needed my inhalers for the past 5 years.'

5 minutes

New condition

Focused history of the presenting complaint and relevant systems enquiry: when were the pneumothoraces, how large were they and what treatment was given?

Screen for other complications of Marfan syndrome, ie lens dislocation, retinal detachment, heart murmurs, abdominal hernias. **Family history** of pneumothorax/joint hypermobility/sudden death aged <50 years or other complications of Marfan syndrome (remember that inheritance is *autosomal dominant*)

Alarm symptoms: syncope, chest pain (aortic root dilatation/dissection)

Investigations/treatments so far: eg video-assisted thoracoscopy

Pre-existing conditions, eg mitral valve prolapse

Drug history, eg inhalers for asthma. **DRUG ALLERGIES**

Social/occupational/family circumstances and impact, eg diving, work at altitude

Other medical conditions: asthma

Begin a **targeted** examination of relevant area/system and continue while taking the history

Expose upper body and inspect

Dolichostenomelia, ie arm span exceeding height

Joint hypermobility

Kyphoscoliosis

Arachnodactyly: Steinberg and Walker–Murdoch signs

Stretch marks over skin, abdominal hernia

Pes planus

Chest

Pectus carinatum or excavatum

Scars from previous chest drains

Listen to lung bases to exclude wheeze

Percuss to exclude current small pneumothorax/partial reinflation

Mouth

High-arched palate, crowding of teeth, retrognathism

Eyes

Ectopia lentis: lens displaced upwards

Iridodonesis, ie tremor of the iris

Other eye signs, ie retinal detachment, heterochromia of the irides, blue discoloration of the sclera

Cardiovascular

Auscultate for mitral valve prolapse and aortic regurgitation

CALLBACK: 'You said at the beginning that the main problem was the lung collapse which gave you quite a shock. Is there anything else troubling you that we haven't covered?'

1–2 minutes

RESPOND TO PATIENT'S CONCERNS (1–2 min)

1. Spontaneous lung collapse is often seen in tall young men but you have some other features of an inherited condition that makes lung collapse more likely. You may have noticed these, for example . . .
2. We can prevent a further collapse by a procedure called pleurodesis. This is similar to the chest drains you've had before but also helps the surface of the lung to stick to the ribcage to stop it collapsing again
3. We will need to do some further tests to exclude problems elsewhere that might trouble you in the future. This includes a scan of the heart and a more detailed examination of the eyes. In many cases these are normal

Thank the patient

Differential diagnosis	Clinical communication skills and managing patient concerns	Physical examination and identifying physical signs	Clinical judgement and maintaining patient welfare
Homocystinuria An autosomal recessive inborn error of amino acid metabolism caused through deficiency of the enzyme cystathionine β-synthase	There may be a history of developmental delay and/or learning difficulties, epilepsy and/or psychiatric illness	The skeletal and ocular features are similar to those of Marfan syndrome, although lens displacement is *downwards* in homocystinuria and *upwards* in Marfan syndrome Structural heart disease is found very rarely in homocystinuria Features present in homocystinuria but **not** typically in Marfan syndrome include: Thromboembolic disease and accelerated atherosclerosis Learning disability and psychiatric disease Seizures Osteoporosis Livedo reticularis	*Investigations* Elevated levels of homocystine in blood or urine (positive cyanide–nitroprusside tests) Reduced levels of cystathionine β-synthase activity on biopsy from tissues of affected patients *Management* High-dose pyridoxine (vitamin B₆), although <50% of patients respond Low-protein diet Betaine (*N,N,N*-trimethylglycine); this converts homocysteine to methionine (which gradually becomes incorporated into protein) Folic acid supplements
MASS phenotype (mitral value prolapse, **a**ortic dilatation, **s**triae atrophica, **s**keletal abnormalities) An autosomal dominant disorder associated with mutations to the *FBN1* gene, with particular features overlapping with Marfan syndrome	Similar presentation to Marfan's disease (often referred for assessment due to body habitus).	Certain features are very similar to those found in Marfan syndrome, including mitral valve prolapse and skeletal abnormalities (scoliosis, chest wall deformities, etc) Key differences between MASS and Marfan syndrome include: The aortic root diameter may be at the upper range of normal in MASS, but does not progress to further dilatation/aneurysms No eye disease in MASS	Diagnosed through genetic analysis and clinical features Management of specific features as per Marfan syndrome
Loeys–Dietz syndrome An autosomal dominant condition related to *TGFBR1* or *TGFBR2* mutations	Usually present in childhood with skeletal abnormalities	This is one example of a large number of familial syndromes associated with a propensity to aortic aneurysm and dissection The syndrome has a very variable phenotype. May have aortic disease very similar to that with Marfan syndrome, but usually lacking the skeletal and ocular features Distinctive clinical features include: Hypertelorism (widely spaced eyes) Cleft palate Premature fusion of the skull	Diagnosed through genetic analysis and clinical features Management of specific features as per Marfan syndrome

Clinical judgement and maintaining patient welfare

Marfan syndrome is an autosomally dominant inherited disorder associated with mutations in the fibrillin-1 (*FBN1*) gene. A quarter of affected patients have no family history, suggesting that these patients have developed the condition through a novel mutation.

Clinical features

As described in the flowchart, Marfan syndrome affects the connective tissue and a large number of organs, although the exact phenotype found is highly variable between individuals. Candidates will be expected to clearly identify connective tissue features of the syndrome (see Figure 5.8); this will include knowledge of the signs that help demonstrate arachnodactyly, including

- *Steinberg's (thumb) sign*: where the thumb protrudes beyond the ulnar border of the hand when held in the clenched palm
- *Walker–Murdoch (wrist) sign*: where the thumb and little finger overlap when wrapped around the wrist of the opposite hand.

The major cause of morbidity and mortality in the syndrome is associated aortic root disease;

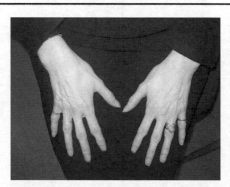
Arachnodactly

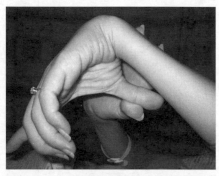
Joint hypermobility

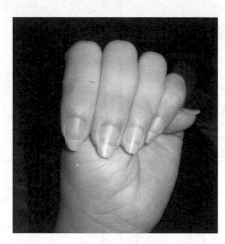
Steinberg's sign

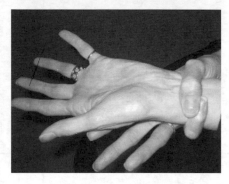
Walker–Murdoch sign

Figure 5.8 Marfan syndrome

the aortic root is prone to dilatation and eventual aortic regurgitation. Over time, patients may also develop aortic root aneurysm and dissection. Patients are also at risk of developing mitral valve disease, particularly mitral valve prolapse.

There are a number of different disorders with features overlapping those of Marfan syndrome, making diagnosis difficult. The diagnosis of Marfan's syndrome is made through the use of a set of diagnostic criteria called the *revised Ghent criteria* (see Resources). These use a combination of clinical features, whether the patient has a family history and the presence of *FBN1* mutations to differentiate Marfan syndrome from other conditions that may mimic it. Note that *FBN1* mutations alone **do not** make the diagnosis. Joint hypermobility may also be assessed using the Beighton 9-point hypermobility scoring scale.

Investigations and management
In addition to those outlined above

- **Cardiac**
  - All patients with Marfan syndrome should undergo regular echocardiograms as surveillance for aortic root disease, because most patients will eventually develop aortic dilatation.
  - There is evidence that lifelong β blockade for patients with Marfan syndrome improves the elasticity of the aorta and slows aortic dilatation.
  - Patients should be advised to limit their levels of physical activity to reduce the risk of dissection.
  - Many centres will arrange elective aortic root replacement when the diameter is wider than 50 mm, or even less if dilatation is occurring at >5 mm/year or there is a family history of dissection.
- **Respiratory**

- Patients with chest wall deformity may develop restrictive lung disease, which may be amenable to surgery.
  - Patients with recurrent pneumothoraces may require pleurodesis.
- **Eye**
  - All patients should be under regular ophthalmological follow-up.
- **Connective tissue**
  - Back pain in patients with Marfan's syndrome may be associated with dural ectasia, diagnosed by MRI.

Maintaining patient welfare
- As for any inherited disease, it is important to be aware of the role of genetic screening and counselling, and the contribution that this may have in particular if a patient with Marfan syndrome hopes to have children.
- Patients with Marfan syndrome in the MRCP (PACES) examination often report chest pain or dyspnoea, and it will be important to thoroughly assess them for cardiac and respiratory disease. This may include a careful explanation of the consequences of aortic root disease.
- Patients with cardiac and eye complications from Marfan's disease may have to discuss this with the DVLA, and may no longer be able to drive.
- There are a number of support groups, including the Marfan Association UK.

Resources
Loeys BL, Dietz HC, Braverman AC, et al. The revised Ghent nosology for the Marfan syndrome. *J Med Genet* 2010;47:476–85.
Marfan Association UK: www.marfan-association.org.uk

SCENARIO 25. OSTEOGENESIS IMPERFECTA

1–2 minutes

Introduce yourself

Confirm the information you've been given: this 34-year-old woman has some discoloration of the eyes which is concerning her. Please assess her.

'What is the main problem from your point of view?' 'The optometrist noticed a smudge on my eyes when I went for an eye test and suggested I see my doctor. She then referred me on to you because she thought it might be related to the fractures I had as a teenager.'

5 minutes

New condition

Focused history of the presenting complaint and relevant systems enquiry: what was the frequency, cause (usually low impact) and location of fractures? Assess for a personal and family history of fractures, hearing loss, short stature, hypermobility and/or cardiac disease

Identify alarm symptoms: syncope, chest pain, dyspnoea (may imply aortic incompetence)

Pre-existing conditions: may have required specialised walking aids in childhood

Current therapy, eg analgesia, NSAIDS and side effects. Any history of previous steroid use?

Impact of new symptoms on daily activities, eg pain of previous fractures, specialised aids for activities of daily living?

Other medical conditions: may have been diagnosed as a child with non-accidental injury, rickets or osteomalacia

Begin a **targeted** examination of relevant area/system and continue while taking the history

Face

Blue sclerae

Dentinogenesis imperfecta (discoloured, translucent teeth)

Hearing aids (reflecting involvement of middle ear bones)

Locomotor

Evidence of multiple previous fractures (may be in a wheelchair, have walking aids nearby or have obvious scars)

Bowing of the long bones

Scoliosis of the spine

Joint hypermobility (eg the ability to oppose the thumb to the ipsilateral forearm by wrist flexion)

Pectus carinatum

Skin

Skin hyperlaxity

Cardiac

Some association with aortic regurgitation

CALLBACK: 'You said at the beginning that the main problem was with your eyes which may have been related to fractures in the past. Is there anything else troubling you that we haven't covered?'

1–2 minutes

RESPOND TO PATIENT'S CONCERNS (1–2 min)

1. I think the issue with your eyes and the fractures you had as child could be connected and may be due to a genetic condition called osteogenesis imperfecta
2. The blue coloration of your eyes is part of the condition and, although there is no specific need to treat this, we can prevent further fractures with medications that increase your bone strength
3. We will need to do some further tests to confirm the diagnosis including a simple radiograph of your bones and a scan to measure their thickness. This is an inherited disorder and there are implications for your (future) children that we need to discuss further if the diagnosis is confirmed

Thank the patient

Differential diagnosis	Clinical communication skills and managing patient concerns	Physical examination and identifying physical signs	Clinical judgement and maintaining patient welfare
Blue sclera			
Marfan syndrome	See Scenario 24. Marfan syndrome flowchart		
Ehlers–Danlos syndrome A group of inherited conditions of the connective tissue associated with defective collagen synthesis	This should be considered wherever there is a family history of multisystem disease, particularly including the soft tissues and skeletal systems	Affected systems include: Skin: fragile, hyperextensible, with large haematomas and 'cigarette-paper' scars at sites of previous injury Connective tissue: hyperextensible joints, epicanthal folds, widely spaced eyes, pes planus Eyes: blue sclera, retinal disease Cardiac: mitral valve prolapse or regurgitation, aortic regurgitation, propensity to aortic aneurysm formation Respiratory: spontaneous pneumothorax GI tract: propensity to GI haemorrhage	*Investigations* Genetic analysis Skin biopsy: diagnosis may be made by analysing collagen activity from cultured skin fibroblasts *Management* Supportive, minimising complications Genetic counselling
Pseudoxanthoma elasticum An inherited condition associated with mutations in the *ABCC6* gene, causing defective calcification of elastic tissues		Affected systems include: Skin: folds of excessive skin, especially in flexural areas and the neck, covered in coalescing yellow–orange papules ('pseudo-xanthomatous plaques'). Skin has a 'plucked chicken'-like appearance Eyes: blue sclera, *angioid streaks* (ie red–brown lines extending from the optic disc, representing breakdown of the elastic fibres around Bruch's membrane) Cardiac: accelerated atherosclerosis, propensity to aneurysm formation, mitral valve prolapse or regurgitation, aortic regurgitation GI tract: propensity to GI haemorrhage	*Investigations* Histology of skin lesions: these will show pseudo-xanthomatous lesions *Management* Supportive, minimising complications Genetic counselling

(continued)

Differential diagnosis	Clinical communication skills and managing patient concerns	Physical examination and identifying physical signs	Clinical judgement and maintaining patient welfare
Hypophosphatasia A rare genetic disorder associated with defective/absent alkaline phosphatase		Multiple connective tissue and musculoskeletal complications, including craniosynostosis, scoliosis and frequent fractures	Diagnosed through finding low serum alkaline phosphatase May be appropriate to limit calcium and vitamin D intake
Alkaptonuria A rare autosomal recessive disorder associated with defective tyrosine metabolism		Blue sclera, ankylosis	Diagnosed through discoloration of urine to black when left exposed Treated through dietary restriction of tyrosine
Frequent fractures			
Osteoporosis A condition of reduced bone mineral density and defective microarchitecture with increased propensity to fracture	The condition is essentially asymptomatic until a fracture occurs. It should particularly be considered in any case of apparent pathological fracture Wherever the condition is suspected, candidates should enquire about risk factors, including: Age Endocrine: female sex (especially if prolonged amenorrhoea or early menopause), hyperparathyroidism, hyperthyroidism, steroid excess (either Cushing syndrome or prolonged use of exogenous steroids), hypogonadism GI: malabsorption Haematological: myeloma Autoimmune: rheumatoid arthritis and primary biliary cirrhosis	Kyphosis Signs of previous hip/pelvic surgery	*Investigations* Blood tests: typically normal bone profile, although often find a rise in ALP after recent fractures DXA scanning: will help distinguish osteoporosis from osteopenia and other metabolic bone disorders *Management* General: treatment of any risk factor, calcium and vitamin D supplementation, exercise, reduction in smoking Pharmacological: bisphosphonates, strontium ranelate, raloxifene, teriparatide (ie recombinant parathyroid hormone) and calcitonin. Hormone replacement therapy still also has a limited role Surgical: treatment of fractures

(continued)

Differential diagnosis	Clinical communication skills and managing patient concerns	Physical examination and identifying physical signs	Clinical judgement and maintaining patient welfare
Osteomalacia and rickets A condition characterised by normal bone density but defective mineralisation Note that strictly speaking, *rickets* refers to skeletal deformities that occur because of defective bone mineralisation in childhood before growth plate fusion, whereas *osteomalacia* refers to ongoing defective mineralisation after the growth plates have fused	Initial symptoms may be non-specific, including generalised pain and weakness The condition particularly occurs in association with reduced vitamin D stores. Where suspected, candidates should enquire about risk factors for vitamin D deficiency, including: Reduced vitamin D intake (lack of sunlight, poor diet) Malabsorption (eg coeliac disease) Defective vitamin D metabolism (eg chronic kidney or liver disease) Vitamin D resistance (eg vitamin D-resistant rickets)	Clinical features may include: Kyphosis Proximal myopathy A 'waddling' gait Skeletal deformities: may include frontal bossing of the skull and bowing of the long bones	*Investigations* Blood tests: typically show low calcium and phosphate, with raised ALP. Vitamin D levels will also be low Radiographs: these will show *Looser's zones*, thin radiolucent lines with sclerotic borders. They are particularly found in the upper femur *Management* Reversal of any risk factor Supplementation of calcium, phosphate and vitamin D
Hypophosphatasia	See above		
Non-accidental injury			

Clinical judgement and maintaining patient welfare

Osteogenesis imperfecta is a rare inherited connective tissue disorder, usually caused through mutations in genes associated with type 1 collagen. The clinical features of the disease vary widely between different patients.

Investigations and diagnosis

The diagnosis may be made clinically based on characteristic clinical features, especially if a family history is present. Genetic tests to identify mutations are available in specialist centres only. DXA scanning will help to confirm or rule out coexisting osteoporosis.

Management

- **Physical therapies**
  - Physiotherapy, orthotics, occupational therapy and exercise classes may help the patient adapt to disability and minimise further fractures.
- **Pharmacotherapy**
  - Calcium and vitamin D supplements to optimise bone mineralisation.
  - Bisphosphonates: cyclical intravenous bisphosphonates have been shown to increase osteoblast activity, allowing cortical thickening and minimising fracture risk.
- **Surgical**
  - Orthopaedic intervention for fractures.

Maintaining patient welfare

- There have been incidences both where osteogeneis imperfecta has been misdiagnosed as non-accidental injury and vice versa, which has caused considerable distress to both patients and their families. Great caution should be taken in distinguishing the two conditions before making a diagnosis.
- Patients need education in the nature of the condition and practical measures that they may take to minimise further fractures. This is not only pharmacotherapy – candidates will be expected to recognise the role of physiotherapy and occupational therapy, and that patients may be entitled to disability allowances. Patients may benefit from input from support groups, such as the UK Brittle Bone Society (see below).
- Candidates will be expected to acknowledge the important role that genetic counsellors may play in patients who wish to have children.

Resources

Brittle Bone Society: www.brittlebone.org

SCENARIO 26. PAGET'S DISEASE

Introduce yourself

Confirm the information you've been given: this 68-year-old man has been experiencing pain in his right leg. His alkaline phosphatase is raised at 530 U/L. Please assess him.

'What is the main problem from your point of view?' 'For a few months I've been getting stabbing pains in my right thigh. Before the pain started, my wife noticed that I was starting to walk with a slight limp. My family doctor did some blood tests and said one of the bony markers was abnormal and so referred me to you.'

New condition

Focused history of the presenting complaint and relevant systems enquiry: differentiate between referred knee or hip pain due to arthritis (occurs secondary to the associated deformity), and the intrinsic bony pain of Paget's disease. Has there been painless bowing of the leg, fractures with minimal trauma, unexplained hearing loss and/or an increase in hat size?

Alarm symptoms: leg swelling and dyspnoea (high-output cardiac failure), sensorimotor symptoms and/or sphincter disturbance (cord compression, spinal stenosis), hearing loss (base of skull disease)

Relevant family history: one in five patients with Paget's disease will have a family history of the condition

Degree of physical impairment/immobility and additional impact of new symptoms: is the current level of care adequate?

Current therapy, eg NSAIDs, analgesia. Is the patient on bisphosphonates already?

Pre-existing conditions predisposing to vitamin D deficiency (risk of hypocalcaemia with bisphosphonate therapy)

Begin a **targeted** examination of relevant area/system and continue while taking the history

Locomotor

- **Examine for deformities**
    - Bowing of the tibia and/or femur
    - Kyphosis
    - Facial deformity: frontal bossing, enlarged maxilla, etc
    - Although bony pain is a feature of Paget's disease, bony tenderness is less common. However, the affected limb may be warmer to the touch, reflecting increased bone turnover and the increased vascular supply
- Assess range of movement and gait; deformity may lead to osteoarthritis of associated joints
- Look for scars from pathological fractures that may have required surgery
- Look for tophi (gout associated with Paget's disease due to higher bone turnover and urate production)

Neurological

- Assess hearing for sensorineural deficit; look for hearing aids
- Exclude proximal myopathy (osteomalacia also presents with bony pain and raised alkaline phosphatase)
- Assess plantar reflexes (cord compression, spinal stenosis)

Cardiovascular

- Signs of congestive (high-output) cardiac failure – although very rare

CALLBACK: 'You said at the beginning that the main problem was the pain in your right leg. Is there anything else troubling you that we haven't covered?'

RESPOND TO PATIENT'S CONCERNS (1–2 min)

1. It does appear that there are changes in the shape of your femur bone that may be associated with a condition called Paget's disease. This can also affect the wear and tear of joints
2. We can address the immediate issue of controlling your pain with effective analgesia. Paget's disease is normally very treatable and we should be able to get the pain under control swiftly
3. We will need to do some radiographs (of the skull, pelvis and long bones) and a blood test to confirm the underlying cause. I'll also need to measure your calcium and vitamin D levels, because low levels can cause similar symptoms

Thank the patient

Differential diagnosis	Clinical communication skills and managing patient concerns	Physical examination and identifying physical signs	Clinical judgement and maintaining patient welfare
Osteomalacia and rickets	See main text, and differential diagnosis table for Scenario 25. Osteogenesis imperfecta.		
Bone metastases	Breast, prostate, lung, renal and thyroid malignancies are the most likely to metastasise to bone Constant pain (particularly at night) and pathological fractures in the context of malignancy should raise suspicion of the condition Other presentations may include Symptomatic hypercalcaemia (eg malaise, constipation, change in mood, pain from renal calculi) Marrow failure from bone metastases (eg lethargy of anaemia, easy bruising from thrombocytopenia) Any associated history of lower limb weakness and change in bladder and bowel function should immediately raise suspicion of cord syndromes	Examination may reveal focal bony tenderness. Bony deformity is unusual unless gross metastases Spinal cord compression will generate upper motor neuron signs below the lesion, whereas cauda equina syndrome presents with lower motor neuron deficits below the lesion. Acute changes in bladder or bowel function and/or loss of anal tone may be found in spinal cord syndromes	*Investigations* Blood tests: may show hypercalcaemia, and cytopenias if bone marrow involvement. Tumour markers (eg PSA) may be of use Imaging: plain radiographs may demonstrate metastatic lesions (generally lytic, although prostatic metastasis is often sclerotic). Bone scintigraphy will demonstrate increased uptake of radioisotope, with results similar to Paget's disease. MR and CT are also useful for identifying metastases and confirming the site of the primary tumour Biopsy: bone biopsy only very rarely indicated, if no tissue from a primary tumour can be obtained *Management* General measures: intravenous fluids and bisphosphonates are needed to treat hypercalcaemia, with the latter also helping to reduce bone pain Radiotherapy is useful for treating the pain of bone metastasis; chemotherapy may also be appropriate In the case of malignant cord syndromes, surgical decompression is the definitive management. Corticosteroids may be used as an adjunct to reduce swelling from cord compression

(continued)

Differential diagnosis	Clinical communication skills and managing patient concerns	Physical examination and identifying physical signs	Clinical judgement and maintaining patient welfare
Renal osteodystrophy	This is a common complication of chronic kidney disease (CKD). The term encompasses all the different forms of bone disease found in CKD, including hyperparathyroidism, osteomalacia, osteosclerosis and osteoporosis The condition is usually asymptomatic, but may present with bony pain, bone deformity and fractures, and thus may be confused with Paget's disease	Distal reabsorption of phalanges may occur in severe untreated cases Evidence of scars from previous surgery may be found on examination	*Investigations* Blood tests: the typical blood profile of untreated secondary/tertiary hyperparathyroidism occurring in renal disease is low plasma calcium, raised plasma phosphate, raised ALP, elevated parathyroid hormone and low vitamin D levels Imaging: this depends on the form of bone disease present; osteosclerosis of the skull and spine may be confused with Paget's disease *Management* Reduction in dietary phosphate and phosphate binders (eg calcium acetate) will reduce plasma phosphate levels. Activated vitamin D analogues (eg alfacalcidol) will help to reduce hyperparathyroidism Cinacalcet binds the calcium receptor on the parathyroid gland and also helps to reduce hyperparathyroidism. Parathyroidectomy may also be considered in severe disease
Fibrous dysplasia A condition in which normal bone is replaced by fibrous tissue	The condition is often asymptomatic and discovered incidentally, but presenting symptoms may include bony pain, bone deformity (sometime very marked) and increased fractures Night or rest pain may suggest development of a tumour in the bone	The condition particularly affects the skull, pelvis and long bones. Bowing of the legs may occur, causing gait abnormalities The combination of precocious puberty (or thyroid, parathyroid or pituitary hormone excess), skin pigmentation (café-au-lait patches) and multiple bony deformities from fibrous dysplasia is suggestive of McCune–Albright syndrome	*Investigations* The condition may be diagnosed clinically or found incidentally on imaging. MRI is the best imaging modality for demonstrating the changes If McCune–Albright syndrome is suspected, a full endocrine screen should be undertaken *Management* General measures: analgesia and physiotherapy Pharmacological: bisphosphonates have been shown to strengthen the medullary bone that is being replaced by fibrous tissue

Clinical judgement and maintaining patient welfare

Paget's disease has a high incidence in Britain and in countries with migrant Britain ancestry (including Australia and New Zealand). This probably reflects a genetic component to the condition, with a fifth of patients with Paget's disease having an affected first-degree relative. There are also environmental triggers, with epidemiological studies identifying an association with paramyxovirus. The incidence has fallen significantly over the past 20 years for reasons that are unclear.

The pathogenesis involves an increase in the activity of osteoclasts, followed by a compensatory increase in osteoblastic bone deposition. This results in a greatly increased rate of bone turnover and remodelling, but the bone that is formed is abnormal in structure and function. Over time, this leads to the generation of deformed, enlarged, weakened bones.

Clinical features

These are as described in the flowchart. It should be noted that the condition may be asymptomatic, with the diagnosis made only because of abnormal investigations initiated for other reasons. Candidates should also have an awareness of complications, particularly osteosarcoma, although this is a rare complication in around 1% of patients who have the condition for >10 years. This should be suspected if patients develop worsening focal bony pain despite optimal treatment.

Investigations

- **Blood tests**
  - Calcium and phosphate levels are usually normal. Alkaline phosphatase is often raised several-fold above the usual upper range of normal and is the most useful marker of disease activity. However, a normal value does not exclude the diagnosis.
  - Vitamin D levels should always be

requested; this helps differentiate the disease from osteomalacia, another condition that may present with bone pain and raised alkaline phosphatase.

- **Imaging**
  - This is usually a combination of radiographs and bone scintigraphy. The pelvis, long bones and skull are those most likely to demonstrate lesions. Classic radiological features of Paget's disease include
    - *Osteoporosis circumscripta* (ie osteolytic lesions) in the occipital bones of the skull
    - 'Cotton-wool' sign: mixed sclerotic areas and osteolytic areas in the skull
    - 'Brim sign': a thickened iliopectineal line in the pelvis
    - V-shaped border between healthy and pagetic bone in the long bones.
  - CT and/or MRI are indicated where osteosarcoma is suspected.

Management

- **General measures**
  - Physiotherapy and occupational therapy to aid mobility and allow the patient to try to retain a normal level of daily function.
- **Pharmacological**
  - Analgesia: NSAIDs are usually the first treatment administered.
  - Bisphosphonates: these dramatically inhibit osteoclast activity. They should always be given with calcium and vitamin D supplements to minimise the risk of hypocalcaemia. Although bisphosphonates were conventionally given only in symptomatic disease, there is now evidence that treatment of asymptomatic base-of-skull disease may avert irreversible deafness, and may reduce the risk of secondary arthritis where the disease involves joint surfaces. The efficacy of treatment is measured by the alkaline phosphatase level and the relief of symptoms. Bisphosphonates may be administered either intravenously or

orally. Gastrointestinal symptoms (especially oesophagitis and heartburn) are common side effects of oral bisphosphonates; patients should be instructed to take tablets in an upright position (not before bed) with plenty of water. A PPI may be necessary to alleviate symptoms.

Maintaining patient welfare

- The pain, deformity, fractures and impaired mobility resulting from the disease may have a profound effect on the patient's ability to undertake normal daily activities. Candidates should show an appreciation of the role that physiotherapy and occupational therapy may potentially play in allowing the patient to maintain his or her normal routine, and understand that patients with associated disability may be eligible for disability benefit.
- Paget's disease is an unusual disorder that few affected patients will have heard of before diagnosis. The potential effects that the condition may have on a patient's physical function may be very marked. As such, patients may benefit from input from a support group, such as the Paget's Association in the UK (see below).

Resources

Paget's Association: www.paget.org.uk

SCENARIO 27. PAPILLOEDEMA

1–2 minutes

Introduce yourself

Confirm the information you've been given and patient details: this 38-year-old woman has presented with headaches and blurred vision. Please assess her.

'What is the main problem from your point of view?' 'I am having increasing headaches for the last few weeks, especially in the morning, with blurred vision on and off.'

5 minutes

New condition

Focused history of the presenting complaint and relevant systems enquiry: identify symptoms with high discriminant value for raised intracranial pressure (ie severe morning headache and nausea, double vision, vomiting, altered consciousness), as opposed to chronic intermittent headache syndromes (ie nausea and neurological symptoms that are intermittent and resolve fully between episodes)

Identify alarm symptoms: diplopia on outward gaze (implies nerve VI palsy – risk of subtentorial herniation)

Pre-existing conditions/risk factors: past meningitis or subarachnoid haemorrhage, haematological disorders, etc

Social/occupational/family circumstances: ask about housing (gas heaters and carbon monoxide poisoning) and occupation (lead poisoning)

Drug history: antihypertensives, recent steroids, and use of medications associated with idiopathic intracranial hypertension (eg oral contraceptive pill). **DRUG ALLERGIES**

Other medical conditions, eg hypertension that has been difficult to treat

Begin a **targeted** examination of relevant area/system and continue while taking the history

General appearance, eg thyroid eye signs (Graves' disease

Examination of the eye

Visual acuity: usually normal, but may be decreased

Fields: increased size of blind spot, concentric field loss ('tunnel vision') if severe

Pupils: may be altered depending on condition

Movement raised ICP may result in cranial neuropathies, eg of cranial nerve VI

Fundoscopy: in papilloedema, stages are

- Stage I: increase in venous calibre/venous engorgement, increase in venous tortuosity with loss of venous pulsation
- Stage II: optic disc less distinct
- Stage III: blurred disc on nasal side (reflects oedema of the nerve fibre layer)
- Stage IV: whole disc unclear and elevated, multiple flame-shaped haemorrhages and cotton-wool spots throughout. The optic nerve head appears swollen (See Figure in Neurological exam)

Extras: ask for blood pressure and urine dipstick (for accelerated hypertension)

CALLBACK: 'You said at the beginning that the main problem was headaches and blurred vision. Is there anything else troubling you that we haven't covered?'

1–2 minutes

RESPOND TO PATIENT'S CONCERNS (1–2 min)

1. I think that your symptoms of headaches and blurred vision are related and may be caused by raised pressure within the skull. Your blurred vision is caused by swelling of the optic nerve head at the back of the eye. This is called papilloedema

2. For your headaches I can give you some painkillers to help you feel better, but it is very important that we find the cause of the raised intracranial pressure

3. You need to be investigated urgently, with a combination of blood tests (eg FBC, coagulation, TFTs), scans of your head (CT scan or MRI) and further investigations depending on these initial results

Thank the patient

Differential diagnosis	Clinical communication skills and managing patient concerns	Physical examination and identifying physical signs	Clinical judgement and maintaining patient welfare
Hypertensive retinopathy	See Scenario 13. Diabetic retinopathy differential diagnosis table		
Papillitis, ie neuritis of the portion of the optic nerve within the orbit	There are a number of different causes, including demyelination, infection (eg toxoplasmosis) and inflammatory diseases (eg vasculitis); clues to these may be present within the history Papillitis should particularly be considered wherever eye movements are painful	This may commonly be confused with papilloedema. Means by which the two may be differentiated include: Papillitis is unilateral, whereas papilloedema is usually bilateral Papillitis is associated with painful eye movements, but this is not found in papilloedema Papillitis is usually associated with an early impairment in visual acuity, but this is only a late finding in papilloedema Papillitis is often associated with disruption of the normal papillary response to light, but this is not found in papilloedema Papillitis may progress over time to optic atrophy, appearances of which may also mimic papilloedema	Diagnosed via clinical findings and fundoscopic appearances Treatment is of the precipitating condition
Congenital disc disease, ie any of a number of congenital disc diseases that may give fundoscopic appearances similar to papilloedema ('pseudo-papilloedema')	These should be considered whenever there is papilloedema and a family history of eye disease	Features that may be seen on fundoscopy to help differentiate these conditions from papilloedema include: *Drusen:* these are yellow–white covered bodies composed of lipid and protein. Although they are most closely associated with age-related macular degeneration, there are also recognised genetic syndromes in which drusen may be deposited at a young age in areas including the disc edges, giving the appearance of papilloedema *Myelinated retinal nerve fibres:* these appear fundoscopically as white, streaky lesions. They may be distributed near to the edge of the optic disc, causing it to blur and making it difficult to distinguish from papilloedema	No treatment necessary Genetic counselling may be appropriate

Clinical judgement and maintaining patient welfare

The term 'papilloedema' describes swelling of the optic disc occurring secondary to raised intracranial pressure (ICP). It may be unilateral or bilateral depending on the underlying aetiology. The causes of papilloedema include those shown in Table 5.14.

Clinical features
Raised ICP may be asymptomatic until late in its course. However, associated symptoms include

- Headache: typically worse in the mornings/ when lying down, and associated with nausea and vomiting
- Visual defects: patients with chronic papilloedema may develop limitation in visual fields, an enlarged blind spot and – in the late phase – loss of visual acuity.

Papilloedema itself is a fundoscopic diagnosis see Station 3, Scenario 17, Figure 3.8(c). It is often divided into four different stages, as described in the flowchart. Papilloedema may be associated with other clinical findings, eg abducens nerve palsy (either unilaterally or bilaterally)

Table 5.14 Causes of papilloedema

Category	Causes
Intracranial space-occupying lesion	Tumour Haemorrhage Oedema, eg post-large cerebral infarct
Excessive CSF production	Choroid plexus papilloma
Excessive CSF protein	Guillain–Barré syndrome Spinal cord tumours
Decreased CSF resorption	Venous sinus thrombosis Inflammatory disease, eg meningitis Haemorrhage, eg subarachnoid Obstructive hydrocephalus
Disrupted venous flow	Haematological causes: retinal vein thrombosis, polycythaemia rubra vera, etc Compression of jugular vein
Idiopathic intracranial hypertension	Idiopathic but can be associated with certain drugs (eg oral contraceptive pill and tetracyclines)
Other	Malignant hypertension Craniosynostosis Graves' disease Metabolic, eg lead poisoning, carbon dioxide retention, steroid withdrawal, vitamin A intoxication

may also be found. The abducens nerve is vulnerable to the effects of raised ICP because it takes a long course from the brain stem to the orbit through the subarachnoid space.

Investigations

This will be influenced by the clinical scenario and the working differential diagnosis, but is likely to include

- Neuroimaging: either CT or MRI of the brain, with venography sequences if indicated, is an appropriate imaging modality.
- Lumbar puncture: to confirm the presence of a raised ICP in the absence of an obvious mass effect on CT, and to provide samples for analysis if there is diagnostic doubt (eg CSF for xanthochromia analysis if suspected subarachnoid haemorrhage).

Management

This involves treating the underlying cause, with regular assessment of visual perimetry during treatment to assess for improvement. Idiopathic intracranial hypertension is treated in a number of ways, including lifestyle changes (losing weight, stopping any precipitant drugs, eg steroids), pharmacologically (eg diuretics, carbonic anhydrase inhibitors) and interventionally (eg serial lumbar punctures, lumboperitoneal shunts, optic nerve sheath fenestration).

Maintaining patient welfare

- Patients may have a number of pre-formed ideas about what might be causing their headaches, including the possibility of brain tumours. It is important for candidates to acknowledge their concerns and give an honest and sympathetic explanation for what the differential diagnosis might be and how they will be investigated.
- Patients may underestimate the degree of impairment in their visual fields and visual acuity, and candidates should emphasise the importance of having this clearly established by an ophthalmologist. Candidates should think broadly about how this visual impairment might affect the patient, eg requiring liaison with the DVLA if still driving.

SCENARIO 28. PEMPHIGUS

Introduce yourself

Confirm the information you've been given and patient details: this 37-year-old woman has presented to out-patients with superficial blisters on her scalp and chest, and lesions within her mouth.
Please assess her.

'What is the main problem from your point of view?' 'I had some mouth ulcers a few months ago that have never completely healed, and now I have painful blisters across my scalp and torso.'

New condition

Focused history of the presenting complaint and relevant systems enquiry: elicit a prodromal history of mucous membrane erosions (>50% patients) before the onset of cutaneous blisters

Differentiate *pemphigus* (younger patients, flaccid superficial blisters) from the major differential diagnosis of *pemphigoid* (elderly patients, with large, tense blisters)

Identify alarm symptoms: secondary infection of blisters, rapid progression of blistering

Pre-existing conditions/risk factors: other autoimmune disorders (ie hypothyroidism, myasthenia gravis) may be found in association with pemphigus

Social/occupational/family circumstances: more common in Ashkenazi Jewish families

Drug history: ask about antihypertensives (ACE inhibitors, nifedipine, propranolol), anti-inflammatories (aspirin, NSAIDs) and other typical drug precipitants.
DRUG ALLERGIES

Other medical conditions: autoimmune disorders (as above).

Begin a **targeted** examination of relevant area/system and continue while taking the history

Examination of the skin

Location: scalp, face, back, chest, flexures, mouth

Description

- Mucous membrane blisters are very flaccid, leaving erosions in the buccal cavity and pharynx
- Skin blisters are flaccid and easily break down. As this happens, they may leave crusted erosions, and secondary infection may occur
- Nikolsky's sign (*to be aware of rather than demonstrated in the examination, as may be painful*): pressure on affected skin from an examining finger causes superficial skin to slide off from deeper layers

CALLBACK: 'You said at the beginning that the main problem was blisters across your chest, back and scalp. Is there anything else troubling you that we haven't covered?'

RESPOND TO PATIENT'S CONCERNS (1–2 min)

1. I think your rash is a rare condition called pemphigus, which is a blistering disorder caused by a problem with an overactive immune system
2. We need to confirm the diagnosis before treating you. If the diagnosis is confirmed, you will need to take steroids and other medication that suppresses the immune system (azathioprine or cyclophosphamide)
3. To make the diagnosis, I will need to refer you to a specialist dermatologist. He or she will want to take a biopsy of the blister and perform a specialist test called immunofluorescence

Thank the patient

Differential diagnosis	Clinical communication skills and managing patient concerns	Physical examination and identifying physical signs	Clinical judgement and maintaining patient welfare
Pemphigoid An autoimmune disorder associated with tense cutaneous bullae developing between the epidermis and dermis		Although pemphigoid and pemphigus are both bullous skin disorders, they have a number of distinctive clinical features to allow their differentiation: Pemphigoid tends to be found in elderly patients, whereas pemphigus is in younger/middle-aged patients Pemphigoid is associated with large, tense bullae that may appear on any aspect of the skin, but particularly on the limbs, torso and flexural areas. Bullae may arise on either normal or erythematous skin. Pemphigus is, however, associated with flaccid blisters that easily break down (very few or no intact lesions may be seen) Pemphigoid may be associated with an urticarial rash that precedes the onset of blisters, but only very rarely with mucosal lesions. Pemphigus is, however, often preceded by mucosal lesions but is not typified by associated urticarial lesions Nikolsky's sign is only rarely detected in pemphigoid, but relatively commonly found in pemphigus	*Investigations* Skin biopsy: direct immunofluorescence will demonstrate IgG deposition in the region of the basement membrane. In contrast, pemphigus is characterised by IgG in the epidermis, but no disruption of the basement membrane ELISA: will detect autoantibodies targeting the antigens BPAg1 and BPAg2 *Management* Corticosteroids are the mainstay of therapy, with the doses required much less than those used in pemphigus. Other immunosuppressants (eg azathioprine) may also be required The disease is self-limiting in approximately 50% of cases
Linear IgA disease A very uncommon bullous disorder of unclear aetiology		Typical clinical features include the presence of bullae and/or urticarial lesions particularly on the back and extensor surfaces. Lesions may be easily confused with those of dermatitis herpetiformis	*Investigations* The condition is diagnosed on skin biopsy, with direct immunofluorescence demonstrating linear IgA deposition at the basement membrane *Management* Dapsone is the mainstay of treatment
Dermatitis herpetiformis	See Scenario 7. Coeliac disease flowchart		

Clinical judgement and maintaining patient welfare

There are a number of different blistering disorders that may appear in MRCP (PACES) and candidates will be expected to distinguish these from each other.

Pemphigus is an uncommon, autoimmune mucocutaneous blistering disorder that tends to affect middle-aged patients. There are several different forms of the condition (including the vulgaris, foliaceus and vegetans variants), but all are characterised pathologically by IgG autoantibodies that target the desmoglein proteins responsible for cellular adhesion within the epidermis.

Investigation and management

The diagnosis is normally suspected clinically but confirmed through skin biopsy. Direct immunofluorescence of the biopsy specimen shows intercellular IgG deposition in the suprabasal epidermis, but no disruption of the basement membrane. ELISA may also be used to detect the autoantibodies associated with the condition, anti-desmoglein-1 and anti-desmoglein-3.

General principles of management include emollients for the skin and avoidance of any precipitating drugs, whereas the definitive treatment is with immunosuppressive therapy. In the first instance, high-dose oral corticosteroids are given. As control of blistering improves, the steroid dose can be reduced and 'steroid-sparing' agents (eg azathioprine) introduced. In particularly severe forms, rituximab, anti-TNF-α therapies (eg infliximab) and intravenous immunoglobulin may be required. Mucosal involvement that has not responded to steroids, for example, may require biologic therapies. Treatment is often continued for many years. Although the disease itself may prove fatal if untreated, the major morbidity and mortality related to the condition now are attributable to complications from immunosuppressive therapy, the cause of death in a quarter of affected patients.

Maintaining patient welfare

- Pemphigus is a chronic disease that may not resolve completely, and which often requires a prolonged course of immunosuppressive therapy to treat effectively. Patients will need to be counselled carefully about the safe use and side effects of the immunosuppressives that they are being given.
- Given that this is a rare disorder that few patients will have heard of before the diagnosis, it may be that they will find the input from a support group (such as the Pemphigus Vulgaris Network – see below) useful.

Resources

Pemphigus Vulgaris Network:
   www.pemphigus.org.uk

SCENARIO 29 PLEURAL EFFUSION

1–2 minutes

Introduce yourself

Confirm the information you've been given and patient details: this 72-year-old man presents with a 2-week history of increasing shortness of breath and weight loss. Please assess him.

'What is the main problem from your point of view?' 'Over the last few weeks I am getting short of breath more easily and climbing the stairs is getting harder. I am also worried because I have lost a stone in weight in 4 weeks.'

5 minutes

New condition

Focused history of the presenting complaint and relevant systems enquiry: differentiate symptoms of pulmonary malignancy (smoker, cough, haemoptysis, occupational risk, etc), pulmonary infection (fever, night sweats, productive cough, etc), congestive cardiac failure (orthopnoea, PND, ankle swelling, etc) and renal disease with fluid overload (known renal impairment with recent decompensation)

Identifying alarm symptoms: unintentional weight loss, haemoptysis, hoarse voice, history of night sweats or fevers

Pre-existing conditions/risk factors: history of COPD, previous cancer; IHD; smoking and/or asbestos history; history of cardiac, renal or liver disease; previous TB

Social/occupational/family circumstances: smoking and occupational history (asbestos exposure). What do the symptoms stop the patient from doing?

Drug history: diuretics stopped/started. **DRUG ALLERGIES**

Other medical conditions: especially cardiac failure, cirrhosis, nephrotic syndrome and thyroid disease

Begin a **targeted** examination of relevant area/system and continue while taking the history

General appearance: cachexia, radiotherapy scars, surgical scars (eg previous mastectomy), cyanosis, autoimmune conditions associated with serositis and effusion (eg SLE)

Hands: clubbing, tar staining on fingers, hypertrophic pulmonary osteoarthropathy

Neck: lymphadenopathy, tracheal deviation away from affected side, raised venous pressure (if cardiac failure)

Chest: reduced chest expansion on affected side, stony dull percussion, decreased vocal fremitus, decreased breath sounds with bronchial breathing above

Extras: look for Horner's syndrome; examine for other features of fluid overload (eg ascites, peripheral oedema); examine available sputum pots or observation charts (temperature and saturations); look for features of paraneoplastic syndromes if indicated in the history, eg cerebellar syndrome

CALLBACK: 'You said at the beginning that the main problem was shortness of breath and weight loss. Is there anything else troubling you that we haven't covered?'

1–2 minutes

RESPOND TO PATIENT'S CONCERNS (1–2 min)

1. I think the cause of your shortness of breath may be a collection of fluid on one side of your lungs, called a pleural effusion that needs to be investigated as soon as possible. Your weight loss may also be associated with this
2. To help with your shortness of breath, we may need to drain this fluid off your lung to make you feel better
3. To try and find the cause of this fluid collection we will need to perform a chest radiograph, and blood tests, and take a sample of fluid from around your lung for analysis. Further scans of your chest may be necessary (eg CT of the chest)

Thank the patient

Differential diagnosis	Clinical communication skills and managing patient concerns	Physical examination and identifying physical signs	Clinical judgement and maintaining patient welfare
Lung collapse	Lung collapse most often occurs secondary to airway obstruction (eg malignancy, inspissated secretions, gross inflammation/oedema, foreign body) Extrinsic compression from a large pneumothorax, pleural effusion or malignancy can generate intrathoracic pressures higher than those within the alveoli	Enquire about known lung pathologies that may increase the patient's vulnerability to developing collapse	Clinical features include: Trachea deviated towards the side of collapse Reduced chest expansion on affected side Dullness to percussion Reduced breath sounds and vocal fremitus in the affected area	The diagnosis is often first suspected clinically, with a chest radiograph usually demonstrating characteristic changes Management is of the underlying condition
Phrenic nerve palsy/ diaphragmatic paralysis	There are a number of causes of this condition, all of which may result in elevation of the diaphragm and give findings that may mimic pleural effusion. Causes include: Neuritis: infective disease (eg pneumonia) or inflammatory disease (eg vasculitis) Extrinsic compression: aortic aneurysm, lung and mediastinal masses Trauma: damage during cardiothoracic surgery, central line insertion, birth trauma Other causes: any cause of peripheral neuropathy, idiopathic	The condition is often asymptomatic, but may give chronic dyspnoea and chest wall discomfort Rarely, patients may present with features of chronic respiratory failure (eg headache and drowsiness relating to chronic carbon dioxide retention)	Clinical features include: Reduced chest expansion on affected side Dullness to percussion Reduced breath sounds and possibly reduced vocal fremitus in the affected area Signs of the underlying disorder (eg scars from previous surgery)	May be diagnosed clinically Often gives a typical 'tented' appearance to the diaphragm that is unchanged on serial imaging The diagnosis may be confirmed through a 'sniff test' (ie failure of the diaphragm to make a normal downward movement on inspiration, as assessed by thoracic ultrasonography) Treatment is of the underlying cause. In cases of respiratory failure, non-invasive ventilation may be required. Diaphragmatic pacing may also be indicated
Hepatomegaly	See also Station 1			

Clinical judgement and maintaining patient welfare

Pleural effusion is a popular case in Station 5, because it is common, has reproducible clinical signs, and is a problem where a focused assessment can quickly narrow down the differential diagnosis (see also Station 1). The major differential diagnoses for a pleural effusion are summarised in Table 5.15.

Investigations

The form and extent of investigation will be guided by the clinical scenario, but will include

- **Blood tests**
  - Biochemistry, including renal function, thyroid function tests, glucose and LDH (see below)
  - Immunology, including an 'autoimmune screen' that includes ANA, rheumatoid

Table 5.15 Major differential diagnoses for pleural effusion

Type of effusion	Category	Examples
Exudate	Malignancy	Lung carcinoma Mesothelioma Metastasis from solid organ malignancy (eg breast carcinoma) Lymphoproliferative disease
	Infection	Primary lung infection: bacterial pneumonia, TB and other mycobacteria Subdiaphragmatic disease: hepatic abscess, subphrenic collection, pancreatitis
	Autoimmune	Rheumatoid arthritis SLE
	Pulmonary infarction	Pulmonary embolism Trauma
	Other	Drugs, eg methotrexate, nitrofurantoin Yellow-nail syndrome Chylothorax Oesophageal rupture Dressler's syndrome
Transudate	Organ failure	Congestive cardiac failure Cirrhosis Nephrotic syndrome Hypothyroidism
	Other	Peritoneal dialysis Hypoalbuminaemia Constrictive pericarditis

factor, anti-CCP, and complement C3 and C4.

- **Chest radiograph**
  - A PA film will hopefully confirm the diagnosis where there is doubt from the clinical examination. At least 200 mL of pleural effusion must accumulate before it can be detected on plain radiography. A lateral decubitus film may help confirm the presence of a small pleural effusion.
- **Ultrasonography**
  - Useful primarily as guidance for aspirating effusions
  - May also help to provide more information about pleural effusion, ie loculated or not, areas of pleural thickening, etc.

Pleural fluid aspiration and analysis: the key diagnostic investigation. Care should be taken in aspirating/draining pleural effusions from patients with possible mesothelioma, because malignant cells may seed into the aspiration track. Fluid should be analysed for

- Appearance
  - Turbid fluid with a putrid smell is suggestive of empyema.
  - Haemorrhagic effusion suggests malignancy, infection (particularly TB) or pulmonary infarction.
  - Cloudy white/yellow fluid suggests chylothorax; the diagnosis may be confirmed by detection of high lipid levels within the fluid.
- Biochemistry
  - Establish where the effusion is an *exudate* or *transudate*. The set of criteria most consistently used for helping to establish this are *Light's criteria* (Table 5.16).
  - Reduced pH (<7.2) is strongly suggestive of empyema, and indicates intercostal drain insertion.
  - Very low glucose concentrations (<2.2 mmol/L) are suggestive of severe infection/empyema, autoimmune rheumatic disease or oesophageal rupture.
  - Very elevated LDH concentrations are

suggestive of severe infection/empyema, malignancy or autoimmune rheumatic disease.
  - Raised pleural fluid amylase is a feature of pancreatitis, although may also be found in bacterial pneumonia.
- Cytology
  - Predominant neutrophilia is suggestive of bacterial infection, whereas lymphocytosis is found most often in malignancy, lymphoproliferative disease and TB.
  - Cytology will be positive in 60% of malignant effusions.
- Microbiology
  - Sputum, pleural fluid and blood should be sent for microscopy (including acid-fast bacilli staining), culture and sensitivity wherever bacterial pneumonia or pulmonary TB is suspected. However, TB is cultured only in approximately 50% of cases where it is the cause of pleuritis. Assays that may be used to increase the diagnostic yield include
    - Mantoux test and interferon-γ release assay (IGRA, eg ELISpot)
    - Adenosine deaminase activity in pleural fluid; this level will be raised in TB pleuritis
    - Pleural biopsy (see below).

Other tests: a number of other tests may be indicated, including

- Echocardiogram: where cardiac failure is suspected.
- CT of the chest: may demonstrate a solid organ malignancy, or enlarged lymph nodes in lymphoproliferative disorders.
- CT pulmonary angiogram: where there is the possibility of pulmonary infarction secondary to pulmonary embolism.
- Bronchoscopy/endobronchial ultrasonography (EBUS): in cases of diagnostic uncertainty (eg lymphadenopathy that may reflect solid organ metastasis or lymphoma), this will help to obtain tissue for histological analysis.
- Pleural biopsy: if pleural fluid analysis is unhelpful but there is evidence of pleural

Table 5.16 Light's criteria

Criterion	Exudate	Transudate
Protein content of effusion (g/L)	>30	<30
Ratio of pleural fluid protein:serum protein	>0.5	<0.5
Ratio of pleural fluid LDH:serum LDH	>0.6	<0.6
Pleural fluid LDH more than two-thirds of the upper limit of normal for serum LDH	Yes	No

fluid thickening on imaging. Often used in the scenario of trying to differentiate malignancy from TB.

Management

Management is treatment of the underlying condition. The risks of intercostal drain insertion for a pleural effusion include pneumothorax, haemothorax and the risk of re-expansion-associated pulmonary oedema if drainage occurs too quickly. In the case of recurrent pleural effusions (most often found in the context of malignancy),

pleurodesis may be considered. This can be achieved by the introduction of talc, doxycycline, bleomycin or other agents into the pleural space, or surgically via thoracoscopy.

Maintaining patient welfare

Even with the full range of investigations outlined above, it may be difficult to ascertain the cause. Patients should be warned that it may be necessary to aspirate fluid more than once for analysis to exclude sinister causes.

SCENARIO 30: PSORIASIS

Introduce yourself

Confirm the information you've been given and patient details: this 32-year-old man presents with itchy scaly plaques on both elbows. Please assess him.

'What is the main problem from your point of view?' 'Over the last 3 months I have developed an itchy rash on both of my elbows.'

New condition

Focused history of the presenting complaint and relevant systems enquiry: description of nature and distribution of rash; whether rash is symmetrical; any obvious precipitating factors (medications, stress, alcohol, streptococcal throat infection); any effect from sunlight; Köbner's phenomenon; pruritus

Identify alarm symptoms: associated arthralgia; rapidly progressive skin disease

Pre-existing conditions: diagnosed with skin disease previously?

Social/occupational/family circumstances: history of alcohol abuse, family history of psoriasis, stress

Drug history: important to check for use of drugs that precipitate psoriasis, including lithium, β blockers, ACE inhibitors and antimalarials.
DRUG ALLERGIES

Other medical conditions: other inflammatory conditions, particularly inflammatory arthropathies

Begin a **targeted** examination of relevant area/system and continue while taking the history

Expose all relevant skin areas and observe

Skin changes

Chronic plaques: white scale above salmon pink plaques. Found particularly over extensor surfaces, scalp, navel and natal cleft

Guttate psoriasis: 'droplet' lesions with silver scaling, especially over limbs and trunks

Palmoplantar pustulosis: sterile pustules overlying plaques, particularly on the palm and sole

Erythrodermic psoriasis: generalised erythema and scaling; may develop superimposed pustules and cause systemic illness

Hands and nails

- Nails: pitting, ridging, onycholysis and subungual hyperkeratosis
- Fingers: dactylitis

Joint and soft-tissue involvement

See Scenario 31. Psoriatic arthropathy flowchart

CALLBACK: 'You said at the beginning that the main problem was an itchy rash on your elbows. Is there anything else troubling you that we haven't covered?'

RESPOND TO PATIENT'S CONCERNS (1–2 min)

1. I think your itchy rash represents a skin condition called psoriasis
2. To help with your itching, I will prescribe some antihistamine medication and some emollient creams
3. To try to improve the rash, I will also prescribe you creams containing a steroid and a chemical related to vitamin D. If these do not work, there are a number of other creams that we can try. If it is still proving difficult to control the rash despite this, I will refer you to a dermatologist; he or she will be able to talk to you about tablet treatments and light therapy which may also be used to treat the condition

Thank the patient

1–2 minutes

5 minutes

1–2 minutes

Differential diagnosis	Clinical communication skills and managing patient concerns	Physical examination and identifying physical signs	Clinical judgement and maintaining patient welfare
Eczema	Particularly Seborrhoeic dermatitis; see Scenario 14. Eczema flowchart		
Rosacea	See Scenario 12. Dermatomyositis differential diagnosis table		
Discoid lupus erythematosus (DLE) A chronic inflammatory skin disease of autoimmune aetiology	Only 5% of affected patients also have SLE	The typical clinical finding is of multiple discrete round plaques that occur on sun-exposed skin (particularly the face and scalp) Plaques are erythematous, and often have scaly centres that may be confused with psoriasis As plaques heal, they may leave hypopigmented skin, or alopecia when occurring on the scalp	*Investigations* Diagnosed clinically *Management* Treated through avoidance of excessive sunlight exposure and with topical steroids Severe disease usually responds to treatment with hydroxychloroquine or systemic steroids
Lupus pernio	This is a dermatological manifestation of sarcoidosis; enquire about other features that may relate to sarcoid, such as dyspnoea from pulmonary involvement	Appears as red- or purple-coloured, indurated plaques or nodules There is no scaling, allowing differentiation from psoriasis Particularly affects the nose, although may affect other parts of the face or fingers	*Investigations* Diagnosed clinically *Management* Often responds to treatment with topical steroids, although systemic steroids/immunosuppressants (eg methotrexate) may be required in severe disease
Granuloma annulare	This is a dermatological condition found in association with diabetes mellitus	Presents as round, erythematous, papular lesions, particularly on the dorsum, face, hands or feet Lesions often cluster and coalesce	*Investigations* Diagnosed clinically *Management* Usually self-resolves within a year of onset without any therapy, although topical or intralesional corticosteroids may be tried in severe cases

(continued)

Differential diagnosis	Clinical communication skills and managing patient concerns	Physical examination and identifying physical signs	Clinical judgement and maintaining patient welfare
Necrobiosis lipoidica (Figure 5.10)	This is a chronic dermatological condition, associated with diabetes mellitus in over two-thirds of cases	The condition is characterised by round or oval red plaques with brown margins. They typically have a shiny surface with yellow-coloured, atrophic centres. They are often also associated with telangiectasia. Over time, lesions may ulcerate. Found on the shins, although may also be found on the face, torso and arms	*Investigations* Appearances may be confused with that of basal cell carcinoma, hence biopsy is useful in confirming the diagnosis *Management* Improved diabetic control probably has no effect in helping to resolve lesions Topical or intralesional steroids may be used, but may worsen the central atrophy Laser therapy and surgery may also be considered in severe cases

Clinical judgement and maintaining patient welfare

Psoriasis is a chronic inflammatory disease of the skin and joints. The aetiology is unknown, but family studies have identified an association between inheritance of particular HLA subtypes and the condition, implying a genetic component. There are also a number of well-recognised environmental associations, including

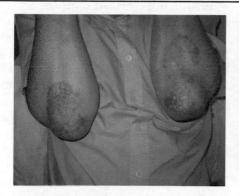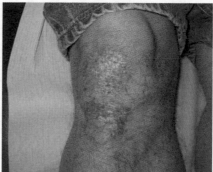

Figure 5.9 Plaque psoriasis

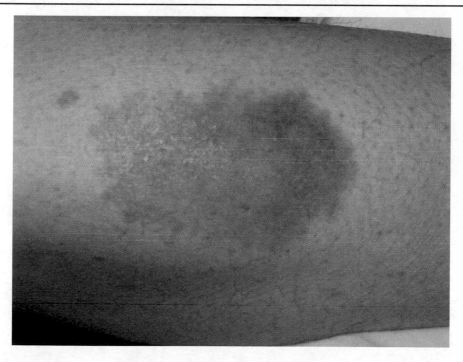

Figure 5.10 Necrobiosis lipoidica

- Medications: see flowchart. Significant changes to a person's alcohol intake or smoking pattern may also affect the condition.
- Infection: in particular, an association between β-haemolytic streptococcal throat infections and guttate psoriasis.
- Sunlight: prolonged sunlight exposure/sunburn may either precipitate or alleviate psoriasis.
- Stress: there is some evidence of psychological stress worsening the condition, although the exact mechanism behind this is unclear.

Investigations

Psoriasis is typically a clinical diagnosis. There are a number of different variations of the condition, as outlined in the flowchart. In cases of diagnostic doubt, a skin biopsy or scraping may be performed; the histology classically demonstrates clubbed rête pegs.

Management

The management of psoriatic skin disease is summarised in Table 5.17.

Maintaining patient welfare

Psoriasis is a chronic disorder that relapses and remits, and may require treatment with medications that have potentially unpleasant side effects. It may involve all areas of the skin including the face. As such, candidates should demonstrate an appreciation of the potential psychological challenges that living with the condition may present, and offer practical advice and support (eg in the UK, the Psoriasis Association).

Resources

The Psoriasis Association: https://www.psoriasis-association.org.uk

Table 5.17 Management of psoriasis

Form of therapy	Specific therapy	Details	Used for which form of psoriasis?
General measures	Education Removal of precipitating factors Emollients Anti-pruritics (eg antihistamines)	These measures should be applied in all cases of the condition	All
Topical therapy	Corticosteroids	Easy to use and often quickly effective However, may be associated with steroid side effects if used for prolonged periods (eg skin atrophy), and psoriasis may 'rebound' and become quickly worse after their withdrawal	Useful in all forms
	Vitamin D analogues	For example, calcipotriol, tacalcitol May be used either by themselves, or in combination/alternating with a topical steroid Their use may be limited by skin irritation	Chronic plaque disease; scalp preparations available
	Retinoids	For example, tazarotene See below for possible side effects	Chronic plaque psoriasis
	Coal tar	May be used together with UVB as the 'Goeckermann regimen', used for erythrodermic psoriasis Unpopular with patients due to the unpleasant smell and messiness in application	Chronic plaque, guttate or erythrodermic psoriasis
	Keratolytics	For example, salicylic acid Particularly useful when scale is very prominent	Most useful for scalp disease
	Dithranol	May be used with UVB and tar baths as part of the 'Ingram regimen' in treatment of severe/erythrodermic disease Can be used only on thick-skinned areas (as may irritate normal skin). Administration must be with care, because stains with a purple colour	Useful for pustular/ severe forms of disease

(continued)

Table 5.17 (*continued*)

Form of therapy	Specific therapy	Details	Used for which form of psoriasis?
Systemic therapies	Phototherapy	Either UVA with a photosensitising agent (eg psoralens – 'PUVA') or UVB. Usually given as a course of therapy, with up to 30 treatments in a course Popular and often effective, but a number of potential complications including symptoms immediately afterwards (nausea, pruritus, etc), and a potential risk of cataracts and skin cancer	Used for severe forms refractory to topical agents
	Systemic steroids	See above	See above
	Retinoids	For example, acitretin May be used either by itself or in combination with phototherapy ('re-PUVA') Many patients may experience minor side effects (eg dry/peeling skin). Severe side effects are rare, but include dyslipidaemia, hepatotoxicity and teratogenicity	Pustular disease
	Methotrexate	Often effective in severe cases Requires monitoring, and a number of potential side effects (eg myelosuppression, hepatotoxicity, teratogenicity)	Severe forms
	Others	A number of other immunosuppressants may also be used, including ciclosporin, azathioprine, mycophenolate mofetil and anti-TNF-α therapies	Pustular or erythrodermic forms

SCENARIO 31. PSORIATIC ARTHROPATHY

Introduce yourself

Confirm the information you've been given: this 48-year-old man has worsening pain and stiffness in both hands. He also has recently developed discomfort in his knees and feet. Please assess him.

'What is the main problem from your point of view?' 'I have had worsening pain and stiffness in my hands for several months. Over the past few weeks, I have also noticed stiffness in my knees, and some discomfort in my feet that is now there every time I walk. My wife noticed that my nails and the skin on my elbows are flaky and dry.'

(margin: 1–2 minutes)

New condition

Focused history of the presenting complaint and relevant systems enquiry: explore the extent of joint involvement – small joints of the hand only, or also involvement of limb and/or spinal joints? Symmetrical or asymmetrical? Has any analgesia been tried? Is there any skin involvement? Any personal or family history of anything similar?

Screen for extra-articular disease, eg nature of nail changes; description of any rash and its distribution; further description of foot pain to establish if consistent with enthesitis

Pre-existing conditions: prior diagnosis of inflammatory arthritis, IBD or psoriatic skin disease

Impact of new symptoms on daily activities, eg do the pain and stiffness affect his ability to work?

Current therapy, eg analgesia and side effects. **DRUG ALLERGIES**

Begin a **targeted** examination of relevant area/ system and continue while taking the history

Establish the pattern of joint involvement

- Asymmetrical oligoarthritis (about 45%)
- Polyarticular, symmetrical, rheumatoid arthritis like (about 35%)
- Distal interphalangeal arthropathy (about 15%, mostly men)
- Spondylitis (about 5%, mostly men)
- Arthritis mutilans (<2%, mostly women)

Assess for extra-articular disease

- Nails: pitting, ridging, onycholysis and subungual hyperkeratosis
- Fingers: dactylitis
- Enthesitis: Achilles tendonitis, plantar fasciitis
- Skin: see Scenario 30. Psoriasis flowchart
- Other features: rarely, may identify the extra-articular manifestations as found in other seronegative diseases, eg anterior uveitis

(margin: 5 minutes)

CALLBACK: 'You said at the beginning that the main problem was the pain and stiffness in your hands, knees and feet, as well as changes to your skin and nails. Is there anything else that we haven't covered?'

RESPOND TO PATIENT'S CONCERNS (1–2 min)

1. The pattern of pain and stiffness you describe and my findings from examining you make me suspect that you have a condition called psoriatic arthropathy
2. To try to help your symptoms, I will today prescribe you some anti-inflammatory painkillers and refer you to the physiotherapist
3. To try to investigate further if you have this condition, I will arrange for some blood tests and radiographs of your hands and knees. If I am able to confirm the diagnosis but am struggling to control your symptoms, I will refer you to a rheumatologist for their advice

Thank the patient

(margin: 1–2 minutes)

Differential diagnosis	Clinical communication skills and managing patient concerns	Physical examination and identifying physical signs	Clinical judgement and maintaining patient welfare
Enteropathic arthritis	Occurs in 10–15% patients with IBD, and a small percentage of those with coeliac and Whipple's diseases The presenting feature is arthralgia, with the number of joints and severity independent of bowel disease activity. This may even precede the onset of bowel disease	Examination usually demonstrates an asymmetrical oligo- or polyarthritis affecting the axial skeleton (sacroiliitis and spondylitis) and lower limbs There are typically no rashes or nail changes present, although erythema nodosum and/or pyoderma gangrenosum may be found Additional examination findings may include clubbing of the digits and anterior uveitis	*Investigations* Blood tests: raised inflammatory markers. Rheumatoid factor negative Imaging: sacroiliitis may be seen on plain radiographs, but is best detected by MRI Endoscopy: to obtain tissue to confirm the diagnosis of IBD *Management* Analgesia: with particular caution in using NSAIDs DMARDs: sulfasalazine is most frequently used, although others (including methotrexate and azathioprine) have also shown efficacy
Juvenile idiopathic arthritis (JIA) This is the most common rheumatic disease of childhood	The condition is defined by a history of persistent arthritis (pain) aged <16 years The symptoms (apart from arthralgia) vary according to different phenotypes, eg fever, weight loss and rash typify Still's disease, whereas a pruritic rash alone may be the predominant feature in the psoriatic form of JIA	Examination findings depend on the phenotype of JIA: Systemic arthritis (Still's disease): 'salmon pink rash', polyarthritis and occasionally lymphadenopathy, hepatosplenomegaly, and/or pleural and pericardial effusions Oligoarthritis (the most common form): often self-limiting Polyarthritis (rheumatoid factor positive): aggressive and destructive, symmetrical Polyarthritis (rheumatoid factor negative): less severe, asymmetrical Psoriatic arthritis: examination findings same as the adult form (see flowchart) Enthesitis-related arthritis: symmetrical lower limb arthritis, enthesitis, anterior uveitis	*Investigations* Blood tests: raised inflammatory markers. Rheumatoid factor positive in some forms and negative in others; ANA often negative in Still's disease Imaging: plain radiographs and MRI are useful to exclude other mimicking diseases (eg bone malignancies) Bone marrow aspiration: this is often performed where systemic arthritis is present to exclude occult haematological malignancy, eg leukaemia *Management* Multidisciplinary, including Physio- and occupational therapy Analgesia: NSAIDs are useful in treating pain and stiffness DMARDs: methotrexate, sulfasalazine, leflunomide and anti-TNF-α treatments have all shown efficacy Glucocorticoids: intra-articular steroids are used in preference to systemic treatment

(continued)

Differential diagnosis	Clinical communication skills and managing patient concerns	Physical examination and identifying physical signs	Clinical judgement and maintaining patient welfare
Rheumatoid arthritis	See Scenario 34. Rheumatoid arthritis flowchart		
Ankylosing spondylitis	See Scenario 3. Ankylosing spondylitis flowchart		
Reactive arthritis (formerly Reiter's syndrome)	See Scenario 3. Ankylosing spondylitis differential diagnosis table		
Septic arthritis	See Scenario 16. Gout differential diagnosis table		

Clinical judgement and maintaining patient welfare

Psoriatic arthropathy is a member of the category of seronegative spondyloarthropathies (see Scenario 3. Ankylosing spondylitis flowchart, page 404, for more details). As with other related diseases, the pattern of arthritis found varies between patients, and different extra-articular manifestations may be found including psoriatic skin disease, as described in a separate flowchart.

Clinical features

Early morning pain and stiffness in joints are the usual initial presentation. As outlined in the flowchart, epidemiological studies have identified five typical patterns of joint extra-articular complications, which may occur either before or after the onset of arthritis.

The prognosis in psoriatic arthropathy is usually better than in other forms of inflammatory arthritis (including rheumatoid arthritis). However, a 20-year cohort study has recently revealed an increased mortality ratio in patients with psoriatic arthropathy, mostly attributable to cardiovascular disease. Men and those with fewer affected joints at presentation tend to have longer periods of remission.

Investigations

As with other seronegative spondyloarthropathies, the diagnosis may be made clinically. There is no single specific diagnostic investigation for the condition. However, a number of investigations may collectively assist the diagnosis

- **Blood tests**
  - Inflammatory markers are raised in active disease and are useful for monitoring the efficacy of treatment.
- **Plain radiographs**
  - Classic changes are those of osteolysis, ie
    - Resorption of the tufts of the distal phalanx

- 'Pencil-in-cup' deformity in the MTP, MCP and DIP joints
    - Complete dissolution of the small bones (as in arthritis mutilans).
  - Other changes on plain radiographs include juxta-articular new bone formation; there are normal joint spaces and no juxta-articular osteopenia (in contrast to rheumatoid arthritis).
- **MRI**
  - Useful at picking up subtle signs of inflammation, particularly in the sacroiliac joints.

The international CASPAR (**ClAS**sification criteria for **P**soriatic **AR**thritis) criteria (CASPAR Study Group, 2006)* provide >90% sensitivity and specificity for diagnosing the condition; a diagnosis of psoriatic arthropathy requires three or more points scored using the following criteria, a combination of clinical, laboratory and radiological factors

- Current psoriasis (2 points) *or* history of psoriasis (1 point) *or* family history of psoriasis only (1 point)
- Dactylitis (1 point)
- Nail dystrophy (1 point)
- Juxta-articular new bone formation on radiographs (1 point)
- Rheumatoid factor negative (1 point).

One common question in MRCP (PACES) is how to distinguish psoriatic arthropathy from rheumatoid arthritis with incidental psoriasis (Table 5.18). Beware the patient without skin lesions but diagnostic nail changes!

Management

Optimal management of psoriatic arthropathy requires a multidisciplinary approach, with input from both primary and secondary care

- **Physical therapies**
  - Exercise, physiotherapy and occupational therapy may reduce pain and stiffness and allow sufferers to adapt to any physical disability.

*Taylor W. *et al.* and CASPAR Study Group (2006). Classification criteria for psoriatic arthritis: development of new criteria from a large international stidy. *Arthritis & Rheumatology*; 54(8), pp. 2665-73.

Table 5.18 Distinction between psoriatic arthropathy and rheumatoid arthritis

Feature	Psoriatic arthropathy	Rheumatoid arthritis
Gender affected	Males = females	Females > males
Joint involvement pattern	Asymmetrical (even in polyarticular disease)	Symmetrical
Joint tenderness	Low	High
Extra-articular manifestations	Includes skin disease No rheumatoid nodules	Often multiple organs involved Rheumatoid nodules in seropositive disease No psoriatic skin disease unless incidentally
Enthesitis	Relatively common	Rare
Dactylitis	Relatively common	Rare
Spondylitis	Relatively common	Rare
Radiology	Features of osteolysis Neither narrowed joint space nor juxta-articular osteopenia	Narrowed joint space Juxta-articular osteopenia
Serology	Approximately 13% rheumatoid factor positive Up to 16% of patients anti-CCP positive	Approximately 75% rheumatoid factor positive Approximately 60% of patients anti-CCP positive

- **Pharmacological**
  - Analgesia/anti-inflammatories: NSAIDs are a useful first-line therapy.
  - Glucocorticoids: intra-articular steroid injection may be used in inflamed peripheral joints. Systemic steroid therapy is usually avoided if there is florid skin disease due to the risk of rebound exacerbations on stopping.
  - DMARDs: sulfasalazine, methotrexate and ciclosporin appear to be the most effective

such therapies, with efficacy against both skin and joint manifestations of the condition. However, there is no clear evidence that these treatments halt either clinical or radiological progression of disease.
  - Anti-TNF-α therapy: there is now evidence that such agents *do* reduce disease progression, both clinically and radiologically. They are now recommended in NICE guidelines to be

used in this condition where there is continued inflammation despite having tried at least two DMARDs.

Maintaining patient welfare

- Patients with psoriatic arthropathy may have a combination of skin disease and arthropathy, which may be disfiguring, painful and functionally limiting. Candidates should show an appreciation that the management of this condition may require physiotherapy, and home and workplace adaptations from occupational therapy, and that patients may be eligible for disability benefit. A support group (such as the Psoriasis Association in the UK – see below) may be helpful.
- Where patients require DMARD or anti-TNF-α therapy, they will need to be counselled carefully on the monitoring required (eg regular full blood count and liver function test assessment) and the range of possible side effects. Young women will need to be informed that many of these treatments are teratogenic, and therefore of the importance of using contraception while taking them.

Resources

The Psoriasis Association: www.psoriasis-association.org.uk

SCENARIO 32. PYODERMA GANGRENOSUM

Introduce yourself

Confirm the information you've been given and patient details: this 36-year-old woman presents with a painful malodorous ulcer on her lower leg. Please assess her.

'What is the main problem from your point of view?' 'I have developed an ulcer on my legs which is getting bigger. I have also had a bit of blood in my stool.'

New condition

Focused history of the presenting complaint and relevant systems enquiry: establish symptoms suggestive of the underlying causes, including IBD, autoimmune liver disease, inflammatory arthropathies and haematological malignancies (approximately 50% of cases are associated with other conditions)

There is often a reported history of an 'insect bite' at the site where the lesion developed

Identify alarm symptoms: B symptoms (weight loss, night sweats, etc) may be suggestive of active lymphoproliferative disease

Social/occupational/family circumstances: impact on lifestyle. Assess with regard to support within the community, eg district nurse visits

Drug history: antibiotics, steroids (oral or steroids), immunosuppression (ciclosporin, azathioprine). **DRUG ALLERGIES**

Other medical conditions: history of associated conditions, as outlined above

Begin a **targeted** examination of relevant area/ system and continue while taking the history

Examination of the skin

Location: lower limbs, trunk and occasionally face

Description: initially a nodulopustular lesion that breaks down to form a tender ulcer; may be up to 10 cm in diameter. These ulcers often have a purplish, necrotic, overhanging edge, with surrounding erythema and a purulent surface. Lesions often heal with scars

Additional examinations

- **Lymph nodes**: if suggestion of lymphoma
- **Abdomen**: if suggestion of IBD, autoimmune liver disease or GI symptoms. There may be splenomegaly if underlying polycythaemia rubra vera. Pyoderma gangrenosum shows Köbner's phenomenon, and may develop around scars from previous abdominal surgery or even around stoma sites
- **Joints**: if arthralgia is described, looking for evidence of active synovitis

CALLBACK: 'You said at the beginning that the main problem was a painful ulcer on your leg and blood in your stool. Is there anything else troubling you that we haven't covered?'

RESPOND TO PATIENT'S CONCERNS (1–2 min)

1. I think the painful ulcer on your leg is a condition called pyoderma gangrenosum. The blood in your stool may be caused by inflammatory bowel disease, which is associated with this type of ulcer
2. To help with the pain, I can give you some painkillers (eg paracetamol). The ulcer needs to be cleaned regularly and you will require antibiotics. However, we need to be sure of the diagnosis before considering other treatments (eg anti-TNF agents). Your bowel symptoms will also need to be investigated
3. To try to help confirm the diagnosis, we will be performing blood tests, swabbing the ulcer and doing a stool culture in the first instance. I will need to refer you to a dermatologist to see if a skin biopsy is necessary and a gastroenterologist to investigate your bowel symptoms

Thank the patient

Differential diagnosis	Clinical communication skills and managing patient concerns	Physical examination and identifying physical signs	Clinical judgement and maintaining patient welfare
Venous/varicose ulcers These are ulcers that develop as a consequence of long-term incompetence of veins in the peripheries	Venous ulcers are usually painless unless complications (such as infection) have developed	These are particularly found over the medial malleolus, as shallow, irregularly shaped ulcers with shelved edges They are associated with brown haemosiderin deposits, lipodermatosclerosis and eczema The base usually contains pink granulation tissue, pale granulations or slough	*Investigations* Diagnosed clinically *Management* Emollients for dry skin and antibiotics if infections The mainstay of treatment is compression bandaging and elevation Skin grafting may be required for very large/non-healing ulcers
Arterial ulcers These are ulcers relating to disrupted arterial blood flow	These often occur in the context of other atherosclerotic disease, eg ischaemic heart disease, stroke These may be first suspected through the presence of intermittent claudication, with severe pain even at rest found in advanced cases	It will often be difficult to palpate arterial pulses, and the limb may be pale and cool. There may be other clinical features of atherosclerotic disease, eg sternotomy scar from previous CABG Ulcers typically affect the shin or lateral malleolus. They often have sharply defined edges and are deep, penetrating down into the fascia. Ulcers are often surrounded by shiny, cyanotic skin with a lack of hair	*Investigations* Often first suspected clinically, with the degree of arterial compromise quantified by measurement of the ankle–brachial pressure indices (ABPIs) and/or arterial Doppler scans *Management* Correction of risk factors for atherosclerosis, eg blood pressure control, lipid management, smoking cessation advice If there is evidence of severe ischaemia, will require revascularisation, ie angioplasty, bypass surgery, etc
Neuropathic ulcer	These may occur in the context of a wide range of neurological conditions as a consequence of the associated sensorimotor deficit	Characteristically found on the base of the foot May quickly develop large, necrotic, ulcerated areas	*Investigations* Diagnosed clinically, after exclusion of other causes for ulcers *Management* Treatment is of the underlying disorder. Where there are few therapeutic options for the neurological condition, the focus will be on dressing the area and avoiding infection or injury
Cutaneous vasculitis	See Scenario 15. Erythema nodosum differential diagnosis table for details of vasculitic ulcers		

(continued)

Differential diagnosis	Clinical communication skills and managing patient concerns	Physical examination and identifying physical signs	Clinical judgement and maintaining patient welfare
Malignancy		A number of different skin malignancies may include ulcers that can mimic pyoderma gangrenosum, including squamous cell carcinoma and malignant melanoma	
Trauma			

Clinical judgement and maintaining patient welfare

Pyoderma gangrenosum is a rare inflammatory disorder characterised by the development of deep ulceration of the skin. It is a popular station in MRCP (PACES), because pyoderma gangrenosum is associated with a number of other conditions; candidates will be expected to perform a focused assessment to identify which of these might be present. These include

- Gastrointestinal: Crohn's disease and ulcerative colitis – <1% of patients with IBD develop pyoderma gangrenosum, but it nevertheless remains the condition with the strongest association
- Hepatological: autoimmune hepatitis
- Rheumatological: including rheumatoid arthritis and seronegative spondyloarthropathies
- Haematological: leukaemia, myeloma, and both lympho- and myeloproliferative diseases.

Investigations

The diagnosis itself is usually first suspected clinically, especially if there are features of other associated conditions present. However, it is a diagnosis of exclusion and a biopsy should be considered in cases of diagnostic uncertainty. Although pyoderma gangrenosum has no highly specific histological changes, biopsy will help to exclude other causes.

Candidates will be expected to formulate an investigative plan that confirms the diagnosis and helps to identify any condition that may have precipitated it, eg if patients also presented with rectal bleeding, then candidates would be expected to consider stool cultures, intestinal imaging, and endoscopy and biopsy as initial investigations for a possible underlying IBD.

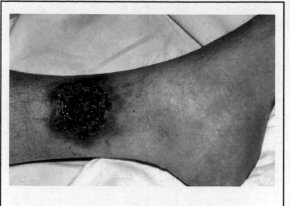

Figure 5.11 Pyoderma gangrenosum

Management

Topical steroids are usually effective for mild cases. More severe cases will require systemic immunosuppressive therapy; high-dose prednisolone (at least 1 mg/kg) is the usual treatment of choice. Other immunosuppressants may be tried in addition to steroids or introduced as steroids are weaned, including ciclosporin, mycophenolate mofetil and azathioprine. In very severe cases, there is also evidence for the efficacy of anti-TNF-α therapies, especially when the condition occurs in association with IBD.

Maintaining patient welfare

In addition to definitive medical treatments, patients may also benefit from the input of a number of other health professionals; this might include the tissue viability team (for slow-healing wounds) and/or the pain clinic (as lesions may be extremely painful, even once healed). Patients may also require follow-up in the community from district nurses for dressing changes.

SCENARIO 33. RETINITIS PIGMENTOSA

1–2 minutes

Introduce yourself

Confirm the information you've been given and patient details: this 33-year-old woman has presented with progressive deterioration in her vision over the last few years. Please assess her.

'What is the main problem from your point of view?' 'Over the last few years, my vision has become progressively worse, particularly at night. Other members of my family also have poor vision.'

5 minutes

New condition

Focused history of the presenting complaint and relevant systems enquiry: establish the exact nature of the visual impairment (whether particularly at night or at all times, the degree of colour vision impairment, whether peripheral or central vision is involved). Ask about a relevant family history

Pre-existing conditions/risk factors: personal or family history of learning disability, subfertility, obesity and polydactyly (consider Bardet–Biedl syndrome); syncope and diplopia (may respectively imply the heart block and ophthalmoplegia found in Kearns–Sayre syndrome)

Social/occupational/family circumstances: family history of blindness, registered blind, aids for daily living, may have white stick

Drug history: may be related to complications of the eponymous disorders. **DRUG ALLERGIES**

Other medical conditions: as above, ensure no other causes of blindness (eg diabetes). Any previous ophthalmological input, eg laser treatment, surgery?

Begin a **targeted** examination of relevant area/system and continue while taking the history

General appearance: obese, polydactyly, short stature (of Bardet–Biedl syndrome); hearing aids (deafness in Usher's, Refsum's and Kearns–Sayre syndromes)

Examination of the eye

Visual acuity: decreased depending on amount of macular damage

Fields: variable, but typically peripheral vision lost first in retinitis pigmentosa

Movement: ophthalmoplegia in Kearns–Sayre syndrome

Fundoscopy: symmetrical and widespread, peripheral, spiculated black pigment in both retinas with pale optic discs is distinctive for retinitis pigmentosa (See Figure 3.8(d) in Neurological Exam)

Additional examination

- Examine for peripheral neuropathy and cerebellar signs (if Bassen–Kornzweig or Refsum's syndrome suspected)
- Ask for plasma glucose/check for fingerprick BM testing (Bardet–Biedl syndrome is associated with diabetes)

1–2 minutes

CALLBACK: 'You said at the beginning that the main problem was progressive loss of vision. Is there anything else troubling you that we haven't covered?'

RESPOND TO PATIENT'S CONCERNS (1–2 min)

1. I think you have a condition called retinitis pigmentosa, which is an inherited disorder
2. As this is an inherited disorder, I am going to refer you for genetic counselling. This will be particularly useful if you are thinking of having children
3. I am also going to refer you to the ophthalmology doctors. Although there is no cure for this condition, there are a number of things that we can do to help you

Thank the patient

Differential diagnosis	Clinical communication skills and managing patient concerns	Physical examination and identifying physical signs	Clinical judgement and maintaining patient welfare
Conditions associated with retinitis pigmentosa			
Bardet–Biedl syndrome A rare inherited disorder, with at least 10 different associated genes	Night blindness may be the first symptom that develops	Clinical features include: Eyes: progressive visual loss secondary to retinitis pigmentosa Genitourinary: interstitial nephritis and renal failure, hypogonadism, congenital abnormalities of the uterus and ovaries Endocrine: diabetes mellitus and diabetes insipidus, obesity Limbs: polydactyly Neurological: learning disability, delayed development of motor skills and autism-like features	*Investigations* Diagnosed on the basis of clinical findings, with genetic tests used to confirm the diagnosis *Management* Supportive treatment Genetic counselling
Bassen–Korzweig syndrome (abetalipo-proteinaemia) A rare autosomal disorder associated with mutations in the microsomal triglyceride transfer protein (MTP) gene	Initial features may be those of the RP-related visual impairment, or of the associated neurological involvement (features of developmental delay, sensorimotor impairment, etc) May also present with steatorrhoea	Other clinical features include: Learning disability Cerebellar ataxia Peripheral neuropathy	*Investigations* Biochemistry: very low/undetectable. LDL in plasma, with associated deficiency in fat-soluble vitamin deficiency Blood film: will demonstrate acanthocytes Genetic testing may confirm the diagnosis *Management* High-dose replacement of fat-soluble vitamins may delay the rate of neurological decline
Kearns–Sayre syndrome A rare mitochondrial myopathy, with symptom onset before age 20	Classically, a triad of: Retinitis pigmentosa: ask about visual impairment Chronic progressive external ophthalmoplegia: may present with either loss of visual acuity or diplopia Cardiac arrhythmia: often high-degree heart block, usually manifesting clinically as palpitations or syncope Sensorineural hearing loss may also be an early feature	Other features may include: Learning disability Cerebellar ataxia Proximal myopathy Endocrine disease: including diabetes, hypoparathyroidism and short stature secondary to growth hormone deficiency	*Investigations* Often first suspected clinically, and diagnosed through detection of mutations in mitochondrial DNA on muscle biopsy *Management* Supportive therapy only

(continued)

Differential diagnosis	Clinical communication skills and managing patient concerns	Physical examination and identifying physical signs	Clinical judgement and maintaining patient welfare
Refsum's disease An autosomal recessive disorder associated with defective phytanic acid metabolism	Visual loss (from RP) and sensorineural hearing loss are often the initial clinical features	Other features include: Cataracts Cerebellar ataxia Peripheral neuropathy Ichthyosis	*Investigations* Diagnosed on genetic testing *Management* Treatment principally involves avoiding foods rich in phytanic acid, ie animal fat, leafy vegetables, etc Plasmapheresis has also been demonstrated to be of benefit
Usher's syndrome An autosomal recessive disease associated with mutations in one of at least 10 genes	This also first presents with RP-associated visual loss and sensorineural hearing loss		*Investigations* Diagnosed on genetic testing *Management* Supportive treatment only
Differential diagnoses			
Laser scars	For example, after treatment for diabetic retinopathy	Normally easily identified on fundoscopy	
Retinal trauma			
Age-related macular degeneration (ARMD)	This presents with progressive loss of visual acuity	As ARMD progresses, there is progressive deposition of the drusen that characterise the disease below the retinal pigment epithelium (RPE). Over time, this will result in loss of the RPE, and the appearance of retinal pigmentation This is particularly found in the 'dry' version of the disease	*Investigations* Diagnosed clinically *Management* There is an ever-growing role for anti-VEGF therapy, eg bevacizumab
Infective disease	There are a number of associated ocular infections, including toxoplasmosis and rubella	Such infections may result in a choroidoretinitis with associated pigment deposition in the retina	*Investigations* Diagnosed clinically *Management* Treatment is of the underlying infection

Clinical judgement and maintaining patient welfare

Retinitis pigmentosa (RP) is an inherited disorder that is characterised by severe visual impairment or blindness. Rather than being a single condition, RP is a feature of a number of different genetic diseases (see differential diagnosis table above). These diseases may be inherited in a variety of ways, and are associated with mutations in a large number of genes. Pathologically, RP is typified by progressive degeneration of photoreceptors (particularly rods, usually spaced at the periphery of the retina); as such cells die, the RPE migrates, causing the formation of the retinal pigment deposits that characterise the disease.

Clinical features

The first sign of the disorder may be night blindness or the development of tunnel vision, both symptoms that reflect degeneration of the rods of the peripheral retina. The clinical signs are variable; although some patients have profound blindness in their early years, others develop any degree of visual impairment only much later in life.

On fundoscopy, the typical appearance is the presence of black-coloured pigmentation in the periphery of the retina, often described as 'bone spiculation'. Optic atrophy may also occur, usually first presenting with a pale optic nerve head. Most patients will also eventually develop cataracts. Clinical assessment may pinpoint the underlying diagnosis (eg polydactyly is suggestive of Bardet–Biedl syndrome; see flowchart and differential diagnosis table).

Investigations and diagnosis

The diagnosis may first be suspected from clinical features and/or a relevant family history. Genetic testing is becoming increasingly available.

The electroretinogram (ERG) is useful for detecting early photoreceptor impairment, and may help in making a diagnosis. It is also a useful tool for following the progression of visual loss once a diagnosis has been made.

Treatment

This is at present supportive. Retinal implants, transplants and stem cell therapy are still only in the pre-clinical/early clinical trial phase.

Maintaining patient welfare

- Genetic counselling will have a useful role in explaining the condition to patients, and in counselling those who are considering having children.
- Candidates will be expected to identify disability benefit, psychological/psychiatric support, liaison with the DVLA (if still driving), visual impairment support (eg walking aids, guide dog) and support groups (eg RP Fighting Blindness – see below) as important aspects of the patient's holistic care.

Resources

RP Fighting Blindness:
    www.rpfightingblindness.org.uk

SCENARIO 34. RHEUMATOID ARTHRITIS

Introduce yourself

Confirm the information you've been given and patient details: this 55-year-old woman presents with 3 months of pain, swelling and stiffness in her hands. Please assess her.

'What is the main problem from your point of view?' 'The joints of my hands have become increasingly painful, swollen and stiff over the past 3 months. My hands are so stiff in the morning that it is now difficult even to make breakfast'.

New condition

Focused history of the presenting complaint and relevant systems enquiry: establish the length of time that symptoms have been present, which joints are involved, whether there is joint stiffness and whether the symptoms are symmetrical. Are there extra-articular symptoms (eg rashes, red and painful eyes)? Ask about dry eyes/mouth (if considering Sjögren's syndrome). Has anything similar occurred in family members?

Identify alarm symptoms: dyspnoea and/or chest pain (may represent cardiorespiratory complications of rheumatoid disease), sensorimotor symptoms (may represent an associated neuropathy), palpable purpura (may suggest rheumatoid vasculitis, with multiple organ disease)

Social/occupational/family circumstances: how do the symptoms affect the patient's daily activities? What is the patient's job (if considering Caplan's disease)?

Drug history: has any analgesia been tried already? **DRUG ALLERGIES**

Other medical conditions: any previous unexplained joint, cardiac, respiratory, neuro-ophthalmological or haematological disease?

Begin a **targeted** examination of relevant area/system and continue while taking the history

General appearance: pallor (anaemia). Look for purpura. There may be disuse atrophy of muscles, especially in the upper limbs

Locomotor

- Symmetrical deforming arthritis affecting the PIPJs and MCPJs but classically sparing DIPJs
- Characteristic deformities including ulnar deviation of the fingers, subluxation at the MCPJs, Boutonnière's deformities, swan-neck deformities and Z deformity of the thumb
- Affected joints are red, hot and swollen

Skin: look for rheumatoid nodules (particularly found on extensor surfaces, especially over the elbows)

Eyes: red eyes suggestive of episcleritis or scleritis. Scleromalacia perforans rarely occurs in severe cases

Chest: stony dull percussion/absent breath sounds if associated pleural effusions; fine late inspiratory crackles in associated pulmonary fibrosis; coarse crackles in associated bronchiectasis

Cardiac: pericardial rub (pericarditis). Auscultate closely for murmurs (particularly associated with mitral valve disease). Look for oedema (may reflect cardiac failure or an associated nephrotic syndrome)

Abdomen: splenomegaly in Felty's syndrome

Neurology: examine if sensorimotor symptoms, assessing for an associated neuropathy.

To finish: check blood pressure and do a urine dipstick (to assess for glomerulonephritis)

CALLBACK: 'You said at the beginning that the main problem was the increasingly severe pain, swelling and stiffness in your hands. It sounds like this is affecting you considerably. Is there anything else that we haven't covered?

RESPOND TO PATIENT'S CONCERNS (1–2 min)

1. I think that the cause of your symptoms is a condition called rheumatoid arthritis. However, there are a number of conditions that can look similar, and we need to do tests to help confirm the diagnosis
2. We can start some anti-inflammatory painkillers. Once they have taken affect, I will also ask the physiotherapist to suggest exercises to strengthen the muscles in your hands
3. I will request some blood tests and radiographs of your hands, take a sample of your urine and refer you to a rheumatologist. There are now many effective therapies available for this condition

Thank the patient

Differential diagnosis	Clinical communication skills and managing patient concerns	Physical examination and identifying physical signs	Clinical judgement and maintaining patient welfare
Psoriatic arthritis	See Scenario 31. Psoriatic arthropathy flowchart		
Ankylosing spondylitis	See Scenario 3. Ankylosing spondylitis flowchart		
SLE	See Scenario 36. SLE flowchart		
Crystal arthropathies	See Scenario 16. Gout differential diagnosis table		
Septic arthritis	See Scenario 16. Gout differential diagnosis table		
Reactive arthritis (formerly Reiter's syndrome)	See Scenario 3. Ankylosing spondylitis differential diagnosis table		
Osteoarthritis	See Scenario 16. Gout differential diagnosis table		
Sjögren syndrome This is an autoimmune condition of exocrine glands, most consistently affecting the lacrimal and salivary glands. The condition typically first presents in the fourth to fifth decades of life, with a female:male ratio of 9:1	Characteristic features of the history include dry eyes (*keratoconjunctivitis sicca*), dry mouth (*xerostomia*), myalgia, arthralgia and fatigue There may also be a history of vaginal dryness, dyspareunia, dysphagia and a dry cough	Examination may demonstrate dry eyes, as well as dryness of other mucosal membranes. Other clinical findings may include a non-deforming polyarthritis, Raynaud's phenomenon, parotid gland swelling and a peripheral neuropathy Lymphadenopathy is a worrying sign – Sjögren syndrome is associated with a significantly increased risk of B-cell lymphoma There may also be features of other associated autoimmune disorders, eg thyroid disease, autoimmune hepatitis, myasthenia gravis	*Investigation* Blood tests: elevated immunoglobulin counts and positive autoantibodies, including rheumatoid factor, ANA (positive in about 70%), anti-Ro (SSA) and anti-La (SSB) (both positive in about 70%) Schirmer's tear test: <10 mm of wetness of filter paper (placed inside the lower eyelid) after 5 min indicates defective tear production Rose Bengal staining of the eyes: shows keratitis on slit-lamp examination Biopsy of salivary glands: demonstrates focal lymphocytic aggregation *Management* Lubrication: eg eye drops, oral lozenges, avoidance of anticholinergic medications Joint aspiration: may help the pain of associated arthralgia NSAIDs and hydroxychloroquine: indicated for arthralgia DMARDs: there is some evidence for their efficacy in severe systemic disease

Clinical judgement and maintaining patient welfare

Rheumatoid arthritis (RA) is a chronic, multi-organ, inflammatory disease. It is a relatively common condition (the UK prevalence is approximately 1%), with the onset typically in the sixth decade of life. The aetiology is complex, but appears to include a genetic component (twin studies have identified an association with particular HLA subtypes) as well as environmental triggers (including cigarette smoking). The high prevalence of the condition and wide range of possible clinical features mean that RA is one of the more common cases found in Station 5.

Clinical features

These are as described in the flowchart. The American College of Rheumatology (ACR; 1987) criteria for the diagnosis of RA are still in use clinically, although they are practically more often applied as a research tool. The criteria require at least four of the following criteria to be able to make a diagnosis of RA

- Morning stiffness >1 hour for ⩾6 weeks
- Symmetrical arthritis for ⩾6 weeks
- Arthritis of three or more joints for ⩾6 weeks
- Arthritis of the small joints of the hands for ⩾6 weeks
- Rheumatoid nodules
- Serum rheumatoid factor
- Radiological evidence of rheumatoid disease.

Candidates should appreciate that the pattern and onset of joint disease may be variable between different patients. Although some patients first present with severe, sudden-onset polyarthritis, other patients may present with an insidious onset of joint disease that has been present for months or even longer. Another unusual but well-recognised presentation is with a pattern of joint involvement that mimics that of polymyalgia rheumatica.

Rheumatoid nodules occur as firm, subcutaneous lesions which occur on particularly bony prominences over extensor surfaces, with the elbows being the region most likely to be affected. They are almost always associated with rheumatoid factor-positive disease.

Investigations

- **Blood tests**
  - Haematology: neutropenia may be suggestive of Felty's syndrome, and the patient should be assessed for splenomegaly. Anaemia is a very common finding in RA and has a number of causes, as described in Table 5.19.
  - Biochemistry: CRP will be raised in active disease. The urinary protein:creatinine ratio is useful where nephrotic syndrome is suspected as a means of accurately assessing renal protein loss.
  - Immunology: *rheumatoid factor* is an antibody, usually IgM, that targets the constant (Fc) portion of the patient's own IgG antibodies. It is positive in approximately 70% of patients with RA, but may also be detected in a number of other conditions. These include other autoimmune conditions (eg Sjögren's syndrome) and bacterial infections (eg endocarditis). The other immunological marker of use is *anti-cyclic citrullinated peptide* (anti-CCP), which appears to have a higher sensitivity and specificity (at least 60% for both) for early rheumatoid disease than rheumatoid factor. Although detection of either of these antibodies is a marker of more severe rheumatoid disease, there is no strong evidence that titres correlate with disease activity.
- **Radiology**
  - Radiographs: the small joints of the hand may be affected early in aggressive disease. Characteristic features include
    - Marginal erosions (this is the most distinguishing feature for RA)
    - Joint space narrowing and subluxation
    - Periarticular osteoporosis
    - Soft-tissue swelling.
- **Synovial fluid analysis**
  - Not performed routinely. This is

particularly of use in cases of diagnostic uncertainty for helping to exclude differential diagnoses, eg septic arthritis, crystal arthritis.

Management

Candidates will be expected to recall poor prognostic factors for the condition. These include

- Male gender
- Multiple joint involvement at presentation
- Anti-CCP positive
- Raised inflammatory markers in early disease
- Higher functional disability score at 1 year
- Erosive joint disease by 3 years after diagnosis.

A generalised approach to management of RA is as follows

- **General measures**
  - Patient education: patients will have the condition for life and may experience a number of complications and changes in therapy, so it is important that they are fully aware of the nature of the condition from the time of diagnosis.
  - Physiotherapy and occupational therapy: the arthritis and fatigue that accompany active disease may cause marked disability. Therapies help minimise the risk of disuse atrophy, and aim to help the patient maintain an optimal level of daily activity.

- **Pharmacological**
  - *NSAIDs*: these are useful analgesic and anti-inflammatory agents, but have no effect on disease progression. Furthermore, they have the associated risks of GI bleeding and renal disease, and so must be used with care.
  - *Corticosteroids*: these have a number of different indications within RA, including use as a interim agent before DMARDs take effect, or as intravenous pulses to treat severe flares in disease. Steroids may also be given intra-articularly for oligoarticular disease.
  - *Disease modifying anti-rheumatic agents (DMARDs)*: these are a diverse range of immunosuppressive therapies that slow down progression of disease as well as reducing complications (eg cardiovascular disease). Combination therapy appears to be more effective than successive monotherapies. Methotrexate-containing combinations have the strongest evidence base for their use, and therefore tend to be the first-line DMARD. More details about commonly used DMARDs are outlined in Table 5.20.
  - *Biologic agents*: there is a growing role for the use of biologic therapies in treating

Table 5.19 Causes of anaemia in rheumatoid arthritis

Mean cell volume	Explanation for anaemia
Low	Iron deficiency (eg GI bleeding secondary to NSAIDs)
Normal	Anaemia of chronic disease Felty's syndrome
High	Coexisting pernicious anaemia Folate deficiency (eg secondary to methotrexate) Haemolytic anaemia (either as a coexisting autoimmune disease, or secondary to medications, eg sulfasalazine)

RA, particularly anti-TNF-α agents such as infliximab and etanercept. The recent recognition of the role of the B cell in the pathogenesis of rheumatoid disease has meant that rituximab (a monoclonal antibody treatment targeting CD20, as found on B cells) is also used increasingly in RA. The UK National Institute for Health and Care Excellence (NICE) recommends the use of biologic agents in RA if there is active synovitis that has failed to respond to methotrexate plus at

Table 5.20 Disease-modifying anti-rheumatic drugs (DMARDs)

DMARD	Details	Side effects	Monitoring
Methotrexate	Inhibits purine metabolism, so reduces cell turnover. Patients must receive folic acid supplements	Myelotoxicity Hepatotoxicity Pneumonitis Nausea and vomiting Mouth ulcers	Chest radiograph before use Regular FBC and liver function monitoring
Sulfasalazine	The precise mechanism of action unknown	Myelotoxicity Hepatotoxicity Nausea and vomiting Mouth ulcers Transient azoospermia	Regular FBC and liver function monitoring
Azathioprine	Inhibits immune cell proliferation	Myelotoxicity Hepatotoxicity Pancreatitis Nausea and vomiting	Requires assay of TPMT levels before use Regular FBC and liver function monitoring
Leflunomide	Inhibits pyrimidine metabolism, and therefore immune cell turnover	Myelotoxicity Hepatotoxicity Diarrhoea Hypertension	Regular FBC and liver function monitoring Blood pressure monitoring
Sodium aurothiomalate (gold)	Available only as an intra-articular preparation	Myelotoxicity Skin rash/flushing ('nitritoid reaction') Mouth ulcers Proteinuria	Test dose before any regular use Monitoring of renal function/urinary protein
Ciclosporin	A calcineurin inhibitor that reduces IL-2 activity	Renal toxicity Hypertension Pancreatitis Hepatotoxicity Gingival hypertrophy	Blood pressure monitoring Therapeutic drug level monitoring

least one other DMARD. However, these are expensive agents with a number of contraindications and side effects (see Scenario 10. Crohn's disease flowchart), so should be used with great care.

Maintaining patient welfare
- Many patients will describe constitutional symptoms (particularly severe fatigue) at the onset of the condition or during disease flares; although they are not part of any diagnostic criteria or validated as a marker of disease severity, they are important to recognise because they may be severely debilitating for the patient and greatly affect day-to-day function.

- RA is associated with a significantly increased risk of cardiovascular disease; this is one of the main causes of morbidity and mortality related to the condition. As such, reversible risk factors for cardiovascular disease (eg smoking, blood pressure, lipid profile) should all be addressed as well as specific treatments for RA.

- DMARD and anti-TNF-α therapies may have a number of serious side effects and patients should be carefully counselled about these (as well as the importance of careful monitoring) before starting. The particular therapy used may depend on patient factors, eg methotrexate is teratogenic, so would be contraindicated in a young woman trying to start a family.

SCENARIO 35 SCLERODERMA

1–2 minutes

Introduce yourself

Confirm the information you've been given: This 54-year-old woman has had intermittent diarrhoea for the past year and has now lost 4 kg. Stool samples are negative and inflammatory markers normal. Her past medical history is unremarkable apart from Raynaud's phenomenon. Please assess her.

"What is the main problem from your point of view?" "I've had diarrhoea and cramping stomach pains for the last year. I was told this was irritable bowel syndrome but I'm concerned about the weight loss. I've been trying to eat more – I have a good appetite – but I've noticed food gets stuck if I don't drink lots of water and chew carefully."

5 minutes

New condition

Take a brief account of new symptoms, then closed questions to characterise the dysphagia (i.e. solids vs liquids, static or progressive, presence of pain, etc) and diarrhoea (malabsorption due to bacterial overgrowth results in frequent, watery stools). Confirm Raynaud's phenomenon (pallor → cyanosis → reactive hyperaemia) and establish duration, severity and triggers.

Screen for other involved sites, i.e. exertional dyspnoea (pulmonary fibrosis, cardiomyopathy), chest pain (ischaemic heart disease, pericarditis), joint/muscle pain (myositis, arthritis), headache (trigeminal neuralgia).

Alarm symptoms: ankle oedema (pulmonary hypertension, heart failure, renal involvement).

Investigations to date: e.g. endoscopy, barium swallow, etc.

Impact of new symptoms on daily activities: e.g. how many days off work?

Current therapy: e.g. anti-diarrhoeals, PPIs.

Pre-existing conditions associated with systemic sclerosis, e.g. hypo-/ hyperthyroidism, ischaemic heart disease, etc.

Begin a **targeted** examination of relevant area/system and continue whilst taking the history

Hands

Sclerodactyly (skin is shiny, smooth and tight).

Atrophy of finger pulps – with or without digital ulceration.

Erosive arthritis – with or without deformity.

Nail fold infarcts.

Raynaud's phenomenon.

Calcinosis.

Face (see Figure 5.12)

Beaked nose.

Perioral puckering.

Telangiectasia.

Small mouth.

Sclerosis of the frenulum, limiting tongue mobility and affecting speech.

Tight, shiny skin.

Examination of the abdomen is appropriate given the symptoms – although the examination is often normal in systemic sclerosis.

Presence/ absence of symptoms indicating involvement of other organs will determine the remainder of the examination.

Ask for blood pressure and urine dipstick to complete assessment.

CALLBACK: "You said at the beginning that the main problem was diarrhoea and weight loss. Apart from the other things we've discussed, is there anything else troubling you that we haven't covered?"

1–2 minutes

RESPOND TO PATIENT'S CONCERNS (1–2 mins)

1. Your symptoms suggest you may not be absorbing your food properly. This, together with the difficulty swallowing and the Raynaud's in your fingers, makes me suspect that you have a condition in which all of these occur together, called systemic sclerosis.
2. We will need to do a number of tests to try and confirm if you really do have this condition (ie nail capillary microscopy, auto- antibodies, chest radiograph, etc).
3. I suspect that your diarrhoea and weight loss may be caused by stagnant growth of bacteria in your gut, which is a problem associated with systemic sclerosis. We will do tests to investigate if this is the case (ie glucose breath test) and to help exclude other causes of your symptoms (ie upper and lower GI endoscopy). If this is the cause, we can treat it easily with antibiotics. We will need to do some further tests to confirm the diagnosis (CXR, nail capillary microscopy, anti-centromere antibodies).

Thank the patient

Differential diagnosis	Clinical communication skills and managing patient concerns	Physical examination and identifying physical signs	Clinical judgement and maintaining patient welfare
Pseudo-scleroderma – the collective term for a number of very rare conditions, i.e.			
Scleroderma-like syndrome – induced by environmental factors.	To be considered if there is history of exposure to dust (silica), hydrocarbons, bleomycin and/ or penicillamine.	Clinically, many of the same features of systemic sclerosis, with the distinction from systemic sclerosis only made because of history and investigation findings.	*Investigations* • Often only distinguishable from scleroderma histologically, on biopsy of skin lesions. *Management* • Treated by avoiding the precipitating factor.
Eosinophilic fasciitis: A condition associated with acute onset bilateral swelling of the extremities.	Typically triggered by trauma or severe exertion.	The condition may have many of the typical clinical features of systemic sclerosis, but also 'woody' induration of the skin. Skin changes are marked on the extremities, with the face, fingers and feet typically spared.	*Investigations* • Blood tests: Peripheral eosinophilia, hypergammaglobulinaemia and raised ESR. • Histology of skin lesions: Eosinophilic and mononuclear infiltrates. *Management* • Usually responds to systemic steroids, often combined with phototherapy. • Methotrexate and ciclosporin are reserved for resistant cases.
Scleromyxoedema: A condition associated with raised smooth skin on the face, limbs and trunk.	This condition has an association with multiple myeloma.	Clinically, may have many typical features of systemic sclerosis, but Raynaud's phenomenon is **not** found. In addition, patients often exhibit firm, smooth papules on limbs, the trunk and face.	*Investigations* • Blood tests: Often will detect paraproteinaemia on serum electrophoresis. • Histology of skin lesions: Mucin in the papillary dermis is typical. *Management* • Plasmapheresis and cyclophosphamide will reduce progression of the condition.
Premature aging syndromes – e.g. acrogeria, progeria.		Patients may have clinical features of systemic sclerosis, but also other soft tissue/musculoskeletal features that help distinguish the condition, e.g in progeria, the presence of prematurely wrinkled skin, alopecia and growth retardation.	*Investigations* • Often diagnoses of exclusion. *Management* • Treatment is often supportive only.

(continued)

Differential diagnosis	Clinical communication skills and managing patient concerns	Physical examination and identifying physical signs	Clinical judgement and maintaining patient welfare
Raynaud's disease	This is a condition where – in response to exposure to particular triggers – digits become first pale, then blue, then red. When the trigger is removed, digits become painful, numb and burning as blood returns to the hands. This reflects peripheral vasospasm. Classical triggers include cold, vibrating tools, emotion, and medications (e.g. beta-blocker, oral contraceptive pill, etc).	*Raynaud's disease* must be distinguished from *Raynaud's phenomenon*. The latter has the same principle clinical feature as Raynaud's disease, but certain other distinguishing features too • Raynaud's phenomenon is associated with a number of other autoimmune diseases (systemic sclerosis, SLE, rheumatoid arthritis, etc.), features of which may be present on clinical assessment. Clinically, this may be suggested by dilated nail fold capillaries, which are not typically present in Raynaud's disease. • Raynaud's phenomenon may be asymmetric, whilst Raynaud's disease is almost always symmetrical. • Raynaud's phenomenon may over time lead to digital necrosis, but this is not a finding in Raynaud's disease. Raynaud's disease may be diagnosed if typical clinical features are present for three months in the absence of any clinical conditions with an association with Raynaud's phenomenon.	*Investigations* • Diagnosed clinically. *Management* • General measures: Hand-warming with gloves, smoking cessation, avoiding any precipitating medications. • Pharmacological – this is principally calcium channel antagonists, with nifedipine the agent typically used. Nebulised iloprost may also be of efficacy. • Surgical – dorsal sympathectomy may be indicated in severe cases.

Clinical judgement and maintaining patient welfare

Scleroderma is an uncommon disorder, but one that appears commonly in MRCP (PACES). The condition is autoimmune in nature, and characterised by collagen deposition in the skin and other organs. It has a highly variable phenotype dependent on the organs affected. Scleroderma is more common in women than men and tends to first present in young or middle-aged people. It is a rare disorder, with the annual incidence of systemic forms in the UK of 2 per million.

Clinical features

The term 'scleroderma' encompasses a number of diverse disorders, all of which feature sclerotic skin lesions. Several different classifications are used, but the simplest of these is into either *localised* or *systemic* sclerodermic disease

- Localised: disease confined to the skin. This may be subdivided into *linear scleroderma* (where sclerotic skin lesions are confined to a limb, the face or scalp, often in a dermatomal distribution) and *morphoea* (either localised or generalised sclerotic skin lesions).
- Systemic: also known as *systemic sclerosis,* this is where disease involves internal

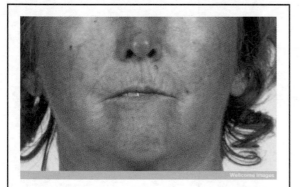

Figure 5.12 Scleroderma facies

organs as well as the skin. This category is often subdivided into a number of smaller categories, the best established of which are *diffuse cutaneous systemic sclerosis (DCSS)* and *limited cutaneous systemic sclerosis (LCSS)*, as described in more detail in Table 5.21.

Diagnostic criteria for systemic sclerosis were devised by the American College of Rheumatology in 1980. These have >95% sensitivity and specificity for histological corroboration. The diagnosis may be made in the presence of either the major criterion itself, or at least two of the three minor criteria. These are

- **Major** criterion
  - Truncal (proximal) skin sclerosis
- **Minor** criteria
  - Sclerodactyly
  - Digital pitting scars, or finger pulp loss
  - Bilateral pulmonary fibrosis.

In addition to these original criteria, two further minor criteria are also commonly acknowledged, namely abnormal nail capillary microscopy and positive anti-centromere antibody.

The flowchart summarises the features of systemic sclerosis on the skin and soft tissues. Table 5.22 outlines some of the manifestations of systemic sclerosis on major organ systems, and their effect on survival.

Overall, it is estimated that patients with systemic sclerosis have a 4.6-fold increased risk of death compared with unaffected individuals. In one Swedish study, 5- and 10-year survival rates were 86% and 69%, respectively. The main causes of death are cardiopulmonary or renal disease. Poor prognostic factors include

- Male gender
- Truncal skin disease
- Internal organ involvement
- Proteinuria
- Low CO diffusion capacity
- High ESR.

Table 5.21 Classification of systemic sclerosis

	Limited cutaneous systemic sclerosis	Diffuse cutaneous systemic sclerosis
Degree of skin and soft-tissue involvement	Only acral skin involvement (ie face, hands, forearms, feet) Rarely tendon involvement	Truncal and acral skin involvement Often tendon friction rubs
Raynaud's phenomenon	Raynaud's phenomenon typically for years before other features of disease	Raynaud's phenomenon typically occurs only at the same time as onset of other features of disease
Degree of organ involvement	Organ involvement often late in disease course Previously described as CREST syndrome (ie calcinosis, Raynaud's phenomenon, oesophageal dysmotility, sclerodactyly, telangiectasia) Also respiratory disease – particularly pulmonary hypertension (approximately 10%), rarely interstitial lung disease Rarely renal disease	Organ involvement often early in disease course Often extensive cardiac, respiratory, gastrointestinal and renal disease Respiratory disease most likely to be interstitial lung disease; only rarely pulmonary hypertension
Antibody profile	Anti-centromere antibody detected in about 70% Anti-PM-Scl and anti-Scl-70 antibodies detected in about 10%	Anti-Scl-70 antibody detected in about 30% Anti-RNA polymerase antibodies detected in about 10%

Investigations
- Laboratory tests
  - Haematology: ESR is raised in active disease.
  - Biochemistry: serum creatinine and urine dipstick/urinary protein:creatinine ratio will give a measure of the degree of renal disease.
  - Immunology: anti-centromere antibody is associated with LCSS, whereas anti-Scl 70 (also known as anti-DNA topoisomerase I) antibody and anti-RNA polymerase I, II and III antibodies are associated with DCSS.
- Other tests: these will depend on the exact balance of organ involvement, but include
  - Cardiac disease: ECG and echocardiogram will establish if there is arrhythmia, cardiomyopathy or evidence of pulmonary hypertension.
  - Respiratory disease: chest radiograph, pulmonary function tests and high-resolution CT will identify pulmonary fibrosis.
  - Renal disease: renal biopsy will confirm systemic sclerosis-related renal disease.
  - Gastrointestinal disease: a glucose breath test will help to confirm small bowel bacterial overgrowth.

Management
Management options for systemic sclerosis vary depending on the organs involved in the disease progress. Options include

Table 5.22 Manifestations of systemic sclerosis

System involved	Common manifestations	Prevalence in systemic sclerosis (%)	Survival impact
Gastrointestinal	Oesophageal dysmotility: associated with dysphagia and reflux-like symptoms Small bowel bacterial overgrowth/malabsorption Colonic diverticula Association with primary biliary cirrhosis	~80	Minimal
Respiratory	Pulmonary fibrosis Pulmonary hypertension Pleural calcification and effusions Bronchoalveolar carcinoma	40–80	Pulmonary hypertension reduces 5-year rate survival by ~40%
Cardiac	Accelerated ischaemic heart disease Pericarditis Myocardial fibrosis: may result in restrictive cardiomyopathy and arrhythmias	20–25	Reduces 5-year rate survival by ~20%
Renal	Sclerodermal renal disease (onion-skin hypertrophy of glomerular arteries): may result in severe glomerulonephritis and accelerated hypertension	~20	Reduces 5-year survival rate by ~80% untreated, 40% treated
Musculoskeletal	Myositis Arthritis: may resemble rheumatoid disease	15–20	Minimal
Neurological	Trigeminal neuralgia Carpal tunnel syndrome	~5	Minimal

- Raynaud's phenomenon
  - General measures: smoking cessation and hand warmers will help reduce frequency and severity of attacks.
  - Calcium channel antagonists: these inhibit endothelial smooth muscle contraction and have an anti-platelet aggregation effect. They reduce the frequency and severity of Raynaud's phenomenon attacks and the number of digital ulcerations after 6 weeks of therapy in double-blind RCTs.
  - Prostacyclin analogues (eg iloprost): when given as an intravenous infusion over 5–10 days, these have a beneficial effect on Raynaud's phenomenon for several weeks.
  - ACE inhibitors/angiotensin II receptor agonists: these reduce the severity and frequency of Raynaud's phenomenon attacks.
  - α-Receptor blockers: induce vasodilatation, but only relieve Raynaud's phenomenon at high doses (thus leading to orthostatic hypotension).
  - Pentoxifylline: reduces digital infarction, but does not reduce the frequency of attacks.
- Renal involvement
  - ACE inhibitors: these are the treatment of choice for renal failure or hypertension associated with systemic sclerosis.
- Respiratory disease
  - Immunosuppression: cyclophosphamide and prednisolone appear to slow down the progression of systemic sclerosis-associated pulmonary fibrosis.
  - Bosentan: this is an endothelin-receptor antagonist that appears to be of benefit in both primary and scleroderma-associated pulmonary hypertension. Traditional therapies such as iloprost infusion are also beneficial.
- Gastrointestinal disease
  - Prokinetics (eg metoclopramide): useful for treating bowel dysmotility.
  - Proton pump inhibitors: useful for treating reflux-like symptoms.
  - Antibiotics: for small bowel bacterial overgrowth.
- Skin sclerosis
  - Benzylpenicillin/D-penicillamine: both these agents probably improve skin softening, but side effects are common, and their efficacy has yet to be proven in large RCTs.
  - Methotrexate: may possibly be of benefit in improving skin sclerosis.

Maintaining patient welfare

- The multisystemic nature of the condition means that patients will require input from a number of different sources. As well as doctors from different specialties, patients will also gain benefit from a number of allied health professionals, eg physiotherapists and occupational therapists, when myositis/arthritis is a dominant factor in their condition.
- As scleroderma is an unusual disorder, many patients will not have heard of the condition at the time of diagnosis. Patients may gain benefit from input from a support group, such as the Scleroderma Society in the UK (see below).

Resources

The Scleroderma Society:
  www.sclerodermasociety.co.uk

SCENARIO 36. SYSTEMIC LUPUS ERYTHEMATOSUS

1–2 minutes

Introduce yourself

Confirm the information you've been given and patient details: this 37-year-old woman presents with a rash on her face. Please assess her.

'What is the main problem from your point of view?' 'I have developed a rash on my face over the last few weeks that looks like I have been sunburnt.'

5 minutes

New condition

Focused history of the presenting complaint and relevant systems enquiry: differentiate the cause of a facial rash, eg palpitations, dizziness, shortness of breath (malar rash of mitral stenosis); paroxysmal flushing, diarrhoea and wheeze (carcinoid syndrome); pustules and flushing (acne rosacea); association with starting ACE inhibitors, ciprofloxacin or isoniazid (drug eruption); pregnancy (chloasma). Establish if there is a history of contact dermatitis or psoriasis

Identify alarm symptoms: easy bruising (thrombocytopenia), arthralgia, chest pain (myo-/pericarditis), pleurisy and dyspnoea (pleural effusion), personality change (psychosis), weakness/paraesthesia (CNS involvement), history of thrombosis/recurrent miscarriage (anti-phospholipid syndrome)

Social/occupational/family circumstances: how do the symptoms affect the patient's daily activities?

Drug history: especially if drug-induced lupus is suspected (isoniazid, hydralazine, phenytoin, etc). **DRUG ALLERGIES**

Other medical conditions: connective tissue disorders, pre-existing skin disorders

Begin a **targeted** examination of relevant area/system and continue while taking the history

General appearance: pale (anaemia), alopecia, purpura, photosensitive rash in sun-exposed regions, livedo reticularis (particularly legs)

Face: oral ulcers, scaly maculopapular malar rash in 'butterfly' distribution that spares nasolabial folds

Hands/nails: nail-fold infarcts, Raynaud's phenomenon, palmar erythema

Cardiac: pericardial rub (pericarditis), cardiac murmurs (sterile (Libman–Sacks) endocarditis). *Exclude* opening snap ± mid-diastolic murmur (mitral stenosis)

Chest: stony dullness to percussion (pleural effusion), fine late inspiratory crackles of interstitial lung disease

Locomotor: arthritis, including symmetrical non-erosive polyarthritis involving MCP and PIP joints in the hands (Jaccoud's arthropathy). Look for arthritis with effusions in large joints

CNS: if history suggests focal neurological signs

Ask to check blood pressure and do a urine dipstick (looking for microscopic haematuria ± proteinuria)

CALLBACK: 'You said at the beginning that the main problem was a rash on your face. Is there anything else troubling you that we haven't covered?

1–2 minutes

RESPOND TO PATIENT'S CONCERNS (1–2 min)

1. I think the cause of your rash is a condition called systemic lupus erythematous, which is a disorder of the immune system that can affect many parts of your body
2. For your facial rash it is very important to apply sunblock, because without this the rash may get worse. However, we need to confirm the diagnosis and ensure that no other parts of your body are affected before more specific treatments can be started
3. To investigate further, I need to perform blood tests (eg FBCs, U+Es, LFTs, CRP, ESR, ANAs, dsDNA, complement, thrombophilia screen) and take a sample of your urine. Once we confirm the diagnosis, you may be started on medications such as steroids or hydroxychloroquine to treat the underlying condition

Thank the patient

Differential diagnosis	Clinical communication skills and managing patient concerns	Physical examination and identifying physical signs	Clinical judgement and maintaining patient welfare
Eczema	A history of isolated skin disease without systemic symptoms (see Scenario 14. Eczema flowchart)	A number of different forms of eczema may mimic the skin changes of SLE, including atopic eczema, contact dermatitis and seborrhoeic dermatitis; see Scenario 14. Eczema flowchart	
Psoriasis	See Scenario 30. Psoriasis flowchart		
Chloasma	See Scenario 39. Vitiligo differential diagnosis table		
Rosacea	See Scenario 12. Dermatomyositis differential diagnosis table		
Dermatomyositis	See Scenario 12. Dermatomyositis flowchart		
Carcinoid syndrome	Patients typically report diarrhoea, palpitations, symptomatic flushing, abdominal pain and wheeze (see Scenario 10. Crohn's disease flowchart)	The facial flushing of carcinoid syndrome may be confused with the skin changes of SLE; see full details in Scenario 19. Hereditary haemorrhagic telangiectasia differential diagnosis table	
Mitral stenosis	See Station 3	Severe mitral stenosis may be associated with a 'malar flush' which may mimic the malar rash of SLE	

Clinical judgement and maintaining patient welfare

Patients with systemic lupus erythematosus (SLE) commonly appear in Station 5 of the MRCP (PACES). SLE is a disorder that particularly affects African–Caribbean women (female:male ratio 9:1) and tends to present first at a young age. The condition has a complex autoimmune basis with no obvious trigger identified in most cases. However, exposure to certain drugs is the precipitant in certain patients, who are described as having *drug-induced lupus*. Such drugs include

- Antibiotics, eg isoniazid, tetracyclines
- Cardiovascular medications, eg procainamide, hydralazine, methyldopa

- Neurological/psychiatric medications, eg chlorpromazine, phenytoin.

Furthermore, certain medications (particularly sulfonamides and the oral contraceptive pill) may worsen SLE without directly triggering the onset of the condition.

Clinical features

SLE is a multisystem disorder with a huge variety of possible presentations, as outlined in the flowchart. There have been various attempts to establish diagnostic criteria – the ACR Criteria for Classification of Systemic Lupus Erythematosus (1997) provide a useful summary of clinical features (Table 5.23).

Table 5.23 Classification of systemic lupus erythematosus

Criterion	Details
Malar rash	Fixed erythema, flat or raised, over the malar eminences, tending to spare the nasolabial folds
Discoid rash	Erythematous raised patches with adherent keratotic scaling and follicular plugging; atrophic scarring may occur in older lesions
Photosensitive rash	Rash as a result of unusual reaction to sunlight, by patient history or physician observation
Oral ulceration	Oral or nasopharyngeal ulceration, usually painless, observed by physician
Arthritis	Non-erosive arthritis involving two or more peripheral joints, characterised by tenderness, swelling or effusion
Serositis	This may be either of the following Pleuritis: convincing history of pleuritic pain, rub heard by a physician or evidence of pleural effusion, *or* Pericarditis: documented by ECG, rub or evidence of pericardial effusion
Renal involvement	This may be either of the following Persistent proteinuria >0.5 g/day, or >3+ if quantitation not performed, *or* Cellular casts: may be red cell, haemoglobin, granular, tubular or mixed

(*continued*)

Table 5.23 (*continued*)

Criterion	Details
Neurological involvement	This may be seizures *or* psychosis, occurring in the absence of offending drugs or known metabolic derangements, eg uraemia, ketoacidosis or electrolyte imbalance
Haematological involvement	This may be any of the following Haemolytic anaemia: with reticulocytosis, *or* Leukopenia: <4000/mm^3 total on two or more occasions, *or* Lymphopenia: <1500/mm^3 on two or more occasions, *or* Thrombocytopenia: <100 000/mm^3 in the absence of offending drugs
Immunological involvement	This may be any of the following Anti-DNA antibody in abnormal titre, *or* Anti-Sm antibody, *or* Positive anti-phospholipid antibody on • An abnormal serum level of IgG or IgM anti-cardiolipin antibodies • A positive test result for lupus anticoagulant using a standard method • A false-positive test result for at least 6 months confirmed by *Treponema pallidum* immobilisation or fluorescent treponemal antibody absorption test (FTA-Abs)
Antinuclear antibody	An abnormal titre of ANA by immunofluorescence or an equivalent assay at any point in time, and in the absence of drugs known to be associated with the 'drug-induced lupus' syndrome

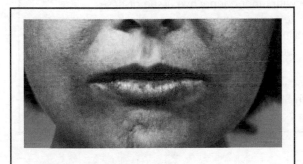

Figure 5.13 Facial rash in SLE

Formally, 4 of the 11 criteria must be present (although not necessarily at the same time) for a diagnosis of SLE to be made. However, active lupus disease is often predominantly characterised by constitutional symptoms that are not found within the ACR diagnostic criteria, eg fever, fatigue, unintentional weight loss.

Investigation
• Laboratory investigations: these are summarised in Table 5.24.
• Cardiological, respiratory and neurological investigations
  • An ECG may demonstrate arrhythmia where there is heart muscle involvement. An echocardiogram may demonstrate pericardial effusion in lupus pericarditis, and/or valvular thickening in the form of sterile endocarditis (Libman–Sacks endocarditis).
  • A chest radiograph and/or CT of the chest

Table 5.24 Laboratory investigations for SLE

Category	Details
Haematology	FBC may show the normocytic/normochromic anaemia of chronic disease, or a macrocytic anaemia associated with haemolysis. There may also be leukopenia and/or thrombocytopenia ESR raised in active disease
Biochemistry	Serum creatinine elevated and variable degrees of urinary blood and protein where there is renal involvement Although ESR is raised in active disease, CRP tends not to be elevated unless there is significant serositis and/or intercurrent infection
Immunology	Complement factors C3 and C4 are consumed in active disease, and are in reduced levels in serum; the complement degradation product C3d is increased Autoantibodies: these include • Antinuclear antibody (ANA): this is a screening test with a sensitivity of 95%, but is not itself diagnostic in the absence of clinical features. ANA is non-specific, and also present in many patients with systemic autoimmune conditions, eg scleroderma, Sjögren's syndrome • Anti-double-stranded DNA (anti-dsDNA) antibody: an antibody with high specificity for SLE, but sensitivity of only approximately 70%. An increased titre of this antibody reflects increased disease activity • Anti-Sm antibody: this is the most specific antibody, but its sensitivity is only approximately 30–40% • Anti-SSA (Ro) or anti-SSB (La) antibodies: these are present in approximately 15% of patients with SLE, as well as those with other connective tissue diseases • Anti-RNP antibody: this may indicate mixed connective tissue disease, with overlap of SLE, systemic sclerosis and myositis • Anti-histone antibodies: these are detectable in the vast majority of patients with drug-induced lupus • Anti-phospholipid antibodies: anti-cardiolipin antibodies and lupus anticoagulant should be checked in patients with SLE, because they are associated with anti-phospholipid syndrome (APS)

may be required where respiratory complications of SLE (including pleural effusions and interstitial lung disease) are suspected.

• Neuroimaging (eg MRI of the brain) is of use where a neuropsychiatric manifestation of SLE is suspected.

• Histology
    • Skin biopsy: biopsy of affected skin lesions is useful in cases of diagnostic uncertainty.
    • Renal biopsy: this is merited in suspected lupus nephritis to establish the degree of renal involvement.

Management

The management of SLE is multidisciplinary. Management includes

- **General measures**
  - Patient education.
  - Minimise exacerbating factors, ie remove precipitating medications in presumed drug-induced lupus.
  - Avoiding excessive sunlight, ie use of sunscreen, hats and long sleeves to minimise progression of the photosensitive rash.
  - Physiotherapy and occupational therapy: useful to aid mobility and help patient to return to normal functional abilities where they have been affected by arthritis.
  - Cardiovascular optimisation: even in the absence of overt cardiac and/or renal disease, SLE is associated with accelerated rates of ischaemic heart disease (this remains the major cause of death in patients with SLE). As such, assessment for and management of other risk factors for cardiovascular disease (including blood pressure and cholesterol control, smoking cessation advice, etc) is crucial.
- **Pharmacological**
  - Analgesics: NSAIDs have particular efficacy for tackling the pain and inflammation associated with arthritis and serositis, but may worsen lupus nephritis.
  - Antimalarials (eg hydroxychloroquine): particularly useful for treating the skin disease associated with lupus. A potential complication of using antimalarials is retinopathy; patients should have a baseline visual assessment, with subsequent reviews at regular intervals.
  - Corticosteroids: these may be used topically (for skin disease), orally (to treat systemic disease, eg arthritis) or intravenously (eg pulsed methylprednisolone for treatment of flares of lupus nephritis).
- Immunosuppressants: agents including cyclophosphamide, azathioprine, mycophenolate mofetil and monoclonal antibody therapies (eg rituximab) may all be used in severe systemic disease.
- **Other**
  - Intravenous immunoglobulin may be used in resistant lupus, especially where concomitant infection makes immunosuppression risky.
  - Autologous stem cell transplantation is a therapeutic option in very severe disease; the treatment-related mortality rate has now fallen to <5%, with a 5-year survival rate of >80%.
  - Other specific treatments will depend on the exact clinical features of disease, eg renal replacement therapy and/or transplantation is indicated for patients with end-stage renal failure secondary to lupus nephritis.

Maintaining patient welfare

- SLE has an unpredictable nature, and may suddenly cause patients considerable disability after long periods of quiescence. The pharmacological treatments available are effective, but may have significant side effects.
- Candidates will be expected to demonstrate awareness that lupus is not a condition just to be managed pharmacologically – the potential input that may be provided by physiotherapists, occupational therapists, social workers (eg for patients requiring disability benefit) and even psychological support will be expected to be highlighted if relevant. Patients may derive benefit from a support group, such as Lupus UK.

Resources

Lupus UK: www.lupusuk.org.uk

SCENARIO 37 TREMOR

Introduce yourself

Confirm the information you've been given and patient details: this 60-year-old man presents with difficulty writing and a tremor. Please assess him.

'What is the main problem from your point of view?' 'Over the last few months, I have developed a tremor in my right hand, and my writing has become like a scrawl. The only thing that seems to help it is having a beer or two.'

New condition

Focused history of the presenting complaint and relevant systems enquiry

Detailed history of the tremor: at rest, postural or related to action? Which part of the body affected: uni- or bilateral? Exacerbating/relieving factors (eg alcohol)? Any sign of rigidity or slow movements, either by patient or by others? Any effect on handwriting? Any sensorimotor deficit? Any suggestion of cerebellar features (eg uncoordinated movements)? Any features of confusion and/or hallucinations (as in Lewy body dementia)? Any features of thyroid disease?

Identify alarm symptoms: symptoms of Parkinson's disease

Pre-existing conditions/risk factors: recreational drug use, change in regular medications, known thyroid disease, relevant family history

Social/occupational/family circumstances: impact on job if driving, or if job dependent on fine motor skills. Any alcohol history? Any features suggestive of anxiety disorder?

Drug history: including salbutamol, antipsychotics, anticonvulsants, lithium, thyroid medications, steroids. **DRUG ALLERGIES**

Other medical conditions: further screen for relevant symptoms, eg symptoms of liver disease in suspected Wilson's disease; heat intolerance in suspected thyrotoxicosis

Begin a **targeted** examination of relevant area/system and continue while taking the history

General appearance: expressionless facies

Nature of tremor: assess whether uni- or bilateral, present at rest and affected by movement. Does it only occur while holding a fixed posture, as in postural tremor?

Check handwriting: any micrographia, as in Parkinson's disease? If present, assess for cogwheel rigidity and bradykinesia (eg ask patient to open and close hands quickly)

Cerebellar features: assess to see 'past pointing', as in intention tremor. Assess for other cerebellar features, including dysdiadochokinesis

Eye movements: nystagmus in cerebellar disease; upgaze palsy in progressive supranuclear palsy

Check speech: monotone and quiet? Dysarthria?

Check gait: postural instability, stooped with a hesitant, shuffling, narrow-based gait with reduced arm swing in Parkinson's disease; negative Romberg's test with broad-based gait and impaired heel–toe walking in cerebellar disease

If suspected thyroid disease, eg goitre, eye signs?

If suspected Wilson's disease: evidence of chronic liver disease?

CALLBACK: 'You said at the beginning that the main problem was difficulty writing and a tremor. Is there anything else troubling you that we haven't covered?'

RESPOND TO PATIENT'S CONCERNS (1–2 min)

1. I think your tremor and difficulty writing may be due to a condition called benign essential tremor. I do not think this is Parkinson's disease
2. The best way to treat this condition is with some medication called β blockers
3. Although I am sure that this is the diagnosis, I would like to check your thyroid gland function with a blood test, because problems with this can give similar features. I am also keen for you to reduce your alcohol intake even though I know that this helps your tremor because the β blockers will now assist with this

Thank the patient

1–2 minutes

5 minutes

1–2 minutes

Differential diagnosis	Clinical communication skills and managing patient concerns	Physical examination and identifying physical signs	Clinical judgement and maintaining patient welfare
Neurological/psychiatric disorders			
Parkinson's disease and Lewy body dementia	See Station 3, Neurological, Scenario 2		
'Parkinson's +' conditions	See Station 3, Neurological, Scenario 2		
Cerebellar syndrome	See Station 3, Neurological, Scenario 2		
Anxiety disorders	A history of panic attacks, palpitations, shortness of breath unrelated to activity, peripheral paraesthesiae, previous depression, use of alcohol to suppress symptoms	Anxiety disorders may give an exaggerated physiological tremor	CBT is the mainstay of therapy, with benzodiazepines delivering diminishing returns with extended use

(*continued*)

Differential diagnosis	Clinical communication skills and managing patient concerns	Physical examination and identifying physical signs	Clinical judgement and maintaining patient welfare
Endocrine and metabolic disorders			
Wilson's disease A rare autosomal recessive disorder associated with excessive copper deposition in the nervous system and liver. It is caused through mutations in the *ATP7B* gene that encodes a copper-transporting ATPase	Neuropsychiatric disease usually precedes liver disease	Clinical features include: Neuropsychiatric disease: often the first features in older children/adults. Features may be those of movement disorder (tremor and other parkinsonian features, dystonia, dysarthria, ataxia, etc) or of psychiatric disease (memory loss, emotional lability, learning disability, etc) Liver disease: often the first features in children. May present with acute liver failure, or features of decompensated chronic liver disease (encephalopathy, jaundice, ascites, variceal bleed, etc) Eyes: Kayser–Fleischer rings are often seen only on slit-lamp examination; these represent copper deposition at Descemet's membrane	*Investigations* Blood and urine: serum copper and ceruloplasmin are reduced, whereas 24-hour urinary copper excretion is increased. Genetic studies may be used to confirm the presence of an *ATP7B* mutation MR of the brain: typically demonstrates atrophy, particularly of the basal ganglia Liver biopsy: increased copper deposition with a variable degree of liver fibrosis *Management* Medical therapies: low copper diet and copper chelation, usually with penicillamine Surgical: liver transplantation in advanced chronic liver disease Genetic counselling/screening
Thyrotoxicosis	See Scenario 17. Graves' disease flowchart		
Hypoglycaemia	The history should establish risk factors for this condition, including diabetes mellitus, use of insulin/oral hypoglycaemic agents, alcohol excess, endocrine disorders (including Addison's and pituitary diseases) and liver disease	Cognitive impairment can develop with repeated episodes of hypoglycaemia but there are no specific clinical signs	During hypoglycaemic episodes, measure plasma glucose, insulin, C-peptide, proinsulin and β-hydroxybutyrate concentrations and screen for oral hypoglycaemic agents Test glucose response to intravenous injection of 1.0 mg glucagon This will distinguish hypoglycaemia caused by endogenous or exogenous insulin from other mechanisms Management: patients may need to carry glucagon (for intramuscular injection) which can be administered if they are unable to take oral carbohydrate when neuroglycopenic

(continued)

Differential diagnosis	Clinical communication skills and managing patient concerns	Physical examination and identifying physical signs	Clinical judgement and maintaining patient welfare
Drugs and toxins			
Alcohol withdrawal	This should be established from the history, and suspected in any case of unexplained rest tremor	The relatively fine tremor of withdrawal should be carefully distinguished from a liver flap and the intention tremor of alcohol-induced cerebellar atrophy. All three may occur together	Chlordiazepoxide is still the mainstay of therapy for withdrawal but this should not be initiated for tremor alone. Gradated alcohol reduction is the current recommended means of alcohol cessation. If the tremor persists after prolonged abstinence cerebellar atrophy may be the cause
Medications: these include: Endocrine medications: excessive thyroxine, corticosteroids, etc Respiratory medications: salbutamol, theophylline, etc Anticonvulsants: phenytoin, sodium valproate, etc Antiemetics: metoclopramide Psychiatric medications: haloperidol, chlorpromazine, lithium Recreational drugs: cocaine, amphetamines	Culprit medications may be established from the history. A detailed history of duration and compliance is key	Fine tremor: β_2 agonists, thyroxine, corticosteroids, theophyllines, lithium, tacrolimus, ciclosporin Associated extrapyramidal signs: antipsychotics	Cessation of suspected culprit medications is usually adequate for diagnosis and treatment
Toxins: including organophosphates and heavy metals (eg mercury)	Tremor is rarely the only symptom; patients will have a history of general deterioration after exposure to insecticides, anthelmintics, herbicides or heavy-metal compounds	Clinical signs vary by toxin but tremor, seizures, slurred speech and anxiety are common themes	The diagnosis is often missed due to inexperience with toxicological conditions in the general medical setting. A high index of suspicion and early liaison with toxicology centres are key

Clinical judgement and maintaining patient welfare

Assessing a patient with tremor may be difficult, because there are a large number of different possible explanations. However, a careful, focused history and examination will often find clues to the underlying aetiology, and will help quickly to narrow the differential diagnosis.

Clinical features

It should be possible from simple questions in the history and a focused examination alone to make the key distinction of category of tremor, ie

- *Postural tremor:* tremor occurring while in a fixed posture, such as found in benign essential tremor, or an exaggerated physiological tremor (eg in anxiety disorders)
- *Rest tremor:* as found in extrapyramidal conditions, eg Parkinson's disease
- *Intention tremor:* as found in cerebellar disease (eg multiple sclerosis).

There are a number of particularly useful questions in the history. One would be about exacerbating and relieving factors; alcohol classically relieves benign essential tremor, whereas exaggerated physiological tremors tend to be exacerbated by anxiety and caffeine. Conversely, patients with alcohol dependence who are beginning to withdraw may describe a rest tremor. It is also important to ask about other relevant medical conditions, eg psychiatric illness may be a feature of Wilson's disease, and bipolar disorder may be treated with antipsychotics, anticonvulsants and lithium, which are all associated with tremor.

Although the major aim of the examination is to establish the nature of the tremor, it may be relevant to extend the assessment beyond the neurological system in trying to establish the aetiology, eg tremor may be a presenting feature of thyrotoxicosis, and examining for other features of the condition (goitre, etc) may be crucial to confirming the diagnosis. Assessment of handwriting may also be useful; patients with Parkinson's disease typically display micrographia, whereas those with benign essential tremor notice that handwriting tends to become poorly legible.

Investigations

Many cases of tremor are diagnosed clinically, such as benign essential tremor as in the scenario here. However, relevant investigations may include

- **Blood tests**
  - Thyroid function tests if suspected thyrotoxicosis and plasma glucose in suspected hypoglycaemia. Liver function tests, clotting profile and copper studies (see differential diagnosis table) are relevant if Wilson's disease is suspected. Assays of drug levels (eg lithium, tacrolimus levels) may be appropriate in cases of suspected drug toxicity.
- **Urinalysis**
  - Urinary copper studies are relevant in suspected Wilson's disease (see differential diagnosis table).
  - Toxicology screen in suspected poisoning.
- **Neuroimaging**
  - Either CT or MR of the brain may be relevant if a structural cause of tremor is suspected (eg demyelinating disease or a space-occupying lesion causing a cerebellar syndrome).
  - Although neuroimaging in itself cannot establish the diagnosis of Parkinson's disease, some centres will use radioactive dopamine transporter (DAT) scans where the diagnosis is suspected; typical findings are of an asymmetrical loss of presynaptic dopaminergic receptors.

Management

This depends on the underlying disorder. In the case of benign essential tremor, the major therapeutic options are pharmacological, with β blockers and anticonvulsants (typically primidone) being the mainstay of treatment. Although alcohol may help in reducing the tremor, patients should be carefully counselled about the medical and psychosocial risks of excessive alcohol use.

Maintaining patient welfare

- Benign essential tremor is rarely benign and can have a devastating effect on a patient's function. As well as pharmacological treatment, candidates should demonstrate an appreciation of the potential importance of physiotherapy, occupational therapy and psychological support among other services in providing assistance to the patient. A support group may be useful, such as the UK National Tremor Foundation (see below).

- The tremor may mean that the patient cannot continue in the same job and may no longer be able to drive, so candidates should appreciate that patients may be eligible for disability benefits and may have to inform the DVLA about their diagnosis.

Resources

National Tremor Foundation: www.tremor.org.uk

SCENARIO 38 TURNER SYNDROME

1–2 minutes

Introduce yourself

Confirm the information you've been given and patient details: this 17-year-old young woman has presented to outpatients with primary amenorrhoea, hypertension and short stature. Please assess her.

'What is the main problem from your point of view?' 'I have not started with periods yet and my doctor has also told me that I have high blood pressure.'

5 minutes

New condition

Focused history of the presenting complaint and relevant systems enquiry: the combination of short stature, hypertension and primary amenorrhoea would suggest Turner's syndrome

Consider different causes of primary amenorrhoea (ie gonadal dysgenesis, approximately 50%; hypothalamic hypogonadism approximately 20%; structural abnormality/absence of female reproductive system approximately 20%; other defects approximately 10%)

Differentiate causes of hypertension: cardiac (previous surgery for coarctation of aorta, bicuspid aortic valve), renal disease (horseshoe kidneys), endocrine

Social/occupational/family circumstances: difficulty forming friendships due to failure of secondary sexual characteristics, and learning disability/developmental delay

Drug history: antihypertensives, hormone replacement therapy. **DRUG ALLERGIES**

Other medical conditions: previous cardiac surgery, known renal disease

---

Begin a **targeted** examination of relevant area/system and continue while taking the history

General appearance: short stature (100%)

Lymph: lymphoedema – puffiness over the fingers and toes may be all that remains in adulthood (80%)

Ear: anomalous auricles (>80%), otitis media in childhood (40%)

Facies: narrow maxilla and/or high arched palate (80%), small, wide mandible (70%), inner canthal folds (40%), ptosis (16%)

Neck: low posterior hairline, short neck (80%), webbed posterior neck (50%), goitre (Hashimoto's thyroiditis in up to 30%)

Cardiac: hypertension (25%, increasing with age), bicuspid aortic valve (10%) or coarctation of the aorta (15%) – four times more common in patients with webbing of the neck

Chest: 'shield chest' with widely spaced nipples (these may be hypoplastic, inverted or both), often pectus excavatum (80%)

Extremities: cubitus valgus or other deformity at elbow (70%), knee anomalies, eg medial tibial exostosis (60%), short fourth metacarpal and/or metatarsal (50%), scars from surgery for fractures (increased risk of osteoporosis)

Nails: narrow, hypoplastic and/or hyperconvex and/or deep set nails (70%). Look for fingerprick marks of BM testing (significantly increased risk of diabetes)

Skin: excessive pigmented naevi (50%), distal palmar axial triradii (40%) and loose skin (especially around the neck in infancy)

CNS: hearing loss (50%)

CALLBACK: 'You said at the beginning that the main problem was a delay in your periods starting and high blood pressure. Is there anything else troubling you that we haven't covered?'

1–2 minutes

RESPOND TO PATIENT'S CONCERNS (1–2 min)

1. I think you have a condition called Turner's syndrome. This can affect your periods and blood pressure, among other things. It is a condition caused by lacking one copy of something called the X chromosome, which is a collection of different genes that should be within every cell of the body
2. I will need to refer you to a hormone specialist because you will require hormone replacement. I will also refer you to a genetics specialist
3. The diagnosis is confirmed by doing a genetic test called karyotyping, which involves a simple blood test. Other investigations include blood tests and scans assessing the degree of function of your pituitary gland and ovaries to see how well developed they are. You will also need investigation into your heart and kidneys, which can be affected in Turner's syndrome, and this could also affect your blood pressure

Thank the patient

Differential diagnosis	Clinical communication skills and managing patient concerns	Physical examination and identifying physical signs	Clinical judgement and maintaining patient welfare
Fragile X syndrome A genetic condition caused through expansion of a trinucleotide repeat (CGG) that is associated with the expression of the fragile X mental retardation 1 (*FMR1*) gene on the X chromosome. This is a gene with a protein product that has a number of roles in neurodevelopment	A history of learning disability and developmental delay, particularly motor skills As the pathology of the condition is based on the X chromosome, the full syndrome is found only in males. Females carrying the mutation may have a variable clinical phenotype (but much less severe)	Neurological/psychiatric: a learning disability is found in almost all patients, but with a wide spectrum of severity. A large proportion of patients have many of the features of autism and/or attention deficit hyperactivity disorder Musculoskeletal: generalised hypotonia, hyperextensible joints, pes planus Head and neck: the typical facial appearance includes enlarged ears, elongation of the face and a high arched palate. Recurrent otitis media is also commonly found Macro-orchidism	*Investigations* Diagnosed through genetic analysis for *FMR1* mutations. This may be done prenatally via chorionic villous sampling or amniocentesis *Management* There is no specific treatment, but useful aspects in management include Behavioural therapies and stimulants may be used to treat neuropsychiatric conditions Clinical genetics input will be helpful for explaining the pathogenesis of the condition, and for pre-conception counselling
Klinefelter syndrome A chromosomal disorder associated with an additional X chromosomes (with karyotype 47,XXY being found in at least 80% of cases)	The condition may first be suspected from learning disability and/or subfertility	General appearance: tall stature Neuropsychiatric: learning disability Endocrine: subfertility, gynaecomastia, reduction in body and facial hair, small genitals and increased osteoporotic fractures as a result of the hypogonadism found in the condition. There is also an association with diabetes mellitus and hypothyroidism Cardiac: mitral valve prolapse is also associated with the condition (found in approximately half of patients)	*Investigations* First suspected based on clinical features, with the diagnosis confirmed through karyotyping Blood tests will show the typical pattern of hypergonadotrophic hypogonadism found in all causes of primary hypogonadism, ie low plasma testosterone levels, with raised LH and FSH *Management* There is no specific treatment, but important management steps include Echocardiography to screen for mitral valve disease Genetic counselling and fertility clinic input for those planning families

(continued)

Differential diagnosis	Clinical communication skills and managing patient concerns	Physical examination and identifying physical signs	Clinical judgement and maintaining patient welfare
Noonan syndrome An autosomal dominant condition with several overlapping phenotypic features with Turner syndrome	A history of learning difficulties and/or impaired motor development, cardiac disease, easy bruising	Clinical features include: General appearance: generalised lymphoedema, short stature, cryptorchidism Face: widely spaced eyes (*hypertelorism*), epicanthal folds of the eyes, low-set ears, flattened nasal bridge, webbed neck Neurological: learning disability, impaired coordination Cardiac disease: pulmonary stenosis, ASD, hypertrophic cardiomyopathy Haematological: reduced platelet count and coagulation factors	*Investigations* First suspected through clinical features, with genetic tests useful in helping to confirm the diagnosis *Management* Treatment is of the complications of the condition
Down syndrome A multisystem condition associated with trisomy of chromosome 21	Usually detected by screening at birth	Clinical features include: General appearance: short stature, single palmar crease on hands Face: low-set ears, epicanthal folds on the eyes, flattened nasal bridge, shortened neck Neurological: learning disability, premature development of dementia Cardiac: atrial and ventricular septal defects, patent ductus arteriosus, tetralogy of Fallot Endocrine: increased propensity to diabetes mellitus and hypothyroidism. Subfertility is also common, particularly in affected men Haematological: increased susceptibility to developing acute leukaemia	*Investigations* Diagnosis usually first suspected based on clinical features, but confirmed through karyotyping *Management* There is no specific treatment; treatment is focused on the underlying complications (eg cardiac surgery for congenital heart disease)

Clinical judgement and maintaining patient welfare

Turner syndrome is a chromosomal disorder affecting women that is characterised by a 45,XO karyotype. This abnormality means that most affected patients experience primary amenorrhoea (with normal ovarian tissue replaced by fibrotic tissue), and hence have high rates of subfertility and failure to develop secondary sexual characteristics. The exact clinical phenotype is variable between patients, with a wide range of recognised clinical features.

The most life-threatening consequence of X chromosome haploinsufficiency involves the cardiovascular system. During fetal development, major defects in cardiac and aortic development result in a significant *in utero* mortality for fetuses with the 45,XO karyotype. In those who survive, patients with a bicuspid aortic valve and/or coarctation of the aorta are at risk of aortic dilatation and dissection. In addition, bicuspid aortic valves may become a nidus for infective endocarditis in adult life.

Investigations

The syndrome may be first suspected through clinical features, as described in the flowchart. The identification of peripheral blood lymphocytes that demonstrate the 45,XO karyotype is required to confirm the diagnosis. A small proportion of patients will demonstrate mosaicism, with evidence of 46X,X or 46X,Y cell types in addition to 45,XO; it is important for this to be recognised, because the former are more likely to have preserved ovarian function, and the latter are at higher risk of developing gonadoblastoma (see below).

Other tests required once the diagnosis is confirmed include

- Endocrine: the typical biochemical pattern found in patients with Turner syndrome is low plasma estradiol with raised FSH and LH levels, ie hypergonadotrophic hypogonadism.

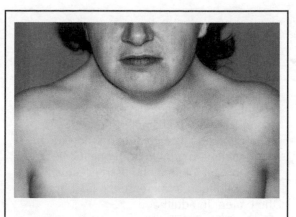

Figure 5.14 Turner syndrome

Patients should also have their thyroid function tests, blood glucose and bone profile/vitamin D levels checked, because patients are at an increased risk of hypothyroidism (particularly from Hashimoto's thyroiditis), diabetes mellitus and osteoporosis.

- Cardiological: patients will require serial echocardiography to assess for the presence of aortic valve disease and/or aortic root dilatation. Patients are also at an increased risk of ischaemic heart disease (thought to represent their increased propensity to diabetes and hypertension), and functional assessment for ischaemia may also be required, eg stress echocardiogram.
- Urinary tract imaging: patients with Turner's syndrome are at an increased risk of structural abnormalities of the urinary tract, particularly a horseshoe kidney; these are best assessed by ultrasonography in the first instance. Those with horseshoe kidney are at an increased risk of hydronephrosis and urinary tract infections.

Management

Management is multidisciplinary, with input from a range of individuals who will be able to provide input with the complex physical and psychological needs that patients may have. Specific medical needs include

- Hormone replacement therapy should be started in the early teenage years in order to aid growth, help patients obtain normal height and encourage development of secondary sexual characteristics.
- Although patients with Turner syndrome are not deficient in growth hormone (GH), recombinant GH may be used effectively from childhood to increase the final height of the patient in adulthood.
- Only a minority (in the order of a few per cent) of patients will develop ovulatory cycles; even among these patients, most will experience early secondary amenorrhoea. Specialist fertility clinic input will be required for patients seeking to have children.
- Input from clinical geneticists is useful for helping to explain the chromosomal nature of the disease. Of the small subgroup who are able to conceive, up to a third will have children with a serious congenital anomaly, and patients will require careful pre-conception counselling.
- As described above, a small proportion of patients will have cells with the karyotype 46X,Y and have a high propensity to develop gonadoblastoma. Such patients should be encouraged either to have prophylactic gonadectomy or to undergo serial ovarian imaging, with surgery undertaken at the earliest sign of development of the condition.

Maintaining patient welfare

- Turner syndrome is a difficult condition to manage for both medical and psychological reasons
  - Patients may have anxiety about their body image and sexuality and regard themselves as 'not as feminine' as other women.
  - It may be difficult for patients to grasp the idea of why they need to continue hormone replacement therapy when they remain unable to conceive.
  - Patients may find it difficult to understand why prophylactic gonadectomy may be appropriate.
  - The underlying chromosomal nature of the disease may be complex to appreciate, and patients will often benefit from input from a genetics team.
- Furthermore, the disease phenotype is somewhat variable between different patients, and the needs of each patient will need to be assessed on an individual basis.
- Patients with Turner syndrome will often benefit from meeting others with the condition for support, and offering them information about support groups (such as the Turner Syndrome Support Society) may be invaluable.

Resources

Turner Syndrome Support Society:
    www.tss.org.uk

SCENARIO 39 VITILIGO

Introduce yourself

Confirm the information you've been given and patient details: this 45-year-old Caribbean woman has presented with areas of hypopigmented skin on her hands and neck. Please assess her.

'What is the main problem from your point of view?' 'For the last few months I have noticed that I have started getting white patches of skin on my hands and my neck'

Focused history of the presenting complaint and relevant systems enquiry: ask specifically about location, symmetry, hyperpigmented borders, hypopigmented hair and the presence of alopecia

Pre-existing conditions/risk factors: other autoimmune conditions (see below)? Ask about a family history of vitiligo (there may be in up to 40% of affected patients)

Social/occupational/family circumstances: there may be embarrassment/distress if vitiligo is visible to friends and family

Drug history: related to other autoimmune diseases. May also occur following exposure to industrial chemicals. **DRUG ALLERGIES**

Other medical conditions: ask about other autoimmune conditions (as found in 30%), including thyroid disease, pernicious anaemia, Addison's disease, diabetes mellitus, alopecia areata, primary biliary cirrhosis, fibrosing alveolitis and coeliac disease

Begin a **targeted** examination of relevant area/system and continue while taking the history

Examination of the skin

Location: can occur anywhere. Often affects the hands, face, neck, extensor surfaces of limbs and dorsum of the feet. Look for scarred areas, as Köbner's phenomenon is also found

Description: symmetrical hypopigmentation macules, often with hyperpigmented borders. Look for hypopigmented hair

Additional examination

- Examine scalp for alopecia
- Inspect for goitre and evidence of thyroid disease
- If chest symptoms, complete full respiratory examination
- If symptoms of liver or GI disease, complete full abdominal examination
- Ask for postural blood pressures and examine for buccal pigmentation
- Ask to test for glycosuria

CALLBACK: 'You said at the beginning that the main problem was white patches on your skin. Is there anything else troubling you that we haven't covered?'

RESPOND TO PATIENT'S CONCERNS (1–2 min)

1. I think you have a condition called vitiligo, which is a condition related to the immune system
2. It is unfortunately difficult to treat vitiligo. One option is to use special make-up to conceal the more obvious patches if that would be helpful. Other treatments require a dermatological specialist to manage, and include creams put directly onto the skin (eg mometasone) or light therapy (eg PUVA)
3. The diagnosis is made from examination of the skin, but I also would like to perform some investigations to see if you have any of the other conditions associated with vitiligo. In the first instance, this will include some simple blood tests

Thank the patient

Differential diagnosis	Clinical communication skills and managing patient concerns	Physical examination and identifying physical signs	Clinical judgement and maintaining patient welfare
Hypopigmentation			
Post-inflammatory Causes include: Chemical exposure, eg phenols, liquid nitrogen, previous cryotherapy	A history of occupational exposure to unusual agents		Treatment is supportive, focused on avoiding further exposure to the precipitant
Endocrine causes Includes Addison's disease and hypopituitarism	See Scenario 2. Addison's disease flowchart (page 400)		
Infection Pityriasis versicolor, a chronic fungal condition caused through infection with the yeast *Malassezia sp.*	Usually asymptomatic, lesions often appear after increased exposure to UV light (due to increased contrast with tanned skin)	Pityriasis versicolor often presents on dark skin as hypopigmented, scaly patches, and is particularly found on the torso and proximal limbs	The diagnosis of pityriasis is confirmed from culture of scrapings of scale from the lesions Treatment is with topical or oral antifungals
Tuberculoid leprosy	This should be suspected in patients who have been to endemic regions who present with hypopigmentation	Features include anaesthetic and anhidrotic hypopigmented macules	The diagnosis of leprosy is often made clinically, but confirmed through biopsy Treatment is with a prolonged course of anti-mycobacterial chemotherapy
Genetic Albinism, ie any of a wide number of autosomal recessive disorders associated with widespread depigmentation		In addition to globally depigmented skin, patients with albinism may have white hair, depigmentation of the iris, impaired visual acuity, photophobia and abnormalities of eye movements (eg nystagmus)	Albinism may be diagnosed clinically, with genetic testing used to confirm the underlying syndrome Genetic counselling may also be indicated
Phenylketonuria (PKU): an autosomal recessive inborn error of metabolism		PKU is often diagnosed on neonatal screening tests. If not, widespread depigmented skin develops, as well as severe learning disability and a movement disorder (choreoathetosis)	PKU is part of the UK neonatal screening tests for inborn errors of metabolism It is treated through avoiding phenylalanine within the diet

(continued)

Differential diagnosis		Clinical communication skills and managing patient concerns	Physical examination and identifying physical signs	Clinical judgement and maintaining patient welfare
Other	Causes include: Morphea: see Scenario 36. Systemic lupus erythematosus flowchart Discoid lupus erythematosus: see Scenario 30. Psoriasis differential diagnosis table Tuberous sclerosis Lichen sclerosis Halo naevus		Tuberous sclerosis is associated with a number of characteristic dermatological changes, including hypopigmented macules, often over the torso and buttocks ('ash leaf' macules), which may be confused with vitiligo	Diagnosis is usually clinical, with treatment depending on the underlying disorder
Hyperpigmentation				
Genetic	Freckles and lentignes		Both are forms of pigmented macules found particularly on the face, but freckles have a normal number of melanocytes (with increased melanin content) whereas lentignes have an increased number of melanocytes (but normal melanin content). Freckles darken on sun exposure, whereas lentignes do not. There are certain genetic syndromes in which distinctive patterns of freckles and lentignes are seen, ie: Neurofibromatosis-1: café-au-lait spots and axillary/inguinal freckling Peutz–Jeghers syndrome: lentignes around the lips, chronic anaemia, intussusception and risk of GI malignancies	Freckles and lentignes may be recognised clinically. No treatment is usually required, although lentignes will respond to cryotherapy Syndromes such as neurofibromatosis and Peutz–Jeghers syndrome are suspected through the pattern of freckling in association with other characteristic clinical features. Genetic testing/counselling is appropriate if suspected
	Haemochromatosis			

(continued)

Differential diagnosis		Clinical communication skills and managing patient concerns	Physical examination and identifying physical signs	Clinical judgement and maintaining patient welfare
Drugs	A large list, including psoralens, amiodarone, phenothiazines and oestrogens			Treatment is supportive, involving limiting further exposure to the precipitating drug
Endocrine	Disorders of cortisol metabolism, including Addison's disease and Nelson syndrome	See Scenario 2. Addison's disease flowchart and Scenario 11. Cushing's disease flowchart		
	Chloasma	This is found particularly in women using the oral contraceptive pill or pregnant women	A condition characterised by symmetrical facial macular hyperpigmented lesions	The condition often improves spontaneously or on discontinuing the oral contraceptive Camouflage and sunscreens may also be useful
Other	Causes include: Melanoma Post-inflammatory, ie eczema, lichen planus Acanthosis nigricans			The diagnosis may be made clinically and confirmed through biopsy Treatment is of the underlying disorder

Clinical judgement and maintaining patient welfare

Vitiligo is a depigmentation disorder affecting approximately 1% of the population, with a male:female ratio of 1:1. The exact aetiology is unclear; familial studies show that there is a genetic component, although the strong association with autoimmune diseases also suggests an immunological element. In PACES, many patients will also have other autoimmune conditions.

Clinical features
The clinical findings are as described on the flowchart. There is often no particular 'trigger', but lesions are often more prominent after scarring or after prolonged exposure to sunlight (where depigmented skin stands out in contrast to tanned skin).

Investigations and management
Vitiligo is a clinical diagnosis. In cases of uncertainty, vitiligo may be confirmed by skin biopsy, where the absence of melanocytes will be noted. Where appropriate, there should be assessment for the presence of associated autoimmune diseases; a basic screen might include FBC, ESR, LFT, TFTs, vitamin B_{12}, folate, 9 am cortisol, fasting glucose, rheumatoid factor and autoantibodies.

Treatment is as summarised in Table 5.25.

Maintaining patient welfare
The psychological impact of vitiligo should not be underestimated. Candidates should appreciate the useful input that a support group might be able to offer, such the Vitiligo Society in the UK (see below).

Resources
The Vitiligo Society: www.vitiligosociety.org.uk

Table 5.25 Treatment of vitiligo

Modality of treatment	Details
General measures	Camouflage of affected areas Sunscreen: reduces tanning, so helps to reduce contrast between skin with and skin without vitiligo
Medical therapies	Potent topical corticosteroids (eg mometasone): may occasionally induce repigmentation Topical tacrolimus: some evidence for inducing repigmentation, although data are limited Monobenzyl ether of hydroquinone: used as a 'last resort' when vitiligo is widespread to induce global depigmentation
Phototherapy	UVB or PUVA (with or without topical or oral psoralens) has been demonstrated to reduce depigmentation. However, this requires a very prolonged course before the benefit may be noticed
Surgery	Mini-grafting may be used, but is not widely available
Other treatments	Tattooing of areas of vitiligo to produce the appearance of pigmented skin may also be considered

Abbreviations

5-ASA	5-aminosalicylic acid		AST	aspartate aminotransferase
5HIAA	5-hydroxyindole acetic acid		ATN	acute tubular necrosis
A&E	accident and emergency department		AV	arteriovenous or atrioventricular
ABG	arterial blood gas		AVM	arteriovenous malformation
ABPI	ankle–brachial pressure index		AVED	ataxia with isolated vitamin E deficiency
ABPA	allergic bronchopulmonary aspergillosis		AVNRT	atrioventricular nodal re-entry tachycardia
AC	air conduction		AVRT	atrioventricular re-entry tachycardia
ACA	anterior cerebral artery		AVSD	atrioventricular septal defect
ACE	angiotensin-converting enzyme		AZT	azidothymidine
ACh	acetylcholine		BAL	bronchoalveolar lavage
ACR	American College of Rheumatology		BBE	Bickerstaff's brain-stem encephalitis
ACTH	adrenocorticotrophic hormone		BC	bone conduction
ADH	antidiuretic hormone		BCG	Bacille Calmette– Guérin
ADL	activities of daily living		BHIVA	British HIV Association
ADPKD	autosomal dominant polycystic kidney disease		BiPAP	bilevel positive airway pressure
AF	atrial fibrillation		BMA	British Medical Association
AFB	acid-fast bacillus		BMD	Becker muscular dystrophy
AIDS	acquired immune deficiency syndrome		BMI	body mass index
			BMS	bone marrow sampling
AIH	autoimmune hepatitis		BNP	brain natriuretic peptide
AIP	acute interstitial pneumonia		BOOP	bronchiolitis obliterans organising pneumonia
ALKMA	anti-liver–kidney microsomal antibody		BP	blood pressure
ALP	alkaline phosphatase		CABG	coronary artery bypass graft
ALS	amyotrophic lateral sclerosis		CAD	coronary artery disease
ALT	alanine aminotransferase		cANCA	cytoplasmic anti-neutrophil cytoplasmic antibody
AMA	anti-mitochondrial antibody			
ANA	anti-nuclear antibody		CAPD	continuous ambulatory peritoneal dialysis
AP	anteroposterior			
AR	atrial regurgitation		CBT	cognitive–behavioural therapy
ARB	angiotensin receptor blocker		CCF	congestive cardiac failure
ARMD	age-related macular degeneration		CCP	cyclic citrullinated peptide
AS	ankylosing spondylitis		CDSC	Communicable Disease Surveillance Centre
ASD	atrial septal defect			
ASLA	anti-soluble liver antigen antibody		CF	cystic fibrosis
ASMA	anti-smooth muscle antibody		CFA	cryptogenic fibrosing alveolitis
ASOT	anti-streptolysin O titre		CFS	cerebrospinal fluid

CK	creatine kinase		EAA	extrinsic allergic alveolitis
CKD	chronic kidney disease		EBUS	endobronchial ultrasonography
CHD	coronary heart disease		EBV	Epstein–Barr virus
CIDP	chronic inflammatory demyelinating polyneuropathy		ECG	electrocardiogram
			EDTA	ethylenediaminetetraacetic acid
CML	chronic myeloid leukaemia		EEG	electroencephalogram
CMT	Charcot–Marie–Tooth disease		ELISA	enzyme-linked immunosorbent assay
CMV	cytomegalovirus			
CN	cranial nerve		EMG	electromyogram
CNS	central nervous system		EN	erythema nodosum
COMT	catechol-*O*-methyl transferase		ENA	extractable nuclear antigen
COP	cryptogenic organising pneumonia		EENT	ear, nose and throat
COPD	chronic obstructive pulmonary disease		EPS	electrophysiological study
			ERCP	endoscopic retrograde cholangiopancreatography
CPEO	chronic progressive external ophthalmoplegia			
			ERG	electroretinogram
CPO	cerebellopontine angle		ESKD	end-stage kidney disease
CPR	cardiopulmonary resuscitation		ESM	early systolic murmur
CPTA	CT pulmonary angiography		ESR	erythrocyte sedimentation rate
CRH	cortisol-releasing hormone		ET	essential tremor
CRP	C-reactive protein		FAPS	functional abdominal pain syndrome
CRT	cardiac resynchronisation therapy		FBC	full blood count
CT	computed tomography		FEV_1	forced expiratory volume in 1 second
CTD	connective tissue disease			
CTS	carpal tunnel syndrome		FH	family history
CV	central venous		FSH	follicle-stimulating hormone
CVA	cerebrovascular accident		FSHD	facioscapulohumeral dystrophy
CYP450	cytochrome P enzymes		FVC	forced vital capacity
DAA	directly acting antiviral agent		GBM	glomerular basement membrane antibody
DC	dilated cardiomyopathy			
DCCT	Diabetes Control and Complications Trial		GCA	giant cell arteritis
			GCS	Glasgow Coma Scale
DCSS	diffuse cutaneous systemic sclerosis		GFR	glomerular filtration rate
*D*LCO	carbon monoxide transfer factor		GGT, γ-GT	γ-glutamyl transpeptidase
DLE	discoid lupus erythematosus		GI	gastrointestinal
DH	drug history		GIST	gastrointestinal stromal tumour
DIP	desquamative interstitial pneumonia/ distal interphalangeal		GOLD	Global Initiative for Chronic Obstructive Lung Disease
DMARD	disease-modifying anti-rheumatic drug		GORD	gastro-oesophageal reflux disease
			GH	growth hormone
DMD	Duchenne muscular dystrophy		GHRH	growth hormone-releasing hormone
DNAR	do not attempt resuscitation		HAART	highly active antiretroviral therapy
dsDNA	double-stranded DNA		HAV	hepatitis A virus
DVLA	Driver and Vehicle Licensing Agency		HbA1c	glycated haemoglobin
			HBsAg	hepatitis B surface antigen
DVT	deep vein thrombosis		HBV	hepatitis B virus
DXA	dual-energy X-ray absorptiometry		HCC	hepatocellular carcinoma

HCV	hepatitis C virus		JFS	jugular foramen syndrome
HDL	high-density lipoprotein		JIA	juvenile idiopathic arthritis
HDV	hepatitis D virus		JVP	jugular venous pressure
HEV	hepatitis E virus		K_{CO}	gas transfer
HH	hereditary haemochromatosis		LA	left atrial
HHT	hereditary haemorrhagic telangiectasia		LABA	long-acting β_2 agonist
HIV	human immunodeficiency virus		LAD	left anterior descending
HMSN	hereditary motor and sensory neuropathy		LAM	lymphangioleiomyomatosis
			LAMA	long-acting muscarinic antagonist
HOCM	hypertrophic cardiomyopathy		LCSS	limited cutaneous systemic sclerosis
HPC	history of the presenting complaint		LDH	lactate dehydrogenase
HPOA	hypertrophic pulmonary osteoarthropathy		LDL	low-density lipoprotein
			LEMS	Lambert–Eaton myasthenic syndrome
HPP	hyperkalaemic periodic paralysis		LFT	liver function test
HRS	hepatorenal syndrome		LGV	lymphogranuloma venereum
HS	hereditary spherocytosis		LH	luteinising hormone
HSAN	hereditary sensory and autonomic neuropathy		LIP	lymphocytic interstitial pneumonia
HSP	Henoch–Schönlein purpura		LMN	lower motor neuron
HSV	herpes simplex virus		LOC	loss of consciousness
HUS	haemolytic–uraemic syndrome		LP	lumbar puncture
IBD	inflammatory bowel disease		LTOT	long-term oxygen therapy
IBS	irritable bowel syndrome		LV	left ventricular
ICA	integrated clinical assessment		LVEF	left ventricular ejection fraction
ICAS	Independent Complaints Advocacy Service		LVESD	left ventricular end-systolic diameter
			LVF	left ventricular failure
ICD	implantable cardioverter defibrillator		LVH	left ventricular hypertrophy
ICE	ideas, concerns, expectations		LVOT	left ventricular outflow tract
ICP	intracranial pressure		LVRS	lung volume reduction surgery
ICS	inhaled corticosteroid		MAI	*Mycobacterium avium intracellulare*
ICU	intensive care unit		MCA	middle cerebral artery
IFN	interferon		MC&S	microscopy, culture and sensitivity
IGF-1	insulin-like growth factor 1		MCPJ	metacarpophalangeal joint
IGRA	interferon-γ release assay		MCV	mean corpuscular volume
IHD	ischaemic heart disease		MD	myotonic dystrophy
IIP	idiopathic interstitial pneumonia		MDRD	Modification of Diet in Renal Diseases
IL	interleukin			
ILD	interstitial lung disease		MDT	multidisciplinary team
INO	intranuclear ophthalmoplegia		MEN	multiple endocrine neoplasia
INR	international normalised ratio		MFS	Miller–Fisher syndrome
IPF	idiopathic pulmonary fibrosis		MGUS	monoclonal gammopathy of unknown significance
IRMA	intraretinal microvascular abnormality			
			MI	myocardial infarction
IUS	intrauterine system of contraception		MLF	medial longitudinal fasciculus
IVDU	intravenous drug user		MMN	multifocal motor neuropathy
IVIG	intravenous immunoglobulin		MRA	magnetic resonance angiography

MMSE	Mini-Mental State Examination	PCD	paraneoplastic cerebellar degeneration
MND	motor neuron disease		
MR	mitral regurgitation	PCP	*Pneumocystis carinii* pneumonia (no longer used)
MRC	Medical Research Council		
MRCP	magnetic resonance cholangiopancreatography	PCR	polymerase chain reaction
		PCOS	polycystic ovarian syndrome
MRI	magnetic resonance imaging	PD	Parkinson's disease
MRSA	meticillin-resistant *Staphylococcus aureus*	PDA	patent ductus arteriosus
		PDE-5	phosphodiesterase-5
MS	multiple sclerosis	PE	pulmonary embolism
MSA	multiple-system atrophy	PEG	percutaneous endoscopic gastrostomy
MTP	metatarsophalangeal		
MuSK	muscle-specific tyrosine kinase	PET	positron emission tomography
MVP	mitral valve prolapse	PFP	pulmonary function test
MVR	mitral valve regurgitation	P-IFN	pegylated interferon-α
nAChR	nicotinic acetylcholine receptor	PIP	proximal interphalangeal
NASH	non-alcoholic steatohepatitis	PJP	*Pneumocystis jirovecii* pneumonia (replaces PCP)
NASS	National Ankylosing Spondylitis Society		
		PKD	polycystic kidney disease
NCS	nerve conduction studies	PKU	phenylketonuria
NF	neurofibromatosis	PM	paramyotonia/post mortem
NICE	National Institute for Health and Care Excellence	PMH	past medical history
		PML	progressive multifocal leukoencephalopathy
NIV	non-invasive ventilation		
NMDA	*N*-methyl-D-aspartate	PMN	polymorphonuclear neutrophil
NMO	neuromyelitis optica	PMR	polymyalgia rheumatica
NNRTI	non-nucleoside reverse transcriptase inhibitor	PMRF	paramedian pontine reticular formation
		PND	paroxysmal nocturnal dyspnoea
NNT	number needed to treat	PNS	peripheral nervous system
NRTI	nucleoside reverse transcriptase inhibitor	PPI	proton pump inhibitor
		PPS	post-polio syndrome
NSAID	non-steroidal anti-inflammatory drug	PR	per rectum
NSCLC	non-small-cell lung cancer	PROMM	proximal myotonic myopathy
NSIP	non-specific interstitial pneumonia	PSM	pansystolic murmur
NYHA	New York Heart Association	PSC	primary sclerosing cholangitis
OA	osteoarthritis	PTH	parathyroid hormone
OCP	oral contraceptive pill	PTHrP	parathyroid hormone-releasing peptide
OGD	oesophagogastroduodenoscopy		
OSA	obstructive sleep apnoea	PTLD	post-transplantation lymphoproliferative disease
OT	occupational therapy		
PALS	Patients' Advice Liaison Service	PRV	polycythaemia rubra vera
PAN	polyarteritis nodosa	PUVA	psoralens + UVA
pANCA	perinuclear anti-neutrophil cytoplasmic antibody	QALY	quality-adjusted life-year
		RA	rheumatoid arthritis
PAP	pulmonary alveolar proteinosis	RAD	right axis deviation
PBC	primary biliary cirrhosis	RAPD	relative afferent papillary defect
PCA	posterior cerebral artery		

RAST	radioallergosorbent test	TAVI	transcatheter aortic valve implantation
RBBB	right bundle-branch block		
RB-ILD	respiratory bronchiolitis–interstitial lung disease	TB	tuberculosis
		TFT	thyroid function test
RCN	Royal College of Nursing	TIA	transient ischaemic accident
RHS	Ramsay Hunt syndrome	TIBC	total iron-binding capacity
RNS	repetitive nerve stimulation	TIMI	thrombolysis in myocardial infarction
RP	retinitis pigmentosa		
RPE	retinal pigment epithelium	TLC	total lung capacity
RUQ	right upper quadrant	TNF	tumour necrosis factor
RVH	right ventricular hypertrophy	tPA	tissue plasminogen activator
RVOT	right ventricular outflow tract	TPMT	thiopurine methyltransferase
SAAG	serum–ascites albumin gradient	TR	tricuspid regurgitation
SABA	short-acting β_2 agonist	TSH	thyroid-stimulating hormone
SACD	subacute combined degeneration of the cord	TTG	transglutaminase antibody
		TVF	tactile vocal fremitus
SAH	subarachnoid haemorrhage	U&Es	urea and electrolytes
SAMA	short-acting muscarinic antagonist	UC	ulcerative colitis
SBE	subacute bacterial endocarditis	UIP	usual interstitial pneumonia
SBP	spontaneous bacterial peritonitis	UKPDS	UK Prospective Diabetes Study
SCC	squamous cell carcinoma	UMN	upper motor neuron
SCLC	small-cell lung cancer	uPCR	urinary protein:creatinine ratio
SIADH	syndrome of inappropriate secretion of antidiuretic hormone	UTI	urinary tract infection
		UV	ultraviolet
SLE	systemic lupus erythematosus	VA	visual acuity
SOB	shortness of breath	VATS	video-assisted thoracoscopic surgery
SPECT	single photon emission computed tomography	VBS	vertebrobasilar system
		VC	vital capacity
SR	systems review	VEGF	vascular endothelial growth factor
SS	systemic sclerosis	VEP	visual evoked potential
SSRI	selective serotonin reuptake inhibitor	VF	vocal fremitus
STI	sexually transmitted infection	VR	vocal resonance
STN	subthalamic nucleus	VSD	ventricular septal defect
SVCO	superior vena caval obstruction	VT	ventricular tachycardia
SVR	sustained viral response	VZV	varicella-zoster virus
SVT	supraventricular tachycardia	WBC	white blood cell
T_3	triiodothyronine	WCC	white cell count
T_4	thyroxine	WHO	World Health Organization
		XDR	extended drug-resistant

Index

This index covers Stations 1–5.